D0162749

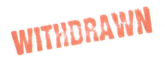

STEM CELL BIOLOGY

**COLD SPRING HARBOR
MONOGRAPH SERIES**

STEM CELL BIOLOGY

Edited by

Daniel R. Marshak
Johns Hopkins University, Baltimore, Maryland and
Cambrex Corp.
Walkersville, Maryland

Richard L. Gardner
University of Oxford
Oxford, United Kingdom

David Gottlieb
Washington University, St. Louis, Missouri

COLD SPRING HARBOR LABORATORY PRESS
Cold Spring Harbor, New York

**STEM CELL
BIOLOGY**

Monograph 40
© 2001 by Cold Spring Harbor Laboratory Press,
   Cold Spring Harbor, New York
All rights reserved
Printed in the United States of America

Project Coordinator: Inez Sialiano
Production Editor: Patricia Barker
Desktop Editor: Danny deBruin
Interior Book Designer: Emily Harste

Library of Congress Cataloging-in-Publication Data

Stem cell biology / edited by Daniel R. Marshak, Richard L. Gardner, David Gottlieb
      p. cm.
   Includes bibliographical references and index.
   ISBN 0-87969-575-7 (alk. paper)
   1. Stem cells. I Marshak, Daniel R. II. Gardner, Richard L. (Richard Lavenham),
   1943- . III. Gottlieb, David (David I.)

   QH587.S72 2000
   571.8'35--dc21

                                                              00-065791

10 9 8 7 6 5 4 3 2

All Cold Spring Harbor Laboratory Press publications may be ordered directly from Cold Spring Harbor Laboratory Press, 500 Sunnyside Boulevard, Woodbury, New York 11797-2924. Phone: 1-800-843-4388 in Continental U.S. and Canada. All other locations: (516) 422-4100. FAX: (516) 422-4097. E-mail: cshpress@cshl.org. For a complete catalog of Cold Spring Harbor Laboratory Press publications, visit our World Wide Web Site http://www.cshlpress.com

Contents

Preface

The field of stem cell research has attracted many investigators in the past several years. Progress in embryology, hematology, neurobiology, and skeletal biology, among many other disciplines, has centered on the isolation and characterization of stem cells. The approaching completion of the sequencing of the human genome has lent further impetus to exploring how gene expression in stem cells relates to their dual functions of self-renewal and differentiation.

Two small meetings held at the Banbury Center of Cold Spring Harbor Laboratory in 1996 and 1999 served to bring together groups of scientists eager to discuss the role of stem cells in development, tissue homeostasis, and regeneration. These meetings highlighted both the quickening pace of discovery relating to the basic biology of stem cells and the increasing scope for their clinical exploitation. They also convinced us that it was timely to assemble a monograph that would help to make the fundamentals of stem cell biology more accessible to those seeking better acquaintance with the subject.

We thank Inez Sialiano, Pat Barker, Danny deBruin, and John Inglis of the Cold Spring Harbor Laboratory Press for enabling this project to be realized. We also acknowledge the efforts of the entire staff of the Press who contributed to the editing and production process. Drs. James Watson, Bruce Stillman, and Jan Witkowski were highly supportive of this enterprise. A particular note of thanks is due Mr. James S. Burns for his encouragement and enthusiasm, as well as his vision and accomplishments, in both the development of stem cell research and its practical exploitation. Finally, we thank our authors for agreeing so generously to take the time to contribute to this volume, and our families for their patience throughout its gestation.

D.R. Marshak
R.L. Gardner
D. Gottlieb

1

Introduction: Stem Cell Biology

Daniel R. Marshak

Cambrex Corp.
Walkersville, Maryland 21793 and
Johns Hopkins School of Medicine
Baltimore, Maryland 21205

David Gottlieb

Department of Anatomy and Neurobiology
Washington University
St. Louis, Missouri 63110

Richard L. Gardner

Department of Zoology
University of Oxford
Oxford, OX1 3PS, United Kingdom

STEM CELLS: AN OVERVIEW

There is still no universally acceptable definition of the term stem cell, despite a growing common understanding of the circumstances in which it should be used. According to this more recent perspective, the concept of "stem cell" is indissolubly linked with growth via the multiplication rather than the enlargement of cells. Various schemes for classifying tissues according to their mode of growth have been proposed, one of the earliest of which is that of Bizzozero (1894). This classification, which relates to the situation in the adult rather than in the embryo, recognizes three basic types of tissues: renewing, expanding, and static. Obvious examples of the first are intestinal epithelium and skin, and of the second, liver. The third category was held to include the central nervous system, although recent studies have shown that neurogenesis does continue in adulthood, for example, with regard to production of neurons that migrate to the olfactory bulbs (Gage 2000). There are various problems with such schemes of classification including, for instance, assignment of organs like the mammary gland which, depending on the circumstances of the individual, may engage in one or more cycles of marked growth, differentiation, and subsequent involution.

Any attempt to find a universally acceptable definition of the term stem cell is probably doomed to fail. Nonetheless, certain attributes can be assigned to particular cells in both developing and adult multicellular organisms that serve to distinguish them from the remaining cells of the tissues to which they belong. Most obviously, these cells retain the capacity to self-renew as well as to produce progeny that are more restricted in both mitotic potential and in the range of distinct types of differentiated cells to which they can give rise. However, kinetic studies support the notion that in many tissues a further subpopulation of cells with a limited and, in some cases, strictly circumscribed self-renewal capacity, so-called "transit amplifying" cells, can stand between true stem cells and their differentiated derivatives (see, e.g., Chapters 19 and 22 by Watt and Winton). This mode of cell production has the virtue of limiting the total number of division cycles in which stem cells have to engage during the life of an organism. Unlimited capacity for self-renewal is therefore not normally demanded of stem cells in vivo and, indeed, in practice, the distinction between stem and transit amplifying cell may be difficult to make.

"Stem cell," like many other terms in biology, has been used in more than one context since its initial appearance in the literature during the 19th century. In the first edition of his great treatise on cell biology, E.B. Wilson (1896) reserved the term exclusively for the ancestral cell of the germ line in the parasitic nematode worm, *Ascaris megalocephala*. Elegant studies by Boveri (1887) on early development in this organism revealed that a full set of chromosomes was retained by only one cell during successive cleavage divisions, and that this cell alone gave rise to the entire complement of adult germ cells. However, what is clear from more recent studies on cell lineage in nematodes is that the developmental potential of the germ-line precursor cell clearly changes with each successive cleavage division (see Sulston et al. 1983). Hence, neither product of early cleavage divisions retains identity with the parental blastomere, arguing that self-renewal, which is now regarded as a signal property of stem cells, is not a feature of this early lineage. In current embryological parlance, what Wilson refers to as a stem cell would be classed as a "progenitor," "precursor," or "founder" cell. Studies on cell lineage in embryos of other invertebrates, particularly various marine species, revealed a degree of invariance in the patterns of cleavage that enabled the origin of most tissues of larvae to be established. In such organisms, somatic tissues were often found to originate from single blastomeres. Thus, in many mollusks and annelids, all mesentoblasts and entoblasts are descended from the 4d blastomere (Davidson 1986). This contrasts with the situation in invertebrates with more variable lineage, like *Drosophila,* and all vertebrates, in which both somatic tissues and the germ line normally originate from several cells rather than just one. In a general sense, all stem cells qualify as progenitor cells although, as noted for the germ line in nematodes, the reverse is not always true.

That tissues in many species really are polyclonal in origin has been demonstrated most graphically by the finding that they can be composed of very variable proportions of cells of two or more genotypes in genetic mosaics and chimeras (Gardner and Lawrence 1986). In the mouse, the epiblast, the precursor tissue of the entire fetal soma and germ line, has recently been found to exhibit an extraordinary degree of dispersal and mixing of the clonal descendants of its modest number of founder cells before gastrulation (Gardner and Cockroft 1998). One consequence of such mixing, especially since it is evidently sustained during gastrulation (Lawson et al. 1991), is that, depending on their progenitor cell number, primordia of fetal tissues and organs are likely to include descendants of many or all epiblast founder cells.

In the remainder of this chapter, we examine the stem cell concept first in the general context of embryogenesis, then more specifically in relation to neurogenesis, before finally considering the situation in the adult.

EMBRYOGENESIS

It is during the periods of embryonic and fetal development that the rate of production of new cells is at its highest. Therefore, in considering the various functions that increasing the number as opposed to the size of cells serve during the life cycle of an organism, it is instructive to begin from an embryological perspective. It has been estimated that an adult vertebrate may be composed of more than 200 different types of cells. As noted earlier, in many organisms each type evidently originates from several progenitor cells rather than just one. Hence, in such organisms, production of a significant number of cells must occur before the process of embryonic differentiation begins.

Development starts with a period of cleavage during which all cells are in cycle but do not engage in net growth between divisions so that their size is approximately halved at each successive mitosis. It is also a period during which S is the dominant phase, even in mammals in which the intervals between cleavages are measured in hours rather than minutes

(Chisholm 1988). In most species, this initial phase of development depends largely or entirely on transcriptional activity of the maternal genome before fertilization. Mammals are an obvious exception in this regard, with transcription from the zygotic genome beginning by, if not before, the 2-cell stage in the mouse (Ram and Schultz 1993), and at most only one or two divisions later in other species, including the human and cow (Braude et al. 1988; Memili and First 1999). Although the number of cleavage divisions is variable even between related species, it seems to be invariant within a species. Furthermore, there is no evidence that the continued proliferation of cells can be uncoupled from the progressive change in their developmental potential or other properties that occurs during the cleavage period. Whether this is related to the lower than normal nuclear cytoplasmic ratio that obtains during cleavage is not clear, although restoration of this ratio to a value typical of somatic cells has been implicated in the onset of transcription of the zygotic genome in amphibians (Newport and Kirschner 1982). The appearance of extended G_1 and G_2 phases of the cell cycle seems to coincide with the end of cleavage in mammals (see, e.g., Chisholm 1988).

Even allowing for the maternal provision of nutrients via yolk, there are limits to the increase in cell number that can be sustained before cell differentiation is required to meet the demands of basic processes such as respiration, excretion, and digestion. Essential for the effective operation of such processes is, of course, the establishment of a heart and circulation, which is therefore invariably one of the earliest systems to function. The onset of differentiation is precocious in relation to cell number in species with small, relatively yolk-free, eggs. Here there is a need for the embryo rapidly to attain independence, or, in the case of eutherian mammals, a stage when it is able to satisfy its increasing metabolic needs through exploiting maternal resources. Hence, viviparity in mammals involves devoting cleavage mainly to the production of cells that will differentiate as purely extraembryonic tissues that are concerned with mediating attachment of the fetus to the mother and its nutrition. These tissues must differentiate precociously, since it is only when they have done so that development of the fetus itself can begin. Eutherian mammals are also unusual in exhibiting the onset of apoptotic cell death as a normal feature of development well before gastrulation. Thus, dying cells are discernible routinely in the blastocyst and, at least in the mouse, belong mainly if not exclusively to the ICM rather than the trophectodermal lineage (El-Shershaby and Hinchliffe 1974; Copp 1978; Handyside and Hunter 1986). One view is that this death reflects cell turnover, because further growth of this internal tissue is not sustainable until implantation has occurred (Handyside and Hunter 1986). A further remarkable feature of the early mammalian conceptus is its impressive ability to adjust its growth following radical loss or gain of cells. Downward size regulation in conceptuses made chimeric by aggregation of pairs or larger numbers of entire morulae occurs immediately following implantation and is invariably completed before gastrulation (Lewis and Rossant 1982; Rands 1986a). Upward regulation following loss of cells, typically removal of one blastomere at the 2-cell stage in the mouse, is not achieved until approximately mid-gestation (Rands 1986b). However, an estimated loss of up to 85% of epiblast cells shortly before gastrulation following a single maternal injection of mitomycin C can also be followed by almost complete restoration of growth and near normal development to term (Snow and Tam 1979). It is interesting in this context that the very early epiblast has proved to be a source of pluripotent cells, so-called embryonic stem (ES) cells. At least in the mouse, these cells retain the capacity to contribute both to all somatic lineages and to the germ line after an indefinite period of proliferation in vitro (for further details, see Chapter 10 by Smith). More recently, cells with a marked ability to self-renew in vitro have also been derived from the trophectoderm and its polar derivatives in the mouse (see Chapter 12 by Kunath et al.). These show restriction to the trophectodermal lineage following reintroduction into the blastocyst and, from the range of tissues to which they contribute, would seem to qualify as multipotential trophoblastic stem (TS) cells. Whereas the successful derivation of ES cells seems to be restricted to a narrow window between the early and late blastocyst stage, that of TS cells is broader, extending from the blastocyst through to well beyond gastrulation (G. Uy, pers. comm.).

Thus, early in development when growth holds primacy, all cells cycle, except for certain precociously specialized ones like those of the mural trophectoderm in the mouse that embark on repeated endoreduplication of their entire genome via polyteny at the late blastocyst stage (Brower 1987; Varmuza et al. 1988; Gardner and Davies 1993). However, once tissue differentiation begins, the proportion of cells engaged in proliferation declines and, as is believed to be the case in the central nervous system, may largely cease postnatally. Other tissues like skin, blood, and intestinal epithelium which are subject to continuous renewal throughout life must maintain an adequate number of cells that retain the potential to proliferate to make good such losses. This is also true of other tissues like the mammary gland that normally engage in more sporadic cycles of differentiation followed by involution during the course of adult life. Hence, during the life of a tissue its growth fraction will be expected to be very high, possibly unity, early on and then to decline to a value that is sufficient to maintain its adult size until aging eventually sets it (see Chapter 5 by Holliday). Therefore, many tissues are envisaged as being composed of two subpopulations of cells, one of which is postmitotic and responsible for their physiological activity and a second that retains the ability to cycle and is responsible for their growth. As an organism approaches its final size, the relative proportions of cells assigned to the two populations shift markedly in favor of the former.

One view as to why such a division of labor exists is that differentiated function is incompatible with engagement in mitosis (for discussion, see Cameron and Jeter 1971; Holtzer et al. 1972). That this is not true universally is evident from the behavior of the extraembryonic endoderm of the murine visceral yolk sac placenta. All cells in this tissue are clearly differentiated morphologically and biochemically by the time that gastrulation is under way. However, notwithstanding their polarized form with apical brush border and system of caveolae, they continue to engage in mitosis until a very advanced stage in gestation (R.L. Gardner, unpubl.). They are, in addition, very susceptible to reprogramming and, following exteriorization of the yolk sac from the uterus, can yield teratomas that rival those derived from ES or embryonal carcinoma cells in the range of differentiated tissues they contain (Sobis et al. 1993). It should be borne in mind, however, that certain differences in the state of the genome between cells of wholly extraembryonic tissues and those derived from the epiblast or fetal precursor tissue have been discerned (see, e.g., Kratzer et al. 1983; Rossant et al. 1986). Hence, there is the possibility that regulation of gene expression differs between the wholly extraembryonic lineages and those originating from the epiblast. However, retention of the capacity to divide by overtly differentiated cells is not unique to extraembryonic tissues. Regeneration of the liver following partial hepatectomy is attributable to resumption of mitosis by differentiated hepatocytes (see Chapter 20 by Grompe and Finegold). Nevertheless, it is conceivable that the nature of their differentiated state is the critical factor in determining whether particular tissues can grow thus rather than depending on the persistence of more primitive precursor cells to enable them to do so. In this context, it has been argued, for example, that because their differentiated products are readily shed, cells with secretory function can easily engage in mitosis, whereas those like muscle that have undergone enduring and complex cytoplasmic differentiation cannot (Goss 1978). Again, this is an area in which generalization is fraught with difficulty since, despite sharing similar functions with visceral endoderm, the adult intestinal epithelium shows obvious partitioning of its growth and differentiation between distinct populations of cells (see Chapter 22 by Winton).

NEUROGENESIS

New technical developments in the 1950s allowed major advances in the analysis of neurogenesis in the vertebrate nervous system. Replicating cells were selectively labeled with tritiated thymidine, and a detailed chronology of their withdrawal from the cell cycle to produce adult neurons and glia was charted. The principal generalization to emerge was that, at least in mammals and birds, neural progenitors replicated in the embryo only, where they generated the vast majority of neurons that would serve the individual throughout adult life. Each region of the CNS had a stereotyped schedule for creating postmitotic neurons. Even the different layers of complex structures such as the cerebral cortex had individuated schedules of progenitor cycling and final mitoses leading to neurons. In a few regions, neurogenesis continued for several weeks after birth. Past that period, the production of new neurons was thought not to happen in most regions of the CNS. The dentate gyrus of the hippocampus and the olfactory bulb were among the exceptional areas where production of new neurons persisted into adulthood. Further studies in vertebrate animals revealed other fascinating exceptions to this rule. In canaries, as in mammals, most regions of adult CNS did not engage in the production of new neurons. However, a small group of nuclei exhibited neurogenesis in the adult (Kirn et al. 1994). The function of these nuclei was especially intriguing (see below). Fish and amphibians were also shown to have extensive neurogenesis in the adult.

The conclusion that mammals receive a fixed allotment of neurons in embryogenesis that must last for life shaped contemporary thinking in two related disciplines. Those concerned with the mechanism of learning, memory, and adaptation of the brain to new experience were compelled to rule out any mechanisms in which new neurons joined neural circuits. Instead, the basis of memory needed to rest on altering in some way the circuits created by neurons present at birth. Interestingly, the neurons generated in the brain of the adult canary were discovered to form new circuits underlying song production. This was treated as a compelling but singular exception to the rule that learning did not involve the production of new neurons. However, it was the medical implications of the "no new neurons" view that had the greatest impact. Injury to the brain and spinal cord from trauma and degenerative processes extracts a devastating toll, whether considered from the perspective of the individual patient or of society as a whole. Usually large-scale death of neurons is involved. Studies of neurogenesis and stem cell function sent a grim message: The CNS lacked progenitors to replace neurons lost to disease and trauma. Loss of function was consequently irreversible.

In the mid-1980s, new technical advances allowed deeper insights into progenitors in the mammalian and avian brain. Until that time there was no reliable method for discovering the fate of daughter cells of individual progenitors. This technical hurdle was overcome by two elegant techniques. One was to infect the developing brain with a replication-defective retrovirus (Sanes et al. 1986; Price et al. 1987). Virus infecting a progenitor would integrate into the genome and be passed on to all descendants. A reporter protein, usually LacZ, was included in the viral genome to allow visualization of descendants of the original infected cell. The other method was to physically inject stable fluorescent dyes into individual progenitor cells. Daughter cells received sufficient dye to be visualized. Lineage-tracing studies with both methods produced largely concordant results. Individual progenitors were shown to give rise to multiple cell types within just a few divisions. For instance, the descendants from two replications of a progenitor might include a glial cell and three separate types of neurons. There are exceptional cases of progenitors having a more restricted range of daughters. However, by and large, fate appears not to be determined by belonging to a pre-specified lineage of replicating progenitors.

The studies reviewed above provided important insights into mammalian CNS stem cells and progenitors at the cellular level. Investigations into the molecular regulation of these events were constrained by the small size and complexity of the embryonic CNS and the difficulty of applying genetic approaches. At this juncture, the genetic power of *Drosophila* proved to be crucial. A large number of mutants exhibiting perturbations of early nervous system development were isolated and analyzed (for review, see Jan and Jan 1994). Some of these proved to be in key genes related to basic aspects of stem cell proliferation, asymmetric division, and choice of cell fates. Because many details of progenitor cell biology differ between vertebrates and invertebrates, it came as something of a surprise that many of the key genes involved were shared across these large evolutionary distances. Vertebrate homologs of genes first identified in *Drosophila* were cloned, thus opening a new chapter in the analysis of neural stem cells and progenitors.

Whereas studies in model organisms revealed many of the genes underlying stem and progenitor cell function, the view that neurogenesis does not occur in adult mammals remained unchallenged until the 1990s. Now there are good reasons for re-examining this basic tenet (see Chapter 18 by Panicker and Rao). First, it has proved possible to culture multipotent progenitor cells directly from the adult rat and human brain and spinal cord. In defined tissue culture medium, these cells grow as compact aggregates termed neurospheres (Reynolds and Weiss 1992; for review, see Gage et al. 1995; Gage 2000; McKay 2000). Cells in neurospheres replicate rapidly for many generations while retaining the characteristics of primitive neuroepithelial cells. Upon plating on an adhesive substratum and altering the culture medium, they give rise to glial cells and neurons. Derivation of neurospheres from adult brain does not, by itself, prove the existence of endogenous progenitors, since the spheres might arise by dedifferentiation of a recognized cell type in the brain, perhaps under the influence of the cell culture environment. This does, however, justify a much closer scrutiny of the evidence behind the concept that new neurons are not produced in the adult brain. Very recently, more direct data suggesting that there is production of neurons in the adult have been published (Gould et al. 1999). They raise a host of questions as to the nature of these adult-acquired neurons. How vigorous is the process? Do these cells replace dying neurons, or is there a net increase in neuronal number? Most crucially, do they form functional circuits, and might these subserve newly acquired abilities? Finally, these recent discoveries have raised new hopes in the clinical arena. If the brain can acquire new neurons in normal life, might this power be harnessed to restore the functions so tragically lost through traumatic injury and degenerative disease?

THE ADULT

As discussed earlier, the notion that stem cells occur during embryogenesis has emerged from both descriptive and experimental studies. The case for the existence of such cells rests on three kinds of evidence. First, one must account for the enormous expansion of cell number that takes place during development to maturity, as well as the hundreds of distinguishable cell types in the adult organism. Second, observations in vivo on embryonic tissues of diverse species show that there are cells which are capable of producing more of themselves as well as yielding differentiated progeny. Third is the finding that multipotent, self-renewing cells can be isolated from embryonic or fetal tissues, and that such cells exhibit the dual properties of expansion and differentiation ex vivo.

That stem cells are also still present in postnatal vertebrates is evident from the observed continuation of tissue growth and differentiation, which is essentially an extension of the latter part of prenatal gestation in eutherian mammals. However, in the adult vertebrate (i.e., following sexual and skeletal maturation), it is somewhat less obvious that stem cells should exist at all. Certainly in the male reproductive organs, mature gametes can be produced in large numbers throughout life, so at least progenitors, if not stem cells, of such gametes must be present to account for the expansion and differentiation. In spermatogenesis, a self-renewing population of premeiotic stem cells does appear to persist throughout adult life (see Chapter 8 by Kiger and Fuller). These are derived from primordial germ cells whose origin and possible mode of specification in mammals are discussed in Chapter 9 by Hogan.

Many somatic tissues, in contrast, do not appear to be growing in a unidirectional, developmental sense in the adult, at least upon gross inspection. Hypertrophy and atrophy of muscle, enlargement or reduction of fat deposits, and cognitive learning in the adult all seem to occur without significant changes in cell number. Rather, these processes are the results of a combination of environmental and genetic factors involving behavioral, dietary, endocrine, and metabolic events. Therefore, to a first approximation, one could doubt any requirement a priori for stem cells in adult somatic tissues. Following a century of investigation, however, the weight of considerable experimental evidence and observation falls in favor of the conclusion that stem cells persist throughout life in many somatic tissues.

Early evidence that stem cells exist in the somatic tissues of animals arose from observations of the regeneration of entire organisms, including the head, from small sections of the *Hydra* soma (for reviews, see Bode and David 1978; Martin et al. 1997). Substantial somatic regeneration also occurs among other invertebrates, including members of relatively highly organized groups such as annelids (Golding 1967a,b; Hill 1970). Limb regeneration can be observed also in insects and, among vertebrates, this property extends to the amphibians, which can regenerate the distal portions of limbs following their amputation (Thornton 1968; Brockes 1997). Limb regeneration does not occur under normal conditions in mammals, but the formation of multiple tissues during wound healing is consistent with the concept that mammals have retained progenitors capable of repairing limited damage to organs. Even a century ago, a seminal monograph on wound healing by Marchand (1901) described the various cell types that appear during the repair process and argued against blood cells serving as progenitors of connective tissues.

Wound repair is a multistep process that involves the formation of blood clots and hematoma to prevent blood loss, immune cell invasion and inflammation to prevent infection and remove tissue debris, and the recruitment of cells from surrounding tissues to form a repair blastema (Allgöwer 1956). Within the blastema, new vasculature and structural tissues re-form to regenerate the site of the original wound. The structural and functional nature of this blastema resembles that of the regenerating amphibian limb. Both serve to provide elements of protection from the external environment and to establish a focus of regenerative cells. Both require the presence of growth factors to effect repair. For example, the amphibian limb must be innervated to be regenerated (for review, see Brockes 1997) whereas, in mammals, the extent of regeneration and scar tissue formation is governed by the age of the animal and availability of polypeptide growth factors belonging to the TGFβ superfamily (see, e.g., Shah et al. 1994). In addition to the parallels between wound healing and limb regeneration, many of the cellular steps of tissue repair in mammals are reminiscent of those occurring in development. For example, the formation of bone at sites of fracture repair entails accumulation of a calcified cartilage that is replaced by bone, much as is seen during endochondral bone formation during development (Aubin 1998). In Chapter 16, Pittenger and Marshak review the evidence for stem cells for various mesenchymal tissues and their relationship with wound healing. Furthermore, Flake reviews the use of the fetal sheep as a host for cellular grafting and the formation of chimeric mesodermal tissues (see Chapter 17). Such observations show that cells isolated from the adult can repopulate developing tissues in the fetus, thus affirming their stem cell nature. Among endodermal tissues, the mammalian liver can regenerate two-thirds of its mass following partial hepatectomy or chemical lesion. However, whereas regeneration following partial hepatectomy occurs through limited resumption of cycling by hepatocytes, that induced by chemical damage is achieved through activation of oval cells associated with the bile ducts. These latter cells, which are uniform morphologically and present in small number, give rise to multiple cell types within the liver. The origin and nature of stem cells in adult liver are reviewed by Grompe and Finegold (Chapter 20), and in pancreatic tissue, which is also a source of hepatic stem cells, by Kritzik and Sarvetnick (see Chapter 21).

Apart from wound healing, the most obvious evidence for the persistence of stem cells in the adult derives from the kinetics of normal tissue turnover. The clearest indications of cell turnover are the diverse kinetics of the cellular components of blood in which neutrophils may survive for hours, platelets for days, erythrocytes for weeks to months, and some lymphocytes for years. The existence of hematopoietic stem cells is supported by the observation that huge numbers of blood cells continue to be produced throughout decades of life, which would be physically impossible if the entire complement of the progenitor cells of blood was fixed at birth or maturity. Furthermore, the production of blood cells occurs successively at defined locations, in the yolk sac of the early, and liver of the later, fetus, and in the bone marrow of the adult, suggesting that there are reservoirs of progenitors (for reviews, see Domen and Weissman 1999;

Weissman 2000). The essential proof of the existence of such cells comes from experiments in which cells derived from bone marrow, mobilized peripheral blood, or cord blood can reestablish the entire hematopoietic compartment of an animal following its ablation by a lethal dose of radiation. Moreover, clonal dilution and stem cell competition analyses demonstrate that a single cell can repopulate the entire spectrum of blood lineages (see Harrison et al., Chapter 6). In Chapter 15, Keller reviews the evidence in mammalian development for the hemangioblast, a common progenitor both for all blood cells and vascular endothelium, whose existence was proposed by Sabin (1920). Orkin (Chapter 13) presents a logical ordering of our current knowledge of the hematopoietic stem cell in the adult. Flake (Chapter 17) also describes experiments for in utero injections of cells into the fetal sheep to trace the fate of both mesenchymal and hematopoietic stem cells.

Other observations of cell turnover in the normal adult mammal have been made in bone remodeling, which occurs throughout life. Although different types of bone turn over at various rates, on average, the entire adult human skeletal mass is replaced every 8–10 years. Gut epithelium and epidermis are replaced much more rapidly than bone, whereas cartilage turnover, in contrast, is extremely slow in the adult. The replacement of brain tissue in the adult, once discounted, has now been demonstrated beyond doubt, as discussed by Panicker and Rao (see Chapter 18). Thus, tissue homeostasis occurs by production of multiple differentiated cell types at very different rates, according to tissue types.

Some tissue types have assigned stem cells and some have multipotent stem cells. For example, skeletal muscle has satellite cells that appear to be committed to muscle cell phenotype upon differentiation in situ. As described by Watt (Chapter 19), certain epithelial cells are regarded as stem cells, but are still evidently committed to epidermal differentiation. Perhaps stem cells are part of larger repair systems in many mammalian tissue types, and possibly in all vertebrate tissues.

A fundamental question facing cell biology in regard to tissue turnover is, Do multiple cell types emerge from predestined cells programmed to proliferate as committed cells or from multipotent, highly plastic, stem cells? Despite the fact that stem cells may have extensive proliferative capacities, as demonstrated in vitro in cell culture, in vivo the cells may be quiescent until injury or tissue degradation stimulates the regenerative signal. Cells that are committed to a particular lineage are often referred to as committed transitional cells. These cells can commit following expansion as blast cells, or alternatively, stem cells can proliferate as multipotent cells. For example, in the hematopoietic system highly differentiated lymphocytes, descendants of stem cells, such as B cells or activated T cells, divide in clonal fashion to produce the large numbers of progeny necessary for their differentiated function (see Chapter 14, Melchers and Rolink). This is distinct from the hematopoietic stem cell expansion that can occur in vivo or ex vivo as relatively undifferentiated cells. Therefore, for each cell and tissue system, understanding the relationship between expansion by proliferation and functional commitment is important to characterizing the level at which stem cells are active. One of the challenges to modern stem cell biology is understanding the molecular basis of lineage commitment when a cell becomes irreversibly locked to a terminal phenotype, despite retaining the full genome.

Recently, several studies have presented evidence to challenge the long-held belief that stem cells which persist after the early embryonic stages of development are restricted in potential to forming only the cell types characteristic of the tissue to which they belong. There are, for example, data showing that oligodendrocyte precursors can revert to the status of mutilineage neural stem cells (Kondo and Raff 2000), and that, depending on the conditions to which they are exposed, neural stem cells retain an even wider range of options (Clarke et al. 2000). In addition, hematopoietic stem cells have been found to have the potential to repopulate liver hepatocyte populations (Lagasse et al. 2000). Both muscle and neural tissue appear to be a source of hematopoietic stem cells (Jackson et al. 1999; Galli et al. 2000), whereas bone marrow may house muscle precursor cells (Ferrari et al. 1998). Moreover, bone marrow stroma, which contains mesenchymal stem cells (Liechty et al. 2000), may also give rise to neurons and glia (Kopen et al. 1999; Mezey and Chandross 2000; Woodbury et al. 2000). Indeed, the breadth of lineage capabilities for both the mesenchymal stem cells and hematopoietic stem cells of bone marrow are subjects of active study and lively debate (Goodell et al. 1997; Lemischka 1999; Deans and Moseley 2000; Huss et al. 2000; Liechty et al. 2000; Weissman 2000). Thus, the field of stem cell biology has entered an exciting new era that raises interesting questions regarding the significance of cell lineage and germ layers for the process of cellular diversification.

REFERENCES

Allgöwer M. 1956. *The cellular basis of wound repair.* C.C. Thomas, Springfield, Illinois.
Aubin J.E. 1998. Bone stem cells. *J. Cell Biochem Suppl.* **30/31:** 73–82.
Bizzozero G. 1894. An address on growth and regeneration of the organism. *Br. Med. J.* **1:** 728–782.
Bode H.R. and David C.N. 1978. Regulation of a multipotent stem cell, the interstitial cell

of *Hydra. Prog. Biophys. Mol. Biol.* **33:** 189–206.

Boveri T. 1887. Ueber Differenzierung der Zellkerne Wahrend der Furchung des Eies von *Ascaris megalocephala. Anat. Anz.* **2:** 688–693.

Braude P., Bolton V., and Moore S. 1988. Human gene expression first occurs between the four- and eight-cell stages of preimplantation development. *Nature* **332:** 459–461.

Brockes J.P. 1997. Amphibian limb regeneration: Rebuilding a complex structure. *Science* **276:** 81–87.

Brower D. 1987. Chromosome organization in polyploid mouse trophoblast nuclei. *Chromosoma* **95:** 76–80.

Cameron I.L. and Jeter J.R. 1971. Relationship between cell proliferation and cytodifferentiation in embryonic chick tissue. In *Developmental aspect of the cell cycle* (ed. I.L. Cameron et al.), pp. 191–222. Academic Press, New York.

Chisholm J. 1988. Analysis of the fifth cell cycle of mouse development. *J. Reprod. Fertil.* **84:** 29–35.

Clarke D.L., Johansson C.B., Wilbertz J., Veress B., Nilsson E., Karlström H., Lendahl U., and Frisén J. 2000. Generalized potential of adult neural stem cells. *Science* **288:** 1660–1663.

Copp A.J. 1978. Interactions between inner cell mass and trophectoderm of the mouse blastocyst. I. A study of cellular proliferation. *J. Embryol. Exp. Morphol.* **48:** 109–125.

Davidson E.H. 1986. *Gene activity in early development*, 3rd edition. Academic Press, Orlando, Florida.

Deans R.J. and Moseley A.B. 2000. Mesenchymal stem cells: Biology and potential clinical uses. *Exp. Hematol.* **28:** 875–884.

Domen J. and Weissman I.L. 1999. Self renewal, differentiation or death: Regulation and manipulation of hematopoietic stem cell fate. *Mol. Med. Today* **5:** 201–208.

El-Shershaby A.M. and Hinchliffe J.R. 1974. Cell redundancy in the zona-intact preimplantation mouse blastocyst: A light and electron microscope study of dead cells and their fate. *J. Embryol. Exp. Morphol.* **31:** 643–654.

Ferrari G., Cusella-De Angelis G., Coletta M., Paolucci E., Stornaiuolo A., Cossu G., and Mavilio F. 1998. Muscle regeneration by bone marrow-derived myogenic progenitors. *Science* **279:** 1528–1530.

Gage F.H. 2000. Mammalian neural stem cells. *Science* **287:** 1433–1438.

Gage F.H., Ray J., and Fisher L.J. 1995. Isolation, characterization, and use of stem cells from the CNS. *Annu. Rev. Neurosci.* **18:** 159–192.

Galli R., Borello U., Gritti A., Minasi M.G., Bjornson C., Coletta M., Mora M., De Angelis M.G., Fiocco R., Cossu G., and Vescovi A.L. 2000. Skeletal myogenic potential of human and mouse neural stem cells. *Nat. Neurosci.* **3:** 986–991.

Gardner R.L. and Cockroft D.L. 1998. Complete dissipation of coherent clonal growth occurs before gastrulation in mouse epiblast. *Development* **125:** 2397–2402.

Gardner R.L. and Davies T.J. 1993. Lack of coupling between onset of giant transformation and genome endoreduplication in the mural trophectoderm of the mouse blastocyst. *J. Exp. Zool.* **265:** 54–60.

Gardner R.L. and Lawrence P.A., Eds. 1986. Single cell marking and cell lineage in animal development. *Philos. Trans R. Soc. Lond. B Biol. Sci.* **313:** 1–187.

Golding D.W. 1967a. Regeneration and growth control in Nereis. I. Growth and regeneration. *J. Embryol. Exp. Morphol.* **18:** 67–77.

———. 1967b. Regeneration and growth control in Nereis. II. An axial gradient in growth potentiality. *J. Embryol. Exp. Morphol.* **18:** 79–90.

Goodell M.A., Rosenzweig M., Kim H., Marks D.F., DeMaria M., Paradis G., Grupp S.A., Sieff C.A., Mulligan R.C., and Johnson R.P. 1997. Dye efflux studies suggest that hematopoietic stem cells expressing low or undetectable levels of CD34 antigen exist in multiple species. *Nat. Med.* **3:** 1337–1345.

Goss R.J. 1978. *The physiology of growth.* Academic Press, New York.

Gould E., Reeves A.J., Graziano M.S., and Gross C.G. 1999. Neurogenesis in the neocortex of adult primates. *Science* **286:** 548–552.

Handyside A.H. and Hunter S. 1986. Cell division and death in the mouse blastocyst before implantation. *Roux's Arch. Dev. Biol.* **195:** 519–526.

Hill S.D. 1970. Origin of the regeneration blastema in polychaete annelids. *Am. Zool.* **10:** 101–112.

Holtzer H., Weintraub H., Mayne R., and Mochan B. 1972. The cell cycle, cell lineage, and cell differentiation. *Curr. Top. Dev. Biol.* **7:** 229–256.

Huss R., Lange C., Weissinger E.M., Kolb H.J., and Thalmeier K. 2000. Evidence of peripheral blood-derived, plastic-adherent CD34(-/low) hematopoietic stem cell clones with mesenchymal stem cell characteristics. *Stem Cells* **18:** 252–260.

Jackson K.A., Mi T., and Goodell M.A. 1999. Hematopoietic potential of stem cells isolated from murine skeletal muscle. *Proc. Natl. Acad. Sci.* **96:**14482–14486.

Jan Y.N. and Jan L.Y. 1994. Genetic control of cell fate specification in *Drosophila* peripheral nervous system. *Annu. Rev. Genet.* **28:** 373–393.

Kirn J., O'Loughlin B., Kasparian S., and Nottebohm F. 1994. Cell death and neuronal recruitment in the high vocal center of adult male canaries are temporally related to changes in song. *Proc. Natl. Acad. Sci.* **91:** 7844–7848.

Kondo T. and Raff M. 2000. Oligodendrocyte precursor cells reprogrammed to become multipotential CNS stem cells. *Science* **289:** 1754–1757.

Kopen G.C., Prockop D.J., and Phinney D.G. 1999. Marrow stromal cells migrate throughout forebrain and cerebellum, and they differentiate into astrocytes after injection into neonatal mouse brains. *Proc. Natl. Acad. Sci.* **96:** 10711–10716.

Kratzer P.G., Chapman V.M., Lambert H., Evans R.E., and Liskay R.M. 1983. Differences in the DNA of the inactive X chromosome of fetal and extraembryonic tissues of mice. *Cell* **33:** 37–42.

Lagasse E., Connors H., Al-Dhalimy M., Reitsma M., Dohse M., Osborne L., Wang X., Finegold M., Weissman I.L., and Grompe M. 2000. Purified hematopoietic stem cells can differentiate into hepatocytes in vivo. *Nat. Med.* **6:** 1229–1234.

Lawson K.A., Meneses J.J., and Pedersen R.A. 1991. Clonal analysis of epiblast fate during germ layer formation in the mouse embryo. *Development* **113:** 891–911.

Lemischka I. 1999. The power of stem cells reconsidered? *Proc. Natl. Acad. Sci.* **96:** 14193–14195.

Lewis N.E. and Rossant J. 1982. Mechanism of size regulation in mouse embryo aggregates. *J. Embryol. Exp. Morphol.* **72:** 169–181.

Liechty K.W., MacKenzie T.C., Shaaban A.F., Radu A., Moseley A.B., Deans R., Marshak D.R., and Flake A.W. 2000. Human mesenchymal stem cells engraft and demonstrate site-specific differentiation after in utero transplantation in sheep. *Nat. Med.* **6:** 1282–1286.

Marchand F. 1901. *Der Prozess der Wundheilung mit Einschluss der Transplantationen.* Enke, Stuttgart, Germany.

Martin V.J., Littlefield C.L., Archer W.E., and Bode H.R. 1997. Embryogenesis in *Hydra*. *Biol. Bull.* **192:** 345–363.

McKay R. 2000. Stem cells—Hype and hope. *Nature* **406:** 361–364.

Memili E. and First N.L. 1999. Control of gene expression at the onset of bovine development. *Biol. Reprod.* **61:** 1198–1207.

Mezey E. and Chandross K.J. 2000. Bone marrow: A possible alternative source of cells in the adult nervous system. *Eur. J. Pharmacol.* **405:** 297–302.

Newport J. and Kirschner M. 1982. A major developmental transition in early *Xenopus* embryos. II. Control of onset of transcription. *Cell* **30:** 687–696.

Price J., Turner D., and Cepko C. 1987. Lineage analysis in the vertebrate nervous system by retrovirus-mediated gene transfer. *Proc. Natl. Acad. Sci.* **84:** 156–160.

Ram P.T. and Schultz R.M. 1993. Reporter gene expression in G2 of the 1-cell mouse embryo. *Dev. Biol.* **156:** 552–556.

Rands G.F. 1986a. Size regulation in the mouse embryo. I. The development of quadruple aggregates. *J. Embryol. Exp. Morphol.* **94:** 139–148.

———. 1986b. Size regulation in the mouse embryo. II. The development of half embryos. *J. Embryol. Exp. Morphol.* **98:** 209–217.

Reynolds B.A. and Weiss S. 1992. Generation of neurons and astrocytes from isolated cells of the adult mammalian central nervous system. *Science* **255:** 1707–1710.

Rossant J., Sandford J.P., Chapman V.M., and Andrews G.K. 1986. Undermethylation of structural gene sequences in extraembryonic lineages of the mouse. *Dev. Biol.* **117:** 567–573.

Sabin F.R. 1920. Studies on the origin of blood vessels and of red corpuscles as seen in the living blastoderm of the chick during the second day of incubation. *Contrib. Embryol.* **9:** 213–262.

Sanes J.R., Rubenstein J.L., and Nicolas J.F. 1986. Use of recombinant retrovirus to study post-implantation cell lineage in mouse embryos. *EMBO J.* **5:** 3133–3142.

Shah M., Foreman D.M., and Ferguson M.W. 1994. Neutralising antibody to TGF-β 1,2, reduces cutaneous scarring in adult rodents. *J. Cell Sci.* **107:** 1137–1157.

Snow M.H.L. and Tam P.P. 1979. Is compensatory growth a complicating factor in mouse teratology? *Nature* **279:** 555–557.

Sobis H., Verstuyf A., and Vandeputte M. 1993. Visceral yolk sac-derived tumors. *Int. J. Dev. Biol.* **37:** 155–168.

Sulston J.E., Schierenberg E., White J.G., and Thomson J.N. 1983. The embryonic cell lineage of the nematode *Caenorhabditis elegans. Dev. Biol.* **100:** 64–119.

Thornton C.S. 1968. Amphibian limb regeneration. *Adv. Morphog.* **7:** 205–249.

Varmuza S., Prideaux V., Kothary R., and Rossant J. 1988. Polytene chromosomes in mouse trophoblast giant cells. *Development* **102:** 127–134.

Weissman I.L. 2000. Stem cells: Units of development, units of regeneration, and units of evolution. *Cell* **100:** 157–168.

Wilson E.B. 1896. *The cell in development and inheritance.* Macmillan, New York.

Woodbury D., Schwarz E.J., Prockop D.J., and Black I.B. 2000. Adult rat and human bone marrow stromal cells differentiate into neurons. *J. Neurosci. Res.* **61:** 364–370.

2

Differentiated Parental DNA Chain Causes Stem Cell Pattern of Cell-type Switching in *Schizosaccharomyces pombe*

Amar J.S. Klar
Gene Regulation and Chromosome Biology Laboratory
NCI-Frederick Cancer Research and Development Center
Frederick, Maryland 21702-1201

According to the rules of Mendelian genetics, sister chromatids are equivalent, and genes are composed of DNA alone. Violations to both of these rules have been discovered, which explain the stem-cell-like pattern of asymmetric cell division in the fission yeast *Schizosaccharomyces pombe*. In this review, I highlight key ideas and their experimental support so that the reader can contrast these mechanisms, which are not based on differential gene regulation, with those discovered in other diverse systems presented in this monograph.

FISSION YEAST AS A MODEL SYSTEM FOR INVESTIGATING CELLULAR DIFFERENTIATION AT THE SINGLE-CELL LEVEL

S. pombe is a haploid, unicellular, lower eukaryotic organism whose genetics has been studied very thoroughly. Its genome comprises only three chromosomes, with DNA content similar to that of the evolutionarily distantly related budding yeast, *Saccharomyces cerevisiae*. This organism has been exploited as a major system for cell cycle studies as well as for studies of cellular differentiation. The single cells of fission yeast express either P (Plus) or M (Minus) mating-cell type and divide by fission of the parental cell to produce rod-shaped progeny of nearly equal size. Yeast cells do not express mating type while growing on rich medium. Only when they are starved, especially for nitrogen, do cells express their mating type and mate with cells of opposite type to produce transient zygotic diploid cells. Normally, the zygotic cell immediately enters into the meiotic cell division cycle and gives rise to four haploid spore segregants, two of P type and two of M type.

The mating type choice is controlled by alternate alleles of the single mating-type locus (*mat1*). Stable diploid lines can be easily constructed by selecting for complementation of auxotrophic markers before the zygotic cells are committed to meiosis. The diploids can then be maintained by growth in rich medium, which inhibits meiosis and sporulation. Once these cells experience nitrogen starvation, they undergo meiosis and sporulation without mating. The sporulation process requires heterozygosity at *mat1*. Strains that switch *mat1* are called homothallic, and those that do not switch are called heterothallic.

Conjugation in cells of homothallic strains occurs efficiently between newly divided pairs of sister cells (Leupold 1950; for review, see Klar 1992). Switching occurs at high frequency (Egel 1977). The most remarkable feature of the system is that switching occurs in a nonrandom fashion within a cell lineage. Miyata and Miyata (1981) followed the pattern of matings between the progeny of a single cell growing under starvation conditions, on the surface of solid medium. They found that among the four granddaughters of a single cell, a single zygote was formed in 72–94% of the cases. In no case did they observe two zygotes. The mating mostly occurred between sister cells, whereas non-sister (cousin) cells mated infrequently. It appeared, therefore, that among the four granddaughters of a single cell, only one had switched. With this procedure, it was not possible to determine switching potential of cells past the four-cell stage since two of them formed a zygote and underwent meiosis and sporulation, so that their future potential could not be ascertained. Subsequent studies used diploid cells instead where one homolog contained a nonswitchable heterothallic *mat1* allele, whereas the other contained a homothallic locus. Such a diploid will not sporulate when it is homozygous (*mat1P/mat1P* or *mat1M/mat1M*) at *mat1*, but will stop growing and initiate sporulation once switching produces *mat1P/mat1M* heterozygosity. Diploid cells keep on switching regardless of their *mat1* constitution. In such diploid pedigrees (Egel and Eie 1987; Klar 1990), the same rules of switching described for haploids were observed. More importantly, one can determine the competence of switching past the four-cell stage by microscopically monitoring the competence of individual cells to sporulate. Such studies have defined the rules of switching as follows (Fig. 1).

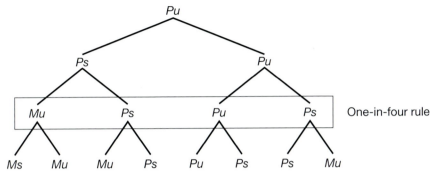

Figure 1. The program of cell-type switching in *S. pombe* cell pedigrees. The subscripts u and s, respectively, reflect unswitchable or switchable cells.

RULES OF SWITCHING

- *The single-switchable-sister rule:* In most cell divisions (80–90% of cases) an unswitchable (e.g., Pu) cell produces one Ps (switching-competent) and one Pu unswitchable cell like the parental Pu cell. Thus, both sisters are never switching-competent.
- *The single-switched-daughter rule:* Switching-competent Ps cell produces one switched and one switching-competent Ps cell in approximately 80–90% of cell divisions. Simultaneous switching of both daughters is never seen.
- *The recurrent switching rule:* Like the parental cell, the sister of the recently switched cell maintains switching competence in 80–90% of cases. Consequently, chains of pedigree result where one daughter in each cell division is switched.
- *The rule of switched allele is unswitchable:* To conform to the one-in-four granddaughter pattern, the newly switched allele must be unswitchable, although this notion has not been experimentally established. It is supported by the Miyata and Miyata (1981) observation, since they never observed two zygotes among four granddaughters of a single cell.
- *The directionality rule:* Since a switchable cell switches to the opposite mating type in 80–90% of cell divisions, it must be that cells show bias in direction of switching such that most switches are productive to the opposite allele rather than undergoing futile switches to the same allele (Thon and Klar 1993; Grewal and Klar 1997; Ivanova et al. 1998).

The same rules also apply when M cells switch to P type. Such rules lead to the following generalizations. First, the switches are presumed to occur in S or G$_2$ phase, such that only one of the two sister chromatids acquires the switched information. Second, most cell divisions are developmentally asymmetric such that one sister is similar to the parental cell, and the other is advanced in its developmental program, a pattern exactly analogous to a stem cell pattern of cell division (Chapters 4 and 13). Third, altogether, starting from an unswitchable cell, two consecutive asymmetric cell divisions must have occurred to produce a single switched cell in four related granddaughter cells.

SWITCHES RESULT FROM GENE CONVERSIONS AT *mat1*

The *mat1* locus is a part of a cluster of tightly linked *mat1-mat2-mat3* genes on chromosome II (Fig. 2). The expressed *mat1* locus contains either *mat1P* or *mat1M* allele. Because cells containing a haploid genome are able to express either mating cell type, both cell types must contain sufficient information to interchange *mat1* alleles. The *mat2P* and *mat3M* alleles are silent and are only used as donors of genetic information for *mat1* switching. The *mat2* gene is located approximately 15 kb distal to *mat1* (Beach and Klar 1984), and *mat3* is located another 11 kb from

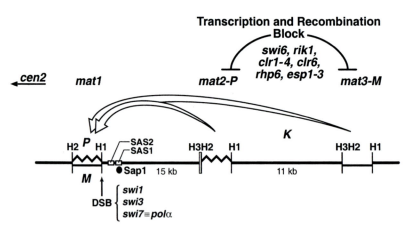

Figure 2. The system of mating-type switching of *S. pombe*. All the *cis*- and *trans*-acting elements have been described in the text. Large arrows reflect unidirectional transfer of genetic information copied from *mat2* or *mat3* to *mat1* by the gene conversion process. DSB reflects a transient double-stranded break that initiates recombination at *mat1*. H1–3 are short DNA sequence homologies shared by *mat* loci. This system shares features with both site-specific and homology-dependent recombination mechanisms.

mat2, separated by the sequence called the K-region (Grewal and Klar 1997). The P-specific region is 1104 bp long, whereas the nonhomologous M-specific region is 1128 bp long. Very short homologies represented by H1, H2, and H3 sequences flank the indicated cassettes (Kelly et al. 1988). Each *mat1* allele codes for two transcripts, one of which is induced during starvation (Kelly et al. 1988). The *mat1* interconversion results from a gene conversion event whereby a copy of *mat2P* or *mat3M* is substituted with the resident *mat1* allele. Consequently, the differentiated state is maintained as a genetic alteration that is subject to further rounds of spontaneous switching.

cis- AND trans-ACTING FUNCTIONS REQUIRED FOR SWITCHING

Southern analysis of yeast DNA indicated that nearly 20–25% of the *mat1* DNA is cut at the junctions of H1 and the allele-specific sequences (Fig. 2) (Beach 1983; Beach and Klar 1984). By analogy to the *MAT* switching system where a *trans*-acting, *HO*-encoded endonuclease cleaves *MAT* to initiate recombination (Strathern et al. 1982), it was proposed that the double-stranded break (DSB) at *mat1* likewise initiates recombination. In support of this proposal, several *cis*- and *trans*-acting mutations were isolated that reduce the level of the DSB and, consequently, reduce the efficiency of switching (Egel et al. 1984). Interestingly, the amount of cut DNA remains constant throughout the cell cycle (Beach 1983), although no study has directly demonstrated that the break actually exists in vivo.

Several *cis*-acting deletion mutations in *mat1* have implicated *mat1*-distal sequences in formation of the DSB. One mutation, C13P11, reduces switching (Egel and Gutz 1981; Beach 1983) and contains a 27-bp deletion that includes 7 bp of the distal end of the *mat1* H1 region (Klar et al. 1991). Another mutation, smt-o, totally blocks switching and contains a larger deletion in the same region (Styrkarsdottir et al. 1993) as well as two sites, called SAS1 and SAS2, which comprise a binding site for a protein called Sap1p (Arcangioli and Klar 1991).

Mutations of three unlinked genes, *swi1, swi3,* and *swi7,* reduce switching by reducing the level of the DSB (Egel et al. 1984; Gutz and Schmidt 1985). The functions of *swi1* and *swi3* remain undefined, but interestingly, *swi7* encodes the catalytic subunit of DNA polymerase α (Singh and Klar 1993). This result implicates the act of DNA replication in generation of the DSB. Nielsen and Egel (1989) mapped the position of the break by genomic sequencing of purified chromosomal DNA. The break was defined with 3′-hydroxyl and 5′-phosphate groups at the junction of H1 and the allele-specific sequences on one strand, but the break on the other strand could not be defined. Of particular note, strains in which both donor loci are deleted and substituted with the *S. cerevisiae LEU2* gene (Δ*mat2,3::LEU2*) exhibit the normal level of the DSB, maintain stable mating type, and surprisingly, are viable.

DSB EFFICIENTLY INITIATES MEIOTIC *mat1* GENE CONVERSION IN DONOR-DELETED STRAINS

When donor-deleted cells of opposite mating type were crossed (*mat1P* Δ*mat2,3::LEU2* × *mat1MΔ mat2,3::LEU2*) and subjected to tetrad analysis, a high rate of *mat1* conversion was observed, such that 10% of the tetrads were of 3P:1M, and another 10% were of the 1P:3M type (Klar and Miglio 1986). When the same cross was repeated with *swi3⁻* strains that lack the DSB, the efficiency of meiotic *mat1* gene conversion was correspondingly reduced. It was suggested that the DSB designed for mitotic *mat1* switching can also initiate meiotic gene conversion such that only one of two sister chromatids is converted, since no 4:0 or 0:4 conversions were observed. This meiotic gene conversion assay tests the switching competence of individual chromosomes and was the key technique in deciphering the mechanism of *mat1* switching in mitotic cells.

COMPETENCE FOR SWITCHING IS CHROMOSOMALLY BORNE

Discovering the mechanism by which sister cells gain different developmental fates is central to understanding eukaryotic cellular differentiation. The single-cell assay for testing *mat1* switching, either by mating or by determining sporulation ability as discussed above, suggests that the developmental decision is imparted to sister cells by cell-autonomous mechanisms. It would therefore seem that the switching potential must be asymmetrically segregated to daughter cells either through the nuclear/cytoplasmic factor(s) or via the DNA template. In the first model, essential components, such as those encoded by *swi* genes, would be unequally expressed, differentially stabilized, or asymmetrically segregated to daughter cells. In the second model, since the DSB seems to initiate recombination required for *mat1* switching and the break may be chromosomally inherited, it may be that only one of two sister chromatids is imprinted in each cell division, thus differentiating sister cells. The term imprinting implies some sort of chromosomal modification such that only one of the two sister chromatids is cleaved to initiate recombination. Any mechanism, however, must explain not only how sisters acquire different development potential, but also how two consecutive asymmetric cell divisions are performed such that only one in four related granddaughter cells ever switches. Since the level of the DSB is highly correlated with the efficiency of switching, it was reasoned that generation of DSB in some cells, but not in other related cells, is the key to defining the program of switching in cell lineage. Should the observed pattern of switching in mitotically dividing cells be the result of chromosomal imprinting, I hypothesized (Klar 1987, 1990) that the likely candidates to catalyze this epigenetic event are the gene functions involved in generating the cut at *mat1*, such as those of *swi1*, *swi3*, and *swi7*. It has not been possible to directly demonstrate the inheritance of the imprint and correlate it to switching in mitotically dividing single cells. However, testing meiotic *mat1* gene conversion potential of individual chromosomes provided a key test of the model.

Meiotic crosses involving Δ*mat2,3::LEU2* strains generate a high rate of *mat1* gene conversion due to *mat1* to *mat1* interaction by which both 3P:1M and 1P:3M asci are produced in equal proportion (Klar and Miglio 1986). Because the spores are haploid and donor-deleted, the recently converted allele is stably maintained in meiotic segregants. We presume that meiotic *mat1* gene conversion events are also initiated by the break resulting from the imprint at *mat1*. With the meiotic gene conversion assay, it became possible to directly test switching potential of individual chromosomes as well as the effect of *swi1*, *swi3*, and *swi7* genotype on switching competence. As *S. pombe* cells mate and immediately undergo meiosis and sporulation, the diploid phase exists transiently. The key result was that a cross between donor-deleted strains *mat1M swi3⁻* and a *mat1P swi3⁺* generated aberrant tetrads, primarily with 3M:1P segregants, in which only *mat1P* converted to *mat1M* (Klar and Bonaduce 1993). On the other hand, if *swi3⁻* mutation was present in the *mat1P* strain, the *mat1M* changed to *mat1P*. Similarly, crosses involving a *swi1⁻* or a *swi7⁻* parent generated meiotic *mat1* conversion in which only the *mat1* allele provided by the *swi⁺* parent gene converted. Thus, clearly (1) the competence for meiotic gene conversion segregates in *cis* with *mat1*; (2) the *swi1⁺*, *swi3⁺*, and *swi7⁺* functions confer that competence; and (3) the presence of these functions in the zygotic cells provided by the *swi⁺* parent fails to confer the gene conversion potential to the *mat1* allele that was previously replicated in the *swi⁻* background. Those meiotic experiments unambiguously showed that chromosomally imprinted functions are catalyzed at *mat1* by the *swi* gene products at least one generation before meiotic conversion. On the basis of these results, we suggest that the same imprinted event may form the basis of mitotic switching, resulting in the specific pattern of switching in cell pedigrees.

NONEQUIVALENT SISTER CELLS RESULT FROM INHERITING DIFFERENTIATED, NONEQUIVALENT PARENTAL DNA CHAINS

If *mat1* switching is initiated by the DSB, it follows that differentiated sister chromatids must be the reason that only one of the sister cells becomes switching-competent or ever switches. Restated another way, How is it that only one of four descendants of a chromosome switches? To explain the one-in-four granddaughter switching rule, we imagined that one of the decisions to make a given switch must have occurred two generations earlier in the grandparental cell (Mu or Pu in Fig. 1). Specifically, a strand-segregation model was proposed in which "Watson" and "Crick" strands of DNA (Watson and Crick 1953) are nonequivalent in their ability to acquire the developmental potential for switching (Klar 1987). It was proposed that some swi^+ gene functions catalyze a strand-specific imprinting event, which in the following cycle will cause switching again in a strand-specific fashion. The proposal was that strand-specific imprinting allows the DNA to be cut in vivo and switching follows. The inherent DNA sequence difference of two strands alone must not be sufficient, because if it were, each cell would produce one switched and one unswitched daughter. To explain the two-generation program of switching, imprinting in one generation and switching in the following generation was imagined (Klar 1987). It was hypothesized that the imprinting event may consist of DNA methylation or some other base modification, an unrepaired RNA primer of Okazaki fragments, a protein complex that segregates with a specific strand, or a site-specific single-stranded nick that becomes DSB in the next round of replication (Klar 1987).

Several follow-up tests of the strand-segregation model have established this model. First, strains constructed to contain an additional *mat1* cassette placed in an inverted orientation approximately 4.7 kb away from the resident *mat1* locus cleaved one or the other *mat1* locus efficiently, but never simultaneously in the same cell cycle, as imprinting occurs only on one specific strand at each cassette (Klar 1987). Second, as opposed to the switching of only one in four related cells in standard strains (Fig. 1), cells with the inverted duplication switched two (cousins) in four granddaughter cells in 34% of pedigrees (Klar 1990). Third, the inverted cassette also followed the one-in-four switching rule and switched in 32% of cases. Clearly, in such a duplication-containing strain, both daughters of the grandparental cell became developmentally equivalent in at least one-third of cell divisions. Thus, all cells are otherwise equivalent, ruling out the factor(s) segregation model, and the pattern is strictly dictated by inheritance of complementary and nonequivalent DNA chains at *mat1*. It was also hypothesized that the strand-specificity of the imprint may result from the inherently nonequivalent replication of sister chromatids due to lagging-versus leading-strand replication at *mat1* (Klar and Bonaduce 1993). Suggestive evidence for this idea came from the finding that *swi7* implicated in imprinting (Klar and Bonaduce 1993) in fact encodes the major catalytic subunit of DNA polymerase α (Singh and Klar 1993). This polymerase provides the primase activity for initiating DNA replication; thus, it is inherently required more for lagging-strand replication than for leading-strand replication. Fourth, more recent observations biochemically established that the imprint is either a single-stranded and strand-specific nick (Arcangioli 1998) or an alkali-labile modification of DNA at *mat1* (Dalgaard and Klar 1999). Both of these studies showed that the observed DSB is an artifact of DNA preparation created from the imprint at *mat1*, since DNA isolated by gentle means from cells embedded in agarose plugs exhibited much-reduced levels of the break. Arcangioli (1998) showed that mung bean nuclease treatment of the DNA results in generation of the DSB. This result, combined with the primer extension experiments, led Arcangioli (1998) to conclude that the imprint is a single-stranded nick which persists at a constant level throughout the cell cycle. In contrast, Dalgaard and Klar (1999) found both strands at *mat1* to be intact while one of the strands breaks after denaturation with alkali, but not with the formaldehyde treatment. Although these biochemical studies are discordant with each other, nonetheless, both support earlier suggestions and the model (Klar 1987, 1990). Combining genetic and biochemical results, the strand-segregation model is now clearly established and, henceforth, would be referred to as a strand-segregation mechanism.

THE IMPRINTING MECHANISM

The DSB was initially discovered when the DNA was prepared with the conventional method, which includes a step of RNase A treatment (Beach 1983; Beach and Klar 1984). All the biochemical studies can be reconciled should the imprint consist of an RNase-labile base(s). Arcangioli (1998) concluded that the imprint must be a single-stranded nick, since mung bean nuclease treatment produces the DSB. It should be noted, however, that this nuclease also has RNase activity, in addition to DNA-cleaving activity at the nick. The alkali-labile site discovered by Dalgaard and Klar (1999) is also consistent with the idea that the imprint is probably an RNA moiety left unrepaired from an RNA primer that has been ligated to form a continuous DNA-RNA-DNA strand. It was previously suggested that lagging- versus leading-strand replication may dictate imprinting (Klar and Bonaduce 1993). Dalgaard and Klar (1999) directly tested this idea by proposing an "orientation of replication model" where it was shown that when *mat1* is inverted at the indigenous location, it fails to imprint/switch. A partial restoration was obtained if origin of replication was placed next to the inverted *mat1* locus. Furthermore, *mat1* was shown to be replicated unidirectionally by centromere-distal origin(s) by experiments defining replication intermediates with the two-dimensional gel analysis. These results, combined with the earlier finding that *swi7* encodes DNA polymerase α (Singh and Klar 1993), led Dalgaard and Klar (1999) to suggest that the imprint is probably an RNA base(s) added only by the lagging-strand replication complex. Alternatively, it may be some other base modification conferring alkali lability to one specific strand. Both these biochemical studies suggest that the DSB is an artifact of the DNA preparation procedure, yet both studies suggest that the imprint leads to transient generation of the DSB at the time of replication of the imprinted strand by the leading-strand replication complex. It is proposed that such a transient DSB initiates recombination required for switching *mat1*. Because meiotic *mat1* conversions are only of 3:1 type (Klar and Miglio 1986) and only one member of a pair of sisters switches (Miyata and Miyata 1981), recombination must occur in S or G_2 such that only one sister chromatid receives the converted allele. Even the transient DSB fails to cause lethality in donor-deleted strains. In principle, the intact sister chromatid may be used to heal the break (Klar and Miglio 1986). Since recombination-deficient (*swi5⁻*) strains can also heal the break (Klar and Miglio 1986), the yeast probably has the capacity to heal the break without recombination. Two *mat1 cis*-acting sites located near the cut site and the cognate binding factor encoded by *sap1* somehow dictate imprinting at *mat1* (Arcangioli and Klar 1991). One possibility is that these elements promote maintenance of the imprint by prohibiting its repair (Klar and Bonaduce 1993). In summary, the biochemical results provide evidence for the notion that DNA replication advances the program of cellular differentiation in a strand-specific fashion (Klar 1987, 1990).

   It remains to be determined exactly how the imprint is made. Dalgaard and Klar (1999) found DNA replication pausing at the site of the imprint. Analysis of DNA replication intermediates around *mat1* revealed another element located to the left of *mat1* where replication terminates in one direction and not in the other to help replicate *mat1* only unidirectionally (Dalgaard and Klar 2000). This study showed that swi1p and swi3p factors act by pausing the replication fork at the imprinting site as well as by promoting termination at the polar terminator of replication. One possibility is that pausing at the fork helps imprinting by providing sufficient time to lay RNA primer at the imprinting site. Using DNA density-shift experiments, Arcangioli (2000) showed that 20–25% of *mat1* DNA is replicated such that both strands are synthesized de novo during S phase. This work also showed directly that the newly switched *mat1* does not have the imprint (i.e., nick), further supporting the strand segregation model (Klar 1987).

SILENCING OF THE *mat2-mat3* REGION IS CAUSED BY AN EPIGENETIC MECHANISM

A mechanistically very different imprinting event has been shown to keep the donor region silent from expression and from mitotic as well as meiotic recombination. Even when another genetic marker, such as *ura4*, was inserted in and around the *mat2-mat3* region, its transcription was highly repressed. Starting with such a Ura⁻ strain, several *trans*-acting factors of *clr1-4* (*clr* for *c*ryptic *l*oci *r*egulator) were identified, mutations of which relieve silencing and recombination prohibition of this interval (Thon and Klar 1992; Ekwall and Ruusala 1994; Thon et al. 1994). Two other previously defined mutations in *swi6* and *rik1* loci likewise compromise unusual properties of this region (Egel et al. 1989; Klar and Bonaduce 1991; Lorentz et al. 1992). Several other newly identified genes, *esp1-3* (Thon and Friis 1997), *rhp6* (Singh et al. 1998), and *clr6* (Grewal et al. 1998), have also been implicated in silencing. Molecular analysis of these *trans*-acting factors and sequence analysis of the 11-kb K-region between *mat2* and *mat3* loci have suggested that this region is silenced due to organization of a repressive heterochromatic structure making this region unaccessible for transcription and recombination. First, 4.3 kb of the 11.0 kb region between *mat2* and *mat3*, called the K-region, shows 96% sequence identity with the repeat sequences present in the chromosome II centromere (Grewal and Klar 1997). A similar silencing occurs when *ura4* is placed in centromeric repeat sequences (Allshire 1996). Second, *swi6* (Lorentz et al. 1994), *clr4* (Ivanova et al. 1998), and *chp1* and *chp2* (Thon and Verhein-Hansen 2000) encode proteins containing a chromodomain motif thought to be essential for chromatin organization (Singh 1994). Third, *clr3* and *clr6* encode homologs of histone deacetylase activities that are certain to influence organization of chromatin structure (Grewal et al. 1998). Fourth, accessibility of *mat2* and *mat3* loci to in vivo expressed *Escherichia coli dam⁺* methylase is influenced by the *swi6* genotype (Singh et al. 1998).

Interestingly, when the 7.5-kb sequence of the K-region was replaced with the *ura4* locus (*K*Δ::*ura4* allele), the *ura4* gene expressed in a variegated fashion (Grewal and Klar 1996; Thon and Friis 1997). Remarkably, both states, designated *ura4-off* and *ura4-on* epistates, were mitotically stable, interchanging only at a rate of approximately 5.6×10^{-4}/cell division. Even more spectacularly, when cells with these states were mated and the resulting diploid was grown for more than 30 generations and then subjected to meiotic analysis, we found that each state was stable and inherited as a Mendelian epiallele of the *mat* region (Grewal and Klar 1996). Thus, the epigenetic state is stable in both mitosis and meiosis as a Mendelian, chromosomal marker.

To explain this kind of inheritance, we advanced a chromatin replication model in which silencing occurs on both daughter chromatids by self-templating assembly of chromatin in the *mat2/3* region (Grewal and Klar 1996). The proposal is that preexisting nucleoprotein complexes presumably segregated to both strands of DNA promote assembly of chromatin on both daughter chromatids to clonally propagate and deliver a specific state of gene expression to both daughter cells. Two recent studies provide support to the chromatin replication model. First, transiently overexpressing *swi6$^+$* in cells with *ura4-on* state efficiently changes them to *ura4-off* state; once changed, overexpression is not required to maintain the altered state (Nakayama et al. 2000). Second, transiently exposing the *ura4-off* cells to histone deacetylase inhibitor trichostatin A efficiently changes them to *ura4-on* state (Grewal et al. 1998). In both of the change-of-state experiments, changes were genetically inherited at the *mat* region and were correlated with the changes in the recruitment of swi6 protein to the *mat* region chromatin (Nakayama et al. 2000). Thus, in this case, the committed states of gene expression are inherited epigenetically rather than through variations in DNA sequence (Klar 1998; Nakayama et al. 2000).

STRAND-SEGREGATION MECHANISM FOR EXPLAINING GENERAL CELLULAR DIFFERENTIATION

Two important lessons learned from the fission yeast system are that (1) by the process of DNA replication developmentally nonequivalent sister chromatids can be produced, and (2) stable patterns of gene expression can be inherited chromosomally over the course of multiple cell divisions akin to the general phenomenon of imprinting so prevalent in mammals. The question arises as to whether the first of these mechanisms is only applicable to yeast. It is impossible to answer this question because in multicellular systems it is not feasible to experimentally test such models because developmental potential and segregation of differentiated chromatids cannot be ascertained at the single-cell level in mitotically dividing cells. In principle, however, it is possible to imagine that the act of DNA replication may modulate activities of developmentally important genes in a strand-specific fashion. It is not necessary to expect that such modulation occurs only through DNA recombination as found in yeast; it could rather be due to differential organization of chromatin structure of sister chromatids from both homologs in diploid organisms. (I never liked the idea of DNA methylation being the primary mechanism of imprinting and gene regulation.) Once established, these states may be maintained through multiple cell divisions akin to the epigenetic control operative in the K-region of *mat2/3* interval (Grewal and Klar 1996). To produce the stem-cell-like pattern, we then propose that the differentiated chromatids from both homologs have to be segregated nonrandomly to daughter cells by yet another mechanism such that one daughter cell will inherit chromosomes with the developmentally important gene in an active state, while the other cell inherits an inactive state. Which daughter will get which sets of chromosomes will have to be influenced by other axes of the developing system, such as a dorsoventral axis. Such a proposal has been made to explain the left–right axis determination of visceral organs of mice (Klar 1994). It is proposed that the *iv* gene (for situs inversus) product functions for nonrandom segregation of sister chromatids to daughter cells at certain cell division during mitosis whenever the left–right decision is distributed during embryogenesis. Interestingly, the iv^- mutant produces randomized mice such that half of the mice have the heart located on the left side, and the other half have situs inversus such that the heart is on the right side of the body (Layton 1976). Recently, it was found that the *iv* gene encodes dynein, which is a molecular motor that functions to move cargo on microtubules (Supp et al. 1997). Of course, the alternate, accepted but not yet proven, model to explain the behavior of the iv^- mutant mice is that the mutation causes random distribution of a hypothetical morphogen-producing center, which in iv^+ mice is localized only to one side of the body (Brown and Wolpert 1990). However, the nature of the morphogen, the mechanism of its graded distribution, and the localization of the morphogen production to only one side remain undefined. Consequently, the morphogen model is only descriptive, because it does not suggest experimental tests to scrutinize its validity. This is not to say that the opportunity for a morphogen-like mechanism does not exist elsewhere in biology. For example, there is ample evidence that such a mechanism operates in the rather unusual development of *Drosophila*. Because the *Drosophila* egg is very large compared to most cells, the graded distribution of egg constituents is required to ensure such a mechanism. In most other developmental systems, decisions are probably made right from the first zygotic cell division such that the sister cells are non-equivalent in their developmental potential. New decisions for regulating developmentally important genes may be made at each cell division. Clearly, investigation of more model systems is needed to ask fundamental questions of specification and distribution of developmental decision in multicellular systems. Another case where such a mechanism may be operative is development of human brain laterality such that in most individuals the left hemisphere of the brain is specified to process language, while the right hemisphere processes emotional information. It is speculated that a genetic function, analogous to that of the iv^+ function for mice visceral specification, may have evolved for nonrandom segregation of Watson and Crick strands of a particular chromosome (Klar 1999). Thus, chromosomal rearrangements or defects in the hypothesized *RGHT* gene may predispose individuals to develop bilaterally symmetrical brains, causing psychiatric disorders such as schizophrenia and manic-depressive disease. In circumstantial support for the strand-segregation mechanism, segregation of sister chromatids in embryonic mouse cells (Lark et al. 1966) and in mouse epithelial cells (Potten et al. 1978) is shown to be nonrandom.

PROGRAM OF CELL-TYPE SWITCHING OF BUDDING YEAST COMPARED WITH THE FISSION YEAST SYSTEM

The stem cell pattern of cell type change is also observed with the evolutionarily distantly related yeast *S. cerevisiae*. Analogous studies with this system have yielded a wealth of knowledge regarding mechanisms of silencing, recombination, cell-type determination, and cell-lineage specification. Both of these yeast systems have become models to address fundamental questions of cellular differentiation. The budding yeast system, in fact, has become a classic textbook case. Most interestingly, the details of the molecular mechanisms of both systems vary in fundamental ways at every level; lessons learned from both systems should be taught to future biologists.

The budding yeast cells inherently divide asymmetrically by budding in which the older (mother) cell pinches off a small (daughter) cell. The daughter cell gains in size by growing in the longer G_1 phase before it starts its division cycle, while the mother cell initiates the next cycle right away. The two sexual types of *S. cerevisiae* are designated **a** and α, which are correspondingly conferred by the *MAT***a** and *MAT*α alleles of the mating-type locus. These two cell types efficiently interchange, and the changed cells of opposite mating type establish a *MATa/MATα* diploid phase in which further switching is prohibited by heterozygosity at *MAT* (for review, see Herskowitz et al. 1992). Cells of the diploid phase under starvation conditions undergo meiosis to produce two **a** and two α spore segregants, which will repeat the switching process to establish diploid colonies. Thus, budding yeast exists primarily in diploid phase, while fission yeast predominantly exists as a haploid culture.

MAT switching also occurs by a gene conversion process where the resident *MAT* allele on chromosome III is replaced by a copy of the donor locus from *HMLα* or from *HMRa*. The donor loci are located more than 120 kb away, one to the left and the other to the right of *MAT,* on opposite arms of chromosome III. Only *MAT* is expressed, while both *HM* loci are kept unexpressed by several *trans*-acting factors encoded by *MAR/SIR* loci (Ivy et al. 1986; for review, see Holmes et al. 1996).

As with any other feature of this system, the program of switching of *S. cerevisiae* is drastically different from that found in *S. pombe*. Notably, only mother cells switch in G_1, with each mother producing both switched daughters. The recombination event is initiated by a transient DSB at *MAT* (Strathern et al. 1982) by the expression of *HO*-gene-encoded site-specific endonuclease only in mother cells. Many *trans*-acting factors are required for expression of *HO*. One such factor is *ASH1* message, which is differentially localized to the daughter cells where it acts as a negative regulator of *HO* expression (Long et al. 1997; Takizawa et al. 1997). Thus, totally different strategies are used by these yeasts to control the program of cellular differentiation; the fission yeast uses a *mat1 cis*-acting strand-specific imprinting mechanism, whereas the budding yeast uses the more conventional differential regulation of the *trans*-acting *HO*-endonuclease gene to initiate recombination required for switching. Likewise, silencing mechanisms are also quite different in these yeasts.

The overall strategy of both yeasts involves DNA recombination, but mechanisms are very different and complementary. Since the sequences of mating-type loci are very different, it is not surprising that these yeasts have evolved very different molecular mechanisms for switching and silencing. I suspect that Darwinian evolution is not only based on divergence of DNA sequence; it may also be based on evolution of biological principles. For example, in the case of evolution of the mating-type system in both yeasts, first duplication of unrelated sequences in different yeasts is required. Once that happens, evolution of any mechanism promoting site-specific initiation of recombination in one and silencing of the other duplicated segment would create the opportunity for a process such as mating-type switching. Once additional model systems are investigated, more strategies will be discovered. For example, haploid cloned lines of malaria parasites produce both male and female haploid gameto-cytes (Alano and Carter 1990). Is sex switching going on there similar to the phenomenon of sex change of yeast?

CONCLUDING REMARKS

In both yeasts, an individual cell serves as a somatic as well as a gametic cell. Thus, it is expected that developmental decisions operative in these systems in both mitosis and meiosis can be investigated with the applica-tion of sophisticated tools at the single-cell level. In both yeasts, the pro-gram of cellular differentiation is due to very different but cell-autonomous controls. Furthermore, the mechanism of silencing is best understood in these systems. From the studies of *S. pombe*, it can be stat-ed that mitotic chromosome replication does not always produce identical daughter chromosomes. This is not to say that Mendel's law of segrega-tion of genes or the law of gene assortment is violated. Rather, Mendel's laws apply only to chromosome and gene segregation during meiotic divi-sion, but production of nonequivalent sister chromatids during replication occurs in mitotically dividing cells of fission yeast. We could consider this as the Law of Nonequivalent Sister Chromatids. Unlike many other systems reported in this monograph, it is worth stressing that production of nonequivalent chromatids or maintenance of specific epigenetic state through cell division does not require differential gene regulation of upstream regulators. Such mechanisms are likely to be prevalent in other systems of cellular differentiation.

ACKNOWLEDGMENTS

It is my pleasure to acknowledge many contributions of the following col-leagues who worked on the *S. pombe* system in my laboratory for two decades and whose work is quoted here: D. Beach, M. Kelly, R. Egel, R. Cafferkey, L. Miglio, M. Bonaduce, B. Arcangioli, G. Thon, A. Cohen, J. Singh, S. Grewal, and J. Dalgaard. J. Hopkins is thanked for manuscript preparation and R. Frederickson for the artwork.

REFERENCES

Alano P. and Carter R. 1990. Sexual differentiation in malaria parasites. *Annu. Rev. Microbiol.* **44:** 429–449.
Allshire R.C. 1996. Transcriptional silencing in the fission yeast: A manifestation of high-

er order chromosome structure and functions. In *Epigenetic mechanisms of gene regulation* (eds.,V.E.A. Russo et al.), pp. 443–466. Cold Spring Harbor Laboratory Press, Cold Spring Harbor, New York.

Arcangioli B. 1998. A site- and strand-specific DNA break confers asymmetric switching potential in fission yeast. *EMBO J.* **17:** 4503–4510.

———. 2000. Fate of *mat1* DNA strands during mating-type switching in fission yeast. *EMBO Rep.* **1:** 145–150.

Arcangioli B. and Klar A.J.S. 1991. A novel switch-activating site (SASI) and its cognate binding factor (SAP1) required for efficient *mat1* switching in *Schizosaccharomyces pombe*. *EMBO J.* **10:** 3025–3032.

Beach D.H. 1983. Cell type switching by DNA transposition in fission yeast. *Nature* **305:** 682–688.

Beach D.H. and Klar A.J.S. 1984. Rearrangements of the transposable mating-type cassettes of fission yeast. *EMBO J.* **3:** 603–610.

Brown N.A. and Wolpert L. 1990. The development of handedness in left/right asymmetry. *Development* **109:** 1–9.

Dalgaard J.Z. and Klar A.J.S. 1999. Orientation of DNA replication establishes mating-type switching pattern in *S. pombe*. *Nature* **400:** 181–184.

———. 2000. *swi1* and *swi3* perform imprinting, pausing, and termination of DNA replication in *S. pombe*. *Cell* **102:** 745–751.

Egel R. 1977. Frequency of mating-type switching in homothallic fission yeast. *Nature* **266:** 172–174.

Egel R. and Eie E. 1987. Cell lineage asymmetry for *Schizosaccharomyces pombe*: Unilateral transmission of a high-frequence state of mating-type switching in diploid pedigrees. *Curr. Genet.* **12:** 429–433.

Egel R. and Gutz H. 1981. Gene activation by copy transposition in mating-type switching of a homothallic fission yeast. *Curr. Genet.* **3:** 5–12.

Egel R., Beach D.H., and Klar A.J.S. 1984. Genes required for initiation and resolution steps of mating-type switching in fission yeast. *Proc. Natl. Acad. Sci.* **81:** 3481–3485.

Egel R., Willer M., and Nielsen O. 1989. Unblocking of meiotic crossing-over between the silent mating-type cassettes of fission yeast, conditioned by the recessive, pleiotropic mutant *rik1*. *Curr. Genet.* **15:** 407–410.

Ekwall K. and Ruusala T. 1994. Mutations in *rik1*, *clr2*, *clr3*, and *clr4* genes asymmetrically derepress the silent mating-type loci in fission yeast. *Genetics* **136:** 53–64.

Grewal S.I.S. and A.J.S. Klar. 1996. Chromosomal inheritance of epigenetic states in fission yeast during mitosis and meiosis. *Cell* **86:** 95–101.

———. 1997. A recombinationally repressed region between *mat2* and *mat3* loci shares homology to centromeric repeats and regulates directionality of mating-type switching in fission yeast. *Genetics* **146:** 1221–1238.

Grewal S.I.S., Bonaduce M.J., and Klar A.J.S. 1998. Histone deacetylase homologs regulate epigenetic inheritance of transcriptional silencing and chromosome segregation in fission yeast. *Genetics* **150:** 563–576.

Gutz H. and Schmidt H. 1985. Switching genes in *Schizosaccharomyces pombe*. *Curr. Genet.* **9:** 325–331.

Herskowitz I., Rine J., and Strathern J.N. 1992. Mating-type determination and mating-type interconversion in *Saccharomyces cerevisiae*. In *The molecular and cellular biology of the yeast* Saccharomyces (eds. E.W. Jones et al.), p. 583–656. Cold Spring Harbor Laboratory Press, Cold Spring Harbor, NY.

Holmes S.G., Braunstein M., and Broach J.R., Jr. 1996. Transcriptional silencing of the yeast mating-type genes. In *Epigenetic mechanisms of gene expression* (eds. V.E.A. Russo et al.), p.467–487. Cold Spring Harbor Laboratory Press, Cold Spring Harbor, New York.

Ivanova A.V., Bonaduce M.J., Ivanov S.V., and Klar A.J.S. 1998. The chromo and SET domains of the Clr4 protein are essential for silencing in fission yeast. *Nat. Genet.* **19:** 192–195.

Ivy J.M., Klar A.J.S., and Hicks J.B. 1986. Cloning and characterization of four *SIR* genes of *Saccharomyces cerevisiae. Mol. Cell. Biol.* **6:** 688–702.

Kelly M., Burke J., Klar A., and Beach D. 1988. Four mating-type genes control sexual differentiation in the fission yeast. *EMBO J.* **7:** 1537–1547.

Klar A.J.S. 1987. Differentiated parental DNA strands confer developmental asymmetry on daughter cells in fission yeast. *Nature* **326:** 466–470.

———. 1990. The developmental fate of fission yeast cells is determined by the pattern of inheritance of parental and grandparental DNA strands. *EMBO J.* **9:** 1407–1415.

———. 1992. Molecular genetics of fission yeast cell type: Mating type and mating-type interconversion. In *The molecular and cellular biology of the yeast* Saccharomyces: *Gene expression.* (ed. E.W. Jones et al.), pp. 583–656. Cold Spring Harbor Laboratory Press, Cold Spring Harbor, New York.

———. 1994. A model for specification of the left-right axis in vertebrates. *Trends Genet.* **10:** 392–396.

———. 1998. Propagating epigenetic states through meiosis: Where Mendel's gene is more than a DNA moiety. *Trends Genet.* **14:** 299–301.

———. 1999. Genetic models for handedness, brain lateralization, schizophrenia and manic-depression. *Schizophr. Res.* **39:** 207–218.

Klar A.J.S. and Bonaduce M.J. 1991. *swi6*, a gene required for mating type switching prohibits meiotic recombination in the *mat2-mat3* 'cold spot' of fission yeast. *Genetics* **129:** 1033–1042.

———. 1993. The mechanism of fission yeast mating-type interconversions: Evidence for two types of epigenetically inherited chromosomal imprinted events. *Cold Spring Harbor Symp. Quant. Biol.* **58:** 457–465.

Klar, A.J.S. and Miglio L.M. 1986. Initiation of meiotic recombination by double-strand DNA breaks in *S. pombe. Cell* **46:** 725–731.

Klar A.J.S., Bonaduce M.J., and Cafferkey R. 1991. The mechanism of fission yeast mating type interconversion: Seal/replicate/cleave model of replication across the double-stranded break site at *mat1. Genetics* **127:** 489–496.

Lark K.G., Consigi R.A., and Minocha H.C. 1966. Segregation of sister chromatids in mammalian cells. *Science* **154:** 1202–1205.

Layton W.M., Jr. 1976. Random determination of a developmental process. Reversal of normal visceral asymmetry in the mouse. *J. Hered.* **50:** 10–13.

Leupold U. 1950. Die vererbung von homothallie und heterothallie bei *Schizosaccharomyces pombe. C.R. Trav. Lab. Carlsberg Ser. Physiol.* **24:** 381–480.

Long R.M. Singer R.H., Meng X., Gonzalez I., Nasmyth K., and Jansen R.P. 1997. Mating type switching in yeast controlled by asymmetric localization of *ASH1* mRNA. *Science* **277:** 383–387.

Lorentz A., Heim L., and Schmidt H. 1992. The switching gene *swi6* affects recombination and gene expression in the mating-type region of *Schizosaccharomyces pombe. Mol. Gen. Genet.* **233:** 436–442.

Lorentz A., Ostermann K., Fleck O., and Schmidt H. 1994. Switching gene *swi6*, involved in repression of silent mating-type loci in fission yeast, encodes a homologue of chromatin-associated proteins from *Drosophila* and mammals. *Gene* **143**: 323–330.

Miyata H. and Miyata M. 1981. Mode of conjugation in homothallic cells of *Schizosaccharomyces pombe. J. Gen. Appl. Microbiol.* **27**: 365–371.

Nakayama J., Klar A.J.S., and Grewal S.I.S. 2000. A chromodomain protein, Swi6, performs imprinting functions in fission yeast during mitosis and meiosis. *Cell* **101**: 307–317.

Nielsen O. and Egel E. 1989. Mapping the double-strand breaks at the mating-type locus in fission yeast by genomic sequencing. *EMBO J.* **8**: 269–276.

Potten C.S., Hume W.J., Reid P., and Cairns J. 1978. The segregation of DNA in epithelial stem cells. *Cell* **15**: 899–906.

Singh P.B. 1994. Molecular mechanisms of cellular determination: Their relation to chromatin structure and parental imprinting. *J. Cell. Sci.* **107**: 2653–2668.

Singh J. and Klar A.J.S. 1993. DNA polymerase α is essential for mating-type switching in fission yeast. *Nature* **361**: 271–273.

Singh J., Goel V., and Klar A.J.S. 1998. A novel function of the DNA repair gene *rhp6* in mating-type silencing by chromatin remodeling in fission yeast. *Mol. Cell. Biol.* **18**: 5511–5522.

Strathern J.N., Klar A.J.S., Hicks J.B., Abraham J.A., Ivy J.M., Nasmyth K.A., and McGill C. 1982. Homothallic switching of yeast mating type cassettes is initiated by a double stranded cut in the *MAT* locus. *Cell* **31**: 183–192.

Styrkarsdottir U., Egel R., and Nielsen O. 1993. The *smt-0* mutation which abolishes mating-type switching in fission yeast is a deletion. *Curr. Genet.* **23**: 184–186.

Supp D.M., Witte D.P., Potter S.S., and Brueckner M. 1997. Mutation of an axonemal dynein affects left-right asymmetry in inversus viscerum mice. *Nature* **96**: 963–966.

Takizawa P.A., Sil A., Swedlow J.R., Herskowitz I., and Vale R.D. 1997. Actin-dependent localization of an RNA encoding a cell-fate determinant in yeast. *Nature* **389**: 90–93.

Thon G. and Friis T. 1997. Epigenetic inheritance of transcriptional silencing and switching competence in fission yeast. *Genetics* **145**: 685–696.

Thon G. and Klar A.J.S. 1992. The *clr1* locus regulates the expression of the cryptic mating-type loci of fission yeast. *Genetics* **131**: 287–296.

———. 1993. Directionality of fission yeast mating-type interconversion is controlled by the location of the donor loci. *Genetics* **134**: 1045–1054.

Thon G. and Verhein-Hansen J. 2000. Four chromo-domain proteins of *Schizosaccharomyces pombe* differentially repress transcription of various chromosomal locations. *Genetics* **155**: 551–558.

Thon G., Cohen A., and Klar A.J.S. 1994. Three additional linkage groups that repress transcription and meiotic recombination in the mating-type region of *Schizosaccharomyces pombe. Genetics* **138**: 29–38.

Watson J.D. and Crick F.H.C. 1953. Molecular structure of nucleic acids. *Nature* **171**: 737–737.

3

On Equivalence Groups and the Notch/LIN-12 Communication System

Domingos Henrique
Instituto de Histologia e Embriologia
Faculdade de Medicina de Lisboa
1649-028 Lisboa, Portugal

The original concept of equivalence groups arose from a series of cell ablation studies in the nematode *Caenorhabditis elegans* (Kimble et al. 1979; Sulston and White 1980; Kimble 1981). One of the organs studied was the vulva, the egg-laying structure of female and hermaphrodite nematodes, which derives from a group of six precursor cells (VPCs, *v*ulva *p*recursor *c*ells) organized in a linear array in the ventral ectoderm (Sulston and Horvitz 1977). Although only three of the VPCs normally give rise to vulval tissue, laser ablation of these cells causes the remaining three, which would become hypodermal cells, instead to adopt a vulval fate and give rise to a normal vulva (Sulston and White 1980; Kimble 1981; Sternberg and Horvitz 1986). Similarly, by ablating each of the VPCs, individually or in combination, and analyzing the behavior of the remaining cells, these studies showed that all six VPCs are capable of becoming any of the three precursor cell types that give rise to the mature vulva. The six VPCs are therefore multipotential, and since they can replace each other, they are defined as an "equivalence group" (Kimble et al. 1979). These studies have also shown that there is a clear hierarchy of cell-fate decisions within an equivalence group, where a default or primary fate has precedence over the other alternative fates: If the cell that would acquire the primary fate is removed, one of the other cells in the equivalence group will replace it and become the primary cell. However, the converse is usually not observed, revealing a clear priority in cell fates within the group (Kimble 1981).

Cell ablation studies in leeches (Weisblat and Blair 1984; Huang and Weisblat 1996), grasshoppers (Doe and Goodman 1985; Kuwada and Goodman 1985), and ascidians (Nishida and Satoh 1989) have demonstrated the existence of equivalence groups with similar properties in these animals. Another example of equivalence groups is the proneural clusters in *Drosophila melanogaster* (Simpson and Carteret 1990), groups of ectodermal cells in the fly embryo with the potential to adopt a neural fate, some of which will indeed become part of the fly nervous system while others give rise to epidermis.

For vertebrate embryologists, the concept of equivalence groups is somewhat different, being defined as groups of cells with similar potential and which are going through a common fate decision process. A good example is the inner cell mass of the mouse embryo, composed of cells that are identically multipotential and that, through intercellular signaling, will diversify to give rise to the different cell lineages in the embryo. The developing embryo can thus be viewed as an organized array of spatial compartments, each composed of cells with similar potential and that constitute equivalence groups. Cells within each group adopt different developmental decisions and possibly give rise to smaller equivalence groups, each with a distinct set of restricted developmental options. However, the members of a given equivalence group are not necessarily clonally related; as the embryo develops, there is extensive cell mixing and migration, and cells with different ancestries can, at a certain point of their developmental history, come to share the same spatial compartment in the embryo and respond to a given signal with a similar set of developmental options.

The vertebrate and invertebrate concepts can be combined into a more comprehensive definition of equivalence group, which should include any group of cells with similar developmental potential but whose members may subsequently adopt different cell-fate decisions. This leads to one of the most interesting questions in developmental biology: How do equivalent cells come to adopt different developmental decisions?

In brief, this can be dictated by lineage or, more often, results from intercellular signaling. If the signals arise from cells within the equivalence group, the process can be described as "lateral signaling," whereas if the signal is provided from cells not belonging to the equivalence group, the process is usually described as "induction" (Greenwald and Rubin 1992). The two processes, lateral signaling and induction, can be coupled, however, as lateral signaling is often used to limit the number of cells in an equivalence group that adopt a given decision in response to an inductive signal.

A DECISION IN CLOSED CIRCUIT: THE AC/VU DECISION

The analysis of a particular cell-fate decision in the developing *C. elegans* gonad, namely the choice between two alternate fates, anchor cell (AC) or ventral uterine precursor cell (VU), provides the simplest example of an equivalence group, with just two cells with identical potential. Signaling between these cells is used to specify different fates without apparent interference from extrinsic signals, and the cell-fate choice seems completely stochastic: In 50% of the cases, one cell becomes AC and the other VU, and in the other 50%, the reverse situation is observed (Kimble and Hirsh 1979). Nevertheless, the primary fate seems to be AC: If one of the two cells is ablated, the other always becomes AC (Kimble 1981). Additionally, if the two precursor cells are separated, both adopt an AC fate (Hedgecock et al. 1990). The acquisition of a VU fate must therefore depend on a signal from AC, involving direct cell–cell contact. Genetic studies led to the conclusion that this signal is mediated through the LIN-12 receptor (Greenwald et al. 1983; Yochem et al. 1988), a molecule belonging to the Notch family of receptors, and its ligand LAG-2 (Lambie and Kimble 1991; Henderson et al. 1994; Tax et al. 1994). In mutants where the LAG-2/LIN-12 signaling fails, both precursor cells become AC, whereas constitutive LIN-12 signaling leads to both becoming VU (Greenwald et al. 1983; Greenwald and Seydoux 1990; Lambie and Kimble 1991; Fitzgerald et al. 1993; Struhl et al. 1993). Furthermore, mosaic analysis where cells with no LIN-12 activity confront wild-type cells has shown that the LIN-12 (–) precursor cell always becomes AC (Seydoux and Greenwald 1989), clearly indicating that LIN-12 is necessary in the VU precursor to receive the VU-specifying signal (mediated by the ligand LAG-2).

Analysis of the expression of the *lin-12* and *lag-2* genes has shown that initially both precursor cells have identical expression levels of the two genes and that, as the decision takes place, the AC cell comes to express only *lag-2*, and the VU cell only *lin-12* (Wilkinson et al. 1994). Thus, from an initially equivalent situation, one reaches a situation where the AC precursor becomes the signaling cell and the VU precursor the receiving cell. This seems to result from the amplification of a small, random fluctuation in the levels of the signal or the receptor (or both) between the two cells, through a feedback mechanism involving the activity of the *lag-2* and *lin-12* genes (Seydoux and Greenwald 1989). This mechanism seems to rely on the fact that LIN-12 activity both increases the transcription of its own gene and represses *lag-2* transcription (Wilkinson et al. 1994). The end result is that the cell with an initially higher level of LIN-12 activity will produce more and more receptor (and less and less signal) and become the receiving cell (VU). Conversely, as the AC precursor receives less signal from the VU precursor, it will have lower levels of LIN-12 and produce more and more LAG-2 signal itself, thus becoming the signaling cell.

The AC/VU decision has been taken as a paradigm for an instructive role of LIN-12 signaling: The AC-derived LAG-2 signal is deemed to specify (instruct) the other cell as VU. Hence the description of LAG-2/LIN-12 signaling as "lateral specification" (Greenwald and Rubin 1992). The alternative view ("lateral inhibition") would be that LAG-2/LIN-12 signaling acts to modulate the competence of the VU precursor cell, restricting its ability to adopt the AC fate and thus driving the cell to the VU fate. Both precursor cells are predetermined to become AC or VU, and the LAG-2 signal is needed merely to select the VU fate from the narrow repertoire of options (AC or VU) that the putative VU precursor is allowed by its developmental history.

This simple equivalence group constitutes a good example of how equivalent cells come to acquire different fates through direct cell–cell interactions, mediated by the Notch/LIN-12 signaling pathway. In this particular case, there seems to be absolutely no programmed difference between the two equivalent cells. A random, small difference in signaling activity between the two precursors suffices to create the initial asymmetry, which is then amplified by the intercellular feedback mechanism. This results in a truly stochastic decision, where the two equivalent cells sort themselves out without any interference from other signals. However, such an indeterminacy is actually very rare in *C. elegans* development, and even in closely related nematode species, the AC/VU decision is not stochastic (Felix and Sternberg 1996). Although in some of these species the two precursor cells still constitute an equivalence group (laser ablation of the presumptive AC cell causes the other cell to alter its normal fate (VU) and become instead AC (Felix and Sternberg 1996), one of the two cells is already biased to become AC. There should therefore exist an earlier asymmetry imposing a bias in signaling and a fixed outcome on the decision, a more common situation throughout development.

THE VULVA EQUIVALENCE GROUP: LATERAL SIGNALING WITH A BIT OF SPICE

The vulval equivalence group is composed of six precursor cells (VPCs, numbered P3.p–P8.p) which are multipotent and can respond to an inductive signal from the somatic gonadal AC cell, adopting any of three fates: 1°, 2°, or 3° (Fig. 1) (Sulston and Horvitz 1977; Sternberg and Horvitz 1986). The initial establishment of the vulva equivalence group seems to be induced by Wnt signaling, acting through the Hox gene *lin-39* to specify the six equivalent VPCs (Eisenmann et al. 1998). These cells are lined up in the ventral epidermis, along the anterior–posterior axis, underlying

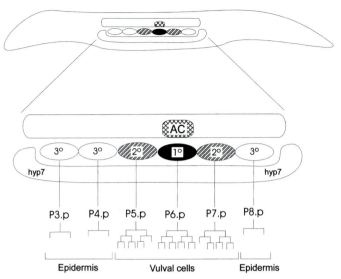

Figure 1 The six cells of the vulva equivalence group are organized in a linear array in the ventral ectoderm, underlying the AC cell. In normal development, the P6.p cell, which is directly under the AC, adopts the primary (1°) fate and gives rise to eight vulval cells, whereas the two immediate neighbors (P5.p and P7.p) adopt the secondary (2°) fate and each generate seven descendants that also make vulval tissue. The three cells more distant from AC (P3.p, P4.p, and P8.p) adopt a non-vulval fate (3°) and become part of the surrounding hypodermis (Sulston and Horvitz 1977).

the AC cell. In normal development, the P6.p cell, which is directly under the AC, adopts the primary (1°) fate and gives rise to eight vulval cells, while the two immediate neighbors (P5.p and P7.p) adopt the secondary (2°) fate and each generate seven descendants that also make vulval tissue. The three cells more distant from AC (P3.p, P4.p, and P8.p) adopt a non-vulval fate (3°) and become part of the surrounding hypodermis (Sulston and Horvitz 1977).

Removal of the AC cell results in a vulvaless worm as P5.p, P6.p, and P7.p all adopt a 3° non-vulval fate (Fig. 2a), revealing the need for a signal from AC to induce vulval fates (Kimble 1981). Genetic screens for vulvaless phenotypes led to the characterization of the signaling cascade responsible for the inducing activity, which involves an activating signal restricted to AC (LIN-3, an EGF-like ligand), a tyrosine-kinase receptor (LET-23), and a downstream RAS-MAP kinase cascade present in all six VPCs (for review, see Horvitz and Sternberg 1991; Kornfeld 1997; Sternberg and Han 1998). Whereas loss-of-function mutations in any of the genes encoding components of this cascade result in vulvaless pheno-

types, constitutive activation of the pathway in the six equivalent cells
leads to multivulva phenotypes, as all six VPCs adopt vulval fates (1° and
2°) (Beitel et al. 1990; Han et al. 1990; Hill and Sternberg 1992). Since
the three most distal VPCs, P3.p, P4.p, and P8.p, don't normally adopt a
vulval fate, this suggests that another signal, most likely derived from the
syncytial hyp7 hypodermal cell which surrounds the VPC equivalence

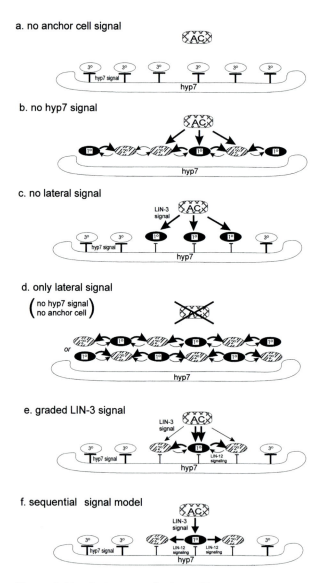

a. no anchor cell signal

b. no hyp7 signal

c. no lateral signal

d. only lateral signal
(no hyp7 signal / no anchor cell)

e. graded LIN-3 signal

f. sequential signal model

Figure 2 (See facing page for legend.)

group, may normally block these three distal VPCs from responding to the AC inducing signal (Fig. 2b) (Herman and Hedgecock 1990). In fact, the presumed hyp7 signal seems to function by negatively regulating a significant basal activity of the LET-23 receptor on the six VPCs, which is overcome only in the three most central cells receiving the LIN-3 activating signal (Ferguson et al. 1987; Clark et al. 1992; Huang et al. 1994b). In this way, by using two opposing signals, a first distinction is made between the six equivalent VPCs, generating two nonequivalent groups of three cells each, the central group giving rise to the actual vulva and the three most lateral cells incorporating into the surrounding hypodermis by fusion with the hyp7 cell. This is a good example of how two signals extrinsic to the equivalence group act to partition it into two smaller groups of cells, each already with a more limited set of developmental options.

The three VPCs in the central equivalence group will then choose between $1°$ and $2°$ fates, ending with a $2°$-$1°$-$2°$ pattern of cells, from which the vulva will develop (Sulston and Horvitz 1977). Contrary to the stochastic AC/VU decision, this is a clearly biased decision in which the cell closest to the AC adopts the $1°$ fate and the neighbors adopt the $2°$ fate. Analysis of various types of mutants affecting vulva development indicate that two signaling events are necessary to correctly pattern the three cells, one arising from outside the equivalence group (LIN-3 from AC) and the other involving lateral signaling between the three equivalent cells, mediated by the LIN-12 receptor (for review, see Horvitz and Sternberg 1991; Kenyon 1995; Kornfeld 1997). As described above, AC removal leads to vulvaless animals due to the absence of $1°$ and $2°$ fates,

Figure 2 The various signals and models to explain the final pattern of cell fates in the *C. elegans* vulva. (*a*) Removal of the AC signaling cell leads to a vulvaless phenotype as all six cells acquire a $3°$ fate. (*b*) In the absence of the vulva-inhibitory signal from the large hyp7 signal, all six VPCs give rise to vulval cells (a multivulva phenotype). (*c*) In *lin-12* mutants, the three central equivalent cells all acquire the default $1°$ fate. (*d*) In the absence of both the hyp7 and AC signals, no initial asymmetry is established, but LIN-12 signaling alone is still able to class the VPCs into different fates and create an ordered, although variable, pattern. (*e*) In the graded signal model, different amounts of the LIN-3 signal cause different cell responses and induce different fates in the three central VPCs. (*f*) In the sequential signal model, the AC signal would specify P6.p to become $1°$ and this cell would then produce another signal, mediated by LIN-12, to specify a $2°$ fate in the neighboring P5.p and P7.p cells. (Adapted from Horvitz and Sternberg 1991.)

indicating that LIN-3/LET-23 signaling is necessary, directly or indirectly, to induce both these fates (Sulston and White 1980; Kimble 1981). On the other side, *lin-12* is necessary only to establish 2° fates: Loss-of-function mutations in *lin-12* have the result that no VPC acquires a 2° fate (Fig. 2c), whereas gain-of-function mutations could lead all VPCs to adopt the 2° fate (in these mutants, AC is absent due to a previous effect of the mutation on the AC/VU decision, as described above) (Greenwald et al. 1983). Expression studies (Wilkinson and Greenwald 1995; Levitan and Greenwald 1998) have shown that the LIN-12 protein is initially present in all six VPCs but is specifically reduced in the P6.p cell acquiring the 1° fate, most likely as a consequence of activation of the RAS signaling cascade in this cell by the AC-derived LIN-3 signal.

Two main models have been put forward to explain the interplay between the LIN-3/LET-23 and LIN-12 signaling pathways and how they contribute to the final pattern of 2°-1°-2° cell fates. In the graded signal model (Fig. 2e) (Sternberg and Horvitz 1986; Horvitz and Sternberg 1991; Katz et al. 1995), LIN-3 is proposed to function as a morphogen, with high levels of LIN-3 inducing a 1° fate on the cell directly underneath the AC (P6.p), whereas neighboring cells (P5.p and P7.p) that receive less signal would acquire a 2° fate. The function of LIN-12 signaling would be to reinforce the initial asymmetry imposed by the LIN-3 graded signal, ensuring that the 1° fate is adopted by only one of the three equivalent cells and that a final 2°-1°-2° pattern is established.

In the sequential signaling model (Fig. 2f) (Sternberg 1988), the AC signal would specify P6.p to become 1° and this cell would then produce another signal, mediated by LIN-12, to specify a 2° fate in the neighboring P5.p and P7.p cells. This model is supported by the analysis of *let-23* genetic mosaics (Koga and Ohshima 1995; Simske and Kim 1995), which revealed that LET-23 signaling in P5.p and P7.p is not necessary for these cells to acquire a 2° fate (a P5.p or P7.p VPC without LET-23 activity can still become 2°, provided that it is flanked by a 1° cell). This constitutes a strong argument against the graded model, where intermediate levels of LIN-3/LET-23 signaling are predicted to induce 2° fates. Instead, LIN-3 will be directly relevant only to the acquisition of a 1° fate, and its requirement for 2° fates (since both 1° and 2° cells are indeed absent in LIN-3 mutants) can be explained by the postulated activity of LIN-3/LET-23 signaling in stimulating the expression of the LIN-12 ligand in the P6.p cell. In this model, LIN-12 activity would have an instructive role in specifying the 2° fate and the interaction between the 1° and 2° cells could be unidirectional, without any need to invoke the intercellular feedback loop provided by the LIN-12 pathway, as described for the AC/VU decision.

RESPECTING THE HIERARCHY

A common characteristic of the AC/VU and the VPC equivalence groups is the striking sequential hierarchy of cell-fate decisions; the VU fate depends on AC and the 2° fate on the 1° fate. This could mean that there is a common pathway to 1° and 2° fate specification and that the 2° decision only happens after the 1° decision. Actually, it is known that the LIN-3 signal acts before the LIN-12 signal, the first during the G_1 phase of the VPC cycle and the second functioning later at G_2 (Wang and Sternberg 1999). LIN-3/LET-23 signaling could therefore be acting to drive the VPCs into a 1°/2° state of competence, which accords with the fact that these cells are equivalent and multipotential (capable of becoming 1° or 2°). What would be the role of LIN-12 signaling in the decision?

A simple way to integrate the two signaling pathways is to suppose that LIN-3/LET-23 signaling positively regulates the expression or activity of the presumed ligand for LIN-12 in the VPCs. Given the graded distribution of the LIN-3 signal between the three VPCs (Katz et al. 1995), the P6.p cell directly underlying the AC would receive more LIN-3 signal and consequently express more LIN-12 ligand than its neighbors P5.p and P7.p. This asymmetry is then amplified through an intercellular feedback mechanism similar to the one acting during the AC/VU decision, whereby the P6.p cell will produce more and more signal (and less receptor), while the flanking cells (P5.p and P7.p) will down-regulate signal production, increase receptor activity, and become net receivers. In this way, small differences in LET-23 activation between the three VPCs are translated into an all-or-none situation where one cell predominantly signals the others, thereby establishing a definitive asymmetry within the equivalence group. The role of LIN-12 signaling in the process would be to selectively repress the 1° fate in the receiving P5.p and P7.p cells, which follow instead the 2° pathway, whereas the P6.p cell escapes LIN-12 signaling and can therefore adopt the 1° fate. Consistent with this mechanism, there is indeed evidence that LIN-12 expression is down-regulated in the P6.p cell acquiring the 1° fate (Levitan and Greenwald 1998).

The integration of the two pathways, mediated by LIN-3/LET-23 and by LIN-12, will therefore result in a correct 2°-1°-2° pattern of cell fates and a normal vulva. The main function of LIN-3/LET-23 signaling would be to drive VPCs into a common 1°-2° pathway of cell-fate specification, where the 2° fate is only possible when the 1° fate is repressed, thus complying with the observed hierarchy of cell fates. As in the AC/VU decision, LIN-12 signaling would again have a selective role, repressing the 1° fate rather than promoting the 2° fate. This is supported by the finding, in the mosaic experiments described above (Koga and Ohshima 1995), that one can obtain 1° cells flanked by 3° cells, which should not happen if LIN-12 is specifying 2° fates.

One can then explain why in the absence of both the hyp7 and AC signals, a pattern of alternated 2° and 1° fates usually occurs (2°-1°-2°-1°-2°-1° or 1°-2°-1°-2°-1°-2°; see Fig. 2d) (Sternberg 1988; Sternberg and Horvitz 1989). In these animals, the basal LET-23 signaling activity would identically affect all six VPCs (since there is no external bias), pushing all of them into the 1°-2° pathway. LIN-12 signaling would then act to amplify any small differences in LET-23 activity (or in LIN-12 activity itself) that might exist between the cells, through its characteristic intercellular feedback loop affecting receptor and ligand transcription (Seydoux and Greenwald 1989; Wilkinson et al. 1994). The final result is that cells alternate in becoming richer in signal and poorer in receptor and vice versa, thus originating a pattern of alternated 1° and 2° cell fates. Therefore, starting from an apparently homogeneous field of six equivalent cells, LIN-12 signaling could still sort these cells into different fates and create an ordered, although variable, pattern.

This process of cell specification in the vulva equivalence group is obviously more complex than the AC/VU decision. Here, six cells have to choose between three unique fates, in a process that involves three different signaling events and has a fixed outcome. Despite the uncertainties about the molecular mechanisms, this equivalence group nevertheless illustrates well how the combined action of inductive signaling and lateral signaling contributes to the nonstochastic assignment of correct fates within the group. In the process, inductive signaling imposes a strong bias on the cells' potential and breaks the asymmetry within the equivalence group. So, contrary to its role in the AC/VU decision process, lateral signaling is not used here to create asymmetry but to implement it, and the final result is a predictable and reproducible patterning of vulval cell fates.

DROSOPHILA PRONEURAL CLUSTERS: A NOTCH IN THE GROUP

In the *Drosophila* embryo, groups of ectodermal cells from which the neural precursors arise are called proneural clusters (PNCs) (Simpson and Carteret 1990) and are thought to constitute equivalence groups: Each cell in a cluster has the potential to become a neural precursor, but only some of them will actually do so. Although no cell ablation studies similar to those done in *C. elegans* have been performed in *Drosophila*, genetic studies in the adult peripheral nervous system have shown that if one neural precursor is prevented from forming, another cell in the neighborhood will replace it (Stern 1954). Cell ablation studies were, however, done in the grasshopper embryo (Doe et al. 1985; Kuwada and Goodman 1985), where neural development seems to be homologous to that of *Drosophila* (Thomas et al. 1984). The results established that neural precursors indeed originate from groups of cells with similar potential: When a given neuroblast was ablated from the ectoderm, it was replaced by one of the neighboring cells. Thus, as expected for an equivalence group, the potential to become a neural precursor is present in several cells, but only a subset of those actually follow a neural fate.

The neural potential of PNC cells is conferred by the activity of genes from the *achaete-scute* complex (AS-C), hence named "proneural genes," which are expressed in all proneural cells (for review, see Skeath and Carroll 1994; Modolell and Campuzano 1998). These genes encode a group of transcriptional regulators of the basic-helix-loop-helix (bHLH) type and are thought to regulate a cascade of downstream genes responsible for the implementation of the neural fate. The phenotypes of flies carrying mutations in proneural genes are revealing about their role in promoting neural competence of ectodermal cells: Whereas loss-of-function mutations lead to a significant reduction of neural cells (Cabrera et al. 1987; Jimenez and Campos-Ortega 1990; Martin-Bermudo et al. 1991), ectopic expression of the AS-C genes can cause the appearance of additional PNCs and consequently of new neural cells (Brand and Campos-Ortega 1988; Rodriguez et al. 1990; Hinz et al. 1994).

Another group of genes, the "neurogenic genes" (Lehmann et al. 1983), seem to control the selection of the cells within a PNC that actually acquire a neural fate. These genes encode components of the Notch signaling pathway and are involved in an active process of cell–cell communication between the proneural cells (lateral inhibition) that results in only one cell, or a few, adopting the neural precursor fate (Simpson 1990; Ghysen et al. 1993). Again, mutations in these genes are revealing about their function. Mutations that inactivate the neurogenic genes cause more neural precursors to be selected from the PNC, leading to an excess of neural cells in the fly nervous system (the "neurogenic" phenotype; Lehmann et al. 1983), whereas gain-of-function mutations suppress the appearance of neural precursors from the PNCs (Lieber et al. 1993; Rebay et al. 1993; Struhl et al. 1993).

Together, these results led to a general model of *Drosophila* neurogenesis where ectodermal cells are first allocated to PNCs by the action of the proneural genes, followed by lateral signaling between the proneural cells to select the neural precursors (Ghysen and Dambly-Chaudiere 1989; Simpson 1990; Ghysen et al. 1993). Once selected, these precursors (neuroblasts in the fly central nervous system and sensory organ precursors [SOPs] in the peripheral nervous system) will divide according to stereotyped cell lineage programs and give rise to the cells in the *Drosophila* nervous system.

The initial establishment of PNCs involves the transcriptional activation of the AS-C genes in well-defined groups of ectodermal cells, in very reproducible locations that anticipate the pattern of neuroblasts and SOPs (for review, see Skeath and Carroll 1994; Modolell and Campuzano 1998). This suggests that the transcription of the AS-C genes must be very precisely controlled, integrating all the information provided by the various positional cues present in the ectoderm, in order to produce such a reproducible and accurate map of PNCs (Ghysen and Dambly-Chaudiere 1988). These cues are globally described as a "prepattern," whose existence was first postulated by Stern (1954). This prepattern must involve various signaling pathways and several transcriptional regulators with different but overlapping distributions in the ectoderm, providing each ectodermal cell with precise coordinates of gene activity that will influence its subsequent development (Huang et al. 1994a; Modolell and Campuzano 1998). As a result, the PNCs will appear only in regions where the exact combinations of these regulators are successful in activating AS-C transcription and thus initiate proneural commitment. Examples of such prepattern transcriptional regulators are the proteins encoded by the genes *extramacrochaetae* (*emc*) (Ellis et al. 1990; Garrell and Modolell 1990; Cubas and Modolell 1992), *pannier* (Ramain et al. 1993), and *iroquois* (Gómez-Skarmeta et al. 1996), the first two being negative regulators and the third a positive regulator of AS-C activity.

Once the PNC is established, the next step in the process of neural specification is the selection of the neural precursor from the PNC. This is controlled by interactions between the proneural cells, in a lateral signaling process that is mediated by the Notch signaling pathway (for review, see Artavanis-Tsakonas et al. 1999). In principle, the situation seems very similar to the selection process in the two *C. elegans* equivalence groups described above, involving homologous molecules from the same signaling pathway (the Notch/LIN-12 pathway) to ensure that equivalent cells adopt different developmental decisions (for review, see Kimble and Simpson 1997). In *Drosophila*, however, the molecular components of this signaling pathway have been better characterized, and one can learn a bit more about its function in controlling the behavior of the cells within an equivalence group.

Essentially, there are two models to explain Notch function and lateral signaling within the PNCs (Fig. 3): the lateral inhibition model and the mutual inhibition model. In the lateral inhibition model (Simpson 1990; Ghysen et al. 1993), one cell becomes selected as a neural precursor and

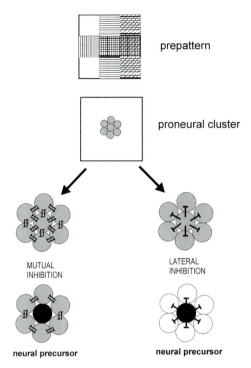

prepattern

proneural cluster

MUTUAL
INHIBITION

LATERAL
INHIBITION

neural precursor

neural precursor

Figure 3 Following the establishment of PNCs in the *Drosophila* ectoderm, in a process controlled by the prepattern genes, a neural precursor is selected through the action of the Notch communication system. Two models were proposed to explain Notch function and lateral signaling within the PNCs. In the mutual inhibition model, all cells within a PNC have identical inhibitory strength and are "frozen" in an inhibited state. Only a predetermined cell would be able to escape this inhibitory field and become a neural precursor, while the remaining cells would continue inhibited. In the lateral inhibition model, one cell becomes selected as a neural precursor and inhibits the other cells within the PNC from adopting the same decision.

inhibits the other cells within the PNC from adopting the same decision. The inhibitory signal is encoded by the *Delta* gene and the receptor by the *Notch* gene. Both Notch and Delta are transmembrane proteins, and their interaction activates a signaling cascade in the receiving cell that leads to the inhibition of its proneural potential, through the down-regulation of the AS-C genes. This signaling cascade (for review, see Weinmaster 1997; Artavanis-Tsakonas et al. 1999) involves the proteolytic release of the intracytoplasmic part of the receptor, its dimerization with the Su(H) protein, and subsequent binding of the complex to specific sites on DNA. This results in the activation of a group of genes from the *Enhancer of Split* complex (Espl-C), seven of which encode related bHLH transcriptional repressors. These seem to function as nuclear effectors of the Notch pathway, repressing the AS-C genes and consequently the neural potential of the cells where Notch signaling is activated.

The selection of the proneural cell that will become the neural precursor and inhibit the other cells in the PNC could happen through two different mechanisms. In the simplest case, small, random variations in the levels of ligand or receptor (or both) between the proneural cells could be amplified through an intercellular feedback mechanism. In this process, one cell becomes richer in signal and poorer in receptor, whereas the neighbors become richer in receptor and poorer in signal; the first cell becomes the neural precursor and signals the others to repress their neural potential (Heitzler and Simpson 1991). This is a very similar situation to the AC/VU decision in *C. elegans* (Seydoux and Greenwald 1989; Heitzler and Simpson 1991), in which there is apparently no initial bias between the cells of the equivalence group and the final outcome looks stochastic: The proneural cell that has initially higher levels of Delta and becomes the neural precursor is selected randomly. This could occur during selection of the SOPs that will give rise to a particular class of sensory organs in the *Drosophila* notum microchaetae, whose number and position can be variable from fly to fly (for review, see Simpson 1997). In contrast, other SOPs that will give rise to macrochaetae, which have a fixed and predictable position in the fly epidermis, seem to be selected through an invariant process, whereby the same proneural cell within the cluster always becomes an SOP. The decision is therefore biased and presumably reflects the existence of different concentrations of AS-C gene products in the proneural cells of a cluster, with a predetermined cell having higher levels from the very beginning. Given the ability of AS-C proteins to regulate positively the transcription of the *Delta* gene (Kunisch et al. 1994), this cell will also have higher levels of Delta activity. This should be enough to trigger the intercellular feedback loop described above and lead to the emergence of this cell as the SOP and consequent inhibition of the other cells in the PNC.

The higher levels of AS-C products in this cell could be intrinsically determined by the action of genes like *emc*, *pannier*, or *iroquois* (for review, see Simpson 1997; Vervoort et al. 1997), which are part of the described prepattern within the ectoderm and have a heterogeneous expression within the PNCs. The *emc* gene works by repressing AS-C function (Van Doren et al. 1991; Cabrera et al. 1994), and therefore cells with higher levels of Emc protein would have less neural competence due to a lower activity of the proneural genes. The Iroquois proteins seem to activate AS-C transcription and thus increase proneural potential in the cells where they are expressed (Gómez-Skarmeta et al. 1996). In both cases, the prepatterning activity of these genes creates an intrinsic bias within the PNC, ensuring that the cell selected as SOP always forms in the same position. This could also be achieved by an extrinsic signal, as seems to be the case with the secreted Wingless molecule that functions during SOP selection in certain PNCs in the *Drosophila* wing disk, causing the proneural cell closest to the source of Wingless signal to become always the SOP (Phillips and Whittle 1993). Thus, as in the developing *C. elegans* vulva, the selection of a cell from an equivalence group would still require lateral signaling and the activation of the intercellular feedback loop mediated by the Notch/LIN-12 pathway, but the decision seems to be biased from the beginning and to lead to a stereotyped pattern of cell fates.

A second model of lateral signaling—mutual inhibition—has been proposed by Mark Muskavitch (Muskavitch 1994; Simpson 1997; Baker 2000). According to this model, the decision about which proneural cell will be selected as neural precursor is also predetermined, but the function of Notch signaling would be completely different. Instead of giving rise to one signaling cell that inhibits the other proneural cells, this model postulates that all cells within a PNC have identical inhibitory strength and are "frozen" in an inhibited state. Only a predetermined cell would be able to escape this inhibitory field and become a neural precursor, while the remaining cells would continue inhibited. This implies that the intercellular feedback mechanism is not at work during the decision; even if there are variations in the transcriptional activities of the *Delta* and *Notch* genes, these cannot be amplified fast enough to overcome the other mechanism of precursor determination. Actually, during neuroblast selection in the fly embryonic neuroectoderm, one cannot detect any differences in *Notch* and *Delta* expression between the proneural cells (Fehon et al. 1991; Kooh et al. 1993). Moreover, experiments where *Notch* and *Delta* transgenes (insensitive to the normal transcriptional controls) were used to replace the endogenous genes resulted in an almost normal segregation of the neuroblasts (Seugnet et al. 1997b), revealing that transcriptional regulation of the receptor and ligand is not necessary for the selection process.

One still needs to explain how one given cell is predetermined to become the neural precursor and how this cell will then overcome the inhibitory field. The first step, involving the nonstochastic choice of a given cell, could be explained by the action of the same intrinsic and extrinsic cues described above, which should tilt the chosen cell to somehow escape the inhibitory field and be able to adopt a neural precursor fate. To do this, that cell has to become insensitive to Notch signaling, but how this happens is not yet known. Several mechanisms are possible, however (for review, see Baker 2000). In a simple scenario, the higher levels of AS-C activity in the predetermined cell should lead to the accumulation of Delta protein, and this could cause a direct down-regulation of Notch receptor activity in this cell. Actually, it has been proposed that Delta and Notch proteins can interact at the membrane of the same cell (*cis* interaction), and this could lead to the formation of an "inactive" Delta/Notch heterodimer, unable to convey any signal (Heitzler and Simpson 1993; Jacobsen et al. 1998). High levels of Delta protein in one cell could therefore make this cell refractory to Notch activation, a mechanism that has been suggested to explain an observed dominant-negative effect due to overexpression of Delta in both flies and vertebrates (Jacobsen et al. 1998). Other mechanisms to make cells insensitive to Notch signaling have come to light recently and involve the activity of the Numb protein, which seems to bind to the intracellular part of the Notch receptor (Guo et al. 1996; Ju et al. 2000) and prevent its activation. However, it is unlikely that these molecules act in the mutual inhibition process during *Drosophila* neural precursor selection, as no anti-neurogenic phenotypes are caused by mutations in the corresponding genes. Other mechanisms to escape Notch signaling are still possible and could work alone or in combination with the other proposed mechanisms (Baker 2000). For instance, the Notch protein could be actively targeted for degradation in the neuroblast, either by promoting its endocytosis into lysosomes (Seugnet et al. 1997a) and subsequent degradation, or by enhancing its ubiquitination (Schweisguth 1999), in both cases resulting in lower levels of Notch activity inside the cell.

Finally, it is still possible that the two processes, lateral inhibition and mutual inhibition, function together within the same PNC to ensure that a single cell emerges as a neural precursor. Actually, in a very careful analysis of the neuroblast selection process, it was observed that within each PNC, two or three cells seem to escape mutual inhibition simultaneously (Huang et al. 1991; Doe 1992), which led to the suggestion that the actual choice of the neural precursor involves a second step of lateral inhibition between these cells so that only one becomes a neuroblast (Seugnet et al. 1997b; Simpson 1997).

What seems to emerge from these models, each supported by a wealth of experimental evidence, is that Notch signaling is a very versatile mechanism to control cell-fate decisions within equivalence groups. This signaling pathway can operate in different ways to select neural precursors in different parts of the fly nervous system, and to produce stochastic or stereotyped outcomes, depending on its interaction with other signaling mechanisms. These molecular strategies accomplish a similar function; namely, forcing equivalent cells to adopt distinct developmental decisions.

CONCLUDING REMARKS

During development, cells experience a more or less gradual loss of potentiality, until final differentiation. Decisions about cell fates are frequently taken collectively by groups of cells, named equivalence groups, and cell–cell communication plays a major role in controlling these decisions. Groups of adjacent cells in the embryo created in this way face similar developmental choices and display similar potential to select any of a set of permitted fates. However, this equivalence is repeatedly broken, and cells within each group may adopt different decisions, giving rise to smaller groups each containing cells that are equivalent but with a different potential. Cell movements also occur, mingling cells of different groups and creating new equivalence groups by bringing together cells with similar developmental potential. The developing embryo can thus be viewed as a constantly evolving mosaic of different equivalence groups, each behaving as an autonomous unit, with a transient existence.

The behavior of equivalence groups has to be based on reliable and versatile communication systems between the equivalent cells, allowing them to respond to signals from outside the group and to interact with their neighbors inside the group, so as to adopt different decisions, despite their identical potential. Actually, the shared use of such communication systems can be regarded as a defining characteristic of an equivalence group. Cells that cannot communicate are logically excluded from the cell-fate decision process and therefore do not belong to the group. Given that equivalence groups are transient and numerous, it would not be surprising that the same communication systems should function repeatedly in the various groups that form during development, independently of the cell-fate decision involved.

The Notch/LIN-12 signaling pathway is an obvious candidate to provide such a cell–cell communication system within equivalence groups. This pathway has been shown to be active in a wide range of cell-fate decisions in both invertebrate and vertebrate organisms, involving groups of cells with the characteristics of equivalence groups. Moreover, mutations that block the function of the Notch/LIN-12 pathway have very pleiotropic phenotypes, affecting a wide variety of cell types in the animal, which reveals the participation of this pathway in a remarkably large proportion of the equivalence groups that form during development (for review, see Artavanis-Tsakonas et al. 1999).

In the three examples described above, Notch/LIN-12 signaling was shown to involve all the cells within the equivalence group, coordinating the different cell-fate decisions taken by adjacent cells within it. In the first case, the AC/VU decision, *lin-12* function alone seems to be enough to force equivalent cells to adopt different fates, whereas in the other two cases, an initial symmetry-breaking step is subsequently amplified by the Notch/LIN-12 pathway, leading to the establishment of different fates within the equivalence group. This communication mechanism is therefore very versatile and robust, being able to interact with other elements of the communication network and still produce very stable outcomes.

What are the molecular characteristics of the Notch/LIN-12 pathway that allow it to play such a basic and fundamental role? It is, first of all, a form of signaling that depends on direct cell-to-cell contact and is therefore suited to creation of fine-grained patterns in which directly neighboring cells are required to become different. From the examples previously discussed, it is clear that the described intercellular feedback mechanism is central to the function of the Notch/LIN-12 pathway in many equivalence groups. Because the feedback loop involves communication between adjacent cells, the behavior of one cell depends intimately, and in a reciprocal fashion, on the behavior of its neighbors. Although the molecular details of such transregulation are not yet fully understood, the mechanism is based on the finding that receptor activation causes a coincident increase in receptor levels and a decrease in ligand levels in the cell (Wilkinson et al. 1994). Thus, the more signal one cell receives, the less signal it can produce and the more receptor it can activate. The end result of this feedback mechanism between adjacent cells is that a cell that comes to have a slightly higher level of signal will become richer and richer in signal and poorer and poorer in receptor, while in the neighboring cells the contrary will happen. The first cell then becomes a net signaler and the neighbors net receivers. At the phenotypic level, the consequence is that the developmental choice taken by the signaling cell precludes the neighbors from adopting a similar decision. The nature of this decision, i.e., the type of cell fate chosen, depends on the intrinsic potential of the cells and/or the influence of inductive signals arising from cells outside the equivalence group. The AS-C proteins are a good example of an intrinsic cell-fate determinant that confers a proneural potential to the equivalent cells of PNCs, and the LIN-3 signal from the AC cell is a good example of an inductive signal that determines two particular cell fates in the *C. elegans* vulva equivalence group. The common theme for these two signals is their role in activating the Notch/LIN-12 communication system in an equivalence group of cells, which are thus enabled to diversify and choose their individual fates in a precisely coordinated fashion.

In recent years, research on the Notch/LIN-12 pathway has highlighted the conservation of this signaling mechanism across many different species, from worms to humans. Functional studies have shown that Notch signaling in higher vertebrates controls many cell-fate decisions, as, for example, the commitment to differentiate as a neuron or remain as a dividing progenitor in the central nervous system, to become an exocrine or an endocrine cell in the pancreas, to differentiate or remain as a dividing progenitor in the hematopoietic system, or to become a hair cell or a supporting cell in the inner ear (for recent reviews, see Artavanis-Tsakonas et al. 1999; Skipper and Lewis 2000). It is also becoming clear that not all Notch functions involve signaling between equivalent cells and that Notch must also play other, perhaps more complex, roles in other biological events, such as neurite arborization (Franklin et al. 1999; Sestan et al. 1999). Nevertheless, the lessons we can learn from studying the role of Notch/LIN-12 signaling in controlling cell-fate decisions within equivalence groups in simpler organisms provide an essential key to help us understand how larger, more complex animals, using more sophisticated communication networks, generate their intricate patterns of cell types.

ACKNOWLEDGMENTS

I thank Julian Lewis, Alain Ghysen, and François Schweisguth for their critical reviews of the original manuscript, which helped to improve it significantly. The author is supported by Fundação Ciência e Tecnologia grants (P/SAU/80/96 and P/SAU/14097/98).

REFERENCES

Artavanis-Tsakonas S., Rand M.D., and Lake R.J. 1999. Notch signaling: Cell fate control and signal integration in development. *Science* **284:** 770–776.

Baker N.E. 2000. Notch signaling in the nervous system. Pieces still missing from the puzzle. *Bioessays* **22:** 264–273.

Beite, G.J., Clark S.G., and Horvitz H.R. 1990. *Caenorhabditis elegans ras* gene *let-60* acts as a switch in the pathway of vulval induction (comments). *Nature* **348:** 503–509.

Brand M. and Campos-Ortega J. 1988. Two groups of interrelated genes regulate early neurogenesis in *Drosophila melanogaster. Roux's Arch. Dev. Biol.* **197:** 457–470.

Cabrera C.V., Alonso M.C., and Huikeshoven H. 1994. Regulation of scute function by extramacrochaete in vitro and in vivo. *Development* **120:** 3595–3603.

Cabrera C.V., Martinez-Arias A., and Bate M. 1987. The expression of three members of the *achaete-scute* gene complex correlates with neuroblast segregation in *Drosophila*. *Cell* **50**: 425–433.

Clark S.G., Stern M.J., and Horvitz H.R. 1992. *C. elegans* cell-signalling gene *sem-5* encodes a protein with SH2 and SH3 domains (comments). *Nature* **356**: 340–344.

Cubas P. and Modolell,J. 1992. The *extramacrochaetae* gene provides information for sensory organ patterning. *EMBO J.* **11**: 3385–3393.

Doe C.Q. 1992. Molecular markers for identified neuroblasts and ganglion mother cells in the *Drosophila* central nervous system. *Development* **116**: 855–863.

Doe C.Q. and Goodman C.S. 1985. Neurogenesis in grasshopper and *fushi tarazu Drosophila* embryos. *Cold Spring Harbor Symp. Quant. Biol.* **50**: 891–903.

Doe C.Q., Kuwada J.Y., and Goodman C.S. 1985. From epithelium to neuroblasts to neurons: the role of cell interactions and cell lineage during insect neurogenesis. *Philos. Trans. R. Soc. Lond. B Biol. Sci.* **312**: 67–81.

Eisenmann D.M., Maloof J.N., Simske J.S., Kenyon C., and Kim S.K. 1998. The beta-catenin homolog BAR-1 and LET-60 Ras coordinately regulate the Hox gene *lin-39* during *Caenorhabditis elegans* vulval development. *Development* **125**: 3667–3680.

Ellis H.M., Spann D.R., and Posakony J.W. 1990. *extramacrochaetae*, a negative regulator of sensory organ development in *Drosophila*, defines a new class of helix-loop-helix proteins. *Cell* **61**: 27–38.

Fehon R.G., Johansen K., Rebay I., and Artavanis-Tsakonas S. 1991. Complex cellular and subcellular regulation of Notch expression during embryonic and imaginal development of *Drosophila*—Implications for Notch function. *J. Cell Biol.* **113**: 657–669.

Felix M.A. and Sternberg P.W. 1996. Symmetry breakage in the development of one-armed gonads in nematodes. *Development* **122**: 2129-2142.

Ferguson E.L., Sternberg P.W., and Horvitz H.R. 1987. A genetic pathway for the specification of the vulval cell lineages of *Caenorhabditis elegans* (erratum *Nature* [1987] **327**: 82). *Nature* **326**: 259–267.

Fitzgerald K., Wilkinson H.A., and Greenwald I. 1993. *glp-1* can substitute for *lin-12* in specifying cell fate decisions in *Caenorhabditis elegans*. *Development* **119**: 1019–1027.

Franklin J.L., Berechid B.E., Cutting F.B., Presente A., Chambers C.B., Foltz D.R., Ferreira A., and Nye J.S. 1999. Autonomous and non-autonomous regulation of mammalian neurite development by Notch1 and Delta1. *Curr. Biol.* **9**: 1448–1457.

Garrell J. and Modolell J. 1990. The *Drosophila extramacrochaetae* locus, an antagonist of proneural genes that, like these genes, encodes a helix-loop-helix protein. *Cell* **61**: 39–48.

Ghysen A. and Dambly-Chaudiere C. 1988. From DNA to form: The *achaete-scute* complex. *Genes Dev.* **2**: 495–501.

———. 1989. Genesis of the *Drosophila* peripheral nervous system. *Trends Genet.* **5**: 251–255.

Ghysen A., Dambly-Chaudière C., Jan L.Y., and Jan Y.N. 1993. Cell interactions and gene interactions in peripheral neurogenesis. *Genes Dev.* **7**: 723–733.

Gómez-Skarmeta J.L., del Corral R.D., de la Calle-Mustienes E., Ferrés-Marcó D., and Modolell J. 1996. *araucan* and *caupolican*, two members of the novel iroquois complex, encode homeoproteins that control proneural and vein-forming genes. *Cell* **85**: 95–105.

Greenwald I. and Rubin G.M. 1992. Making a difference: The role of cell-cell interactions in establishing separate identities for equivalent cells. *Cell* **68:** 271–281.

Greenwald I. and Seydoux G. 1990. Analysis of gain-of-function mutations of the *lin-12* gene of *Caenorhabditis elegans. Nature* **346:** 197–199.

Greenwald I.S., Sternberg P.W., and Horvitz H.R. 1983. The *lin-12* locus specifies cell fates in *Caenorhabditis elegans. Cell* **34:** 435–444.

Guo M., Jan L.Y., and Jan Y.N. 1996. Control of daughter cell fates during asymmetric division: Interaction of Numb and Notch. *Neuron* **17:** 27–41.

Han M., Aroian R.V., and Sternberg P.W. 1990. The *let-60* locus controls the switch between vulval and nonvulval cell fates in *Caenorhabditis elegans. Genetics* **126:** 899–913.

Hedgecock E.M., Culotti J.G., and Hall D.H. 1990. The *unc-5*, *unc-6*, and *unc-40* genes guide circumferential migrations of pioneer axons and mesodermal cells on the epidermis in *C. elegans. Neuron* **4:** 61-85.

Heitzler P. and Simpson P. 1991. The choice of cell fate in the epidermis of *Drosophila. Cell* **64:** 1083–1092.

———. 1993. Altered epidermal growth factor-like sequences provide evidence for a role of Notch as a receptor in cell fate decisions. *Development* **117:** 1113–1123.

Henderson S.T., Gao D., Lambie E.J., and Kimble J. 1994. *lag-2* may encode a signaling ligand for the GLP-1 and LIN-12 receptors of *C. elegans. Development* **120:** 2913–2924.

Herman R.K. and Hedgecock E.M. 1990. Limitation of the size of the vulval primordium of *Caenorhabditis elegans* by *lin-15* expression in surrounding hypodermis. *Nature* **348:** 169–171.

Hill R.J. and Sternberg,P.W. 1992. The gene *lin-3* encodes an inductive signal for vulval development in *C. elegans* (comments). *Nature* **358:** 470–476.

Hinz U., Giebel B., and Campos-Ortega J.A. 1994. The basic-helix-loop-helix domain of *Drosophila* lethal of scute protein is sufficient for proneural function and activates neurogenic genes. *Cell* **76:** 77–87.

Horvitz H.R. and Sternberg P.W. 1991. Multiple intercellular signalling systems control the development of the *Caenorhabditis elegans* vulva. *Nature* **351:** 535–541.

Huang F., Dambly-Chaudiere C., and Ghysen A. 1991. The emergence of sense organs in the wing disc of *Drosophila. Development* **111:** 1087–1095.

———. 1994a. Position-reading and the emergence of sense organ precursors in *Drosophila. Prog. Neurobiol.* **42:** 293–297.

Huang F.Z. and Weisblat D.A. 1996. Cell fate determination in an annelid equivalence group. *Development* **122:** 1839–1847.

Huang L.S., Tzou P., and Sternberg P.W. 1994b. The *lin-15* locus encodes two negative regulators of *Caenorhabditis elegans* vulval development. *Mol. Biol. Cell* **5:** 395–411.

Jacobsen T.L., Brennan K., Arias A.M., and Muskavitch M.A. 1998. *Cis*-interactions between Delta and Notch modulate neurogenic signalling in *Drosophila. Development* **125:** 4531–4540.

Jimenez F. and Campos-Ortega J.A. 1990. Defective neuroblast commitment in mutants of the *achaete-scute* complex and adjacent genes of *D. melanogaster. Neuron* **5:** 81–89.

Ju B.G., Jeong S., Bae E., Hyun S., Carroll S.B., Yim J., and Kim J. 2000. Fringe forms a complex with Notch. *Nature* **405:** 191–195.

Katz W.S., Hill R.J., Clandinin T.R., and Sternberg P.W. 1995. Different levels of the *C. elegans* growth factor LIN-3 promote distinct vulval precursor fates (comments). *Cell*

82: 297–307.

Kenyon C. 1995. A perfect vulva every time: Gradients and signaling cascades in *C. elegans* (comment). *Cell* **82:** 171–174.

Kimble J. 1981. Alterations in cell lineage following laser ablation of cells in the somatic gonad of *Caenorhabditis elegans*. *Dev. Biol.* **87:** 286–300.

Kimble J. and Hirsh D. 1979. The postembryonic cell lineages of the hermaphrodite and male gonads in *Caenorhabditis elegans*. *Dev. Biol.* **70:** 396–417.

Kimble J. and Simpson P. 1997. The LIN-12/Notch signaling pathway and its regulation. *Annu. Rev. Cell Dev. Biol.* **13:** 333–361.

Kimble J., Sulston J.E., and White J.G. 1979. Regulative development in the post-embryonic lineages of *Caenorhabditis elegans*. In *Cell lineage, stem cells and cell determination* (ed. A.M.N. Le Douarin), pp. 59–68. Elsevier, The Netherlands.

Koga M. and Ohshima Y. 1995. Mosaic analysis of the *let-23* gene function in vulval induction of *Caenorhabditis elegans*. *Development* **121:** 2655–2666.

Kooh P.J., Fehon R.G., and Muskavitch M.A. 1993. Implications of dynamic patterns of Delta and Notch expression for cellular interactions during *Drosophila* development. *Development* **117:** 493–507.

Kornfeld K. 1997. Vulval development in *Caenorhabditis elegans*. *Trends Genet.* **13:** 55–61.

Kunisch M., Haenlin M., and Campos-Ortega J.A. 1994. Lateral inhibition mediated by the *Drosophila* neurogenic gene *delta* is enhanced by proneural proteins. *Proc. Natl. Acad. Sci.* **91:** 10139–10143.

Kuwada J.Y. and Goodman C.S. 1985. Neuronal determination during embryonic development of the grasshopper nervous system. *Dev. Biol.* **110:** 114–126.

Lambie E.J. and Kimble J. 1991. Two homologous regulatory genes, *lin-12* and *glp-1*, have overlapping functions. *Development* **112:** 231–240.

Lehmann R., Jiménez F., Dietrich U., and Campos-Ortega J.A. 1983. On the phenotype and development of mutants of early neurogenesis in *Drosophila melanogaster*. *Roux's Arch. Dev. Biol.* **192:** 62-74.

Levitan D. and Greenwald I. 1998. LIN-12 protein expression and localization during vulval development in *C. elegans*. *Development* **125:** 3101–3109.

Lieber T., Kidd S., Alcamo E., Corbin V., and Young M.W. 1993. Antineurogenic phenotypes induced by truncated Notch proteins indicate a role in signal transduction and may point to a novel function for Notch in nuclei. *Genes Dev.* **7:** 1949–1965.

Martin-Bermudo M.D., Martinez C., Rodriguez A., and Jimenez F. 1991. Distribution and function of the *lethal of scute* gene product during early neurogenesis in *Drosophila*. *Development* **113:** 445–454.

Modolell J. and Campuzano S. 1998. The *achaete-scute* complex as an integrating device. *Int. J. Dev. Biol.* **42:** 275–282.

Muskavitch M.A. 1994. Delta-notch signaling and *Drosophila* cell fate choice. *Dev. Biol.* **166:** 415–430.

Nishida H. and Satoh N. 1989. Determination and regulation in the pigment cell lineage of the ascidian embryo. *Dev. Biol.* **132:** 355–367.

Phillips R.G. and Whittle J.R. 1993. *wingless* expression mediates determination of peripheral nervous system elements in late stages of *Drosophila* wing disc development. *Development* **118:** 427–438.

Ramain P., Heitzler P., Haenlin M., and Simpson P. 1993. *pannier*, a negative regulator of *achaete* and *scute* in *Drosophila*, encodes a zinc finger protein with homology to the vertebrate transcription factor GATA-1. *Development* **119:** 1277–1291.

Rebay I., Fehon R.G., and Artavanis-Tsakonas S. 1993. Specific truncations of *Drosophila* Notch define dominant activated and dominant negative forms of the receptor. *Cell* **74:** 319–329.

Rodriguez I., Hernandez R., Modolell J., and Ruiz-Gomez M. 1990. Competence to develop sensory organs is temporally and spatially regulated in *Drosophila* epidermal primordia. *EMBO J.* **9:** 3583–3592.

Schweisguth F. 1999. Dominant-negative mutation in the β2 and β6 proteasome subunit genes affect alternative cell fate decisions in the *Drosophila* sense organ lineage. *Proc. Natl. Acad. Sci.* **96:** 11382–11386.

Sestan N., Artavanis-Tsakonas S., and Rakic P. 1999. Contact-dependent inhibition of cortical neurite growth mediated by notch signaling (comments). *Science* **286:** 741–746.

Seugnet L., Simpson P., and Haenlin M. 1997a. Requirement for dynamin during Notch signaling in *Drosophila* neurogenesis. *Dev. Biol.* **192:** 585–598.

———. 1997b. Transcriptional regulation of Notch and Delta: Requirement for neuroblast segregation in *Drosophila*. *Development* **124:** 2015–2025.

Seydoux G. and Greenwald I. 1989. Cell autonomy of *lin-12* function in a cell fate decision in *C. elegans*. *Cell* **57:** 1237–1245.

Simpson P. 1990. Lateral inhibition and the development of the sensory bristles of the adult peripheral nervous system of *Drosophila*. *Development* **109:** 509–519.

———. 1997. Notch signalling in development: On equivalence groups and asymmetric developmental potential. *Curr. Opin. Genet. Dev.* **7:** 537–542.

Simpson P. and Carteret C. 1990. Proneural clusters: Equivalence groups in the epithelium of *Drosophila*. *Development* **110:** 927–932.

Simske J.S. and Kim S.K. 1995. Sequential signalling during *Caenorhabditis elegans* vulval induction. *Nature* **375:** 142–146.

Skeath J.B. and Carroll S.B. 1994. The *achaete-scute* complex: Generation of cellular pattern and fate within the *Drosophila* nervous system. *FASEB J.* **8:** 714–721.

Skipper M. and Lewis J. 2000. Getting to the guts of enteroendocrine differentiation (news). *Nat. Genet.* **24:** 3–4.

Stern C. 1954. Two or three bristles. *Am. Sci.* **42:** 213–247.

Sternberg P.W. 1988. Lateral inhibition during vulval induction in *Caenorhabditis elegans*. *Nature* **335:** 551–554.

Sternberg P.W. and Han M. 1998. Genetics of RAS signaling in *C. elegans*. *Trends Genet.* **14:** 466–472.

Sternberg P.W. and Horvitz H.R. 1986. Pattern formation during vulval development in *C. elegans*. *Cell* **44:** 761–772.

———. 1989. The combined action of two intercellular signaling pathways specifies three cell fates during vulval induction in *C. elegans*. *Cell* **58:** 679–693.

Struhl G., Fitzgerald K., and Greenwald I. 1993. Intrinsic activity of the Lin-12 and Notch intracellular domains in vivo. *Cell* **74:** 331–345.

Sulston J.E. and Horvitz H.R. 1977. Post-embryonic cell lineages of the nematode, *Caenorhabditis elegans*. *Dev. Biol.* **56:** 110–156.

Sulston J.E. and White J.G. 1980. Regulation and cell autonomy during postembryonic development of *Caenorhabditis elegans*. *Dev. Biol.* **78:** 577–597.

Tax F.E., Yeargers J.J., and Thomas J.H. 1994. Sequence of *C. elegans lag-2* reveals a cell-signalling domain shared with *Delta* and *Serrate* of *Drosophila*. *Nature* **368:** 150–154.

Thomas J.B., Bastiani M.J., Bate M., and Goodman C.S. 1984. From grasshopper to

Drosophila: A common plan for neuronal development. *Nature* **310:** 203–207.

Van Doren M., Ellis H.M., and Posakony J.W. 1991. The *Drosophila* extramacrochaetae protein antagonizes sequence-specific DNA binding by daughterless/achaete-scute protein complexes. *Development* **113:** 245–255.

Vervoort M., Dambly-Chaudiere C., and Ghysen A. 1997. Cell fate determination in *Drosophila. Curr. Opin. Neurobiol.* **7:** 21–28.

Wang M. and Sternberg P.W. 1999. Competence and commitment of *Caenorhabditis elegans* vulval precursor cells. *Dev. Biol.* **212:** 12–24.

Weinmaster G. 1997. The ins and outs of notch signaling. *Mol. Cell. Neurosci.* **9:** 91–102.

Weisblat D.A. and Blair S.S. 1984. Developmental interdeterminacy in embryos of the leech *Helobdella triserialis. Dev. Biol.* **101:** 326–335.

Wilkinson H.A. and Greenwald I. 1995. Spatial and temporal patterns of *lin-12* expression during *C. elegans* hermaphrodite development. *Genetics* **141:** 513–526.

Wilkinson H.A., Fitzgerald K., and Greenwald I. 1994. Reciprocal changes in expression of the receptor *lin-12* and its ligand *lag-2* prior to commitment in a *C. elegans* cell fate decision. *Cell* **79:** 1187–1198.

Yochem J., Weston K., and Greenwald I. 1988. The *Caenorhabditis elegans lin-12* gene encodes a transmembrane protein with overall similarity to *Drosophila* Notch. *Nature* **335:** 547–550.

4

Cell Cycle Control, Checkpoints, and Stem Cell Biology

Gennaro D'Urso

Department of Biochemistry and Molecular Biology
University of Miami School of Medicine
Miami, Florida 33101-6129

Sumana Datta

Department of Biochemistry and Biophysics
Texas A&M University
College Station, Texas 77843-2128

During the past decade, we have seen remarkable advances in our understanding of how the eukaryotic cell cycle is regulated. As a result, we now have a detailed molecular description of the cell cycle machinery that controls both the G_1/S and G_2/M-phase transitions. Moreover, we have also seen the discovery of checkpoint controls that delay the cell cycle in response to intracellular perturbations including DNA damage, incomplete DNA replication, or a defective mitotic spindle. These allow time for repairs to be completed prior to chromosome segregation and cell division. Finally, the cell cycle can be regulated in response to extracellular signals generated by changes in nutrient status, pheromones, and mitogens.

Although we have made significant progress in our understanding of how the cell cycle is controlled in a variety of different organisms, little has been established on how the cell cycle is regulated in stem cells. Stem cells have an unlimited capacity for both self-renewal and production of differentiated progeny, and both processes must be tightly regulated to ensure the survival of the organism. Although it is still not clear what controls the decision to either self-renew or differentiate, or how the fate of a differentiating daughter cell is determined, the regulation of the cell cycle appears to play a key role in these processes. In this chapter, we provide a general overview of checkpoints and other cell cycle controls that operate in eukaryotic cells. This is followed by a discussion of how the cell cycle provides not only a means for controlling the numerical output of stem cells, but also a mechanism to regulate and implement developmental decisions.

REGULATION OF THE EUKARYOTIC CELL CYCLE

The eukaryotic cell cycle consists of alternating rounds of DNA replication (S phase) and cell division (M phase) separated by the gap phases G_1 and G_2 (Fig. 1). Progression through the cell cycle is controlled by the periodic activation of cyclin-dependent kinases (Cdks). Multiple Cdks have been identified in mammalian cells (Hunter and Pines 1994; Sherr 1994), whereas a single Cdk is required for cell cycle progression in yeast (Nurse 1994; see Table 1). In general, Cdks can be regulated by at least three independent mechanisms. First, Cdk kinase activity is dependent on its association with distinct cyclin proteins, and formation of these complexes is driven by cycles of cyclin synthesis and degradation (Hunter and Pines 1994; Sherr 1994). Second, phosphorylation of Cdk kinase at a conserved threonine residue by Cdk activating kinase (CAK) is required for activity (Morgan 1995), whereas inhibitory phosphorylation within the ATP-binding site is regulated by the combined action of the Wee1 kinase and Cdc25 phosphatase (Nurse 1990). Finally, Cdk activity can be regulated by binding to a specific class of Cdk inhibitors (CKIs) (Sherr and Roberts 1995). As we discuss below, these multiple modes of Cdk regulation are involved in controlling cell cycle progression in response to cell cycle checkpoints and extracellular signals that regulate cell proliferation.

The first step in the cell division cycle is to replicate the genetic material. Initiation of DNA replication requires the activity of Cdk kinase (Cdk2 in mammalian cells), which is dependent on expression and accumulation of G_1-specific cyclins (Sherr 1993). Other posttranslational modifications of Cdk may be important during its activation at the G_1-to-S-phase transition, but the details of this regulation are still not clear (Gu et al. 1992; Russo et al. 1992; Sebastian et al. 1993). As cells proceed through S phase, B-type cyclins begin to accumulate in preparation for M phase. Accumulation of B-type cyclins and their association with Cdk1 kinase is essential, but not sufficient, to drive cells into mitosis. Activation of Cdk1 also requires dephosphorylation within the ATP-binding site (Dunphy and Kumagai 1991; Gautier et al. 1991) and phosphorylation by CAK (Fesquet et al. 1993; Poon et al. 1993; Solomon et al. 1993; Fisher and Morgan 1994; Makela et al. 1994; Tassan et al. 1995). Finally, exit from mitosis and entry into the G_1 phase of the next cell cycle requires inactivation of Cdk kinase activity, which is brought about by tar-

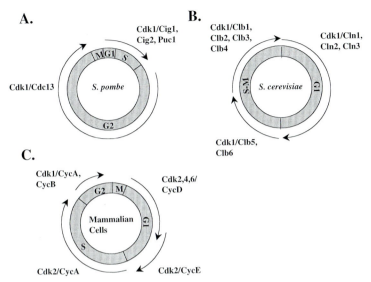

Figure 1 Cell cycle regulation in yeast and mammalian cells. (*A*) *S. pombe*. (*B*) *S. cerevisiae*. (*C*) Mammalian cells. The cell cycle is controlled by the periodic activation of cyclin-dependent kinases. Note that in *S. cerevisiae*, S and M phase temporally overlap and therefore the regulation of the cell cycle in response to DNA damage differs from that of *S. pombe* or mammalian cells. See text for details.

Table 1 Cyclin-dependent protein kinases in yeast and mammalian cells

CdkI	Associated cyclins	Cell cycle phase
S. pombe		
Cdc2 (Cdk1)	Puc1, Cig1, Cig2	G_1 to S-phase transition; S phase
	Cdc13	G_2 to M-phase transition
S. cerevisiae		
Cdc28 (Cdk1)	Cln1, Cln2, Cln3	G_1 to S-phase transition
	Clb5, Clb6	S phase
	Clb1, Clb2, Clb3, Clb4	M phase
Mammalian		
Cdc2	cyclins D1, D2, D3	G_1 phase
	cyclin E	
	cyclin A	
Cdk3	?	?
Cdk4	cyclins D1, D2, D3	G_1 phase
Cdk5	cyclins D1, D2, D3	G_1 phase
Cdk1	cyclins A and B	S phase; G_2 to M transition

geting B-type cyclins for degradation via ubiquitin-mediated proteolysis (Hunt et al. 1992).

The cell cycle is also regulated by checkpoint controls that ensure the normal order of cell cycle events (Hartwell and Weinert 1989; Murray 1994). Checkpoints were first identified in yeast as signaling pathways that delay cell cycle progression in response to DNA damage (Weinert and Hartwell 1988). Most of what we currently understand regarding the molecular basis of checkpoint controls is the result of genetic and bio-chemical analysis in yeast, where a number of checkpoint genes have been identified (Weinert 1998). These genes are highly conserved among all eukaryotic organisms, indicating that the basic checkpoint mecha-nisms have been preserved throughout evolution (see Table 2). In the fol-lowing two sections, we describe the mechanisms of two checkpoint sur-veillance systems that monitor two fundamental cell cycle processes, DNA replication/repair and chromosome segregation.

DNA DAMAGE-DEPENDENT CHECKPOINT IN YEAST AND MAMMALIAN CELLS

In the fission yeast, *Schizosaccharomyces pombe*, at least nine genes have been identified that are essential for the checkpoint control in response to DNA damage (Bentley and Carr 1997). Their gene products are thought to participate in a signal transduction pathway that inhibits activation of Cdk1 kinase at the G_2/M transition (Fig. 2A). Activation of the checkpoint pathway is thought to involve recognition and processing of a DNA lesion by "sensor proteins" generating a "checkpoint signal." This signal is then transmitted via the Rad3 kinase to two additional kinases, Chk1 and Cds1(Walworth et al. 1993; Murakami and Okayama 1995). Both Chk1 and Cds1 phosphorylate and inhibit the Cdc25 phosphatase, which is required for activation of Cdk1 kinase and entry into mitosis (Zeng et al. 1998; Furnari et al. 1999). There is also evidence suggesting that Chk1 can stimulate the Wee1 kinase, a direct inhibitor of Cdk1 (Raleigh and O'Connell 2000). Although it initially appeared that Cds1 and Chk1 function redundantly, closer examination has revealed an interesting specificity regarding their activation during the cell cycle. Cds1 is only activated in response to DNA damage during S phase, whereas Chk1 is activated following DNA damage in G_2. Recently, it has been suggested that Cds1 inhibits Chk1 activity, which may explain why Chk1 remains inactive during S phase (Boddy et al. 1998; Brondello et al. 1999). What determines this specificity is not yet clear, but it has been suggested that Cds1 may be coupled to or activated by specific DNA structures that only

Table 2 Checkpoint genes in yeast and mammalian cells

Gene name			
S. pombe	*S. cerevisiae*	mammalian	Proposed function
DNA damage checkpoint genes			
hus1	?	*HUS1*	DNA damage sensor protein
rad1	*RAD17*	*RAD1*	DNA damage sensor protein; potential nuclease
rad9	?	*RAD9*	DNA damage sensor protein
rad17	*RAD24*	*RAD17*	DNA damage sensor protein; RF-C like
rad26			
crb2/rph9	*RAD9*	*BRCA1*	DNA damage sensor protein
rad3	*MEC1*	*ATM/ATR*	member of PI-3 lipid kinase family
chk1	*CHK1*	*CHK1*	Ser/Thr protein kinase
cds1	*RAD53*	*CHK2*	Ser/Thr protein kinase
?	?	*P53*	transcription factor
Spindle checkpoint genes			
bub1	*BUB1*	*BUB1*	Ser-Thr protein kinase
bub2	*BUB2*	*BUB2*	GTPase-activating protein
bub3	*BUB3*	*BUB3*	forms a complex with Bub1
mad1	*MAD1*	*MAD1*	coiled-coil phosphoprotein
mad2	*MAD2*	*MAD2*	complexed with Mad1 and 3
mad3	*MAD3*	*MAD3*	complexed with Mad1 and 2
mps1	*MPS1*	*MPS1*	Ser-Thr kinase, required for SPB duplication
Other cell cycle regulators that play a role in checkpoint controls			
rum1	*SIC1*	*p21* (other CKIs)	Cdk inhibitor
wee1	*WEE1*	*WEE1*	tyrosine kinase; Cdk inhibitor
cdc25	*CDC25*	*CDC25 A, B, C*	phosphatase; Cdk activator

form during DNA synthesis (Brondello et al. 1999). Interestingly, Cds1 was originally identified as a multicopy suppressor of a temperature-sensitive mutant in DNA polymerase α, suggesting that these two proteins interact (Murakami and Okayama 1995). Therefore, it is possible that Cds1 is directly associated with the replication machinery. Why Cds1 would inhibit Chk1 activation during S phase is not yet known. However, one possibility is that Chk1 might be required for a DNA repair process that is normally restricted to the G_2 phase.

In most eukaryotic cells, DNA damage delays cell cycle progression by inhibiting Cdk kinase activation at either the G_2-to-M (as discussed above) or G_1-to-S-phase transition (see below). However, depending on the organism or how the cell cycle is regulated, other mechanisms can be used to prevent segregation of damaged chromosomes. For example, in the budding yeast *Saccharomyces cerevisiae*, where S phase and certain mitotic events are initiated simultaneously early in the cell cycle, cells respond to DNA damage by inhibiting the metaphase-to-anaphase transition rather than by blocking entry into mitosis (Elledge 1996). Although this represents a very different physiological response to DNA damage, the checkpoint signaling pathway involved remains highly conserved (Fig. 2B). Activation of the checkpoint is still dependent on a DNA damage signal that is generated by sensor proteins, leading to the stimulation

A. *S. pombe*

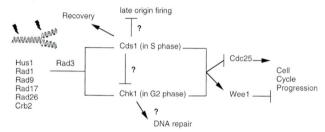

B. *S. cerevisiae*

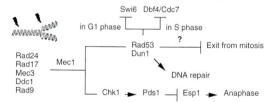

C. *H. sapiens*

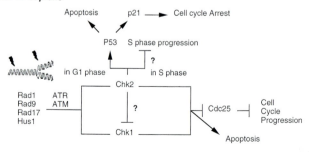

Figure 2 (See facing page for legend.)

of the Rad3 homolog Mec1 (Weinert 1998). Mec1 then activates two independent parallel pathways blocking cell division (Gardner et al. 1999; Sanchez et al. 1999). One pathway involves activation of the Chk1 kinase, which phosphorylates and stabilizes the metaphase-to-anaphase inhibitor, Pds1 (Sanchez et. al. 1999). The second pathway leads to activation of the Rad53 and Dun1 kinases, both of which contribute to the cell cycle delay by unknown mechanisms (Gardner et al. 1999; Sanchez et al. 1999).

In addition to arresting cells in either G_2 or M phase, DNA damage can also delay entry into S phase. In *S. cerevisiae*, this checkpoint, sometimes referred to as the G_1 checkpoint, is also dependent on Mec1 and Rad53 (Siede and Friedberg 1990). Cell cycle arrest is thought to occur via Rad53 phosphorylation and inhibition of the transcription factor, Swi6, which is required for expression of G_1 cyclins (Fig. 2B) (Sidorova and Breeden 1997).

In multicellular organisms, DNA damage activates a checkpoint control pathway that leads to either cell cycle arrest in G_1 or G_2, or programmed cell death, i.e., apoptosis (Evan and Littlewood 1998). A key

Figure 2 Activation of checkpoint pathways in response to DNA damage. (*A*) In fission yeast, the sensor proteins Rad1, Rad9, Rad17, and Crb2 transmit the damage signal to the protein kinase Rad3, which then phosphorylates the downstream kinases Chk1 and Cds1 in a cell-cycle-dependent manner. Cds1 is activated specifically in response to DNA damage in S phase, and Chk1 is activated when DNA damage occurs during G_2. Both Cds1 and Chk1 prevent entry into mitosis by phosphorylating and inhibiting the mitotic activator Cdc25. (*B*) In budding yeast, activation of the Rad3 homolog Mec1 is dependent on the sensor proteins Rad17/24, Rad9, Ddc1, and Mec3. However, in contrast to fission yeast, Mec1 targets regulators of the metaphase–anaphase transition, and exit from mitosis. Mec1 activates the Chk1 kinase, which then phosphorylates and stabilizes the anaphase inhibitor Pds1. Mec1 also activates the Rad53 and Dun1 kinases; Rad53 delays the cell cycle by interfering with S-phase progression, and exit from mitosis. Dun1 is required for expression of genes involved in DNA repair, but also contributes to the cell cycle delay by unknown mechanisms. (*C*) In human cells, homologous checkpoint pathways exist to block entry into S phase and mitosis. Following DNA damage, the Rad3 homologs ATM and ATR kinases phosphorylate and activate the downstream kinases Chk1 and Chk2. It is not yet known whether the activity of these kinases is restricted to specific cell cycle phases as has been observed in fission yeast. If DNA damage occurs in G_2, Chk1 and possibly Chk2 phosphorylate and inhibit Cdc25C, which is required for entry into mitosis. If damage occurs during G_1, P53 is phosphorylated by either Chk1 or Chk2, which stabilizes the protein leading to expression of a number of effector genes including P21, a potent inhibitor of Cdk1 kinase.

regulator in the decision to either arrest the cell cycle or undergo apoptosis is P53 (Lane 1992, 1993). P53 is a sequence-specific DNA-binding protein that activates the transcription of a variety of downstream effector genes (Cox and Lane 1995). Stabilization of P53 following DNA damage is required for cell cycle arrest in G_1, or apoptosis from G_1 or G_2 (Ashcroft et al. 2000). Mammalian cells also arrest the cell cycle in G_2 in response to DNA damage, but this can occur independently of P53 (Kastan et al. 1991; Kuerbitz et al. 1992; O'Connor et al. 1993). Similar to *S. pombe*, arrest in G_2 involves inhibition of Cdc25 phosphatase by Chk1 and Chk2 kinases (Sanchez et al. 1997; Matsuoka et al. 1998; Chaturvedi et al. 1999).

DNA damage-induced P53 stabilization requires a protein kinase cascade similar to one activated in response to DNA damage in both budding and fission yeast (Fig. 2C) (Westphal 1997). In this case, the Rad3 homologs ATR and ATM phosphorylate and activate the downstream kinases Chk2 and possibly Chk1 (Chk2 is homologous to Cds1/Rad53; Matsuoka et al. 1998; Chaturvedi et al. 1999). Both kinases have been shown to phosphorylate P53, leading to stabilization of the protein (Chehab et al. 2000; Shieh et al. 2000). P53 can then *trans*-activate a number of genes, including CIP1/WAF1/p21, a potent inhibitor of CDK activities required for the G_1-to-S-phase transition (el-Deiry et al. 1993; Harper et al. 1993; Xiong et al. 1993; Noda et al. 1994). The proposed role for p21 in cell cycle arrest is twofold; in addition to blocking CDK activity, p21 is also known to bind proliferating cell nuclear antigen (PCNA), a protein required for both DNA replication and DNA repair (Prelich et al. 1987a,b; Shivji et al. 1992; Flores-Rozas et al. 1994; Luo et al. 1995). Although p21 has been shown to inhibit SV40 replication in vitro (Flores-Rozas et al. 1994; Waga et al. 1994; Luo et al. 1995), it is not yet known whether this is a primary function of the protein during DNA damage. Although P53-induced expression of p21 provides an attractive model for how cells arrest in G_1 following DNA damage, in at least some cell types, it is not the sole mediator of the checkpoint response (Brugarolas et al. 1995; Deng et al. 1995). Other potential candidates that might participate in P53-dependent G_1 arrest include the Gadd45 (Kastan et al. 1992; Zhan et al. 1998), WIP1 (Fiscella et al. 1997), Cyclin D1 (Pagano et al. 1994; Chen et al. 1995), and ABL genes (Yuan et al. 1996; Nie et al. 2000).

It is still a mystery as to why, in multicellular organisms, some cells arrest the cell cycle in response to DNA damage whereas others undergo apoptosis. Although the basis for this difference is poorly understood, P53 has been shown to be essential for both G_1 arrest following DNA damage and apoptosis from G_1 or G_2. Apoptosis occurs through a pathway that involves activation of proteases of the ICE/ced3 class and its regulation by members of the Bcl2/ced9 family (Korsmeyer 1995). P53 is known to induce expression of genes that promote apoptosis, including Bax (Miyashita and Reed 1995), FAS (Owen-Schaub et al. 1995), and insulin-like growth factor-1-binding protein-3 (IGF-BP3; Buckbinder et al. 1995). However, there is also evidence that P53 can induce apoptosis in the complete absence of its transcriptional activity, suggesting that P53 is likely to have multiple functions (Ko and Prives 1996). Interestingly, the Rad3 homolog ATM that is required for cell cycle arrest following DNA damage is not required for apoptosis (Meyn et al. 1994). This suggests that the checkpoint pathways leading to cell cycle arrest or apoptosis, which are both dependent on P53 stabilization, are distinct processes. One model proposes that low-level DNA damage may signal cell cycle arrest via the ATM-dependent checkpoint, whereas more extensive damage may activate P53 by an alternative pathway, the latter leading to apoptosis (Enoch and Norbury 1995).

Finally, the DNA damage checkpoint can also inhibit DNA replication initiation and S-phase progression. For example, in budding yeast, treatment of cells with DNA alkylating agents can slow DNA replication in a Mec1, Rad53-dependent manner (Paulovich and Hartwell 1995; Paulovich et al. 1997). Whether this reflects inhibition of initiation or elongation is not yet known. Similarly, human cells defective for the ATM gene no longer delay S phase in response to DNA-damaging agents (Painter and Young 1987). This suggests that in addition to blocking mitosis, the checkpoint pathway can also target components directly involved in DNA synthesis. There is also evidence that the checkpoint control can delay initiation of DNA replication from late origins when cells are arrested in early S phase by treatment with hydroxyurea (Santocanale and Diffley 1998; Shirahige et al. 1998). This delay is dependent on expression of both Mec1 and Rad53 (Santocanale and Diffley 1998), similar to what is observed following treatment of cells with DNA alkylating agents (Paulovich and Hartwell 1995). In this case, the target of Rad53 is believed to be the Cdc7/Dbf4 kinase that has been directly implicated in replication origin firing (Dowell et al. 1994; Hardy et al. 1997; Lei et al. 1997; Owens et al. 1997; Jiang et al. 1999; Pasero et al. 1999; Weinreich and Stillman 1999).

THE SPINDLE CHECKPOINT

Checkpoints are not only involved with coupling DNA metabolic events to mitosis, but are also required to ensure the normal order of mitotic events. Segregation of chromosomes during cell division requires that all replicated chromosomes properly align themselves on the mitotic spindle during metaphase. In the presence of a disrupted or incomplete mitotic spindle, a checkpoint is activated that blocks the metaphase-to-anaphase transition and exit from mitosis (Hardwick 1998; Amon 1999; Burke 2000). The so-called spindle assembly checkpoint was first characterized at the molecular level in budding yeast following the isolation of mutants that failed to arrest the cell cycle in response to microtubule-depolymerizing drugs. Seven genes were found to be essential for the checkpoint; these included *BUB1–3*, *MAD1–3*, *MPS1,* and *PDS1* (Hoyt et al. 1991; Li and Murray 1991; Weiss and Winey 1996; Yamamoto et al. 1996). Homologs for most of these genes have been found in several other organisms, including *S. pombe* (He et al. 1997, 1998; Bernard et al. 1998), *Drosophila melanogaster* (Basu et al. 1998, 1999), *Caenorhabditis elegans* (Kitagawa and Rose 1999), and vertebrates (Chen et al. 1996; Li and Benezra 1996; Pangilinan et al. 1997; Taylor et al. 1998; Jin et al. 1999). Similar to the DNA damage checkpoint, the spindle checkpoint is also thought to involve generation of a signal, in this case from the kinetochore that senses the existence of unattached chromosomes (Chen et al. 1996; Li and Benezra 1996; Taylor and McKeon 1997; Taylor et al. 1998). Before discussing the mechanism of cell cycle arrest induced by the spindle checkpoint, we first briefly review how the later stages of cell division are regulated.

Separation of sister chromatids during anaphase relies on the activity of the anaphase-promoting complex (APC) (Zachariae and Nasmyth 1999). This protein complex has a ubiquitin ligase activity that regulates the destruction of a specific set of proteins by ubiquitin-mediated proteolysis. Sister chromatids are held together by a protein complex known as cohesin (Guacci et al. 1997; Michaelis et al. 1997; Losada et al. 1998; Yanagida 2000), which is released from chromosomes upon anaphase entry. A key step in this process appears to be APC-dependent degradation of a protein called Pds1 (Cohen-Fix et al. 1996), which binds to and inactivates a protein called ESP1 (Ciosk et al. 1998). Esp1 is essential for the proteolytic cleavage of a component of cohesin, a necessary step in the metaphase–anaphase transition (Uhlmann et al. 1999). In addition to the degradation of Pds1, the B-type cyclin-dependent kinases are also targeted for degradation via the APC, and this is required for exit from mitosis.

Two pathways are activated in response to damaged spindles (Fig. 3). One pathway involves the products of the *MAD1–3* and *BUB1* genes and is required for the inhibition of an APC accessory factor Cdc20, which normally targets the Pds1 protein for degradation (Alexandru et al. 1999). The second pathway requires the *BUB2* gene, which is thought to be a

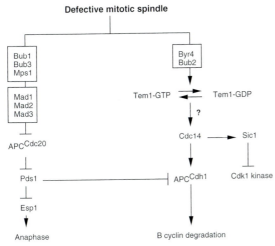

Figure 3 The spindle assembly checkpoint. Failure to align chromosomes on the mitotic spindle during metaphase triggers a checkpoint that blocks chromosome segregation and exit from mitosis. In vertebrate cells, homologs of Mad2, Bub1, and Bub3 have been shown to associate with the kinetochore, suggesting this structure is important for checkpoint signaling. Two pathways are activated in response to detached chromosomes. The first pathway requires the products of the *Bub1*, *Bub3*, *Mps1*, and *Mad1–3* genes. These proteins function in a signal transduction pathway that inhibits APCcdc20, which normally targets the metaphase-to-anaphase inhibitor Pds1 for degradation. The second pathway requires Byr4 and Bub2, which function as a two-component GAP (GTPase activating protein) that maintains the Tem1-GTPase in an inactive (GDP) form, thereby preventing release of Cdc14 from the nucleolus (Shou et al. 1999; Visintin et al. 1999). In the absence of Cdc14 activity, APCcdh1 remains in a phosphorylated inactive state, and therefore cells are prohibited from exiting mitosis (Visintin et al. 1998; Jaspersen et al. 1999).

part of a two-component GTPase activating protein (GAP). In the presence of a damaged or an incomplete mitotic spindle, Bub2 is thought to stimulate the GTPase, Tem1. This leads to an accumulation of Tem1 in the inactive (GDP) form. In the absence of the active (GTP) form of Tem1, the Cdc14 phosphatase remains sequestered in the nucleolus, and cells are inhibited from exiting mitosis (Alexandru et al. 1999).

CELL CYCLE CHECKPOINTS IN A CHANGING CELL CYCLE

Analysis of stem cell divisions in the developing *Drosophila* embryo suggest at least three different checkpoint mechanisms are functioning during early fly development. During the first 13 cell divisions that occur in syncytium, DNA damage activates a checkpoint that blocks anaphase (Fogarty et al. 1997). During cycle 14, the *chk1* and *rad3* homologs *grapes* (*grp*) and *mei-41*, respectively, are required to coordinate completion of DNA replication to chromosome segregation (Sibon et al. 1997,1999), and following cycle 14, DNA damage results in the inhibition of entry into mitosis (Su et al. 2000). Therefore, multicellular organisms like *Drosophila* appear to use a wide variety of checkpoint controls to maintain genome stability during development. These checkpoints share striking similarity to those used by both *S. pombe* and *S. cerevisiae*. However, whereas in yeast the checkpoint response differs depending on how the cell cycle is regulated, in *Drosophila*, the checkpoint response depends on the developmental stage at which DNA damage occurs. Additional studies will be required to clarify whether similar checkpoints function in other organisms during development.

ENVIRONMENTAL REGULATION OF CELL CYCLE PROGRESSION: LESSONS FROM UNICELLULAR ORGANISMS

Extracellular signals can also have a dramatic effect on the regulation of cell division and differentiation. The mating pathway in yeast represents one of the best-understood examples of a how a eukaryotic cell can differentiate in response to changes in its environment (Zhou et al. 1993; Bardwell et al. 1996). This pathway shares many similarities with those used by growth factors to regulate cell proliferation in higher eukaryotic organisms (Cooper 1994; Marshall 1994).

In the yeast, *S. pombe*, the mating pathway is initially triggered by nutritional starvation, which causes cells to arrest in the G_1 phase of the cell cycle (Yamamoto 1996). An important determinant during cell cycle arrest involves decreasing cAMP levels. The decrease in cAMP leads to increased expression of the *ste11* gene, which encodes a key transcription factor required for expression of genes required for cell cycle arrest, conjugation, and meiosis (Mochizuki and Yamamoto 1992). Mutational analyses of *S. pombe* genes encoding components of the cAMP cascade have shown that *S. pombe* cells stay in the mitotic cell cycle as long as the level of cAMP-dependent protein kinase activity remains high, but are committed to mating and meiosis if this activity is lowered. Mating pheromone, which is thought to activate a protein kinase cascade homologous to the MAP kinase cascade in mammalian cells, also contributes to the G_1 arrest (Imai and Yamamoto 1994).

In contrast to fission yeast, in *S. cerevisiae* the first step in the mating pathway does not require nutritional starvation, but only the presence of pheromone. The binding of pheromone to a cell-surface receptor is believed to induce a conformational change in a membrane-associated G (GTP-binding) protein complex that activates a mitogen-activated (MAP) kinase cascade required for gene activation, G_1 arrest, recovery from pheromone arrest, and nuclear and cellular morphological changes (Klein et al. 2000). Following formation of the diploid zygote, cells can resume vegetative growth. The second step in the mating pathway requires nutritional starvation, which triggers G_1 arrest, meiosis, and sporulation. As in *S. pombe*, cell cycle arrest in response to nutritional starvation is thought to involve regulation of cAMP-dependent kinase (Kronstad et al. 1998).

RESPONDING TO THE CELLULAR MILIEU

We have seen how yeast cells respond to external cues such as starvation or mating pheromone by arresting their cell cycle at G_1 preparatory to changing their cellular program. Although it is clear that stem cells (SCs) also respond to environmental factors by undergoing cell cycle arrest or activation, surprisingly little is known about the molecular mechanisms that regulate cell proliferation. The control of SC proliferation is especially critical given SCs' virtually unlimited capacity for the production of new cells and their role as the ultimate source of differentiated cells for the assembly and maintenance of multicellular organisms.

Organismal-level Signals

Numerous organismal-level physiological stimuli have been identified that result in the induction or inhibition of cell cycle progression in SCs. However, since cell cycle status has frequently been monitored through production of genetically marked progeny or BrdU incorporation, the cell cycle phase from which proliferative entry and exit may take place is rarely known. In addition, changes in cellular output or BrdU incorporation could represent either changes in the length of a specific cell cycle phase or canonical cell cycle arrest/activation. Yet, in a few systems we are beginning to see the outlines of pathways that begin with organismal-level cues and terminate in changes in the activity of the cell cycle machinery.

Activation or increase in SC division has been shown to take place under various conditions: transplantation into irradiated hosts; depletion of cycling cells by cytotoxins; in response to developmental programming; and even as a result of physical activity. The best-characterized system for transplantation and depletion studies is the hematopoietic SC or HSC (see Chapters 13, 14, 15, and 17). Both mammalian and human primitive HSCs give rise to long-term repopulation of all blood cell lineages and can be isolated from bone marrow as relatively quiescent G_0/G_1 cells. Upon injection into lethally irradiated mice, these HSCs provide multilineage long-term reconstitution of the peripheral blood. The large percentage of donor-derived cells present in the blood 30 days after transplantation indicates that the rate of primitive HSC cell division must dramatically increase upon transplantation (Fleming et al. 1993). This increase in HSC cell cycle activity is presumably required to replace the more mature lineage-restricted cycling precursors that die as a result of radiation damage. Whether the increase in HSC division occurs as a direct consequence of the loss of the precursors is not yet clear. The relative resistance of primitive HSCs to cycle-active cytotoxic agents suggests that most of these cells are dividing slowly, and indeed, long-term labeling with BrdU of up to 30 days is required before the vast majority of HSCs are observed to incorporate the S-phase label (Cheshier et al. 1999). This implies that primitive HSCs have an extremely elongated cell cycle resulting either from greatly extending at least one cell cycle phase or from undergoing a stop–start cell cycle mode with rounds of transient cell cycle arrest followed by cell division (Fig. 4).

Division of HSCs produces lineage-restricted precursors that in turn give rise to differentiated blood cells. Detection of donor-derived blood cells indicates unequivocally that quiescent HSCs have activated cell division upon transplantation. However, loss of donor-derived blood cell pro-

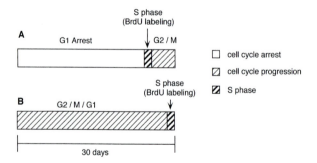

Figure 4 Single stop–start versus slow cell cycle period. (*A*) Stop–start cell cycle shown with a long period of G_1 arrest followed by progression through S, G_2, and M. Stop–start cycles with G_0 or G_2 arrest are also possible. (*B*) Slow or extended cell cycle progression. Note that the length of S phase when the cells would incorporate BrdU remains the same for both models. Either cell cycle arrest or extended G_1/G_2 phases would allow repair of DNA caused by cytotoxic agents.

A. Repopulation by transplanted HSC

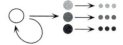

B. Mitotic arrest of HSC

C. Apoptosis of lineage-restricted precursors

Figure 5 Loss of donor-derived peripheral blood cells posttransplantation. (*A*) Multilineage reconstitution from a single transplanted HSC. (*B*) Loss of donor-derived peripheral blood cells due to mitotic arrest of the transplanted HSC. (*C*) Loss of donor-derived peripheral blood cells due to apoptosis of lineage-restricted precursors produced by division of the transplanted HSC.

duction could be due to either return of HSCs to mitotic quiescence or apoptosis of lineage-restricted precursors (Fig. 5). Definitive studies to determine whether primitive HSCs return to their previously quiescent state after a period of rapid mitoses have yet to be performed.

Studies on the effect of depleting cycling precursors on SC division have also been carried out in the mammalian brain (Morshead et al. 1994). The results suggest that forebrain neuroblasts transiently enter a more active mitotic state upon depletion of cycling progenitor cells; these conditions, however, do not address whether the transition is one between cell cycle arrest and activation, or between a very long and a very short cell cycle period.

The activation and arrest of SC division in response to developmental cues has been investigated primarily in mammalian and insect neuroblasts. In *Drosophila*, a number of lineage (Prokop and Technau 1991) and BrdU (White and Kankel 1978; Truman and Bate 1988; Hofbauer and Campos-Ortega 1990) studies have shown that a subset of neuroblasts undergo two bursts of mitotic activity, once in embryos and later during larval stages. The double burst of BrdU incorporation indicates initial embryonic division followed by relative quiescence, then reactivation for larval mitoses and a final arrest concomitant with differentiation. In this proliferation program, "relative mitotic quiescence" entails cell cycle arrest or passage through one very elongated cell cycle period.

Detailed genetic analyses in *Drosophila* have identified a number of genes required to control the temporal pattern of "on and off again" SC division (Fig. 6). The first quiescence is achieved by inhibition of an initial mitogenic signal by the product of the *ana* gene, thus preventing neuroblasts from beginning S phase prematurely (Ebens et al. 1993). The initiation of S phase at the appropriate time for larval division requires the product of the *trol* gene (Datta 1995) and the transcription repressor Even-skipped (Park et al. 1998). Induction of S phase by *trol* occurs at a later stage of G_1 than the G_0/G_1 arrest mediated by *ana* (Caldwell and Datta 1998), suggesting that *Drosophila* neuroblasts may activate cell division in a stepwise fashion reminiscent of the G_1 subphases described for mammalian cells (for review, see Pardee 1989). More complex control of G_1 progression is also observed during differentiation of mouse embryonic SCs. This involves up-regulation of cyclin D and E (two G_1-specific cyclins), Cdk 2 and 4, and the Cdk inhibitors p21 and p27, leading to an elongation of the G_1 period (Savatier et al. 1995). For *Drosophila* neuroblasts, the transition to mitotic arrest is mediated by the developmental transcription factor Prospero (Li and Vaessin 2000). The molecular mechanisms by which some of these *Drosophila* genes regulate cell cycle progression are discussed below.

Finally, experiential cues have also been suggested to alter the mitotic activity of SCs in the adult mammalian brain. Enriched or complex environmental stimuli increased BrdU incorporation in the mouse hippocampus (Kempermann et al. 1998), as did increased physical activity (van Praag et al. 1999). Interestingly, mice that score well in learning paradigms and normally have high levels of neurogenesis do not show increased BrdU incorporation in a more complex environment (Kempermann et al. 1997). These intriguing studies represent the beginning of a new line of investigation that will address whether experiential stimuli increase SC, precursor cell division, or both. Currently, we have no understanding of the molecular events connecting behavior to changes in the cell cycle.

Molecular Signaling

For many of the organismal-level changes described above, the molecular basis underlying the phenomenology and how those changes are translated into molecular signals that can affect the cell cycle machinery in SCs are beginning to be addressed. Signal transduction pathways link many organismal-level changes to alterations in transcriptional or enzymatic activity. This robust area of research has been extensively reviewed (Aza-

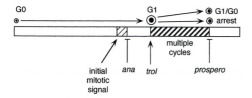

Figure 6 Control of "on and off again" neuroblast division in *Drosophila*. Neuroblasts are assumed to be arrested in G_0 (*open box*) upon larval hatching. An initial mitotic signal activates cell cycle progression (*lightly hatched box)* which is either inhibited by *ana* in G_0 or early G_1 or greatly slowed. Cell cycle progression is reinitiated from late G_1, or the rate of progression is greatly increased by *trol*. The neuroblast begins several rounds of cell division. Cell cycle progression in daughter cells is arrested through the action of *prospero*.

Blanc and Kornberg 1999; Dierick and Bejsovec 1999; Tan and Kim 1999; Zhang and Derynck 1999); however, most of the studies occur in non-SC systems. Which signal transduction pathways operate specifically in stem cells and how they translate extrinsic signals into cell cycle arrest or activation remain to be determined. This is especially critical, since many extrinsic signals are known to produce a variety of different responses depending on cell type. Much of the SC-specific information at this level comes from in vitro analyses of cultured SCs and molecular genetic studies in *Drosophila*.

Studies in vitro have shown that the rate of cell division of freshly isolated G_0/G_1 primitive HSCs or the amplification of HSC-like cells increases upon addition of specific cytokines (Reddy et al. 1997; Zandstra et al. 1997). HSC-like murine cells begin division in vitro in response to cytokines with the same kinetics as observed post implantation in vivo (Oostendorp et al. 2000). These data suggest that cytokines may be directly linked to the increase in HSC mitotic activity in vivo. An interesting possibility is that cytokine signaling may couple decreasing lineage-restricted precursor pools to their regeneration by transplanted HSCs (Fig. 7A–C). Cytokines have been shown to activate a number of signal transduction pathways, prominent among them the Janus kinase/signal transducer and activator of transcription (Jak/Stat) pathway (for review, see Blalock et al. 1999; Heim 1999). Although the Jak/Stat pathway is commonly considered to stimulate cell division, studies of SC proliferation suggest that it may function instead to maintain SC division or identity (Fig. 7D,E) (Datta 1999 and unpubl.; A. Kiger and M. Fuller, unpubl.).

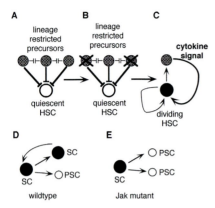

Figure 7 Signal transduction and stem cell division. (*A–C*) Possible model for mammalian HSC division stimulated by cytokine signaling from a diminished lineage-restricted precursor pool. (*A*) Inhibition of HSC division by unknown signals from lineage-restricted precursors. Lateral inhibition would also prevent production of specific cytokines or alter the level of cytokine production by progenitor cells. (*B*) Shrinkage of the precursor pool. (*C*) Lateral inhibition of cytokine production by progenitor cells is removed by the decrease in the number of lineage-restricted precursors. The appropriate combination/level of cytokines is released, resulting in HSC division and repopulation of the progenitor pool. (*D,E*) Effect of Jak mutations on SC fate in *Drosophila*. (*D*) In normal animals, male germ-line SCs divide asymmetrically to generate a primary spermatogonial cell and regenerate the germ-line SC. (*E*) In Jak mutants, germ-line SCs are lost after a few cell divisions, presumably due to loss of SC identity in both daughter cells. This may result from conversion of the normal asymmetric division to a symmetric division.

In vitro analyses of mammalian neuroblasts (Weiss et al. 1996) have also identified a number of factors such as epidermal growth factor (EGF) and basic fibroblast growth factor and their signaling pathways (for review, see Hackel et al. 1999; Moghal and Sternberg 1999; Szebenyi and Fallon 1999) that are necessary to increase or decrease SC division. In vitro cultures of *Manduca* and *Drosophila* central nervous systems have identified the hormone ecdysone as a potential activator of neuroblast cell division through an as-yet-unidentified mechanism (Champlin and Truman 1998; Datta 1999). However, as before, it should be noted that it is not clear whether these factors activate cell cycle progression in an arrested cell or dramatically increase the rate of cell division of cells progressing very slowly through the cell cycle.

Given that it is not always clear whether SCs are cycling between cell cycle arrest and cell cycle activation or between short and very long cell cycle periods, a related issue is how the length of the SC cell cycle is regulated. Genetic studies of female *Drosophila* germ-line development have identified at least two signaling pathways that regulate the rate of SC division. The novel gene *piwi* is required both within an adjacent cell and in the SC itself to increase the division rate of germ-line SCs (Cox et al. 2000). In addition, inhibition of signaling by Dpp, a transforming growth factor-β-like molecule, results in slower cell cycles in germ-line SCs (Xie and Spradling 1998 and Chapter 7).

Linking Molecular Signals to Cell Cycle Phase and the Cell Cycle Machinery

We have surprisingly little information about the cell cycle phase in which signaling pathways function, let alone how they affect the cell cycle machinery to induce or inhibit cell cycle progression in SCs. Thus far, the best-understood system is the mitotic activation of *Drosophila* neuroblasts by *trol*. Preliminary evidence suggests that *trol* encodes the *Drosophila* perlecan, a coreceptor for FGF (S. Datta, M. Caldwell, M. Reynolds, C. Rangel, Y. Park, and S. McDermott, unpubl.). In the absence of *trol* function, neuroblasts arrest in G_1 as indicated by decreased *cyclin E* mRNA levels and are able to enter S phase upon induced expression of either *cyclin E* or *E2F/DP* but not *cyclin B* (Caldwell and Datta 1998). Genetic and molecular analyses suggest that the activity of Cyclin-Cdk complexes may also be stimulated by the Cdc25 protein phosphatase homolog string to promote the G_1-to-S-phase transition (Y. Park and S. Datta, unpubl.).

Cell cycle arrest of *Drosophila* neuroblast progeny in G_1 also occurs prior to differentiation (Fig. 8) (Li and Vaessin 2000). The dividing neuroblasts synthesize Prospero, which becomes asymmetrically localized into the ganglion mother cell upon cell division and is later translocated into the nucleus. Nuclear Prospero activates expression of *asense* and inhibits expression of *deadpan*, which encode two basic helix-loop-helix proteins. Altered levels of these two proteins result in the expression of *dacapo*, which encodes the *Drosophila* p21 homolog. An extrapolation from embryonic function (de Nooij et al. 1996; Lane et al. 1996) would suggest that Dacapo then inhibits CyclinE-Cdk2 activity, thus arresting the immature neuron or glial cell in G_1. Studies of rat oligodendrocyte precursors also show cell cycle arrest in G_1 prior to differentiation by up-regulation of p21 and p27 through a cAMP-mediated pathway (Ghiani et al. 1999).

Although the molecular mechanisms through which organismal-level cues regulate SC proliferation are far from clear, the central portion of the framework, which includes the signal transduction pathways activated by

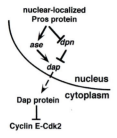

Figure 8 Model for Prospero-mediated cell cycle arrest. Arrows indicate interactions based on genetic analysis and are not meant to imply direct regulation at the molecular level. Arrows within the nucleus represent control at the transcriptional level. Expression of *dacapo* (*dap*) results in the increase in Dacapo (Dap) protein in the cytoplasm (shown by the dashed arrow) where it is thought to act by inhibiting the kinase activity of cyclin E-cdk2 complexes.

molecular signals, has been well characterized. However, large gaps still exist in our understanding of how organismal changes, such as transplantation, translate into molecular signals that will activate the signal transduction pathways (Fig. 9). Other gaps exist at the output end of the pathway: How do changes in the activity of multiple signal transduction pathways result in coordinated changes in cell cycle activity? Are there specific windows of opportunity during cell cycle progression in which signals must effect these changes? Are the input points where cell cycle progression is controlled the same as those used by canonical cell cycle checkpoints? These are just a few of the questions that still need to be addressed.

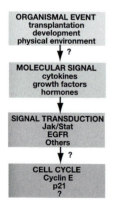

Figure 9. General flow of information from organismal-level cues to changes in cell cycle machinery.

CHANGING THE PROGRAM: WHERE CELL CYCLE REGULATES DEVELOPMENT

We have seen ample evidence for changes in cell cycle activity as a result of environmental cues. However, it is also true that the cell cycle progression itself plays an important role directly and indirectly in determining the potency of a SC and the fate of its progeny.

Cell Cycle and Renewal of Multipotency

One of the most intriguing notions is that passage through the cell cycle can set the developmental fate of cells derived from SC division and renew SC multipotency (McConnell and Kaznowski 1991). Transplantation studies suggest that shortly after S phase, the cell fate of the soon-to-be-born SC progeny is restricted by environmental factors, but passage through the next S phase restores SC multipotency, allowing new cues to dictate the identity of the resulting daughter. How might S phase renew SC multipotency? One hypothesis invokes changes in chromatin structure during DNA replication (Fig. 10) that can have dramatic effects on levels of gene expression and therefore cell fate. Recent studies in yeast (Cosma et al. 1999; Krebs et al. 1999) reveal that chromatin remodeling factors are recruited during M/G$_1$ and the chromatin is remodeled during S phase, resulting in changes in transcriptional programs in the subsequent G$_1$. This suggests that changes that occur at a specific cell cycle phase can affect decisions at a later time.

Direct Cell Cycle Regulation of Gene Expression

In the context of cell cycle control over development, it is reasonable to ask whether cell cycle progression is required for the normal develop-

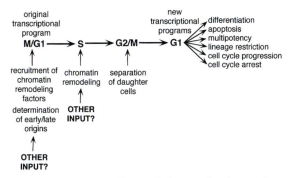

Figure 10 Possible effects of changes in chromatin structure determined at earlier cell cycle phases on stem cell fates at later times.

mental program of gene expression, or whether temporal patterning of gene expression will continue in cell-cycle-arrested cells. This question can be further subdivided to ask whether cytokinesis itself, the physical separation of two daughter cells, is sufficient or whether rounds of DNA synthesis are also essential. Much of our information here comes from analysis of *Drosophila* neuroblasts.

In vitro and in vivo studies show that some genes require neither cytokinesis nor cell cycle progression to achieve normal patterns of expression, whereas others require only cytokinesis, and a few require both. Surprisingly, the cell cycle dependence for expression of a certain gene in the same animal varies with the lineage examined. Analysis of neuroblasts in culture revealed that inhibition of M phase did not alter the expression of neurotransmitter synthetic pathway enzymes (Huff et al. 1989). Studies in vivo identified multiple cell cycle regulation patterns of neuroblast gene expression (Cui and Doe 1995). Therefore, although cell cycle progression is required for the correct expression of some developmentally important genes, the inputs from cell cycle to gene expression are varied, and not all developmental genes require such input for their expression. Whether other cell cycle phases or events also trigger changes in the pattern of gene expression, and what the molecular mechanisms for such controls are, still remain to be elucidated.

Indirect Regulation of Gene Expression

Cell division can also affect gene expression, and therefore cell fate, in an indirect fashion. These types of divisions are generally defined as asymmetric divisions, either in the physical sense that they produce two cells of different size or in the developmental sense that they produce two cells of different identity. The differentiation between two cell types can take place as a result of extrinsic or intrinsic cues. Changes in extrinsic cues might occur when the plane of cell division physically places the two daughter cells in two different microenvironments, whereas changes in intrinsic cues may reflect unequal partitioning of internal factors between the two daughters.

The effect of microenvironment on cell fate is implied by in vitro studies where SC production is altered by different culture conditions and in vivo studies that correlate cell–cell interactions with cell fate. In vitro culture of HSCs demonstrates that the balance between the production of lineage-restricted progenitors versus HSCs depends on the relative concentration of cytokines in the media (Zandstra et al. 1997). Time-lapse microscopy studies of mammalian cerebral cortex show that changes in division plane, and therefore cell–cell or cell–extracellular matrix contacts, change the fate of the daughters (Fig. 11A,B) (Chenn and McConnell 1995). The change in division plane also correlates with symmetric or asymmetric distribution of the signaling molecule Notch1. In vivo studies of the *Drosophila* male and female germ line also correlate changes in SC niche with changes in the fate of SC progeny. Removal of surrounding somatic cells by ablation or by alteration of the expression of signaling molecules such as *piwi* (Cox et al. 2000), *fs(1)Yb* (King and Lin 1999), and *Dpp* (Xie and Spradling 1998 and Chapter 7) leads to the conversion of asymmetric to symmetric daughter cell fate (Fig. 11A,C). Similarly, stimulation or inhibition of the externally activated EGF receptor pathway can also lead to changes in cell fate (Chapter 8).

Asymmetric distribution of internal factors upon SC division has been shown to affect the identities of resulting daughter cells. Perhaps the best-characterized examples of asymmetrically localized cell fate determinants in SCs are the analyses of Prospero and Numb in *Drosophila* neuroblasts (for review, see Fuerstenberg et al. 1998; Jan and Jan 1998). Both Prospero and Numb proteins are segregated into the lineage-restricted cell upon neuroblast division, where they are required for daughter cell fate as assayed by the identity of the progeny produced. Prospero and Numb asymmetric distribution is dependent on the Inscutable protein that is also responsible for spindle orientation during neuroblast division. Thus, the act of mitosis creates two cells with different levels of Prospero and/or Numb and ultimately leads to changes in daughter cell fate.

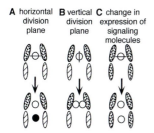

Figure 11 Cell division effects on microenvironment and stem cell fate. (*A*) Horizontal cleavage plane results in one daughter (*top white cell*) maintaining the original cell–cell interactions and retaining SC fate while the second daughter (*bottom black cell*) is displaced into a new microenvironment resulting in a different cell fate. (*B*) Vertical cleavage plane results in both daughters retaining cell–cell interactions similar to those of the original SC and thus retaining SC characteristics. (*C*) Altering the expression of a signaling molecule results in both daughters receiving cues that result in the maintenance of SC fate in both cells.

CANONICAL CELL CYCLE REGULATORS AND DEVELOPMENT

Given that cell cycle progression affects SC gene expression both directly and indirectly, it seems reasonable that delay or arrest of the cell cycle by canonical cell cycle regulators such as starvation and DNA damage may also affect developmental events.

Serum starvation is a classic phenomenon that causes the arrest of mammalian tissue culture cells in early G_1 (for review, see Pardee 1989). The organismal correlate is nutrient starvation in *Drosophila*, which leads to cell cycle arrest of larval neuroblasts (Britton and Edgar 1998) and slowing of division in somatic SCs of the germ line (D. Drummond-Barbosa and A. Spradling, unpubl.). Nutrient-mediated arrest of larval neuroblasts occurs upstream and independent of *trol/ana* developmental regulation and late G_1 events (see above), consistent with an early G_1 arrest. Cell culture experiments have shown that starvation-arrested neuroblasts can be activated by coculture with fat body (Britton and Edgar 1998), possibly by fat-body-derived growth factors that affect proliferation of imaginal disc cells (Kawamura et al. 1999). However, the signaling mechanism and cell cycle machinery targeted by nutritional arrest are not yet known.

As described above, in response to DNA damage, a checkpoint control can delay cell cycle progression in G_1 or G_2, followed by either DNA repair or apoptosis. In mice, overexpression of the *BCL2* gene can prevent apoptosis in HSC populations following irradiation or treatment with DNA-damaging agents (Domen et al. 1998). It is widely accepted that apoptosis offers a level of protection to the organism in providing a mechanism to remove unwanted damaged cells from circulation. It will be interesting to see how HSC development is affected by defects in the apoptosis or checkpoint pathways.

STEM CELLS AND CELL CYCLE CONTROL

With a few notable exceptions, our understanding of the mechanisms governing cell cycle regulation in SCs and the effect of mitotic control on SC development and biology currently centers on cues such as cytokine/growth factor-triggered signal transduction pathways and asymmetric distribution of intrinsic cell fate determinants. For the most part, the fascinating questions of how phenomena translate into distinct molecular signals and how those signals mesh with the intricacies of cell cycle phase and specific components of the cell cycle machinery have yet to be answered.

ACKNOWLEDGMENTS

The authors thank Ted Weinert, John Diffley, Fulvia Verde, Jerry Spangrude, Craig Peterson, Prasanta Datta, and Milton Datta for helpful discussions. We also thank Minx Fuller, Amy Kiger, Allan Spradling, Daniela Drummond-Barbosa, and Youngji Park for sharing unpublished data. S.D. is supported by National Institutes of Health grant R01-NS-36737. G.D. is supported by ACS RPG-00-262-01-GMC.

REFERENCES

Alexandru G., Zachariae W., Schleiffer A., and Nasmyth K. 1999. Sister chromatid separation and chromosome re-duplication are regulated by different mechanisms in response to spindle damage. *EMBO J.* **18:** 2707–2721.

Amon A. 1999. The spindle checkpoint. *Curr. Opin. Genet. Dev.* **9:** 69–75.

Ashcroft M., Taya Y., and Vousden K.H. 2000. Stress signals utilize multiple pathways to stabilize p53. *Mol. Cell. Biol.* **20:** 3224–3233.

Aza-Blanc P. and Kornberg T. 1999. Ci: A complex transducer of the hedgehog signal. *Trends Genet.* **15:** 458–462.

Bardwell L., Cook J.G., Chang E.C., Cairns B.R., and Thorner J. 1996. Signaling in the yeast pheromone response pathway: Specific and high-affinity interaction of the mitogen-activated protein (MAP) kinases Kss1 and Fus3 with the upstream MAP kinase kinase Ste7. *Mol. Cell. Biol.* **16:** 3637–3650.

Basu J., Bousbaa H., Logarinho E., Li Z., Williams B.C., Lopes C., Sunkel C.E., and Goldberg M.L. 1999. Mutations in the essential spindle checkpoint gene bub1 cause chromosome missegregation and fail to block apoptosis in *Drosophila*. *J. Cell Biol.* **146:** 13–28.

Basu J., Logarinho E., Herrmann S., Bousbaa H., Li Z., Chan G.K., Yen T.J., Sunkel C.E., and Goldberg M.L. 1998. Localization of the *Drosophila* checkpoint control protein Bub3 to the kinetochore requires Bub1 but not Zw10 or Rod. *Chromosoma* **107:** 376–385.

Bentley N.J. and Carr A.M. 1997. DNA structure-dependent checkpoints in model systems. *Biol. Chem.* **378:** 1267–1274.

Bernard P., Hardwick K., and Javerzat J.P. 1998. Fission yeast bub1 is a mitotic centromere protein essential for the spindle checkpoint and the preservation of correct ploidy through mitosis. *J. Cell Biol.* **143:** 1775–1787.

Blalock W., Weinstein-Oppenheimer C., Chang F., Hoyle P., Wang X., Algate P., Franklin R., Oberhaus S., Steelman L., and McCubrey J. 1999. Signal transduction, cell cycle regulatory, and anti-apoptotic pathways regulated by IL-3 in hematopoietic cells: Possible sites for intervention with anti-neoplastic drugs. *Leukemia* **13:** 1109–1166.

Boddy M.N., Furnari B., Mondesert O., and Russell P. 1998. Replication checkpoint enforced by kinases Cds1 and Chk1. *Science* **280:** 909–912.

Britton J.S. and Edgar B.A. 1998. Environmental control of the cell cycle in *Drosophila*: Nutrition activates mitotic and endoreplicative cells by distinct mechanisms. *Development* **125:** 2149–2158.

Brondello J.M., Boddy M.N., Furnari B., and Russell P. 1999. Basis for the checkpoint signal specificity that regulates Chk1 and Cds1 protein kinases. *Mol. Cell. Biol.* **19:** 4262–4269.

Brugarolas J., Chandrasekaran C., Gordon J.I., Beach D., Jacks T., and Hannon G.J. 1995. Radiation-induced cell cycle arrest compromised by p21 deficiency. *Nature* **377:** 552–557.

Buckbinder L., Talbott R., Velasco-Miguel S., Takenaka I., Faha B., Seizinger B.R., and Kley N. 1995. Induction of the growth inhibitor IGF-binding protein 3 by p53. *Nature* **377:** 646–649.

Burke D.J. 2000. Complexity of the spindle checkpoint. *Curr. Opin. Genet. Dev.* **10:** 26–31.

Caldwell M. and Datta S. 1998. Expression of *cyclin E* or *DP/E2F* rescues the G_1 arrest of *trol* mutant neuroblasts in the *Drosophila* larval central nervous system. *Mech. Dev.* **79:** 121–130.

Champlin D.T. and Truman J.W. 1998. Ecdysteroid control of cell proliferation during optic lobe neurogenesis in the moth *Manduca sexta*. *Development* **125:** 269–277.

Chaturvedi P., Eng W.K., Zhu Y., Mattern M.R., Mishra R., Hurle M.R., Zhang X., Annan R.S., Lu Q., Faucette L.F., Scott G.F., Li X., Carr S.A., Johnson R.K., Winkler J.D., and Zhou B.B. 1999. Mammalian Chk2 is a downstream effector of the ATM-dependent DNA damage checkpoint pathway. *Oncogene* **18:** 4047–4054.

Chehab N.H., Malikazy A., Appel M., and Halazonetis T.D. 2000. Chk2/hCds1 functions as a DNA damage checkpoint in G(1) by stabilizing p53. *Genes Dev.* **14:** 278–288.

Chen R.H., Waters J.C., Salmon E.D., and Murray A.W. 1996. Association of spindle assembly checkpoint component XMAD2 with unattached kinetochores. *Science* **274:** 242–246.

Chen X., Bargonetti J., and Prives C. 1995. p53, through p21 (WAF1/CIP1), induces cyclin D1 synthesis. *Cancer Res.* **55:** 4257–4263.

Chenn A. and McConnell S. 1995. Cleavage orientation and the asymmetric inheritance of Notch1 immunoreactivity in mammalian neurogenesis. *Cell* **82:** 631–641.

Cheshier S., Morrison S., Liao X., and Weissman I. 1999. In vivo proliferation and cell cycle kinetics of long-term self-renewing hematopoietic stem cells. *Proc. Natl. Acad. Sci.* **96:** 3120–3125.

Ciosk R., Zachariae W., Michaelis C., Shevchenko A., Mann M., and Nasmyth K. 1998. An ESP1/PDS1 complex regulates loss of sister chromatid cohesion at the metaphase to anaphase transition in yeast. *Cell* **93:** 1067–1076.

Cohen-Fix O., Peters J.M., Kirschner M.W., and Koshland D. 1996. Anaphase initiation in *Saccharomyces cerevisiae* is controlled by the APC-dependent degradation of the anaphase inhibitor Pds1p. *Genes Dev.* **10:** 3081–3093.

Cooper J.A. 1994. MAP kinase pathways. Straight and narrow or tortuous and intersecting? *Curr. Biol.* **4:** 1118–1121.

Cosma M., Tanaka T., and Nasmyth K. 1999. Ordered recruitment of transcription and chromatin remodeling factors to a cell cycle- and developmentally regulated promoter. *Cell* **97:** 299–311.

Cox D., Chao A., and Lin H. 2000. *piwi* encodes a nucleoplasmic factor whose activity modulates the number and division rate of germline stem cells. *Development* **127:** 503–514.

Cox L.S. and Lane D.P. 1995. Tumour suppressors, kinases and clamps: How p53 regulates the cell cycle in response to DNA damage. *BioEssays* **17:** 501–508.

Cui X. and Doe C.Q. 1995. The role of the cell cycle and cytokinesis in regulating neuroblast sublineage gene expression in the *Drosophila* CNS. *Development* **121:** 3233–3243.

Datta S. 1995. Control of proliferation activation in quiescent neuroblasts of the *Drosophila* central nervous system. *Development* **121:** 1173–1182.

———. 1999. Activation of neuroblast proliferation in explant culture of the *Drosophila* larval CNS. *Brain Res.* **818:** 77–83.

Deng C., Zhang P., Harper J.W., Elledge S.J., and Leder P. 1995. Mice lacking p21CIP1/WAF1 undergo normal development, but are defective in G1 checkpoint control. *Cell* **82:** 675–684.

de Nooij J.C., Letendre M.A., and Hariharan I.K. 1996. A cyclin-dependent kinase inhibitor, *Dacapo*, is necessary for timely exit from the cell cycle during *Drosophila* embryogenesis. *Cell* **87:** 1237–1247.

Dierick H. and Bejsovec A. 1999. Cellular mechanisms of wingless/Wnt signal transduction. *Curr. Top. Dev. Biol.* **43:** 153–190.

Domen J., Gandy K., and Weissman I. 1998. Systemic overexpression of BCL-2 in the hematopoietic system protects transgenic mice from the consequences of lethal irradiation. *Blood* **91:** 2272–2282.

Dowell S.J., Romanowski P., and Diffley J.F. 1994. Interaction of Dbf4, the Cdc7 protein kinase regulatory subunit, with yeast replication origins in vivo. *Science* **265:** 1243–1246.

Dunphy W.G. and Kumagai A. 1991. The cdc25 protein contains an intrinsic phosphatase activity. *Cell* **67:** 189–194.

Ebens A.J., Garren H., Cheyette B.N.R., and Zipursky S.L. 1993. The *Drosophila anachronism* locus: A glycoprotein secreted by glia inhibits neuroblast proliferation. *Cell* **74:** 15–28.

el-Deiry W., Tokino T., Velculescu V.E., Levy D.B., Parsons R., Trent J.M., Lin D., Mercer W.E., Kinzler K.W., and Vogelstein B. 1993. WAF1, a potential mediator of p53 tumor suppression. *Cell* **75:** 817–825.

Elledge S.J. 1996. Cell cycle checkpoints: Preventing an identity crisis. *Science* **274:** 1664–1672.

Enoch T. and Norbury C. 1995. Cellular responses to DNA damage: Cell-cycle checkpoints, apoptosis and the roles of p53 and ATM. *Trends Biochem. Sci.* **20:** 426–430.

Evan G. and Littlewood T. 1998. A matter of life and cell death. *Science* **281:** 1317–1322.

Fesquet D., Labbe J., Devancourt J., Capony J., Galas S., Girand F., Lorca T., Shuttleworth J., and Doree M. 1993. The MO15 gene encodes the catalytic subunit of a protein kinase that activates cdc2 and other cyclin-dependent kinases (CDKs) through phosphorylation of T161 and its homologues. *EMBO J.* **12:** 3111–3121.

Fiscella M., Zhang H., Fan S., Sakaguchi K., Shen S., Mercer W.E., Vande Woude G.F., O'Connor P.M., and Apella E. 1997. Wip1, a novel human protein phosphatase that is induced in response to ionizing radiation in a p53-dependent manner. *Proc. Natl. Acad. Sci.* **94:** 6048–6053.

Fisher R.P. and Morgan D.O. 1994. A novel cyclin associates with MO15/CDK7 to form the CDK-activating kinase. *Cell* **78:** 713–724.

Fleming W.H., Alpern E.J., Uchida N., Ikuta K., Spangrude G.J., and Weissman I.L. 1993. Functional heterogeneity is associated with the cell cycle status of murine hematopoietic stem cells. *J. Cell Biol.* **122:** 897–902.

Flores-Rozas H., Kelman Z., Dean F.B., Pan Z.Q., Harper J.W., Elledge S.J., O'Donnell M., and Hurwitz J. 1994. Cdk-interacting protein cip1 directly binds with proliferating cell nuclear antigen and inhibits DNA replication catalysed by the DNA polymerase delta holoenzyme. *Proc. Natl. Acad. Sci.* **91:** 8655–8659.

Fogarty P., Campbell S.D., Abu-Shumaya R., Phalle B.S., Yu K.R., Uy G.L., Goldberg M.L., and Sullivan W. 1997. The *Drosophila grapes* gene is related to checkpoint gene chk1/rad27 and is required for late syncytial division fidelity. *Curr. Biol.* **7:** 418–426.

Fuerstenberg S., Broadus J., and Doe C. 1998. Asymmetry and cell fate in the *Drosophila* embryonic CNS. *Int. J. Dev. Biol.* **42:** 379–383.

Furnari B., Blasina A., Boddy M.N., McGowan C.H., and Russell P. 1999. Cdc25 inhibited in vivo and in vitro by checkpoint kinases Cds1 and Chk1. *Mol. Biol. Cell* **10:** 833–845.

Gardner R., Putnam C.W., and Weinert T. 1999. RAD53, DUN1 and PDS1 define two parallel G2/M checkpoint pathways in budding yeast. *EMBO J.* **18:** 3173–3185.

Gautier J., Solomon M.J., Booher R.N., Bazan J.F., and Kirschner M.W. 1991. cdc25 is a specific tyrosine phosphatase that directly activates p34^{cdc2}. *Cell* **67:** 197–211.

Ghiani C., Eisen A., Yuan X., DePinho R., McBain C., and Gallo V. 1999. Neuro-transmitter receptor activation triggers p27(Kip1)and p21(CIP1) accumulation and G1 cell cycle arrest in oligodendrocyte progenitors. *Development* **126:** 1077–1090.

Gu Y., Rosenblatt J., and Morgan D.O. 1992. Cell cycle regulation of cdk2 activity by phosphorylation of Thr160 and Tyr15. *EMBO J.* **11:** 3995–4005.

Guacci V., Koshland D., and Strunnikov A. 1997. A direct link between sister chromatid cohesion and chromosome condensation revealed through the analysis of MCD1 in *S. cerevisiae*. *Cell* **91:** 47–57.

Hackel P., Zwick E., Prenzel N., and Ullrich A. 1999. Epidermal growth factor receptors: Critical mediators of multiple receptor pathways. *Curr. Opin. Cell Biol.* **11:** 184–189.

Hardwick K.G. 1998. The spindle checkpoint. *Trends Genet.* **14:** 1–4.

Hardy C.F., Dryga O., Seematter S., Pahl P.M., and Sclafani R.A. 1997. mcm5/cdc46-bob1 bypasses the requirement for the S phase activator Cdc7p. *Proc. Natl. Acad. Sci.* **94:** 3151–3155.

Harper J.W., Adami G.R., Wei N., Keyomarsi K. and Elledge S.J. 1993. The p21 cdk-interacting protein cip1 is a potent inhibitor of G1 cyclin-dependent kinases. *Cell* **75:** 805–816.

Hartwell L. and Weinert T. 1989. Checkpoints: Controls that ensure the order of cell cycle events. *Science* **246:** 629–634.

He X., Patterson T.E., and Sazer S. 1997. The *Schizosaccharomyces pombe* spindle checkpoint protein mad2p blocks anaphase and genetically interacts with the anaphase-promoting complex. *Proc. Natl. Acad. Sci.* **94:** 7965–7970.

He X., Jones M.H., Winey M., and Sazer S. 1998. Mph1, a member of the Mps1-like family of dual specificity protein kinases, is required for the spindle checkpoint in *S. pombe*. *J. Cell Sci.* **111:** 1635–1647.

Heim M. 1999. The Jak-STAT pathway: Cytokine signalling from the receptor to the nucleus. *J. Recept. Signal Transduct. Res.* **19:** 75–120.

Hofbauer A. and Campos-Ortega J.A. 1990. Proliferation pattern and early differentiation of the optic lobes in *Drosophila melanogaster*. *Roux's Arch. Dev. Biol.* **198:** 264–274.

Hoyt M.A., Totis L., and Roberts B.T. 1991. *S. cerevisiae* genes required for cell cycle arrest in response to loss of microtubule function. *Cell* **66:** 507–517.

Huff R., Furst A., and Mahowald A. 1989. *Drosophila* embryonic neuroblasts in culture: Autonomous differentiation of specific neurotransmitters. *Dev. Biol.* **134:** 146–157.

Hunt T., Luca F.C., and Ruderman J.V. 1992. The requirements for protein synthesis and degradation, and the control of destruction of cyclins A and B in the meiotic and mitotic cell cycles of the clam embryo. *J. Cell Biol.* **116:** 707–724.

Hunter T. and Pines J. 1994. Cyclins and cancer II: CyclinD and CDK inhibitors come of age. *Cell* **79:** 573–582.

Imai Y. and Yamamoto M. 1994. The fission yeast mating pheromone P-factor: Its molecular structure, gene structure, and ability to induce gene expression and G1 arrest in the mating partner. *Genes Dev.* **8:** 328–338.

Jan Y. and Jan L. 1998. Asymmetric cell division. *Nature* **392:** 775–778.

Jaspersen S.L., Charles J.F., and Morgan D.O. 1999. Inhibitory phosphorylation of the APC regulator Hct1 is controlled by the kinase Cdc28 and the phosphatase Cdc14. *Curr. Biol.* **9:** 227–236.

Jiang W., McDonald D., Hope T.J., and Hunter T. 1999. Mammalian Cdc7-Dbf4 protein kinase complex is essential for initiation of DNA replication. *EMBO J.* **18:** 5703–5713.

Jin D.Y., Kozak C.A., Pangilinan F., Spencer F., Green E.D., and Jeang K.T. 1999. Mitotic checkpoint locus MAD1L1 maps to human chromosome 7p22 and mouse chromosome 5. *Genomics* **55:** 363–364.

Kastan M.B., Zhan Q., and el-Diery W.S. 1992. A mammalian cell cycle checkpoint pathway utilizing *p53* and GADD45 is defective in ataxia-telangiectasia. *Cell* **71:** 587–597.

Kastan M.B., Onyekwere O., Sidransky D., Vogelstein B., and Craig R.W. 1991. Participation of *p53* protein in the cellular response to DNA damage. *Cancer Res.* **51:** 6304–6311.

Kawamura K., Shibata T., Saget O., Peel D., and Bryant P.J. 1999. A new family of growth factors produced by the fat body and active on *Drosophila* imaginal disc cells. *Development* **126:** 211–219.

Kempermann G., Brandon E., and Gage F. 1998. Environmental stimulation of 129/SvJ mice causes increased cell proliferation and neurogenesis in the adult dentate gyrus. *Curr. Biol.* **8:** 939–942.

Kempermann G., Kuhn H., and Gage F. 1997. Genetic influence on neurogenesis in the dentate gyrus of adult mice. *Proc. Natl. Acad. Sci.* **94:** 10409–10414.

King F. and Lin H. 1999. Somatic signaling mediated by *fs(1)Yb* is essential for germline stem cell maintenance during *Drosophila* oogenesis. *Development* **126:** 1833–1844.

Kitagawa R. and Rose A.M. 1999. Components of the spindle-assembly checkpoint are essential in *Caenorhabditis elegans*. *Nat. Cell Biol.* **1:** 514–521.

Klein S., Reuveni H., and Leitzki A. 2000. Signal transduction by a nondissociable heterotrimeric yeast G protein. *Proc. Natl. Acad. Sci.* **97:** 3219–3223.

Ko L.J. and Prives C. 1996. p53: Puzzle and paradigm. *Genes Dev.* **10:** 1054–1072.

Korsmeyer S.J. 1995. Regulators of cell death. *Trends Genet.* **11:** 101–105.

Krebs J.E., Kuo M.H., Allis C.D., and Peterson C.L. 1999. Cell cycle-regulated histone acetylation required for expression of the yeast HO gene. *Genes Dev.* **13:** 1412–1421.

Kronstad J., DeMaria A.D., Funnell D., Laidlaw R.D., Lee N., de Sa M.M., and Ramesh M. 1998. Signaling via cAMP in fungi: Interconnections with mitogen-activated protein kinase pathways. *Arch. Microbiol.* **170:** 395–404.

Kuerbitz S.J., Plunkett B.S., Walsh W.V., and Kastan M.B. 1992. Wildtype *p53* is a cell cycle checkpoint determinant following irradiation. *Proc. Natl. Acad. Sci.* **89:** 3988–3992.

Lane D. 1992. Cancer. p53, guardian of the genome. *Nature* **358:** 15–16.

———. 1993. Cancer. A death in the life of p53. *Nature* **362:** 786–787.

Lane M.E., Sauer K., Wallace K., Jan Y.N., Lehner C.F., and Vaessin H. 1996. *Dacapo*, a cyclin-dependent kinase inhibitor, stops cell proliferation during *Drosophila* development. *Cell* **87:** 1225–1236.

Lei M., Kawasaki Y., Young M.R., Kihara M., Sugino A., and Tye B.K. 1997. Mcm 2 is a target of regulation by Cdc7-dbf4 during the initiation of DNA synthesis. *Genes Dev.* **11:** 3365–3374.

Li L. and Vaessin H. 2000. Pan-neural Prospero terminates cell proliferation during *Drosophila* neurogenesis. *Genes Dev.* **14:** 147–151.

Li R. and Murray A.W. 1991. Feedback control of mitosis in budding yeast. *Cell* **66:** 519–531.

Li Y. and Benezra R. 1996. Identification of a human mitotic checkpoint gene: hsMAD2. *Science* **274:** 246–248.

Losada A., Hirano M., and Hirano T. 1998. Identification of *Xenopus* SMC protein complexes required for sister chromatid cohesion. *Genes Dev.* **12:** 1986–1997.

Luo Y., Hurwitz J., and Massague J. 1995. Cell-cycle inhibition by independent CDK and PCNA binding domains in p21cip1. *Nature* **375:** 159–161.

Makela T.P., Tassan J.P., Nigg E., Frutiger S., Hughes G.J., and Weinberg R.A. 1994. A cyclin associated with the CDK-activating kinase MO15. *Nature* **371:** 254–257.

Marshall C.J. 1994. MAP kinase kinase kinase, MAP kinase kinase and MAP kinase. *Curr. Opin. Genet. Dev.* **4:** 82–89.

Matsuoka S., Huang M., and Elledge S.J. 1998. Linkage of ATM to cell cycle regulation by the Chk2 protein kinase. *Science* **282:** 1893–1897.

McConnell S. and Kaznowski C. 1991. Cell cycle dependence of laminar determination in developing neocortex. *Science* **254:** 282–285.

Meyn M.S., Strasfeld L., and Allen C. 1994. Testing the role of p53 in the expression of genetic instability and apoptosis in ataxia-telangiectasia *Int. J. Radiat. Biol.* (suppl.) **44:** 141–149.

Michaelis C., Ciosk R., and Nasmyth K. 1997. Cohesins: Chromosomal proteins that prevent premature separation of sister chromatids. *Cell* **91:** 35–45.

Miyashita T. and Reed J.C. 1995. Tumor suppressor p53 is a direct transcriptional activator of the human bax gene. *Cell* **80:** 293–299.

Mochizuki N. and Yamamoto M. 1992. Reduction in the intracellular cAMP level triggers initiation of sexual development in fission yeast. *Mol. Gen. Genet.* **233:** 17–24.

Moghal N. and Sternberg P. 1999. Multiple positive and negative regulators of signaling by the EGF-receptor. *Curr. Opin. Cell Biol.* **11:** 190–196.

Morgan D.O. 1995. Principles of CDK regulation. *Nature* **374:** 131–134.

Morshead C.M., Reynolds B.A., Craig C.G., McBurney M.W., Staines W.A., Morassutti D., Weiss S., and van der Kooey D. 1994. Neural stem cells in the adult mammalian forebrain: A relatively quiescent subpopulation of subependymal cells. *Neuron* **13:** 1071–1082.

Murakami H. and Okayama H. 1995. A kinase from fission yeast responsible for blocking mitosis in S phase. *Nature* **374:** 817–819.

Murray A. 1994. Cell cycle checkpoints. *Curr. Opin. Cell Biol.* **6:** 872–876.

Nie Y., Li H.H., Bula C.M., and Liu X. 2000. Stimulation of p53 DNA binding by c-Abl requires the p53 C-terminus and tetramerization. *Mol. Cell. Biol.* **20:** 741–748.

Noda A., Ning Y., Venable S.F., Pereira-Smith O.M., and Smith J.R. 1994. Cloning of senescent cell-derived inhibitors of DNA synthesis using an expression screen. *Exp. Cell Res.* **211:** 90–98.

Nurse P. 1990. Universal control mechanism regulating onset of M-phase. *Nature* **344:** 503–508.

————. 1994. Ordering S phase and M phase in the cell cycle. *Cell* **79:** 547–550.

O'Connor P.M., Jackman J., Jondle D., Bhatia K., Magrath I., and Kohn K.W. 1993. Role of the *p53* tumor suppressor gene in cell cycle arrest and radiosensitivity of Burkitt's lymphoma cell lines. *Cancer Res.* **53:** 4776–4780.

Oostendorp R., Audet J., and Eaves C. 2000. High-resolution tracking of cell division suggests similar cell cycle kinetics of hematopoietic stem cells stimulated in vitro and in vivo. *Blood* **95:** 855–862.

Owens J.C., Detweiler C.S., and Li J.J. 1997. CDC45 is required in conjunction with CDC7/DBF4 to trigger the initiation of DNA replication. *Proc. Natl. Acad. Sci.* **94:** 12521–12526.

Owen-Schaub L.B., Zhang W., Cusack J.C., Angelo L.S., Santee S.M., Fujiwara T., Roth J.A., Deisseroth, A.B., Zhang W.W., and Kruzel E. 1995. Wild-type human p53 and a temperature-sensitive mutant induce Fas/APO-1 expression. *Mol. Cell. Biol.* **15:** 3032–3040.

Pagano M., Theodoras A.M., Tam S.W., and Draetta G.F. 1994. Cyclin D1-mediated inhibition of repair and replicative DNA synthesis in human fibroblasts. *Genes Dev.* **8:** 1627–1639.

Painter R.B. and Young B.R. 1987. DNA synthesis in irradiated mammalian cells. *J. Cell Sci. Suppl.* **6:** 207–214.

Pangilinan F., Li Q., Weaver T., Lewis B.C., Dang C.V., and Spencer F. (1997). Mammalian BUB1 protein kinases: Map positions and in vivo expression. *Genomics* **46:** 379–388.

Pardee A.B. 1989. G1 events and regulation of cell proliferation. *Science* **246:** 603–608.

Park Y., Fujioka M., Jaynes J., and Datta S. 1998. The *Drosophila* homeobox gene *eve* enhances *trol*, an activator of neuroblast proliferation in the larval CNS. *Dev. Genet.* **23:** 247–257.

Pasero P., Duncker B.P., Schwob E., and Gasser S.M. 1999. A role for the Cdc7 kinase regulatory subunit Dbf4p in the formation of initiation-competent origins of replication. *Genes Dev.* **13:** 2159–2176.

Paulovich A.G. and Hartwell L.H. 1995. A checkpoint regulates the rate of progression through S phase in *S. cerevisiae* in response to DNA damage. *Cell* **82:** 841–847.

Paulovich A.G., Margulies R.U., Garvik B.M., and Hartwell L.H. 1997. RAD9, RAD17, and RAD24 are required for S phase regulation in *Saccharomyces cerevisiae* in response to DNA damage. *Genetics* **145:** 45–62.

Poon R.Y.C., Yamashita K., Adamczewski J.P., Hunt T., and Shuttleworth J. 1993. The cdc2-related protein p40^{MO15} is the catalytic subunit of a protein kinase that can activate p33^{cdk2} and p34^{cdc2}. *EMBO J.* **12:** 3123–3132.

Prelich G., Kostura M., Marshak D.R., Mathews M.B., and Stillman B. 1987a. The cell-cycle regulated proliferating cell nuclear antigen is required for SV40-DNA replication *in vitro*. *Nature* **326:** 471–475.

Prelich G., Tan C.K., Kostura M., Mathews M.B., So A.G., Downey K.M., and Stillman B. 1987b. Functional identity of proliferating cell nuclear antigen and a DNA polymerase-delta auxiliary protein. *Nature* **326:** 517–520.

Prokop A. and Technau G.M. 1991. The origin of postembryonic neuroblasts in the ventral nerve chord of *Drosophila melanogaster*. *Development* **111:** 79–88.

Raleigh J.M. and O'Connell M.J. 2000. The G(2) DNA damage checkpoint targets both Wee1 and Cdc25. *J. Cell Sci.* **113:** 1727–1736.

Reddy G.P., Tiarks C.Y., Pang L., Wuu J., Hsieh C.C., and Quesenberry P.J. 1997. Cell cycle analysis and synchronization of pluripotent hematopoietic progenitor stem cells. *Blood* **90**: 2293–2299.

Russo G.L., Vandenberg M.T., Yu I.T., Bae Y.S., Franza, Jr., B.R., and Marshak D.K. 1992. Casein kinase II phosphorylates p34cdc2 kinase in G1 phase of the HeLa cell division cycle. *J. Biol. Chem.* **267**: 20317–20325.

Sanchez Y., Bachant J., Wang H., Hu F., Liu D., Tetzlaff M., and Elledge S.J. 1999. Control of the DNA damage checkpoint by chk1 and rad53 protein kinases through distinct mechanisms. *Science* **286**: 1166–1171.

Sanchez Y., Wong C., Thoma R.S., Richman R., Wu Z., Piwnica-Worms H., and Elledge S.J. 1997. Conservation of the Chk1 checkpoint pathway in mammals: Linkage of DNA damage to Cdk regulation through Cdc25. *Science* **277**: 1497–1501.

Santocanale C. and Diffley J.F. 1998. A Mec1- and Rad53-dependent checkpoint controls late-firing origins of DNA replication. *Nature* **395**: 615–618.

Savatier P., Lapillonne H., van Grunsven L.A., Rudkin B.B., and Samarut J. 1995. Withdrawal of differentiation inhibitory activity/leukemia inhibitory factor up-regulates D-type cyclins and cyclin-dependent kinase inhibitors in mouse embryonic stem cells. *Oncogene* **12**: 309–322.

Sebastian B., Kakizuka A., and Hunter T. 1993. Cdc25 activation of cyclin-dependent kinases by dephosphorylation of threonine-14 and tyrosine-15. *Proc. Natl. Acad. Sci.* **90**: 3521–3524.

Sherr C.J. 1993. Mammalian G1 cyclins. *Cell* **73**: 1059–1065.

———. 1994. G1 phase progression: Cycling on cue. *Cell* **79**: 551–555.

Sherr C.J. and Roberts J.M. 1995. Inhibitors of mammalian G1 cyclin-dependent kinases. *Genes Dev.* **9**: 1149–1163.

Shieh S.Y., Ahn J., Tamai K., Taya Y., and Prives C. 2000. The human homologs of checkpoint kinases Chk1 and Cds1 (Chk2) phosphorylate p53 at multiple DNA damage-inducible sites. *Genes Dev.* **14**: 289–300.

Shirahige K., Hori Y., Shiraishi K., Yamashita M., Takahashi K., Obuse C., Tsurimoto T., and Yoshikawa H. 1998. Regulation of DNA-replication origins during cell-cycle progression. *Nature* **395**: 618–621.

Shivji K.K., Kenny M.K., and Wood R.D. 1992. Proliferating cell nuclear antigen is required for DNA excision repair. *Cell* **59**: 367–374.

Shou W., Seol J.H., Shevchenko A., Baskerville C., Moazed D., Chen Z.W., Jang J., Shevchenko A., Charbonneau H., and Deshaies R.J. 1999. Exit from mitosis is triggered by Tem1-dependent release of the protein phosphatase Cdc14 from nucleolar RENT complex. *Cell* **97**: 233–244.

Sibon O.C., Stevenson V.A., and Theurkauf W.E. 1997. DNA-replication checkpoint control at the *Drosophila* midblastula transition. *Nature* **388**: 93–97.

Sibon O.C., Laurencon A., Hawley R., and Theurkauf W.E. 1999. The *Drosophila* ATM homologue Mei-41 has an essential checkpoint function at the midblastula transition. *Curr. Biol.* **9**. 302–312.

Sidorova J.M. and Breeden L.L. 1997. Rad53-dependent phosphorylation of Swi6 and down-regulation of CLN1 and CLN2 transcription occur in response to DNA damage in *Saccharomyces cerevisiae*. *Genes Dev.* **11**: 3032–3045.

Siede W. and Friedberg E.C. 1990. Influence of DNA repair deficiencies on the UV sensitivity of yeast cells in different cell cycle stages. *Mutat. Res.* **245**: 287–292.

Solomon M.J., Wade-Harper J., and Shuttleworth J. 1993. CAK, the p34^{cdc2} activating kinase, contains a protein identical or closely related to p40^{MO15}. *EMBO J.* **12**: 3133–3142.

Su T.T., Walker J., and Stumpff J. 2000. Activating the DNA damage checkpoint in a developmental context. *Curr. Biol.* **10:** 119–126.

Szebenyi G. and Fallon J. 1999. Fibroblast growth factors as multifunctional signaling factors. *Int. Rev. Cytol.* **185:** 45–106.

Tan P. and Kim S. 1999. Signaling specificity: The RTK/RAS/MAP kinase pathway in metazoans. *Trends Genet.* **15:** 145–149.

Tassan J.P., Jaquenoud M., Léopold P., Schultz S.J., and Nigg E.A. 1995. Identification of human cyclin-dependent kinase 8, a putative protein kinase partner for cyclin C. *Proc. Natl. Acad. Sci.* **92:** 8871–8875.

Taylor S.S. and McKeon F. 1997. Kinetochore localization of murine Bub1 is required for normal mitotic timing and checkpoint response to spindle damage. *Cell* **89:** 727–735.

Taylor S.S., Ha E., and McKeon F. 1998. The human homologue of Bub3 is required for kinetochore localization of Bub1 and a Mad3/Bub1-related protein kinase. *J. Cell Biol.* **142:** 1–11.

Truman J.W. and Bate M. 1988. Spatial and temporal patterns of neurogenesis in the central nervous system of *Drosophila melanogaster*. *Dev. Biol.* **125:** 145–157.

Uhlmann F., Lottspeich F., and Nasmyth K. 1999. Sister-chromatid separation at anaphase onset is promoted by cleavage of the cohesin subunit Scc1. *Nature* **400:** 37–42.

van Praag H., Christie B., Sejnowski T., and Gage F. 1999. Running enhances neurogenesis, learning, and long-term potentiation in mice. *Proc. Natl. Acad. Sci.* **96:** 13427–13431.

Visintin R., Hwang E.S., and Amon A. 1999. Cfi1 prevents premature exit from mitosis by anchoring Cdc14 phosphatase in the nucleolus. *Nature* **398:** 818–823.

Visintin R., Craig K., Hwang E.S., Prinz S., Tyers M., and Amon A. 1998. The phosphatase Cdc14 triggers mitotic exit by reversal of Cdk-dependent phosphorylation. *Mol. Cell* **2:** 709–718.

Waga S., Hannon G.J., Beach D., and Stillman B. 1994. The p21 inhibitor of cyclin-dependent kinases controls DNA replication by interaction with PCNA. *Nature* **369:** 574–578.

Walworth N., Davey S., and Beach D. 1993. Fission yeast *chk1* protein kinase links the rad checkpoint pathway to *cdc2*. *Nature* **363:** 368–371.

Weinert T. 1998. DNA damage and checkpoint pathways: Molecular anatomy and interactions with repair. *Cell* **94:** 555–558.

Weinert T. and Hartwell L. 1988. The RAD9 gene controls the cell cycle response to DNA damage in *Saccharomyces cerevisiae*. *Science* **241:** 317–322.

Weinreich M. and Stillman B. 1999. Cdc7p-Dbf4p kinase binds to chromatin during S phase and is regulated by both the APC and the RAD53 checkpoint pathway. *EMBO J.* **18:** 5334–5346.

Weiss E. and Winey M. 1996. The *Saccharomyces cerevisiae* spindle pole body duplication gene MPS1 is part of a mitotic checkpoint. *J. Cell Biol.* **132:** 111–123.

Weiss S., Dunne C., Hewson J., Wohl C., Wheatley M., Peterson A., and Reynolds B. 1996. Multipotent CNS stem cells are present in the adult mammalian spinal cord and ventricular neuroaxis. *J. Neurosci.* **16:** 7599–7609.

Westphal C.H. 1997. Cell-cycle signaling: Atm displays its many talents. *Curr. Biol.* **7:** 789–792.

White K. and Kankel D.R. 1978. Patterns of cell division and cell movement in the formation of the imaginal nervous system in *Drosophila melanogaster*. *Dev. Biol.* **65:** 296–321.

Xie T. and Spradling A. 1998. decapentaplegic is essential for the maintenance and division of germline stem cells in the *Drosophila* ovary. *Cell* **94:** 251–260.

Xiong Y., Hannon G.J., Zhang H., Casso D., Kobayashi R., and Beach D. 1993. p21 is a universal inhibitor of cyclin kinases. *Nature* **366:** 701–704.

Yamamoto A., Guacci V., and Koshland D. 1996. Pds1p, an inhibitor of anaphase in budding yeast, plays a critical role in the APC and checkpoint pathway(s). *J. Cell Biol.* **133:** 99–110.

Yamamoto M. 1996. Regulation of meiosis in fission yeast. *Cell Struct. Funct.* **21:** 431–436.

Yanagida M. 2000. Cell cycle mechanisms of sister chromatid separation: Roles of Cut1/separin and Cut2/securin. *Genes Cells* **5:** 1–18.

Yuan Z.-M., Huang Y., and Whang Y.E.A. 1996. Role for c-Abl tyrosine kinase in growth arrest response to DNA damage. *Nature* **382:** 272–274.

Zachariae W. and Nasmyth K. 1999. Whose end is destruction: Cell division and the anaphase-promoting complex. *Genes Dev.* **13:** 2039–2058.

Zandstra P., Conneally E., Petzer A., Piret J., and Eaves C. 1997. Cytokine manipulation of primitive human hematopoietic cell self-renewal. *Proc. Natl. Acad. Sci.* **94:** 4698–4703.

Zeng Y., Forbes K.C., Wu Z., Moreno S., Piwnica-Worms H., and Enoch T. 1998. Replication checkpoint requires phosphorylation of the phosphatase Cdc25 by Cds1 or Chk1. *Nature* **395:** 507–510.

Zhan Q., Chen I.T., Antinore M.J., and Fornace A.J.J. 1998. Tumor suppressor p53 can participate in transcriptional induction of the GADD45 promoter in the absence of direct DNA binding. *Mol. Cell. Biol.* **18:** 2768–2778.

Zhang Y. and Derynck R. 1999. Regulation of Smad signalling by protein associations and signalling crosstalk. *Trends Cell Biol.* **9:** 274–279.

Zhou Z., Gartner A., Cade R., Ammerer G., and Errede B. 1993. Pheromone-induced kinases. *Mol. Cell. Biol.* **13:** 2069–2080.

5

Senescence of Dividing Somatic Cells

Robin Holliday
CSIRO Molecular Science
North Ryde
Sydney, Australia

GENERAL FEATURES OF SENESCENCE

The senescence of normal diploid cells was first revealed in detailed studies of cultured human fibroblasts (Hayflick and Moorhead 1961; Hayflick 1965). Fibroblasts are connective tissue cells that have a characteristic morphology and synthesize collagen. After a long period of normal growth, the yield of cells per flask began to decrease, and finally reached a very low level, with no further proliferation. These investigators referred to the establishment of a primary culture of normal cells as Phase I, the long period of normal growth as Phase II, and the senescent period as Phase III. Previously, it had been generally assumed that cultured mammalian cells grew indefinitely, but this was based on the growth of neoplastic or transformed cells, and such cell populations are generally known as permanent lines. Saksela and Moorhead (1963) were the first to show that human fibroblasts retain a diploid karyotype during the long period of normal growth, but chromosome abnormalities appear with increasing frequency as cells enter senescence.

There is some controversy about the relationship between senescence, aging, and cell death. If the cells are cultured to a stage where they remain subconfluent, abnormalities in cell morphology are clearly visible. The cells vary in size and shape; the cytoplasm is granular, with many cell inclusions; and debris is formed in the medium. Some of the cells detach to form debris, whereas others remain attached to the substrate. At an earlier stage when the cells still become confluent, these abnormalities are less apparent. However, the cells do not form the "whorls" of growth that are characteristic of younger cultures, and the monolayer of cells is distinctly grainy in appearance. With regular changes of medium, these confluent cells remain attached to the substrate for long periods and continue metabolism (Smith and Lincoln 1984) with occasional cell division

(Matsumura et al. 1979). Innumerable studies of cellular senescence have depended on the use of such cell populations, in comparison to early-passage cells. These studies have documented a large number of changes in physiological, biochemical, or molecular parameters that occur during the aging of human fibroblasts (Holliday 1995). Hayflick lists 167 parameters that have been examined; of these, 117 change during senescence (Hayflick 1980). More recently, a single "biomarker" of aging has been extensively used. This is the formation of β galactosidase (Dimri et al. 1995), but the reason for its appearance is not known; nor is it clear why this particular biomarker is usually preferred to many others that are available. The actual age of a culture is normally recorded in population doublings (PDs), and, typically, human fibroblasts reach 50–70 PDs. In some studies, PDs are broadly equivalent to passages, provided a 1:4 split is recorded as two passages and a 1:8 split as three. However, in many studies, passages are simply the number of subcultures, and they may not correspond at all to PDs.

Following the demonstration of the limited growth potential of human fibroblasts, the same or similar limited life span has been demonstrated in many other cultured somatic cells. These studies are listed in Table 1. With the exception of T lymphocytes, the cells listed typically have a shorter in vitro life span than fibroblasts. Studies of other species also demonstrate the limited growth potential of normal diploid cells (Röhme 1981), and there is a rather clear relationship between the longevity of the donor species and the growth potential of its fibroblasts in culture. From all these studies, the strong conclusion can be drawn that specialized dividing cells eventually become senescent and cease growth in culture.

Table 1 Studies demonstrating the limited growth potential in culture of human or bovine cell types, other than fibroblasts

Cell type	Reference
Glial cells	Ponten and McIntyre (1968)
Smooth muscle cells	Bierman (1978)
Endothelial cells	Mueller et al. (1980)
Thyrocytes	Davies et al. (1985)
Bronchial epithelial cells	Lechner et al. (1981)
Keratinocytes	Rockwell et al. (1987)
Lymphocytes	McCarron et al. (1987)
Breast epithelial cells	Stampfer (1985)
Osteoblasts	Kassem et al. (1997)
Adrenocortical cells[a]	Hornsby et al. (1979)

[a] Bovine cells; all others are human.

Whereas human cells do not transform to permanent cell lines (with the exception of lymphoblastoid cells from lymphocytes previously infected with Epstein-Barr virus), cells from short-lived animals, such as rodents, do commonly give rise to permanent lines with abnormal karyotypes.

VARIABILITY IN GROWTH POTENTIAL OF HUMAN FIBROBLASTS

Human fibroblasts are usually stored at early passage in liquid nitrogen. It is evident that cultures obtained from different ampoules of the same cell strain have very different life spans in PDs. The ranges for the well-known strains WI-38 and MRC-5 are 38–60 PDs and 55–75 PDs, respectively (Holliday et al. 1977). It should be noted that a difference of 10 PDs represents a thousandfold difference in cell mass (if all the cells were grown to senescence), so the range demonstrated is a very substantial variability in growth potential. The studies of clones of cells also demonstrate a very substantial variability in growth potential, and even the daughters of individual cells have different longevities (Smith and Whitney 1978; Smith et al. 1978). It is evident that stochastic events have an important role in determining the life span of somatic cells. The variability in the growth potential of populations and clones of cells can complicate the interpretation of experiments designed to uncover possible causes of senescence.

THEORIES OF CELLULAR SENESCENCE

The key feature of the senescence of dividing cells is the fact that a long period of normal growth is followed by cessation of growth. Therefore, events must be occurring and accumulating through a life span that culminate in senescence. This immediately gives rise to the concept of a molecular clock. At present, most attention has been directed to the loss of telomeric DNA. In the absence of the enzyme telomerase, telomeres gradually get shorter as cell division proceeds, and shortening of telomeres throughout the life span is well documented (Harley et al. 1990; Alsopp et al. 1992; Alsopp and Harley 1995). The consequence may be the inactivation of genes closest to the telomere sequences, either directly, or indirectly by a position effect, perhaps involving the formation of heterochromatin. This would happen at the ends of all 46 chromosomes. Since the lengths of telomeric DNAs could vary, as well as could the loss of the number of DNA base pairs per cell division, this interpretation of cell senescence could probably accommodate the observed variability in life spans. A prediction of the theory is that the introduction of DNA coding for telomerase should immortalize the cell population. This prediction has been verified (Bodnar et al. 1998; Vaziri and Benchimol 1998), although a number of questions about the generality of the loss-of-telomerase theory of cellular senescence remain unanswered and are discussed below.

A second general type of theory proposes that during the normal cell division in Phase II, molecular defects gradually accumulate. This is most easy to envisage at the DNA level, but it is also possible that defects could occur in proteins, membranes, or organelles, provided that their natural dilution by growth and cell division is not sufficient to produce a steady-state level of defects. This theory, in its most general form, is broadly supported by the finding that a large number of genetic, biochemical, or physiological parameters are affected during aging (Hayflick 1980; Holliday 1995). With time, some indispensable cellular component or function may fail, but a more attractive possibility is that a given level of defects triggers a checkpoint control mechanism. This could block DNA synthesis or introduce some irreversible inhibition of cell division. This was first suggested by Rosenberger et al. (1991), and in the last few years has been confirmed by the discovery of checkpoint controls. Thus, there are many studies of genes and proteins involved in one way or another in the regulation of the cell cycle in senescent cells, including the tumor suppressor genes, p53, Rb, and p16, and the p21 cell cycle regulator gene (for review, see Wynford-Thomas 1997, 1999; Reddel 1998). It is generally agreed that senescent cells are irreversibly blocked in cell division, but they are still capable of many other cell functions. According to the telomere theory of cellular senescence, the shortening of chromosome ends would itself trigger a cell cycle block.

The commitment theory of cellular aging dealt with the population dynamics of senescence and did not depend on any specific molecular mechanism (Holliday et al. 1977). It proposed that in the founder population of human fibroblasts there are cells that have unlimited division potential; that is, they are potentially immortal. These cells give rise during division, at probability P, to cells that become committed to eventual senescence after M cell divisions. Provided P is sufficiently high (in the range 0.25–0.275) and M sufficiently long, the immortal cells are gradually lost during routine subculture. The final loss of all uncommitted or immortal cells is a stochastic process, which determines the final life span of the whole culture. The model predicts that the population size, N, is an important parameter and, in particular, that an extremely large population (unfortunately too large to handle in a laboratory) would grow indefinitely. It also predicts that reducing population size at critical times during the life span would have significant life-shortening effects, and this was confirmed by experiment (Holliday et al. 1977, 1981). The commitment the-ory also receives support from the study of immunoglobulin molecules in populations of T lymphocytes. As the cells approach the end of their life span, the population can often be shown to be clonal, suggesting that all these cells are derived from the last remaining uncommitted cell, many cell generations earlier (McCarron et al. 1987). It should be noted that the conversion of uncommitted or immortal cells, at rate P, to committed mor-tal cells could be due to the loss of telomerase activity.

SENESCENCE OF SOMATIC CELLS IN VIVO

There is indirect evidence that somatic cells in their normal environment use up some of their proliferative potential, although they may not actual-ly reach the senescent state. It was shown that the growth potential of human fibroblasts was inversely related to donor age (Martin et al. 1970; Smith et al. 1978), although a contrary result has recently appeared (Cristofalo et al. 1998). The results of Martin et al. (1970) suggested that the cells, on average, underwent 0.2 PDs per year of chronological life. Moreover, cells from the premature aging syndrome, Werner's syndrome, have a very short in vitro life span. The gene has now been cloned and been shown to belong to a family of DNA helicases (Gray et al. 1997). The most clear-cut evidence that cell life span is inversely related to donor age comes from studies of Syrian hamster dermal fibroblasts (Bruce et al. 1986). Fetal cells, at 13 days gestation, grew for 30 PDs, whereas cells for a 24-month adult grew for only 9 PDs. Those from a 3-day-old animal had a life span of 19 PDs, and those from a 6-month young adult, 14 PDs. These results strongly suggest that dermal fibroblasts continually turn over in vivo, and that cells from old animals have "used up" most of their growth potential. Tissue transplantation experiments also indicate that in vivo aging is a reality. For example, mouse mammary tissue can be trans-planted between isogenic animals but eventually becomes senescent and is unable to proliferate further (Daniel et al. 1968; Daniel and Young 1971).

It is widely believed that somatic stem cells have unlimited growth potential. Although this may be so, it is hard to prove experimentally. The population of stem cells may be structured in such a way that a relatively small pool of cells can give rise to a very large number of descendants. Alternatively, there could be a pool of potentially immortal cells that give rise to stem cells with finite growth. Telomerase is present in hematopoi-etic stem cells, suggesting they are immortal, but a discussion of the growth potential of the various components of this stem cell system is outside the scope of this review. Many aspects are discussed elsewhere in this volume (see especially Chapter 6).

ENVIRONMENTAL INFLUENCES ON POPULATION LIFE SPANS

In addition to the intrinsic variability of culture life spans, there are also well-documented examples of an induced decrease or increase in longevity of human fibroblasts. In one of the earliest experiments, the incubation temperature was varied (Thompson and Holliday 1973). Interestingly, a reduction of the normal temperature of 37°C to 34°C had no effect on growth potential. However, an increase to 40°C appeared to have a severe life-shortening effect, which could not be reversed by returning the cultures to 37°C. The antibiotic paramycin reduces the fidelity of ribosomal translation in eukaryotes. At concentrations that did not affect growth rate, the life span of human fibroblasts was significantly reduced, provided treatment was continuous (Holliday and Rattan 1984). A more dramatic result was obtained with the pyrimidine analogs 5-aza-cytidine (5-aza-C) or 5-aza-deoxycytidine (5-aza-dC). These are both incorporated into DNA and are known to inhibit DNA methyl transferase activity (Santi et al. 1984; Jones 1985). It is well known that a single treatment with either analog will significantly reduce the total level of 5-methyl-cytosine in the genome. It is also well established that the level of DNA methylation declines during serial passaging (Wilson and Jones 1983; Fairweather et al. 1987; Matsumura et al. 1989a). The striking result is that a single treatment of 5-aza-C or 5-aza-dC to young cells, followed by full growth recovery, produces a population of cells with a greatly reduced life span in comparison to untreated controls (Holliday 1986; Fairweather et al. 1987). The significance of this result is that the single treatment is "remembered" by the cells, and the final effect is seen only many generations later. The results suggest that artificially reducing the level of 5-methyl-cytosine in DNA, followed by further natural decline, leads to the critical level seen in senescent cells. This in turn suggests that the gradually decreasing level of DNA methylation may be an important molecular clock in its own right, which induces senescence. Other studies with primary mouse, hamster, and human fibroblasts support this view. Wilson and Jones (1983) found that mouse primary cells lose DNA methylation at a very high rate, and they have a short life span. Syrian hamster cells lose DNA methylation at a rate intermediate between mouse and human, and their life span is intermediate as well. In the same and other studies (Matsumura et al. 1989a), it was shown that two permanent lines maintain DNA methylation at a constant level, which is what one might expect. Additionally, when 5-aza-C was used to repeatedly drive down the level of DNA methylation in the mouse permanent line, C3H 10T1/2, it was found that it could not be reduced to zero (0.45% was the lowest achieved), so presumably some DNA methylation is essential for viability of these cells (Flatau et al. 1984).

Many years ago, it was discovered that hydrocortisone significantly increases the growth potential of normal human fibroblasts, but the mechanism remains unknown (Cristofalo and Kabakjian 1975; Macieira-Coelho 1996). More recently, it was found that physiological concentrations of the natural dipeptide L-carnosine (β-alanyl-L-histidine) also increases culture life span (McFarland and Holliday 1994, 1999). Moreover, when division finally ceases, the cells have a normal rather than a senescent morphology. Switching senescent cells to a high concentration of carnosine produces a rejuvenated phenotype, and removal of the dipeptide causes the cells to revert to senescence. Again, the specific mechanism of action of carnosine is not known, but it has been suggested that it may have an important role in cell maintenance in vivo (Holliday and McFarland 2000).

SOME PROBLEMS WITH THE TELOMERE THEORY OF SENESCENCE

Comparative studies strongly indicate that somatic cells from different species have a limited life span in culture, and it is reasonable to suppose that all these cells have the same or similar mechanism of senescence. It is therefore a surprise to find that Syrian hamster cells, which have very clear-cut senescence, have long telomeres, an active telomerase, and maintain their telomere lengths (Carman et al. 1998; Russo et al. 1998). Furthermore, mouse cells also have very long telomeres (Kipling and Cooke 1990), and yet they only divide about 10 times before becoming senescent (Todaro and Green 1963; Wilson and Jones 1983).

The fact that environmental treatments can significantly increase or reduce culture life span suggests that telomeres can be lost at different rates under different conditions. This need not be a serious problem for the theory, but a study of the effect of increased oxygen is harder to explain. It was found that cells incubated in 40% oxygen soon stopped growing and, at the same time, had shortened telomeric DNA. This shows that telomeric DNA can be lost without cell division, perhaps by the introduction of single-strand breaks in DNA (von Zglinicki et al. 1995; von Zglinicki 1998).

DNA methylation poses another problem. What happens in diploid cells immortalized by the introduction of telomerase activity? Presumably, the DNA methylation does not decline to zero, so one must suppose that the DNA methylation is stabilized at a constant level. If this is so, it implies that DNA methylation is in some way coupled to telomere maintenance. In normal cells, both DNA methylation and telomere length decline in concert. When normal human fibroblasts are infected by SV40, the large-T antigen transforms these cells so that they lose contact inhibition and have an abnormal karyotype and an extended life span. These cells eventually enter a nonproliferative phase known as crisis. SV40-infected cells maintain their DNA methylation level (Matsumura et al. 1989b), but they do not maintain their telomeres, which continue to shorten until crisis is reached (Counter et al. 1992). It is well established that crisis occurs later than senescence and is distinct from it (Reddel 1998; Wei and Sedivy 1999). Immortalized cells that emerge from crisis either have telomerase or maintain telomeres by another mechanism known as alternative lengthening of telomeres (ALT) (Bryan et al. 1995). These observations suggest that it may be the loss of telomeres that precipitates crisis, and this is later than the senescence of normal cells. The interesting observation is that senescent cells have telomere lengths which are significantly longer than those of cells entering crisis. Perhaps, then, it is the loss of DNA methylation that precipitates senescence, as outlined in Figure 1. How then should one explain the results of Bodnar et al. (1998) and Vaziri and Benchimol (1998), namely, that normal cells are immortalized by telomerase? One could conclude they are in a steady state both with regard to telomere length and DNA methylation and, furthermore, that telomerase in some way restores maintenance of DNA methylation. However, the reverse could not be true, at least in pre-crisis cells, because they maintain DNA methylation but continue to lose telomeric DNA.

IS CELL SENESCENCE A BARRIER TO THE EMERGENCE OF MALIGNANT TUMOR CELLS IN VIVO?

Tumor cell lines are immortal, so it has often been asserted that the senescence of normal diploid cells is a barrier, or defense mechanism, to the emergence of neoplastic cells. In other words, overcoming this barrier is an essential step in tumor progression. This hypothesis is not as simple and straightforward as it may seem. It is probably rare for somatic cells to reach senescence in vivo. Skin fibroblasts from 90-year-old individuals are capable of 20–40 PDs in vitro (Martin et al. 1970), and much the same residual growth is probably true for other types of dividing cells. Therefore, the initiation of early steps in carcinogenesis is occurring in cells with considerable remaining growth potential. Let us assume that

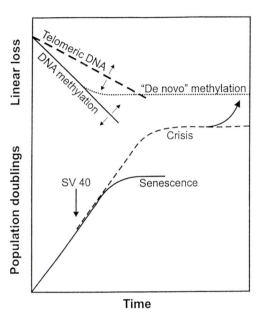

Figure 1 During serial passaging of human diploid fibroblasts, telomeric DNA and DNA methylation are lost linearly with time. Senescence of these cells can be bypassed by SV40 infection and the expression of large-T antigen. These cells are capable of de novo methylation. They enter crisis at a higher population doubling level than senescence. Immortalization is a rare event (*large arrow on right*) and depends on the acquisition of telomerase, or an alternative mechanism for lengthening telomeric DNA. The small arrows at the top indicate that certain environmental treatments could alter the rate of loss of telomeric DNA or DNA methylation (see text for references).

these cells proliferate with a transformed, or perhaps partially transformed, phenotype. It is probable that they already have abnormal karyotypes and may also be mutator strains (Loeb 1991). Thus, while growing, these cells are generating considerable genetic diversity, and it is generally agreed that cell selection is very important during tumor progression. This leads to the formation of a primary tumor (note that a tumor of 1 gm contains about 10^9 cells, after about 30 PDs from a single cell). These cells would not be expected to enter senescence, in the normal sense, but they may enter the period of growth arrest known as crisis. In transformation experiments in vitro, crisis is demonstrably different from senescence. For example, cells in crisis have a high mitotic index, and the cells regularly detach from the substrate (Wei and Sedivy 1999). Nevertheless, it is quite possible that crisis is due to the loss of telomeric

DNA, and the emergence of permanent lines depends on the acquisition of the means to maintain telomeres. With regard to primary tumors in vivo, it is well known that tissue biopsies from them rarely give rise to permanent cell lines. However, by the time secondary tumors have appeared, it is somewhat easier to obtain such cell lines. Thus, this scenario suggests that many small primary tumors consist of transformed pre-crisis cells. This crisis could be a barrier to the emergence of metastatic malignant cells, but it is not clear that senescence, in the normal sense, is involved. Primary tumors in many, but not all, cases can give rise to immortalized cells, following rare mutations or epigenetic events. These cells are fully transformed and malignant.

It should be noted that cultured human diploid cells do not spontaneously give rise to transformed pre-crisis cells. They are very resistant to transformation, irrespective of senescence. It is possible to regard the senescence that is regularly seen in vitro as simply a result of imperfect cell maintenance. It benefits the organism to down-regulate or turn off maintenance mechanisms that are not required during the lifetime of the individual. Thus, many human somatic cells no longer synthesize telomerase if their telomeres are long enough for many sequential divisions. They also presumably reduce DNA methyl transferase activity, which results in a continual decline in total DNA methylation. They may turn off other activities, such as DNA repair mechanisms, which may be only fully maintained in germ-line cells. It is now well recognized that the efficiency of cell maintenance mechanisms is related to the longevity of mammalian species, and the resources invested must be at some optimum value for each species (Holliday 1995). It is also well known that the incidence of tumorigenesis per cell in short-lived animals such as rodents is enormously higher than in humans, and also that rodent cells spontaneously transform in vitro (for review, see Holliday 1996). The rare emergence of human tumors may have nothing to do with cell senescence, but may instead be related to an intrinsic resistance to transformation.

CONCLUSIONS

Specialized mammalian cells that are capable of division normally have a finite life span in vitro, and there is evidence that the extent of proliferation is related to the longevity of the donor species. Cells from long-lived species do not become transformed in vitro, but instead enter an irreversible nonproliferative state known as senescence. Senescence of human cells can be bypassed if certain tumor suppressor genes are inactivated, or if appropriate oncogenes are present (for review, see Reddel

1998; Wynford-Thomas 1999). These cells characteristically proliferate to a higher PD level than senescence and then enter a period of growth arrest known as crisis. The emergence of immortalized transformed cell lines depends on the ability to maintain telomeres either by telomerase activity or by an alternative mechanism known as ALT (Bryan et al. 1995). It is reported that the introduction into normal cells of a gene coding for the catalytic subunit of telomerase known as hTERT results in a greatly extended life span (Bodnar et al. 1998; Vaziri and Benchimol 1998). These cells have reached at least 400 PDs and can be regarded as immortal (W.E. Wright, pers. comm.). However, there is no published information about their karyotypes, cell morphology, or other phenotypic characteristics, such as contact inhibition. It is possible that events other than the acquisition of telomerase are necessary to establish immortalization. This is known to be the case in immortalized keratinocytes, where loss of the Rb/p16^{INK4a} cell cycle control mechanism is also necessary (Kiyono et al. 1998; Dickson et al. 2000; Chapter 4).

Normal human diploid fibroblasts have at least two molecular clocks, and possibly there are others (Reddel 1998). The loss of telomeric DNA has received the most attention, but it is also well established that total DNA methylation steadily declines during the serial passaging of human fibroblasts. In contrast, immortalized cells maintain both telomeres and DNA methylation. Therefore, if maintenance of telomeres is the essential event, it must also be linked to maintenance of DNA methylation. Little is known about the regulatory mechanism that silences the gene(s) for telomerases in many normal somatic cells, or about the events that have activated it in many immortalized cells. Similarly, nothing is known about the control or maintenance of total DNA methylation.

Normal Syrian hamster fibroblasts have a very clear-cut senescence in vitro, from which transformed lines emerge rather rarely. These cells have telomerase activity and maintain their telomeres (Carman et al. 1998; Russo et al. 1998). In contrast, they steadily lose DNA methylation during serial subculture (Wilson and Jones 1983). This suggests that the molecular clock for senescence may be loss of DNA methylation. In addition, it is known that artificially reducing the level of DNA methylation in young human fibroblasts significantly reduces their final life span. These results indicate that senescence may be triggered by the loss of methylation. Oncogenes, or the loss of tumor suppressors, can lead to the bypass of senescence, and de novo methylation to maintain a constant level (Matsumura et al. 1989b). These cells continue to lose telomeric DNA (Counter et al. 1992), and it may well be that this precipitates crisis, at a greater PD level than senescence, as shown in Figure 1. Many more studies are necessary to unravel the respective roles of different molecular clocks for senescence, or to discover whether an accumulation of cellular defects is responsible. Whatever precipitates senescence, it is widely agreed that this is related to an interference with normal cell cycle controls that results in an irreversible block in cell division.

ACKNOWLEDGMENTS

I thank Roger Reddel and Lily Huschtscha for helpful comments, and Jenny Young for preparing the manuscript.

REFERENCES

Allsopp R.C. and Harley C.B. 1995. Evidence for a critical telomere length in senescent human fibroblasts. *Exp. Cell Res.* **219:** 130–136.

Allsopp R.C., Vaziri H., Patterson C., Goldstein S., Younglai E.V., Futcher A.B., Greider C.W., and Harley C.B. 1992. Telomere length predicts replicative capacity of human fibroblasts. *Proc. Natl. Acad. Sci.* **89:** 10114–10118.

Bierman E.L. 1978. The effect of donor age on the in vitro life span of cultured human arterial smooth-muscle cells. *In Vitro* **14:** 951–955.

Bodnar A.G., Ouellette M., Frolkis M., Holt S.E., Chiu C.-P., Morin G.B., Harley C.B., Shay J.W., Lichtsteiner S., and Wright W.E. 1998. Extension of life-span by introduction of telomerase into normal human cells. *Science* **279:** 349–352.

Bruce S.A., Deamond S.F., and Ts'o P.O. 1986. In vitro senescence of Syrian hamster mesenchymal cells of fetal to aged adult origin. Inverse relationship between in vivo donor age and in vitro proliferative capacity. *Mech. Ageing Dev.* **34:** 151–173.

Bryan T.M., Englezou A., Gupta J., Bacchetti S., and Reddel R.R. 1995. Telomere elongation in immortal human cells without detectable telomerase activity. *EMBO J.* **14:** 4240–4248.

Carman T.A., Afshari C.A., and Barrett J.C. 1998. Cellular senescence in telomerase-expressing Syrian hamster embryo cells. *Exp. Cell Res.* **244:** 33–42.

Counter C.M., Avilion A.A., LeFeuvre C.E., Stewart N.G., Greider C.W., Harley C.B., and Bacchetti S. 1992. Telomere shortening associated with chromosome instability is arrested in immortal cells which express telomerase activity. *EMBO J.* **11:** 1921–1929.

Cristofalo V.J. and Kabakjian J. 1975. Lysosomal enzymes and aging in vitro: Subcellular enzyme distribution and effect of hydrocortisone on cell life-span. *Mech. Ageing Dev.* **4:** 19–28.

Cristofalo V.J., Allen R.G., Pignolo R.J., Martin B.G., and Beck J.C. 1998. Relationship between donor age and the replicative lifespan of human cells in culture: A reevaluation. *Proc. Natl. Acad. Sci.* **95:** 10614–10619.

Daniel C.W. and Young L.J. 1971. Influence of cell division on an aging process. Life span of mouse mammary epithelium during serial propagation in vivo. *Exp. Cell Res.* **65:** 27–32.

Daniel C.W., De Ome K.B., Young J.T., Blair P.B., and Faulkin Jr., L.J. 1968. The in vivo life span of normal and preneoplastic mouse mammary glands: A serial transplantation study. *Proc. Natl. Acad. Sci.* **61:** 53–60.

Davies T.F., Platzer M., Schwartz A.E., and Friedman E.W. 1985. Short- and long-term evaluation of normal and abnormal human thyroid cells in monolayer culture. *Clin. Endocrinol.* **23:** 469–479.

Dickson M.A., Hahn W.C., Ino Y., Ronfard V., Wu J.Y., Weinberg R.A., Louis D.N., Li F.P., and Rheinwald J.G. 2000. Human keratinocytes that express hTERT and also bypass a p16^{INK4a}-enforced mechanism that limits life span become immortal yet retain normal growth and differentiation characteristics. *Mol. Cell. Biol.* **20:** 1436–1447.

Dimri G.P., Lee X.H., Basile G., Acosta M., Scott C., Roskelley C., Medrano E.E., Linskens M., Rubelj I., Pereira-Smith O., Peacocke M., and Campisi J. 1995. A biomarker that identifies senescent human cells in culture and in aging skin in vivo. *Proc. Natl. Acad. Sci.* **92:** 9363–9367.

Fairweather D.S., Fox M., and Margison G.P. 1987. The in vitro lifespan of MRC-5 cells is shortened by 5-azacytidine-induced demethylation. *Exp. Cell Res.* **168:** 153–159.

Flatau E., Gonzales F.A., Michalowsky L.A., and Jones P.A. 1984. DNA methylation in 5-aza-2′-deoxycytidine-resistant variants of C3H 10T1/2 C18 cells. *Mol. Cell. Biol.* **4:** 2098–2102.

Gray M.D., Shen J.-C., Kamath-Loeb A.S., Blank A., Sopher B.L., Martin G.M., Oshima J., and Loeb L.A. 1997. The Werner syndrome protein is a DNA helicase. *Nat. Genet.* **17:** 100–103.

Harley C.B., Futcher A.B., and Greider C.W. 1990. Telomeres shorten during ageing of human fibroblasts. *Nature* **345:** 458–460.

Hayflick L. 1965. The limited *in vitro* lifetime of human diploid cell strains. *Exp. Cell Res.* **37:** 614–636.

———. 1980. Cell aging. *Annu. Rev. Gerontol. Geriatr.* **1:** 26–67.

Hayflick L. and Moorhead P.S. 1961. The serial cultivation of human diploid cell strains. *Exp. Cell Res.* **25:** 585–621.

Holliday R. 1986. Strong effects of 5-azacytidine on the in vitro lifespan of human diploid fibroblasts. *Exp. Cell Res.* **166:** 543–552.

———. 1995. *Understanding ageing.* Cambridge University Press, Cambridge, United Kingdom.

———. 1996. Neoplastic transformation: The contrasting stability of human and mouse cells. *Cancer Surv.* **28:** 103–115.

Holliday R. and McFarland G.R. 2000. A role for carnosine in cellular maintenance. *Biochemistry (Moscow)* **65:** 991–996.

Holliday R. and Rattan S.I.S. 1984. Evidence that paromomycin induces premature aging in human fibroblasts. *Monogr. Dev. Biol.* **17:** 221–233.

Holliday R., Huschtscha L.I., and Kirkwood T.B.L. 1981. Further evidence for the commitment theory of cellular ageing. *Science* **213:** 1505–1508.

Holliday R., Huschtscha L.I., Tarrant G.L., and Kirkwood T.B.L. 1977. Testing the commitment theory of cellular ageing. *Science* **198:** 366–372.

Hornsby P.J., Simonian M.H., and Gill G.N. 1979. Aging of adrenocortical cells in culture. *Int. Rev. Cytol.* (suppl.), pp. 131–162.

Jones P.A. 1985. Altering gene expression with 5-azacytidine. *Cell* **40:** 485–486.

Kassem M., Ankersen L., Eriksen E.F., Clark B.F., and Rattan S.I. 1997. Demonstration of cellular aging and senescence in serially passaged long-term cultures of human trabecular osteoblasts. *Osteoporos. Int.* **7:** 514–524.

Kipling D. and Cooke H.J. 1990. Hypervariable ultra-long telomeres in mice. *Nature* **347:** 400–402.

Kiyono T., Foster S.A., Koop J.I., McDougall J.K., Galloway D.A., and Klingelhutz A.J. 1998. Both Rb/p16^{INK4a} inactivation and telomerase activity are required to immortalize human epithelial cells. *Nature* **396:** 84–88.

Lechner J.F., Haugen A., Autrup H., McClendon I.A., Trump B.F., and Harris C.C. 1981. Clonal growth of epithelial cells from normal adult human bronchus. *Cancer Res.* **41:** 2294–2304.

Loeb L.A. 1991. Mutator phenotype may be required for multistage carcinogenesis. *Cancer Res.* **51:** 3075–3079.

Macieira-Coelho A. 1966. Action of cortisone on human fibroblasts in vitro. *Experientia* **22:** 390–391.

Martin G.M., Sprague C.A., and Epstein C.J. 1970. Replicative life-span of cultivated human cells. Effect of donor's age, tissue, and genotype. *Lab. Invest.* **23:** 86–92.

Matsumura T., Malik F., and Holliday R. 1989a. Levels of DNA methylation in diploid and SV40 transformed human fibroblasts. *Exp. Gerontol.* **24:** 477–481.

Matsumura T., Zerrudo Z., and Hayflick L. 1979. Senescent human diploid cells in culture: Survival, DNA synthesis and morphology. *J. Gerontol.* **34:** 328–334.

Matsumura T., Hunter J.L., Malik F., and Holliday R. 1989b. Maintenance of DNA methylation level in SV40-infected human fibroblasts during their in vitro limited proliferative life span. *Exp. Cell Res.* **184:** 148–157.

McCarron M., Osborne Y., Story C.J., Dempsey J.L., Turner D.R., and Morley A.A. 1987. Effect of age on lymphocyte proliferation. *Mech. Ageing Dev.* **41:** 211–218.

McFarland G.A. and Holliday R. 1994. Retardation of the senescence of cultured human diploid fibroblasts by carnosine. *Exp. Cell Res.* **212:** 167–175.

———. 1999. Further evidence for the rejuvenating effects of the dipeptide L-carnosine on cultured human diploid fibroblasts. *Exp. Gerontol.* **34:** 35–45.

Mueller S.N., Rosen E.M., and Levine E.M. 1980. Cellular senescence in a cloned strain of bovine fetal aortic endothelial cells. *Science* **207:** 889–891.

Ponten J. and Macintyre E.H. 1968. Long term culture of normal and neoplastic human glia. *Acta Pathol. Microbiol. Scand.* **74:** 465–486.

Reddel R. 1998. A reassessment of the telomere hypothesis of senescence. *BioEssays* **20:** 977–984.

Rockwell G.A., Johnson G., and Sibatani A. 1987. In vitro senescence of human keratinocyte cultures. *Cell Struct. Funct.* **12:** 539–548.

Röhme D. 1981. Evidence for a relationship between longevity of mammalian species and life spans of normal fibroblasts in vitro and erythrocytes in vivo. *Proc. Natl. Acad. Sci.* **78:** 5009–5013.

Rosenberger R.F., Gounaris E., and Kolettas E. 1991. Mechanisms responsible for the limited lifespan and immortal phenotypes in cultured mammalian cells. *J. Theor. Biol.* **148:** 383–392.

Russo I., Silver A.R.J., Cuthbert A.P., Griffin D.K., Trott D.A., and Newbold R.F. 1998. A telomere-independent senescence mechanism is the sole barrier to Syrian hamster cell immortalization. *Oncogene* **17:** 3417–3426.

Saksela E. and Moorhead P.S. 1963. Aneuploidy in the degenerative phase of serial cultivation of human cell strains. *Proc. Natl. Acad. Sci.* **50:** 390–395.

Santi D.V., Norment A., and Garrett C.E. 1984. Covalent bond formation between a DNA-cytosine methyltransferase and DNA containing 5-azacytosine. *Proc. Natl. Acad. Sci.* **81:** 6993–6997.

Smith J.R. and Lincoln D.W. 1984. Aging of cells in culture. *Int. Rev. Cytol.* **89:** 151–177.

Smith J.R. and Whitney R.G. 1980. Intraclonal variation in proliferative potential of human diploid fibroblasts: Stochastic mechanism for cellular aging. *Science* **207:** 82–84.

Smith J.R., Pereira-Smith O.M., and Schneider E.L. 1978. Colony size distributions as a measure of in vivo and in vitro aging. *Proc. Natl. Acad. Sci.* **75:** 1353–1356.

Stampfer M.R. 1985. Isolation and growth of human mammary epithelial cells. *J. Tissue Cult. Methods* **9:** 107–115.

Thompson K.V. and Holliday R. 1973. Effect of temperature on the longevity of human fibroblasts in culture. *Exp. Cell Res.* **80:** 354–360.

Todaro G.J. and Green H. 1963. Quantitative studies of the growth of mouse embryo cells in culture and their development into established lines. *J. Cell Biol.* **17:** 299–313.

Vaziri H. and Benchimol S. 1998. Reconstitution of telomerase activity in normal human cells leads to elongation of telomeres and extended replicative life span. *Curr. Biol.* **8:** 279–282.

von Zglinicki T. 1998. Telomeres: Influencing the rate of aging. *Ann. N.Y. Acad. Sci.* **854:** 318–327.

von Zglinicki T., Saretzki G., Döcke W., and Lotze C. 1995. Mild hyperoxia shortens telomeres and inhibits proliferation of fibroblasts: A model for senescence? *Exp. Cell Res.* **220:** 186–193.

Wei W. and Sedivy J.M. 1999. Differentiation between senescence (M1) and crisis (M2) in human fibroblast cultures. *Exp. Cell Res.* **253:** 519–522.

Wilson V.L. and Jones P.A. 1983. DNA methylation decreases in aging but not in immortal cells. *Science* **220:** 1055–1057.

Wynford-Thomas D. 1999. Proliferative life span checkpoints: Cell-type specificity and influence on tumour biology. *Eur. J. Cancer* **33A:** 716–726.

———. 1997. Cellular senescence and cancer. *J. Pathol.* **187:** 100–111.

6

Repopulating Patterns of Primitive Hematopoietic Stem Cells

David E. Harrison, Jichun Chen, and Clinton M. Astle

The Jackson Laboratory
Bar Harbor, Maine 04609-1500

SIGNIFICANCE AND CLINICAL RELEVANCE

Primitive hematopoietic stem cells (PHSC) are the self-renewing precursors that regenerate myeloid and lymphoid cells throughout the life span, and they are required for successful long-term bone marrow transplantation. PHSC are found in bone marrow cells (BMC), spleen, blood, and newborn or fetal liver and blood. PHSC will be vital for putative therapeutic measures such as human gene transfer via autologous marrow cell transplantation. PHSC proliferation is required for the long-term success of clinical grafts, yet it cannot be fully defined clinically because 10–20 years may be required to recognize long-term functional cells in human beings. Fortunately, mouse PHSC appear to provide a good model for human PHSC function, and since mice are short-lived, aging about 30 times faster than humans, PHSC function over much of the life span can be studied directly.

Cells, obtained from bone marrow, cord blood, or mobilized peripheral blood of healthy donors, are clinically useful for transplantation (Barnett et al. 1994). After transplantation, donor PHSC compete with residual host PHSC for engraftment; thus, high levels of donor PHSC function are essential since host PHSC remain functional in many clinical conditions. Unfortunately, donor PHSC are often damaged by clinical manipulations, so that they repopulate less well than residual host cells. Often the most primitive cells are the most damaged (Gardner et al. 1997; Miller and Eaves 1997). Competitive repopulation directly models the donor and host stem cell competition for engraftment. One of the most important and demanding problems in hematology is regulating and maximizing the levels of donor PHSC function.

PHSC REPOPULATE, SELF-RENEW, AND FUNCTION LONG TERM

PHSC repopulate both the lymphoid and myeloid systems (Harrison et al. 1989, 1990; Morrison and Weissman 1994; Spangrude et al. 1995). The same PHSC produces erythrocytes, platelets, granulocytes, macrophages, B cells, and T cells proportionally, with high correlations between all these cell types (Harrison and Zhong 1992; Zhong et al. 1996).

Demonstrating both lymphoid and myeloid function is not adequate to identify a cell as a PHSC, since most precursors that repopulate both lymphoid and myeloid lineages soon after transplantation are short-lived (Jordan and Lemischka 1990; Harrison and Zhong 1992; Morrison and Weissman 1994; Spangrude et al. 1995; Zhong et al. 1996). The length of time that such short-term multilineage precursors function appears to be proportional to the life span of the species. Short-term precursors disappear 3–4 months after transplantation in mice, but persist for 1–4 years in cats (Abkowitz et al. 1995). Human short-term multilineage precursors might function for 10–20 years. Thus, long-term functional determination is essential in defining the biology of the PHSC. This makes mouse models more practical than human models for studying PHSC function.

Competitive repopulation assay evaluates primitive PHSC in vivo by testing the defining characteristics of PHSC directly (Harrison 1980). Donor cells must seed/home and then proliferate and differentiate to continuously form both myeloid and lymphoid cells during large portions of the life span. Function is tested relative to normally functional standard competitor cells. Figure 1 illustrates that as donor PHSC numbers increase fourfold, from 2 to 8, with a constant competitor dose of 4, percentages of donor cells only double, from 33% to 66%, if all PHSC repopulate equally. Since use of percentages understates alterations in donor function, we calculate repopulating units (RU), where 1 RU is the repopulating ability of 100,000 standard competitor BMC. Numbers of RU from each donor are calculated from the percentage of donor cells where the number of competitor marrow cells used divided by $10^5 = C$. By definition, $\% = 100 \ (RU \ / \ RU + C)$, so $RU = \% \ (C) \ / \ (100\text{-}\%)$.

PHSC self-renewal is tested most rigorously after long-term serial transplantation. Effects of age on PHSC self-renewal after serial transplantation were shown by the results from competitive repopulation. By measuring retransplanted RUs in carrier BMC, we compare the amount of expansion from PHSC in the original dose of donor marrow cells received by each carrier. Since the same competitor was used with old and young donors of the same strain, the total RU per carrier is directly comparable between each strain's young and old donors.

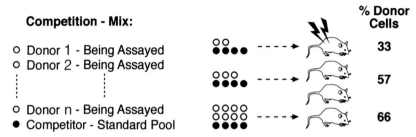

Figure 1 In the competitive repopulation assay, donor cells being tested are mixed with doses of genetically distinguished standard competitor BMC and grafted into irradiated recipients. Thus, each donor is compared to the common standard in identical recipients, whose percentage of donor-type cells measures donor PHSC function relative to the standard. Donor "1" has half the repopulating ability of the standard. Donor "2" has repopulating ability equal to the standard. Donor "n" has twice the repopulating ability of the standard.

Competitive dilution assays use limiting dilution with the addition of a standard dose of competitor marrow. This measures relative repopulating abilities of individual genetically marked PHSC without the stress to the cells of enrichment or to the recipients of inadequate numbers of precursors. Low enough numbers of PHSC and standard competitor cells (0.5×10^5 to 5×10^5) are used so that variance in percentage of repopulation depends on relative repopulating abilities of the individual clones, with numbers of clones distributed according to the Poisson equation.

PHSC concentrations per 10^5 B6 marrow cells measured by two different competitive dilution experiments are 0.7–1.1 and 1.0–1.6 (95% confidence limits) (Zhong et al.1996), which confirm previous results using other models (Harrison et al. 1993). PHSC numbers in BALB are similar to those in B6 and far less than shown by the long-term culture-initiating cell (LTC-IC) assay, with the best estimates for fetal, young, or old cells being 1 PHSC per 100,000 BMC. Unlike B6, BALB relative repopulating abilities change with age; each fetal PHSC repopulates 50–100% better than a young adult PHSC. Old BALB PHSC repopulate about 66% as well as young adult PHSC (Chen et al. 1999).

Szilvassy et al. (1990) reported concentrations more than 10 times as high as we find from limiting dilution studies of PHSC. The conflict probably is due to their practice of using defective competitors. This illustrates the relative nature of cell competition within a mixture and emphasizes the need for normally functional standard competitors.

The competitive repopulation and dilution assays complement each other, as the former measures normally functioning PHSC populations and the latter focuses on behavior of individual clones. Importantly, competitive dilution overcomes the limitation of describing results of competitive repopulation with a binomial model where donor and competitor PHSC must contribute equally (Chen et al. 1999). To calculate expected percentages of donor cells in each recipient in the competitive dilution, a distribution based on a Poisson model is used to estimate contributions from donor PHSC to the differentiated cell populations, while hypothesizing that donor cell contributions can be a multiple of those from competitor cells.

WAYS TO MEASURE HEMATOPOIETIC STEM CELLS

Differences between short-term and long-term multilineage repopulating precursors are deterministic, since they can be separated using cell surface markers (Morrison and Weissman 1994). Spangrude et al. (1988) were the first to use specific cell surface markers to enrich PHSC. By this strategy, PHSC have been enriched very highly, and used in limiting dilution assays (Morrison et al.1995; Spangrude et al. 1995), even engrafting a small proportion of lethally irradiated recipients long term using a single donor cell (Osawa et al. 1996). However, problems with enrichment still exist. It may severely reduce repopulating ability. Some markers are strain-specific, or are effective for fetal but not adult cells (Jordan et al. 1990; Morrison et al. 1995). Most seriously, enrichment markers fail to predict PHSC function, since cells carrying all the markers associated with long-term reconstitution proliferate greatly in vivo (Spangrude et al. 1995) or in vitro (Rebel et al. 1994) without a proportionate increase in PHSC function.

Spleen colonies in vivo or myeloid cell colonies in vitro are measured to test precursor differentiation. Many types of colony-forming cells can be separated from PHSC (Ploemacher and Brons 1989; Jones et al. 1990; Morrison and Weissman 1994; Spangrude et al. 1995), and colony assays often fail to predict PHSC function (Bertoncello et al. 1988; Jones et al. 1989).

LTC-IC populations contain precursors capable of long-term repopulation in vivo, although they may not compete with normal BMC (Cho and Müller-Sieburg 2000). The cobblestone area forming cell (CAFC) assay measures clusters of tightly packed rounded cells on stromal layers evaluated after 3–5 weeks by a limiting dilution assay (Ploemacher et al. 1989). Müller-Sieburg and Riblet (1996) found that long-term CAFC gave results similar to LTC-IC. B6 mice gave the lowest levels of stem cells in marrow, BALB/c were about 5 times higher, and D2 gave the highest levels, 11 times more than B6. However, after serial transplantation, two million BMC from young B6, BALB, or D2 donors expanded to 276, 147, and 98 total RU, respectively (Chen et al. 2000a). Thus, the strain pattern for self-renewal is the opposite of that for LTC-IC. Furthermore, by competitive dilution, PHSC numbers in BALB are similar to those in B6, far less than in the LTC-IC assay, with the best models having 1 PHSC per 100,000 BMC (Chen et al. 1999).

LTC-IC assays may measure an early step in PHSC differentiation. Perhaps B6 cells respond better to stimuli to self-renew, whereas BALB or D2 cells respond better to stimuli to differentiate. This would explain why D2 precursor cells cycle faster than those of B6 (Van Zant et al. 1990), as they are responding better to stimuli to differentiate, giving an initial competitive advantage in allophenic mice. However, B6 cells respond better to stimuli to self-renew, giving them the advantage for long-term maintenance (Chen et al. 2000a).

SUMMARY OF METHODS USED

Mice

To distinguish donor and competitor (or recipient) cell types, we use mice carrying electrophoretically differing hemoglobin (Hbb^s or Hbb^d) and $Gpi1$ isoenzymes ($Gpi1^a$ or $Gpi1^b$), as detailed below. For the competitive repopulation and self-renewal studies from Chen et al. (2000a), young (2–6 months) and old (20–24 months) mice of normal inbred strains—B6 (Hbb^s and $Gpi1^b$), BALB (Hbb^d and $Gpi1^a$), and D2 (Hbb^d and $Gpi1^a$)— were used as donors. We used congenics differing at the Hbb and $Gpi1$ loci as competitors, and young mice of the normal inbred strain were used as recipients. Thus, standard competitors were young congenic B6 (Hbb^d and $Gpi1^a$), BALB (Hbb^s and $Gpi1^b$), and D2 (Hbb^s and $Gpi1^b$), respectively. These congenic inbred mice were produced from single stocks that were each back-crossed for more than 18 generations (Harrison et al. 1993). In all cases, young and old donors were compared with portions from the same pools of standard competitor BMC from young congenics differing from the donors at the Hbb and $Gpi1$ loci.

For the competitive dilution studies from Chen et al. (2000b), recombinant inbred (Bailey 1981; Taylor 1996) mice of the CXB-12 line were used as donors. Hybrid CByB6F1 ($Gpi1^a/Gpi1^b$) were used as recipients, since the hybrid $Gpi1$ band readily identifies recipient cells. Recipients were given sublethal irradiation with 500 rads 14 days before transplantation and intraperitoneally injected with 100 µg/mouse of a natural killer (NK) cell antibody (anti-NK1.1, clone PK 136) 3 days before transplantation to deplete NK cells (NK-cell-depleted recipients). In this study, standard competitors were young CByB6F1 (Hbb^s and $Gpi1^b$) mice, produced by mating congenic BALB (Hbb^s and $Gpi1^b$) with normal B6.

All mice were produced at The Jackson Laboratory where they had free access to an NIH-31 (4% fat) diet and acidified water and were maintained under standard pathogen-free animal husbandry conditions (for details, see JAX Report 1997). Before each experiment, old mice were examined to exclude those with abnormal circulating white blood cell (WBC) concentrations (WBC > 18×10^9/l or > 5×10^9/l), or with grossly visible subcutaneous, intestinal, liver, spleen, lung, lymph node, or thymus tumors.

Competitive Repopulation

BMC were extracted from two femurs and two tibias of each donor or carrier mouse through a 23-gauge needle into 2.0 ml of Iscove's Modified Dulbecco's Medium (IMDM) and filtered through a 100-µm mesh, sterile, nylon cloth to remove debris. Nucleated cells were counted using a model ZBI Coulter Counter (Coulter Electronics, Inc., Hialeah, Florida). BMC from each donor or carrier were mixed with BMC from a competitor pool in a 1:1 (donor:competitor) ratio, and then iv (intravenously) injected into lethally irradiated strain- and gender-matched recipients. Irradiation doses were 11 Gy for B6, 8.5 Gy for BALB, 10 Gy for D2, and were delivered at 1.6 Gy per minute using a Shepard Mark 1 ^{137}Cesium gamma source (J.L. Shepherd and Associates, Glendale, California). Standard competitor BMC were distinguishable from donor BMC by different electrophoretic alleles at the $Gpi1$ and Hbb loci. In each experiment, the original bone marrow donors were defined as old/young pairs at transplantation. The same competitor pool of BMC was used by each donor pair, so repopulating functions of old and young donors were measured relative to the same competitor standard (Harrison et al. 1993). This allows the calculation of an old/young RU ratio for each donor pair, so variances can be demonstrated. In each experiment, with inbred strains, a group of control mice received only competitor BMC and were monitored to ensure that irradiated host PHSC did not produce detectable numbers of circulating erythrocytes and lymphocytes.

Serial Transplantation and Competitive Repopulation

To test PHSC self-renewal by serial transplantation, 2×10^6 BMC from each of the young and old B6, BALB, or D2 donors was injected into separate lethally irradiated, strain- and gender-matched, young carrier mice, using five carriers per donor. After 10 months, BMC were pooled from two healthy carriers of each original donor, mixed with BMC from congenic standard competitors as detailed above, and re-transplanted into lethally irradiated recipients. This was done to measure PHSC proliferation in the carriers by competitive repopulation as detailed in the previous section, except that BMC from each carrier were mixed with BMC from its competitor pool in a 5:1 (carrier:competitor) ratio. Carriers differed from donors at the *Gpi1* and *Hbb* markers, but were matched with the competitors used in the assay stage of the experiment. Thus, any host cell function from the carrier would reduce the number of donor cells measured.

Analyses of Donor Engraftment in Carriers

Recipients were bled at time points specified in each experiment. At each bleeding, three microhematocrit tubes of blood (75 µl/tube) were obtained from each recipient through the orbital sinus and were mixed in 2 ml of IMDM with 3.8% sodium citrate. Each sample was then layered onto 2 ml of lymphocyte separation medium and centrifuged at $500g$ for 50 minutes at room temperature to separate lymphocytes (middle layer) from erythrocytes (sediment at the bottom of the tube). Cell lysates were analyzed by cellulose acetate gel electrophoresis to separate isoforms of *Gpi1* and *Hbb*. Percentages of donor-type lymphocytes were calculated based on the proportion of their *Gpi1* after electrophoretic gel bands were quantitatively analyzed using a Helena Cliniscan 2 densitometer. Percentages of donor-type erythrocytes were calculated from the proportion of donor-type *Hbb* in each sample after electrophoretic separation of the two *Hbb* types. These methods have been detailed previously (Harrison et al. 1993). After each sampling, percentages of donor-type blood cells (mean of donor erythrocytes and lymphocytes) of the four or five recipients for each donor were averaged to calculate RU of donor BMC, using the formula: RU = % donor × C / (100 − % donor). One RU is defined as the repopulating ability of 100,000 standard competitor BMC, where % donor is the mean percentage of donor-type erythrocytes and lymphocytes, and C is the number of repopulating units of competitor BMC, so that for 20×10^5 standard competitor BMC, C = 20. The RU:carrier ratio was calculated assuming that the two femurs and two tibias sampled from each carrier contained 25% of its total marrow cells.

Competitive Dilution Using Poisson Modeling

Portions containing 5×10^4 CXB-12 donor BMC (*Gpi1^a/Gpi1^a*) and 5×10^5 CByB6F1 standard congenic competitor BMC (*Gpi1^b/Gpi1^b*) were injected into each of 38 NK-cell-depleted CByB6F1 ($Gpi1^a/Gpi1^b$) recipients. The Poisson function, $P_i = e^{-N} \times (N^i/i!)$, gives the probability (P_i) that a recipient gets a certain number (i) of PHSC, where N is the average number of PHSC injected to each recipient (Zhong et al. 1996; Chen et al. 1999). The proportion of recipients with 0% CXB-12 type cells 6 months after reconstitution was used to compute the number of PHSC (N) in CXB-12 BMC using the $i = 0$ term of the Poisson function; $P_0 = e^{-N}$ or $N = -\ln P_0$. This gave $N = 1.2$ for 5×10^4 CXB-12 donor BMC. Then the probabilities (P_i) of having 0, 1, 2, 3, or 4 donor PHSC in a recipient were, according to the Poisson function: 0.3012, 0.3614, 0.2169, 0.0867, or 0.0260, respectively. Since 5×10^5 competitor cells were used, $N = 5.0$ for the competitor, giving probabilities of having 0, 1, 2, 3, 4, 5, 6, 7, 8, or 9 competitor PHSC in a recipient as 0.0067, 0.0337, 0.0842, 0.1404, 0.1755, 0.1755, 0.1462, 0.0653, 0.0363, or 0.0181, respectively. In practice, we calculated two arrays of probabilities, one for the donor and one for the competitor, with $i = 0$–15 for 16 probabilities in each case. These form a 16 × 16 matrix of 256 combined probabilities, and each is associated with a donor:competitor PHSC ratio that can be used to predict a value representing donor contribution. In the current study, we used the highest 37 probability values since there were 37 recipients available 6 months after transplantation.

We used the 37 corresponding donor:competitor ratios in the Poisson modeling to estimate repopulating ability per cell for CXB-12 PHSC by comparing three hypothesized levels of repopulating abilities (F) per cell for CXB-12 PHSC: $F = 1$, $F = 1.4$, and $F = 2$, each relative to a repopulating ability per CByB6F1 standard PHSC of $F = 1$. From the value of F, a predicted percentage donor value was calculated for each of the 37 donor:competitor ratios associated with the 37 highest probabilities. This produced three sets of predicted donor percentage values, which were each ranked from low to high and compared to the 37 ranked observed values in a paired t test. The hypothesized F values that generated predictions significantly different from observed data were rejected. The F value whose predictions were not significantly different from the observed data was accepted to represent repopulating ability per cell for CXB-12 donor PHSC relative to those of the CByB6F1 standard.

Effects of strain and age on RU concentrations and total RUs per carrier were analyzed through variance analyses. For Poisson modeling, differences between ranked predicted values and ranked observed data were analyzed through paired t tests using the JMP statistical discovery software on "Fit Y by X" and "Fit Model" platforms, respectively (SAS Institute Guide 1998).

RESULTS AND DISCUSSION

Competitive Repopulation

Competitive repopulation demonstrates that PHSC senescence is strain-specific. We tested PHSC senescence by comparing PHSC function in young and old B6, BALB, or D2 mice through competitive repopulation in vivo. Within each strain, 2×10^6 genetically marked congenic standard competitor BMC were mixed with 2×10^6 BMC from each of four young and four old donors, and each mixture was used to engraft four irradiated recipients per donor. The % donor-type erythrocytes and lymphocytes in recipient peripheral blood measured the functional ability of PHSC from each young or old donor relative to the standard competitor. Throughout this study, percentages of lymphocytes and erythrocytes were closely correlated, so they were averaged in each recipient to calculate RU numbers. By definition, 10^5 competitor BMC produced one RU of functional ability (Harrison et al. 1993).

RU numbers/10^5 BMC at 8 months after reconstitution were significantly higher in old than in young B6 mice, and were significantly lower in old than in young BALB and D2 mice (Fig. 2), indicating that PHSC become senescent in BALB and D2 mice, but not in B6 mice. Measurements at 1, 3, 6, and 8 months all showed similar differences between young and old (Chen et al. 2000a), so functional abilities of both short-term precursors and long-term PHSC were affected similarly by aging. The old/young RU ratio, the PHSC senescence phenotype, showed that BALB (0.57 ± 0.24) and D2 (0.48 ± 0.07) BMC decline in function with age, whereas B6 (2.52 ± 0.88) increase (Fig. 2).

In a preliminary experiment, old/young RU ratios for BALB and D2 were 0.27 and 0.50, respectively, after 9 months. The gain in repopulating ability with age had already been shown in B6 mice (Harrison et al. 1989; 1993; Morrison et al. 1996), as had the loss with age in BALB mice (Chen et al. 1999). Figure 2 shows that these strain-specific patterns of PHSC senescence are repeatable. Furthermore, these data are very interesting when they are compared to the results of long-term self-renewal of PHSC in other portions of BMC from the same donors that were serially transplanted. They show that PHSC senescence is not tested as rigorously by this competitive repopulation assay as by an assay after serial transplantation and long-term self-renewal.

PHSC Self-renewal

Portions of the BMC samples taken from the donors in Figure 2 were also transplanted into lethally irradiated, strain-matched, carrier mice, using

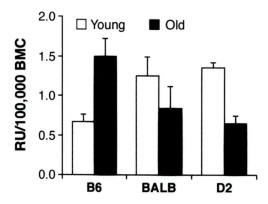

Figure 2 Effects of age on PHSC function. RU (repopulating unit) concentrations from old and young B6, BALB, and D2 mice were measured by competitive repopulation. BMC from each donor were mixed with BMC from a strain-matched young *Gpi1* and *Hbb* congenic standard competitor pool. Mixtures of 2 x 10^6 donor and 2 x 10^6 competitor BMC were iv injected into four lethally irradiated strain-matched recipients per donor. Percentages of donor-type erythrocytes and lymphocytes were analyzed in recipient blood 8 months after reconstitution using the *Gpi1* and *Hbb* markers, respectively. Their averages were used to calculate the RU concentration for each donor, where one RU was the functional ability of 1 x 10^5 cells from the standard competitor BMC. Data are presented as mean with standard error bars from four old/young donor pairs in each strain (Chen et al. 2000a).

2 x 10^6 BMC per carrier and five carriers per donor. After 10 months, BMC from two of the five carriers were pooled and re-transplanted to lethally irradiated secondary recipients in competitive repopulation assays to measure RU concentration in carrier BMC. Mixtures of 5 x 10^6 carrier BMC plus 1 x 10^6 competitor BMC were re-transplanted to each of the secondary recipients, which were tested after 1, 3, 6, and 8 months. RU concentrations for carrier BMC were less than 10% of those for fresh donor BMC (Table 1). Similar results were previously reported for young B6 donors (Harrison et al. 1990).

The difference between total numbers of donor RU per carrier and numbers in the 2 x 10^6 donor BMC originally injected in each carrier represents RU expansion (Table 1). However, the initial RU measures (Fig. 2) apparently included PHSC that failed to expand as well as they functioned in the initial assay. Therefore, the most meaningful measure of

Table 1 Effects of strain and age on bone marrow RU self-renewal

Strains	Donor age	RU injected[1]	RU per 10^6 carrier BMC[2]	Total BMC per carrier[3]	Total RU per carrier	RU expansion
B6	young	13.8	1.1 ± 0.3	224 ± 37	276 ± 52	20
	old	30.6	0.7 ± 0.2	199 ± 28	169 ± 71	5.5
BALB	young	26.0	1.2 ± 0.5	149 ± 11	147 ± 45	5.7
	old	14.2	0.2 ± 0.2	119 ± 13	35 ± 29	2.5
D2	young	26.2	0.9 ± 0.4	100 ± 4	96 ± 5	3.7
	old	12.6	0.4 ± 0.1	87 ± 8	30 ± 6	2.4

Data given as mean ± S.D. Based on Chen et al. 2000a.

[1] RU injected calculated from pooled donor lymphocyte and erythrocyte % after 8 months (in which $P<.01$ that old and young groups are the same in each strain) in the original competitive repopulation measures on portions of the original donor BMC samples that were injected into each carrier mouse.

[2] RU per 10^6 carrier BMC are calculated from pooled donor lymphocyte and erythrocyte % after 8 months (in which $P<.01$ that old and young groups are the same in BALB and D2; $P<.05$ in B6 for erythrocytes, but old and young % in B6 did not differ for lymphocytes) in new competitive repopulation measures on BMC from carriers 10 months after they were given BMC from original donors.

[3] Average BMC per carrier calculated assuming that two tibiae and two femurs contain 25% of the total BMC.

functional ability after long-term serial transplantation appears to be the total donor RU per carrier, each produced from a dose of 2×10^6 donor BMC. These values can be used to compare expansion in the three different genotypes, giving results in terms of RU produced in each carrier by the two million donor cells. PHSC self-renewal declined with donor age in BALB and D2. The strain differences were large with the following old/young ratios of total RU produced: 0.61 in B6, 0.24 in BALB, and 0.31 in D2 (Table 1).

Strain differences were most obvious comparing old donors. Old B6 donors with 30 RU produced 169 RU, while the 13 and 14 RU from old BALB or D2 donors produced only 35 and 30 RU, respectively. The B6 advantage was evident even comparing young donors: PHSC expansion in young B6 BMC (to 276 RU) was 1.9 times as high as in young BALB BMC (to 147 RU), and 2.9 times as high as in young D2 BMC (to 96 RU). The same genetic differences that retard PHSC senescence in the B6 strain may also increase PHSC self-renewal.

Measuring PHSC Senescence In Vivo

Studies in vivo that continue for a substantial fraction of the life span are required to test PHSC, since their most important feature is long-term function. Multilineage repopulation alone fails to demonstrate PHSC function, since short-term precursors can be multilineage; in fact, most of the multilineage precursors assayed over the short term are more differentiated than PHSC (Zhong et al. 1996). In the current study, in Figure 2, competitive repopulation directly measures how well PHSC produce mature lymphocytes and erythrocytes for about a third of the murine life span. Normal PHSC function in vivo is tested, while avoiding potentially confusing effects from unnatural environments in vitro or from cell manipulations used for enrichment.

PHSC Senescence Is Genetically Regulated

The decline in PHSC repopulating ability with increasing donor age seen in BALB and D2 mice suggests that PHSC from these strains become senescent. This agrees with results from inbred CBA mice (Harrison 1983) and B6 ↔ D2 allophenic mice (Van Zant et al. 1990) and fits well with the classic idea that cellular function decreases with donor age (Hayflick 1965). Our observation that PHSC from old B6 donors repopulate recipients better than those from young B6 is also consistent with previous reports (Harrison et al. 1989; Van Zant et al. 1990; Morrison et al. 1996).

Effects of age on PHSC self-renewal were shown by the results from competitive repopulation after serial transplantation (Table 1). By measuring re-transplanted RUs in carrier BMC, we compare the amount of expansion from PHSC in the original dose of donor marrow cells received by each carrier. Since the same competitor was used for old and young donors of the same strain, the total RU per carrier is directly comparable between each strain's young and old donors. In BALB and D2 mice, both repopulation (Fig. 2) and self-renewal (Table 1) declined with age, although measures of self-renewal showed a greater decline. In B6 mice, self-renewal declined slightly, but not significantly, with age (Table 1), differing from competitive repopulation where B6 PHSC repopulation increased with age (Fig. 2).

We suggest two possible mechanisms to explain the genetic differences. First, old PHSC may have a homing defect (Morrison et al. 1996), and this defect may be much more severe in BALB and D2 than in B6 cells. Serial transplantation followed by competitive repopulation requires original donor PHSC to home twice, so effects of the homing deficiency would be amplified. Second, B6 PHSC may have a proliferative limit but at a much higher level than the limits of BALB and D2 PHSC. Serial transplantation requires extra proliferation and thus shows more of a functional decline with age. Such a decline is consistent with results reported in human hematopoietic stem cell candidates (Landsdorp et al. 1994).

B6 Genes Are Dominant in PHSC Senescence

The old/young RU ratio for the BALBxB6 F_1 was larger than 1, as with B6 (Chen et al. 2000a). Old/young RU ratios calculated from data in Harrison (1983) for the B6xCBA and WBxB6 F_1 hybrids are also larger than 1, whereas ratios for the CBA/CaJ parent strain are less. Thus, in different F_1 hybrids between B6 and a parent strain showing PHSC senescence, the B6 pattern is dominant.

Genetic Effects on PHSC Aging

The strain comparisons and genetic analyses reported here lead to the following model: PHSC self-renewal is limited in BALB and D2 mice, so PHSC from 20–24-month-old donors show functional defects. Far more self-renewal can occur in B6 PHSC, so that in old age, PHSC function increases to compensate for other aging defects; thus old donors have more PHSC function than young donors. This B6 phenotype is genetically dominant since it is shown by F_1 hybrids. However, when self-renewal is rigorously tested and PHSC from old and young B6 donors are serially transplanted into lethally irradiated carriers, even in the B6 strain there is a small decline with age. The decline with age in BALB and D2 is far greater; these strain differences in RU expansion in the carriers demonstrate an enormous range of PHSC proliferative potentials.

Competitive Dilution

An important step in defining the biology behind increased PHSC function is to test whether the increase is in numbers of PHSC, function per PHSC, or both. CXB-12 mice have more PHSC as well as more repopulating ability per PHSC. This is detailed in Figure 3. Each of the F_1 recipients is given 5×10^4 CXB-12 donor BMC mixed with 5×10^5 F_1 competitor BMC. After 6 months, 11 of the 37 recipients have 0% CXB-12 type ($Gpil^a$) blood cells. This gives the average PHSC number as $N = -\ln(11/37)$, so $N = 1.2$ PHSC in 5×10^4 BMC, or 2.4 PHSC in 10^5 BMC in CXB-12 mice.

To compare relative repopulating functions F of individual CXB-12 PHSC, we produce three sets of predictions. Of these, $F = 1.4$ times the function of the standard fits the real data almost exactly (Fig. 3), and the differences between predicted and observed values for $F = 1$ or $F = 2$ are significantly larger than those for $F = 1.4$. Thus, each CXB-12 PHSC is 1.4 times as efficient as each F_1 PHSC in engrafting F_1 recipients. Doses of CXB-12 BMC are very low, so hybrid resistance is not saturated, and

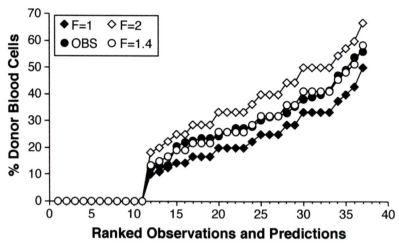

Figure 3 CXB-12 cell numbers and repopulating abilities per cell. The observed donor cell percentages after 6 months for the 37 recipients in the competitive dilution assay described in the text are ranked from low to high and shown as OBS (*filled circles*). We hypothesized three levels of repopulating potential, F, for each CXB-12 donor PHSC relative to $F = 1$ for each CByB6F1 competitor PHSC: $F = 1$ (*filled diamond*), $F = 2$ (*open diamond*), and $F = 1.4$ (*open circle*), and generated three sets of predictions based on combined Poisson probabilities as described in the text. The predictions from models $F = 1$ and $F = 2$ were significantly different from actual observations, thus, models $F = 1$ and $F = 2$ were rejected. Predictions from model $F = 1.4$ were not significantly different from actual observations. Thus, $F = 1.4$ best represents the repopulating ability of a CXB-12 PHSC relative to that of a CByB6F1 PHSC (Chen et al. 2000b).

thus it reduces PHSC numbers and increases the advantage of the F_1 hybrid competitor cells. Concentrations of 2.4 PHSC per 10^5 BMC, and functions of 1.4 times the standard, are minimum estimates.

CXB-12 BMC Do Not Kill Competitor PHSC

Since the model calculates data with the normal condition of 1 PHSC per 10^5 cells for the F_1 competitor, the extremely good fit between the model and real data in Figure 3 suggests that there is no killing of standard competitor F_1 PHSC by CXB-12 BMC. Thus, the CXB-12 repopulating advantage does not result from an immune reaction or other destruction of the standard competitor cells. The degree of killing required would have reduced competitor numbers so the model failed to fit with the expected F_1 concentration of 1.0 PHSC per 10^5 competitor BMC. Additionally, if the F_1 standard PHSC N had been reduced by reaction with CXB-12 BMC, we would expect some recipients to have 100% donor-type cells. However, none of the recipients in this experiment had 100% donor-type cells.

The very high number and function of CXB-12 PHSC may be maintained by alterations in a receptor that regulates this cell type, or in its ligand. Increases in numbers of PHSC could result from changes in either ligand or receptor; however, the increased proliferative capacity of CXB-12 cells after transplantation in normal recipients suggests that the change is intrinsic to the PHSC, perhaps an altered receptor. Understanding the CXB-12 phenotype may eventually lead to improved clinical transplantation procedures to enhance the effectiveness of PHSC in marrow transplantation.

ACKNOWLEDGMENTS

The authors thank Ms. Karen Davis, Ms. Avis Silva, and Ms. Bee Stork for technical assistance. This work was supported by postdoctoral grant AG-05754 to JC, plus RO1 grants HL-58820 and HL-58705 to DEH from the National Institutes of Health. Portions of this review are taken from Chen et al.(2000a,b).

REFERENCES

Abkowitz J.L., Persik M.T., Shelton G.H., Ott R.L., Kiklevich J.V., Catlin S.N., and Guttorp P. 1995. Behavior of hematopoietic stem cells in a large animal. *Proc. Natl. Acad. Sci.* **92:** 2031–2035.

Bailey D.W. 1981. Recombinant inbred strains and bilineal congenic strains. In *The mouse in biomedical research*, vol. 1., pp. 223–239. Academic Press, New York.

Barnett M.J., Eaves C.J., Phillips G.L., Gascoyne R.D., Hogge D.E., Horsman D.E., Humphries R.K., Klingemann H.G., Lansdorp P.M., Nantel S.H., et al. 1994. Autografting with cultured marrow in chronic myeloid leukemia: Results of a pilot study. *Blood* **84:** 724–732.

Bertoncello I., Hodgson G.S., and Bradley T.R. 1988. Multiparameter analysis of transplantable hemopoietic stem cells. II. Stem cells of long-term bone marrow-reconstituted recipients. *Exp. Hematol.* **16:** 245–249.

Chen J., Astle C.M., and Harrison D.E. 1999. Development and aging of primitive hematopoietic stem cells in BALB/cBy mice. *Exp. Hematol.* **27:** 928–935.

———. 2000a. Genetic regulation of primitive hemopoietic stem cell senescence. *Exp. Hematol.* **28:** 442–450.

———. 2000b. Primitive hemopoietic stem cell function in vivo is uniquely high in the CXB-12 mouse strain. *Blood* **96:** 4124–4131.

Cho R.H. and Müller-Sieburg C.E. 2000. A high frequency of LTC-IC retain in vivo repopulation and self-renewal capacity. *Exp. Hematol.* **28:** 1080–1086.

de Haan G., Nijhof W., and Van Zant G. 1997. Mouse strain-dependent changes in frequency and proliferation of hematopoietic stem cells during aging: Correlation between lifespan and cycling activity. *Blood* **89:** 1543–1550.

Gardner R.V., Astle C.M., and Harrison D.E. 1997. Hematopoietic precursor cell exhaustion is a cause of proliferative defect in primitive hematopoietic stem cells (PHSC) after chemotherapy. *Exp. Hematol.* **25:** 495–501.

Harrison D.E. 1980. Competitive repopulation: A new assay for long-term stem cell functional capacity. *Blood* **55:** 77–81.

———. 1983. Long-term erythropoietic repopulating ability of old, young, and fetal stem cells. *J. Exp. Med.* **157:** 1496–1504.

Harrison D.E. and Zhong R.K. 1992. The same exhaustible multilineage precursor produces both myeloid and lymphoid cells as early as 3–4 weeks after marrow transplantation. *Proc. Natl. Acad. Sci.* **89:** 10134–10138.

Harrison D.E, Astle C.M., and Stone M. 1989. Numbers and functions of transplantable primitive immunohemopoietic stem cells: Effects of age. *J. Immunol.* **142:** 3833–3840.

Harrison D.E., Stone M., and Astle C.M. 1990. Effects of transplantation on the primitive immunohematopoietic stem cell (PSC). *J. Exp. Med.* **172:** 431–437.

Harrison D.E., Jordan C.T., Zhong R.K., and Astle C.M. 1993. Primitive hemopoietic stem cells: Direct assay of most productive populations by competitive repopulation with simple binomial, correlation, and covariance calculations. *Exp. Hematol.* **21:** 206–219.

Hayflick L. 1965. The limited in vitro lifetime of human diploid cell strains. *Exp. Cell Res.* **37:** 614–635.

JAX Report. 1997. Animal health and genetic quality control report. *Jackson Laboratory Handbook,* 5th edition (available quarterly from: Director, Laboratory Animal Health, The Jackson Laboratory, Bar Harbor, Maine 04609).

Jones R.J., Celano P., Sharkis S.J., and Sensenbrenner L.L. 1989. Two phases of engraftment established by serial bone marrow transplantation in mice. *Blood* **73:** 397–401.

Jones R.J., Wagner J.E., Celano P., Zicha M.S., and Sharkis S.J. 1990. Separation of pluripotent haematopoietic stem cells from spleen colony forming cells. *Nature* **347:** 188–189.

Jordan C.T. and Lemischka I.R. 1990. Clonal and systemic analysis of long-term hematopoiesis in the mouse. *Genes Dev.* **4:** 220–232.

Jordan C.T., McKearn J.P., and Lemischka I.R. 1990. Cellular and developmental properties of fetal hematopoietic stem cells. *Cell* **61:** 953–963.

Lansdorp P.M., Dragowska W., Thomas T.E., Little M.T., and Mayani H. 1994. Age-related decline in proliferative potential of purified stem cell candidates (comments). *Blood Cells* **20:** 376–381.

Miller C.L. and Eaves C.J. 1997. Expansion in vitro of adult murine hematopoietic stem cells with transplantable lympho-myeloid reconstituting ability. *Proc. Natl. Acad. Sci.* **94:** 13648–13653.

Morrison S.J. and Weissman I.L. 1994. The long-term repopulating subset of hematopoietic stem cells is deterministic and isolatable by phenotype. *Immunity* **1:** 661–663.

Morrison S.J., Hemmati H.D., Wandycz A.M., and Weissman I.L. 1995. The purification and characterization of fetal liver hematopoietic stem cells. *Proc. Natl. Acad. Sci.* **92:** 10302–10306.

Morrison S.J., Wandycz A.M., Akashi K., Globerson A., and Weissman I.L. 1996. The aging of hematopoietic stem cells. *Nat. Med.* **2:** 1011–1016.

Müller-Sieburg C.E. and Riblet R. 1996. Genetic control of the frequency of hematopoietic stem cells in mice: Mapping of a candidate locus to chromosome 1. *J. Exp. Med.*

183: 1141–1150.

Osawa M., Hanada K., Hamada H., and Nakauchi H. 1996. Long-term lymphohematopoietic reconstitution by a single CD34-low/negative hematopoietic stem cell. *Science* **273:** 242–245.

Ploemacher R.E. and Brons R.H. 1989. Separation of CFU-S from primitive cells responsible for reconstitution of the bone marrow hemopoietic stem cell compartment following irradiation: Evidence for a pre-CFU-S cell. *Exp. Hematol.* **17:** 263–266.

Rebel V.I., Dragowska W., Eaves C.J., Humphries R.K., and Lansdorp P.M. 1994. Amplification of SCA-1+ Lin- WGA+ cells in serum-free cultures containing steel factor, interleukin-6 and erythropoietin with maintenance of cells with long-term in vivo reconstituting potential. *Blood* **83:** 128–136.

SAS Institute Guide. 1998. JMP statistics and graphics guide, version 3. SAS Institute Inc. Cary, North Carolina.

Spangrude G.J., Brooks D.M., and Tumas D.B. 1995. Long-term repopulation of irradiated mice with limiting numbers of purified hematopoietic stem cells: In vivo expansion of stem cell phenotype but not function. *Blood* **85:** 1006–1016.

Spangrude G.J., Heimfeld S., and Weissman I.L. 1988. Purification and characterization of mouse hematopoietic stem cells (erratum *Science* [1989] **244:** 1030]). *Science* **241:** 58–62.

Szilvassy S.J., Humphries R.K., Lansdorp P.M., Eaves A.C., and Eaves C.J. 1990. Quantitative assay for totipotent reconstituting hematopoietic stem cells by a competitive repopulation strategy. *Proc. Natl. Acad. Sci.* **87:** 8736–8740.

Taylor B.A. 1996. Recombinant inbred strains. In *Genetic variants and strains of the laboratory mouse,* 3rd edition (eds. M.F. Lyon et al.), vol. 2, pp. 1597–1633. Oxford University Press, New York.

Van Zant G., Holland B.P., Eldridge P.W., and Chen J.J. 1990. Genotype-restricted growth and aging patterns in hematopoietic stem cell populations of allophenic mice. *J. Exp. Med.* **171:** 1547–1565.

Zhong R.K., Astle C.M., and Harrison D.E. 1996. Distinct developmental patterns of short-term and long-term functioning lymphoid and myeloid precursors defined by competitive limiting dilution analysis in vivo. *J. Immunol.* **157:** 138–145.

7

The Drosophila Ovary: An In Vivo Stem Cell System

Ting Xie
Stowers Institute for Medical Research
Kansas City, Missouri 64110

Allan Spradling
Howard Hughes Medical Institute
Department of Embryology
Carnegie Institution of Washington
Baltimore, Maryland 21210

STEM CELLS: A SPECIAL CASE OF PATTERNED GROWTH REGULATION

Adult multicellular organisms are massively larger than the eggs from which they arise. To a significant degree, the final shapes of tissues, organs, and, ultimately, bodies are dictated by highly regulated cell growth processes that spatially and temporally control the rates of cell division within tissue primordia. Biologists have made great advances in understanding this fundamental problem during the last ten years. The molecular regulation of the cell cycle has been largely deciphered, and many aspects of intercellular signaling, which regulate growth spatially, have also been clarified. Now, in favorable systems such as the *Drosophila* embryo and larval imaginal discs (for review, see Edgar and Lehner 1996), as well as in vertebrate organ primordia (see Clarke and Tickle 1999), complex mechanisms that integrate patterning and growth-promoting signals are being learned. The major signaling systems mediated by hedgehogs, epidermal growth factors, bone morphogenetic proteins, fibroblast growth factors, and wingless/wnts frequently stimulate, modulate, or repress the growth rates of receptive cells. Eventually, proliferation ceases when a programmed size and morphology has been achieved, presumably due to changes in the signals and in cellular responsiveness.

On the basis of the studies described below, we have come to regard adult stem cells as a special case of developmental growth regulation, albeit a particularly interesting and potentially informative one. We define an adult stem cell as a cell residing within an adult tissue that divides, either autonomously or in response to regulated signals, to produce cells that contribute to organismal homeostasis. Stem cells make it possible for tissues to recover from injuries and to continue functioning well beyond the average lifetime of their component cells. They make possible organ systems such as epithelial and germinal tissues which regularly produce progeny that are shed from the body. Our studies of *Drosophila* stem cells suggest that as the adult form is realized and most cells cease division and complete their differentiation, stem cells continue to receive and respond to internal or external growth-promoting signals. Moreover, differentiation has contrived to stabilize the anatomical context and signaling environment experienced by these cells. Daughter cells move away, leaving the microenvironment within and around the stem cells unchanged, ensuring that their activity will continue.

This view of stem cells raises a variety of obvious questions. Do the cells that become adult stem cells require a particular developmental history, or can they be selected from among a wide variety of relatively undifferentiated embryonic cells? Do they express characteristic stem cell genes, or do they simply reside in a special anatomical context or niche? Are there special signals that act in the permanent context of an adult stem cell, or do they utilize the same growth-promoting signals as in developing tissues? Other than the requirement to disperse and differentiate to avoid tumor formation, do stem cell progeny play any role in regulating their activity? Likewise, do processes internal to stem cells such as differential divisions play a necessary role in programming daughter cells to take on different fates? How long do individual stem cells live, and can they be replaced during adult life? How variable are the mechanisms that program and maintain stem cells? Are some common to stem cells in different tissues, or between related tissues of evolutionarily distant species? To address all these questions, it is necessary to have systems where stem cells and their neighbors can be identified and genetically perturbed. In this review, we describe studies on one such system, the stem cells of the *Drosophila* ovariole, which can be studied with a high level of anatomical precision and genetic sophistication.

THE OVARY: A STEM CELL-BASED TISSUE

The ovary requires highly active stem cells because it is a large-scale egg production machine. *Drosophila* females are able to produce massive numbers of eggs continuously (more than half the adult's weight per day) during adult life (for general reviews, see King 1970; Spradling 1993). The prodigious reproductive capacity of ovaries results from a highly parallel design. Each of the paired ovaries contains about 16 ovarioles that each independently produce eggs (see Fig. 1A). At its anterior end, every ovariole contains a special region known as the germarium, where permanent germ-line stem cells (GSCs) and somatic stem cells (SSCs) reside, followed by increasingly older and more mature germ cells, followed by a string of progressively older ovarian follicles (see Fig. 1B). Young females of most strains contain two or three GSCs at the anterior tip of the germarium (Lin and Spradling 1993; Margolis and Spradling 1995; Xie and Spradling 2000). *Drosophila* follicles contain not just an oocyte, but a cyst of 16 interconnected germ cells. Cysts form near the anterior of the germarium, and then move posteriorly, first in a double file and then a single file, until they finish acquiring a somatic follicular layer and bud off the posterior end of the germarium. Throughout life, follicles continue to mature, move posteriorly in the ovariole, and, when complete, exit the ovariole at its posterior end. The loss of completed oocytes is balanced by the continued production of new follicles in the germarium, and the entire process from stem cell to mature egg requires only about 8 days to complete.

The distinctive cell biology of early germ cell development greatly aids the study of ovarian stem cells and their progeny, which would otherwise be hard to distinguish in the germarium. After a GSC divides, one daughter remains as a stem cell at the tip while the other daughter differentiates into a cystoblast. Cystoblasts subsequently undergo four rounds of synchronized cell division without cytokinesis to form 16-cell cysts, whose individual germ cells are interconnected by ring canals and a fusome. Fusomes are specialized vesicular organelles that are known to be present primarily in germ cells (for reviews, see Telfer 1975; de Cuevas et al. 1997). They contain membrane skeletal proteins including α- and β-spectrins, and Hu-li Tai Shao (Hts), that may form a cytoskeletal meshwork to retain the vesicles (for review, see McKearin 1997; de Cuevas et al. 1997). Completed 16-cell cysts become wrapped with somatic follicle cells as they pass through the middle portion of the germarium. These somatic cells are produced by exactly two SSCs located on opposite sides near the middle of the germarium that divide about every 9.6 hours (Margolis and Spradling 1995). So far, neither fusomes nor any other distinctive cytoplasmic structures have been observed in somatic stem cells.

The ovariole provides at least two major advantages for stem cell studies. First, the linear organization and steady posterior movement of cells in the ovariole allows the past activity of the stem cells to be deduced for many days after it has occurred. Second, individual stem cells can be

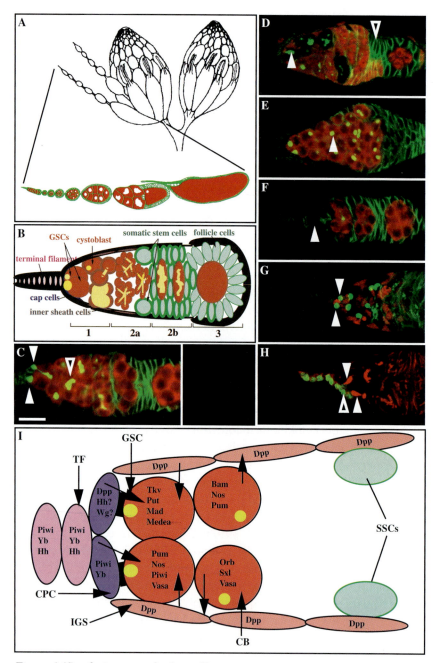

Figure 1 (See facing page for legend.)

Figure 1 The *Drosophila* ovariole is a model system to study stem cells and their niches. (*A*) Explanatory diagram of ovaries (*top*) and a colored ovariole (*bottom*). Every wild-type female has a pair of ovaries, and each ovary has 12–16 ovarioles that represent egg assembly lines. In the ovariole, germ-line cells (*red*) are wrapped inside by somatic cells (*green*). (*B*) Explanatory diagram of a wild-type germarium. The germarium is divided into four regions, 1, 2a, 2b, and 3, based on germ-line development stages. In region 1, germ-line stem cells and all mitotic germ-line cysts reside. In region 2a, all germ-line cysts are 16-cell cysts but not surrounded by somatic follicle cells, whereas all region 2b cysts are lens-shaped and start to be wrapped by somatic follicle cells. In region 3, stage 1 egg chambers are ready to bud off. (*C*) Micrograph of a wild-type germarium after immunofluorescent labeling with anti-Vasa (*red*) and anti-Hts (*green*) antibodies. Two germ-line stem cells at the anterior contain spectrosomes (*closed arrowheads*), and developing cysts at the posterior are connected by branched fusomes (*open arrowhead*). (*D*) Wild-type germarium showing a germ-line stem cell clone and a somatic stem cell clone (for experimental procedures for generating the clones, see Xie and Spradling 1998). This germarium is immunostained with anti-lacZ (*red*) and anti-Hts (*green*) 1 week after heat shock treatment. Marked stem cell clones can be identified by their absence of LacZ expression. The closed arrowhead indicates a marked germ-line stem cell, and its progeny are also marked and lie at the posterior, whereas the open arrowhead indicates the progeny of a marked somatic stem cell clone. (*E*) Tumorous germarium from a *hs-gal4/UAS-dpp* female generated after 4 days of heat shock treatments. In the germarium stained with anti-Vasa (*red*) and anti-Hts (*green*), all germ-line cells are single cells with spectrosomes (one indicated by *closed arrowhead*) that resemble germ-line stem cells. This phenotype is identical to those of mutant *bam* and *bgcn* germaria. (*F*) Germarium losing all germ-line stem cells. This is a 2-week-old *sax* mutant germarium stained with anti-Vasa (*red*) and anti-Hts (*green*), showing that no germ-line stem cells exist in the germarial tip (*closed arrowhead*). Mutations in many genes such as *pum, nos, piwi, Yb,* and *dpp* cause similar stem cell loss phenotypes. (*G*) Enhancer trap line labeling cap cells and inner sheath cells. The germarium stained with anti-LacZ (*red*) and anti-Hts (*green*) antibodies shows inner germarial sheath cells and cap cells (*red*, nuclei) covering regions 1 (two spectrosomes indicated by *closed arrowheads*) and 2a. (*H*) Germarium with labeled terminal filament and cap cells. The germarium stained with anti-Lamin C (*green*, labeling nuclear membrane of both TFs and CPCs) and anti-Hts (*red*) antibodies shows germ-line stem cells (their spectrosomes indicated by *closed arrowheads*) contacting cap cells (indicated by *open arrowhead*). (*I*) Explanatory diagram for germ-line stem cell niche structure and function. The scale bar in *C* represents 10 μm, and all micrographs are shown at the same scale. Abbreviations: (TF) Terminal filament; (GSCs) germ-line stem cells; (CPC) cap cells; (IGS) inner germarial sheath cells; (CB) cystoblasts; (SSCs) somatic stem cells.

precisely recognized, and distinguished from subsequent developmental stages. Ovarian GSCs can be distinguished from neighboring cells by their size, location, and the precise structure of their fusome (see Fig. 1B,C). GSCs are the largest and most anterior germ-line cells in the germarium. GSCs and cystoblasts contain a round fusome (also called a spectrosome), whereas germ cells in developing and completed cysts contain branched fusomes. The exact structure of the fusome in stem cells and cystoblasts can even indicate their cell cycle stage (see de Cuevas and Spradling 1998). A round fusome accompanied by a small "plug" of fusome material in the ring canal joining it with its daughter cystoblast indicates a G_1 or early S-phase stem cell. Later in G_1 and S phase, the stem cell fusome extends to join old and new fusome components, creating an elongated fusome (de Cuevas and Spradling 1998). Finally, in late S or G_2 phase, the fusome breaks in two, reverts to a round shape, and the stem cell and daughter cystoblast lose cytoplasmic contact. During G_1 and early S phase, cystoblasts resemble stem cells in their fusome morphology, but can be recognized since they are located more posteriorly and do not contact the cap cells. Later in their cell cycle, cystoblasts never display an elongated fusome; the old fusome and newly synthesized plug simply fuse and the ring canal does not break down. Still older germ cells are easily distinguished from stem cells and each other by fusome morphology and location.

It is equally important that the somatic cells surrounding GSCs and SSCs have been well defined by their unique morphologies and locations, and by using molecular markers, which allow the relationships between GSCs and their surroundings to be precisely studied (Fig. 1G,H) (for review, see Spradling et al. 1997; Lin 1998).

EXPERIMENTAL METHODS FOR STUDYING STEM CELLS

Before describing the molecular biology of ovarian stem cells in detail, it is worthwhile to briefly mention the techniques that allow their properties to be characterized. The major experimental approaches used for studying stem cells are the same ones that make *Drosophila* a premier system for studying many other aspects of cell and developmental biology. The *Drosophila* genome has been completely sequenced (Adams et al. 2000), and mutations in thousands of different genes have been identified (see Flybase Consortium 1999). Large-scale genetic screens can be carried out that have the potential to identify any *Drosophila* gene by a loss-of-function or gain-of-function phenotype (see Greenspan 1997; Rørth et al. 1998). Special techniques have been developed to misexpress genes in a regulated manner, to construct mosaic animals that lack gene function in special cell subgroups, and recently, for homologous gene knockouts. These resources can be applied more quickly and with less expense than in vertebrate models. Finally, a large cadre of *Drosophila* researchers have already generated extensive knowledge about fundamental processes likely to be relevant for understanding stem cell regulation.

Several techniques are used heavily in stem cell studies. One is the ability to mark cells genetically using site-specific recombination to activate a *lacZ* gene within random members of cell populations (Harrison and Perrimon 1993). GSCs can be unambiguously marked, and the number and development of their labeled progeny can be studied so that the self-renewal capacity and division rate of stem cells can be measured quantitatively (Fig. 1D) (Margolis and Spradling 1995; Xie and Spradling 1998). By creating marked stem cells that are also homozygous for a known mutation, it is possible to test the role of specific genes in stem cell function (Xie and Spradling 1998). Mutants that have defects in stem cell maintenance and differentiation can be identified among collections of candidate mutations isolated in genetic screens using this test (Fig. 1E,F) (Spradling et al. 1997; Lin 1998). A second important technique is the ability to visualize the stem cells and their surrounding cells by confocal microscopy.

Somatic stem cells are more difficult to identify than GSCs. SSCs strongly resemble the flattened, inner germarium sheath (IGS) cells among which they reside. Currently, there are no known morphological or molecular markers that distinguish SSCs from their neighboring IGS cells. SSCs do not contain a detectable fusome or other cytological specialization. However, SSCs can be genetically marked using the same techniques described above for GSCs, and the division and differentiation of their marked progeny can be studied (Fig. 1D) (Margolis and Spradling 1995). Under these conditions, an SSC can be recognized as the most anterior *lacZ*-positive cell of a somatic stem cell clone, and its precise location relative to nearby cells can be tested by double labeling using appropriate markers. SSC behavior can then be tested by observing how SSCs marked with *lacZ* are affected by genetic or environmental perturbation.

REGULATION OF GERM-LINE STEM CELLS

Internal Versus External Regulatory Mechanisms

A major issue in understanding ovarian stem cell regulation has been to distinguish whether regulation occurs primarily as a result of internal or external mechanisms. In the *Drosophila* embryo, neuroblasts, progenitors of the central nervous system, clearly undergo asymmetric divisions to regulate the cell fates of both progenitors and their progeny (for review, see Matsuzaki 2000). Interestingly, in the *Drosophila* ovary, the asymmetry of germ-line stem cell division is revealed by the asymmetric segregation of their spectrosomes, as described above. However, spectrosomes can be completely eliminated by *hts* gene mutations without affecting the maintenance and division of germ-line stem cells at all, although cyst development and the cyst asymmetry are affected (Lin and Spradling 1997; Deng and Lin 1997). These results indicate that spectrosomes and the asymmetry associated with them are not essential for the germ-line stem cell maintenance and division, but instead, set the asymmetry for later germ cell development.

There are two major issues concerning external mechanisms that act on stem cells. The first is to identify the signals and their cellular sources that act on stem cells. During development, cells frequently send and receive information from neighboring cells that critically affect their subsequent behavior. Signals may initiate steps on differentiation pathways that change the cells' internal properties and subsequent responsiveness to additional signals. Moreover, as noted above, many signals regulate cell proliferation rates. Consequently, understanding the signals that affect stem cell differentiation and growth lies at the heart of understanding stem cell function. A number of genes have been identified that are strong candidates for encoding products that directly or indirectly control signals sent from somatic cells and received by GSC (see below). At present, the best evidence exists for Dpp, and in addition, mutations in at least four genes outside the known *dpp* pathway also seem to act via changes in external signaling. However, there are still some uncertainties regarding how each of these genes acts on GSC.

A second issue regarding external signals provided by surrounding somatic cells concerns their stability in the absence of a stem cell target. In mammalian systems, stromal cells have been hypothesized to form special microenvironments or niches for stem cells (for review, see Potten and Loeffler 1990). Some recent evidence from diverse organisms and tissue types supports the existence of stem cell niches (for review, see Kimble and Simpson 1997; Morrison et al. 1997; Mayer et al. 1998; Gage 2000; Schoof et al. 2000; Slack 2000; Watt and Hogan 2000; Weissman 2000). However, the difficulty in studying and manipulating these stem cells and their surroundings in vivo has so far made it impossible to define the structure and function of any specific stem cell niches. *Drosophila* ovarian stem cells have recently been shown to reside in a functional stem cell niche. Investigations into how it operates are beginning to reveal interesting regulatory principles that may pertain more widely.

Extracellular Regulation of GSC: The Existence
of a Stem Niche

The cells surrounding ovarian stem cells are organized into an asymmetric structure. In principle, this asymmetry would allow the two daughters of a stem cell to find themselves in different microenvironments whose differing signals would lead them to adopt different cell fates. The anterior tip of the germarium contains three differentiated somatic cell types: terminal filament cells, cap cells, and inner germarial sheath cells (Fig. 1) (for review, see Spradling et al. 1997; Lin 1998). GSCs directly contact cap cells anteriorly and inner sheath cells laterally. In contrast, cystoblasts are closer to inner sheath cells than to cap cells. Somatic stem cells also experience an asymmetric environment. SSCs reside in region 2a, near the boundary with region 2b, where they touch inner sheath cells anteriorly. However, the progeny of SSC division move posteriorly where they are no longer in direct contact with IGS cells. The asymmetry in the organization of the cells surrounding ovarian stem cells may ensure that two stem cell daughters interact with different sets of cells, and potentially receive different signals, which makes the existence of the stem cell niches possible. In the *Drosophila* testis, germ-line stem cells and somatic stem cells are anchored to the terminally differentiated somatic hub cells, and their differentiated progeny also move away from the hub cells, suggesting that both ovaries and testes use similar strategies to regulate their stem cells (see Chapter 8).

Some or all of these cell types appear to produce signals that are required for the normal functioning of the GSCs. Presently, the BMP pathway is the only characterized signaling pathway that is required to maintain GSCs. Genetic studies of downstream components in the pathway show that a BMP signal must be received in the GSC itself (Xie and Spradling 1998). This signal is most likely encoded by *decapentaplegic (dpp)*, a *Drosophila* homolog of human *bmp 2* and *4*, and is directly received by germ-line stem cells (Xie and Spradling 1998). Dpp and BMP2 and 4 are transforming growth factor-β (TGFβ)-like secreted growth factors. Overexpression of *dpp* in somatic cells prevents germ cell differentiation and results in the formation of stem cell-like tumors, whereas reductions in *dpp* expression cause germ-line stem cells to differentiate and exit the germarium (see Fig. 1E,F) (Xie and Spradling 1998). Interestingly, BMP4 is also implicated in the proliferation and formation of primordial germ cells in the mouse, suggesting that the ability of TGFβ-like growth factors to regulate germ-line stem cells has been conserved (Lawson et al. 1999; also see Chapter 9). Dpp mRNA is expressed in cap cells, IGS cells, and the SSC lineage, and levels appear to be relatively uniform in the neighborhood of the GSCs. Unfortunately, the lack of a suitable anti-Dpp antibody means that it remains uncertain whether Dpp protein levels are also uniform. Finally, until a genetic function can be demonstrated in somatic clones of cup cells or IGS cells, it cannot be completely ruled out that a low level of *dpp* expression takes place in germ cells themselves and that it is this expression which is essential for stem cell maintenance.

Two other growth factors, *wingless* (*wg*) and *hedgehog* (*hh*), often function together with *dpp* synergistically or antagonistically to regulate cell growth and differentiation during embryonic and larval development. Both Wg and Hh are also produced in the germarium (for review, see Lawrence and Struhl 1996). *wg* is highly expressed in cap cells, and *hh* is expressed highly in terminal filament and cap cells (Forbes et al. 1996a,b). The presence of Hh, for example, a known inducer of Dpp and/or Wg signaling molecules, suggests that some of the same pathways that signal embryonic and larval cell growth might be used in the ovary. At least some of the interactions among these players appear to differ between the embryo and the ovariole. For example, increasing Hh up-regulates Ptc, but does increase *wg* expression, at least as measured by a *wg-lacZ* reporter (Forbes et al. 1996b). Roles for *wg* and *hh* in GSC regulation remain to be determined.

Two other genes, *fs(1)Yb* (*Yb*) and *piwi,* also contribute to GSC maintenance (Cox et al. 1998; King and Lin 1999). Unlike *dpp*, the biochemical function of these proteins is unclear. Whereas the structure of Yb is novel, Piwi is part of a highly conserved protein group found in plants, worms, *Drosophila*, mice, and humans. Both genes act in somatic cells, because mutations in either gene cause GSC loss, but clones of germ cells lacking either Yb or Piwi can complete differentiation (Cox et al. 1998; King and Lin 1999). Piwi is highly expressed in the somatic cells including cap cells that adjoin GSCs, and may influence maintenance signals (including possibly Dpp) from these cells. When *piwi* was overexpressed in somatic cells using a hs-GAL4 driver and an EP-piwi responder, additional GSC-like cells accumulated in region 1 of the germarium (Cox et al. 2000), similar to the effects of somatically overexpressing *dpp* (Xie and Spradling 1998). In addition, *piwi* is expressed at a high level in GSCs and at lower levels in cystoblasts and dividing cysts. GSCs lacking *piwi* are maintained but divide slowly (Cox et al. 2000). Piwi is localized to the nucleoplasm, and to explain these effects, Piwi is hypothesized to influence the production of gene transcripts that have different targets in somatic cells and GSCs (Cox et al. 2000).

The differentiated somatic cells surrounding the GSCs send important signals that help maintain and regulate these cells. However, if the surrounding somatic cells form a true GSC niche, a functional niche should exist without resident stem cells, and an empty niche should allow other undifferentiated cells to occupy it and become stem cells. This prediction has been directly tested by generating marked GSCs mutant for *dpp* downstream components in the ovary (Xie and Spradling 2000). Removal of *dpp* downstream components increases germ-line stem cell loss rates and generates more empty stem cell niches. Interestingly, these empty stem cell niches are efficiently repopulated. Wild-type GSCs have a half-life of 4–5 weeks, indicating that stem cells also turn over naturally (Xie and Spradling 1998). Because stem cell replacement also happens naturally, stem cell loss is much slower than is predicted by its half-life of 4–5 weeks. In this way, the functional life of the ovary has been prolonged, and the number of stem cells can be stable for an extended period of time.

The way germ-line stem cells are replaced is also very interesting. Normally, a germ-line stem cell divides along the anterior–posterior axis of the germarium so that one daughter remains in contact with cap cells and the other daughter moves away and differentiates. After a GSC is lost, one of its neighboring stem cells changes its division plane by about 90°, and the usually differentiating daughter occupies the empty stem cell niche and both stem cell daughters gain stem cell identity. This change in the division plane is reminiscent of the cleavage orientation change of neuronal stem cells in the mammalian brain (Chenn and McConnell 1995). Vertical cleavages produce identical daughters that resemble stem cells, which may serve to maintain the stem cell pool. In contrast, horizontally dividing cells produce basal daughters that behave like differentiated neurons and apical daughters that remain as stem cells. Therefore, the existence of stem cell niches not only explains how stem cell self-renewal versus differentiation is regulated, but also how a stable stem cell number is maintained.

Different Roles for Different Somatic Cell Types at the Ovariole Tip

The germarium also provides an excellent system to study the structure and function of niches. Developmental studies implicate the cap cells as one key component of the GSC niche (Xie and Spradling 2000). Normally, approximately 6 cap cells are organized into a cap-like structure at the germarial tip, some of which form special junctions with GSCs (Xie and Spradling 2000). In addition, cell junctions are known to be important for cell–cell communication. Cap cells may serve to anchor GSCs and/or directly signal to them. Interestingly, the number of stem cells in the germarium is significantly correlated with the number of cap cells. Germaria with one GSC have an average of 4.2 cap cells, germaria with two GSCs have an average of 5.3 cap cells, germaria with three GSCs have an average of 6.6 cap cells (Xie and Spradling 2000). Thus, cap cells most likely determine niche size and stem cell number. The genes *dpp, piwi,* and *Yb,* which are known to be essential for germ-line stem cell maintenance, are expressed in cap cells, supporting an important role of cap cells in the regulation of germ-line stem cells.

Both inner germarial sheath cells (IGSs) and terminal filament cells (TFs) could also be an integral part of the germ-line stem cell niche. In young females, approximately 9 terminal filament cells are tightly packaged linear disc-shaped cells in which the most posterior one makes extensive contact with a cap cell, whereas inner germarial sheath cells (IGSs) consist of approximately 35 stretched somatic cells covering the regions from region 1 to region 2a. When females age, TFs start to detach from the cap cells and form ball-like structures, and their number dramatically reduces, while the number of IGS cells also decreases with age (Xie and Spradling 2000). No good correlations between TFs and GSCs or between IGSs and GSCs have been detected in aging females. Therefore, the role of TFs and IGSs in the GSC niche could be very complex, and merits further study in the future.

Inner germarial sheath cells are a very interesting group of somatic cells in terms of their regulation. IGS cells do not exist in a germarium derived from an embryonic gonad lacking primordial germ cells, suggesting that germ cells are required for the formation or maintenance of IGSs (Margolis and Spradling 1995). Furthermore, complete elimination of germ-line cells in the adult ovary by overexpression of Bam protein in GSCs also causes the complete loss of IGS cells, indicating an essential role of germ-line cells in the maintenance of IGS cells (Xie and Spradling 2000). There is also a strong correlation between the number of IGSs and the number of germ-line cysts in aging females, further supporting the notion that germ-line cells maintain IGS cells. Because all germ cells are generated by GSCs, the mitotic activity of GSCs directly regulates the number of IGS cells by undefined signals. Therefore, the integrity of the GSC niche structure is likely controlled by both functional GSCs and niche cells.

INTRACELLULAR MECHANISMS TO REGULATE OVARIAN STEM CELLS

The identification of intrinsic factors will greatly help in understanding how extrinsic signals from the niche are interpreted in germ-line stem cells, and also how asymmetric signaling is translated into intrinsic asymmetry, which regulates stem cell self-renewal and differentiation. Screens for female-sterile mutations have identified two major classes of genes with opposite effects on germ-line stem cells. Mutations in stem cell maintenance genes, such as *pumilio* (*pum*), *nanos* (*nos*), and *vasa* (*vas*), cause the differentiation of germ-line stem cells and result in stem cell loss (Lin and Spradling 1998; Forbes and Lehmann 1997; Styhler et al. 1998). They seem to be also required for the differentiation of early germ-line cysts since these mutant ovaries accumulate ill-differentiated early germ cells. Nos functions cooperatively with Pum as a translational repressor in posterior patterning of the early embryo and in pole cell migration (Murata and Wharton 1995; Kobayashi et al. 1996). Vas is a functional homolog of human eIF-4A, a major translation initiation factor, and is expressed throughout cell development of the germ line, including in GSCs (Hay et al. 1988; Lasko and Ashburner 1988). Therefore, Nos, Pum, and Vas must function in germ-line stem cells and early germ cells to regulate gene expression at the level of translation, but their targets remain to be identified. *piwi* has been reported to regulate germ-line stem cell division but not maintenance in a cell-autonomous manner, besides its non-cell-autonomous role in the regulation of germ-line stem cell self-renewal (Cox et al. 2000). Its gene product is present in the nuclei of germ-line stem cells, but its function in the nucleus remains unclear.

Mutations in early germ cell differentiation genes, such as *bag-of-marbles* (*bam*), *benign germ cell neoplasia* (*bgcn*), *orb*, and *Sex-lethal* (*Sxl*), cause the accumulation of many GSC-like germ cells or early germ-line cysts. The *bam* and *bgcn* mutant ovaries accumulate a population of single germ cells that resemble GSCs, suggesting that both genes function in the same pathway to promote cystoblast differentiation (McKearin and Spradling 1990; Lavoie et al. 1999). Bam is a novel protein with two different functional forms, fusome-associated and cytoplasmic (McKearin and Ohlstein 1995). It can also interact with one of the vesicle transport proteins, Ter94, an AAA ATPase protein, suggesting that Bam may be involved in membrane trafficking (León and McKearin 1999). The cytoplasmic form of Bam is present in cystoblasts and is required for their differentiation. Forced expression of *bam* in GSCs results in their loss (Ohlstein and McKearin 1997). Ectopic expression of *bam* in *bgcn* mutants will not cause germ-line stem cells to differentiate, suggesting that *bgcn* functions downstream of *bam* (Lavioe et al. 1999). Fusome-associated Bam but not its mRNA is affected in *bgcn* mutants, indicating that *bgcn* must regulate *bam* function at posttranslational levels. It remains to be determined how *bgcn* regulates *bam* molecularly. Mutations in *orb* and *Sxl* cause the excessive accumulation of mixed early germ cells that fail to form 16-cell cysts. Orb and Sxl are expressed in both germ-line stem cells and developing cysts (Christerson and McKearin 1994; Lantz et al. 1994). Orb is structurally related to vertebrate cytoplasmic polyadenylation element binding protein (CPEB) (Hake and Richter 1994). CPEB regulates the translation of stored mRNAs after fertilization in *Xenopus*. Sxl is localized in the cytoplasm of germ-line stem cells, cystoblasts, and two-cell and four-cell cysts (Bopp et al. 1993). The cytoplasmic form of Sxl can bind to U-rich sequences in the untranslated regions of mRNAs and regulates their translation (Kelley et al. 1997). Likely, Sxl is also involved in translational regulation of some mRNAs in early developing germ cells in the ovary.

As mentioned earlier, *dpp* directly signals to germ-line stem cells and regulates their maintenance and normal cell division (Xie and Spradling 1998). Many known signaling components in the *dpp* pathways have been shown to be required in germ-line stem cells to transduce the signal. Germ-line stem cells mutant for *punt*, *thick veins* (*tkv*), *saxophone* (*sax*), *mothers against dpp* (*mad*), *Medea* (*Med*), and *schnurri* (*shn*) have significantly shorter life spans and divide significantly more slowly than wild-type cells (Xie and Spradling 1998, 2000). Mutations in *Daughters against dpp* (*Dad*), a negative regulator of the *dpp* pathway, can prolong the life span of germ-line stem cells. Mutations in these genes do not affect the normal development of cystoblasts and early developing cysts, indicating that the *dpp* pathway is very specific to germ-line stem cells. *punt*, *tkv,* and *sax* encode transmembrane serine-threonine kinase receptors, whereas *mad*, *Med*, and *shn* encode DNA-binding proteins (for review, see Padgett et al. 1998; Padgett 1999). Dad is related to Mad and Med, and prevents Mad phosphorylation by receptors and further nuclear translocation. Likely, the *dpp* pathway transcriptionally regulates the expression of other genes, which are important for germ-line stem cell maintenance and division. Identifying these *dpp* target genes, and revealing the relationships between *dpp* signaling and the two classes of genes discussed above will greatly aid in understanding how germ-line stem cell maintenance and division are controlled intracellularly.

SSC REGULATION

Less is known about the intrinsic factors for somatic stem cells. One of the important signals controlling follicle cell production is the *hh* pathway (Forbes et al. 1996a). *patched* (*ptc*)-mutant somatic follicle cells overproliferate as in *hh*-overexpressing ovaries because *ptc,* encoding a seven-transmembrane protein, is a negative regulator of the *hh* signaling pathway. Thus, SSCs or early follicle progenitors may directly receive the IGS-produced *hh* signal. *Notch* (*N*) is known to regulate differentiation of somatic follicle cells (Xu et al. 1992; Larkin et al. 1996). Mutations in *N* cause the fusion of egg chambers because of ill-differentiated follicle cells (Xu et al. 1992). N starts its expression at the region 2a/2b junction, suggesting that it could also function in somatic stem cells. Overexpression of activated N and its ligand Delta prevents the proper differentiation of somatic stalk cells and causes the accumulation of excessive somatic cells in stalks (Larkin et al. 1996). Notch family members have been known to regulate stem cell proliferation in different organisms (Kimble and Simpson 1997). It is still unclear whether the mitotic activity and number of SSCs are affected in loss-of-function and gain-of-function *N* mutants.

Little is known about the structure and function of the SSC niche. However, circumstantial evidence suggests that posterior IGS cells form the SSC niche. Hh is expressed at low levels in IGSs, which is revealed by one enhancer trap line. Interestingly, overexpression of *hh* or removal of a negative regulator of the *hh* pathway, *patched* (*ptc*), from SSCs and their progeny can lead to overproduction of somatic follicle cells (Forbes et al. 1996a,b). This overproliferation takes place near the 2a/2b junction where SSCs and their immediate daughters are located, suggesting that it could be caused either by increasing stem cell number or activity. In order to study SSCs and their niche effectively, SSC molecular markers and the IGSs surrounding SSCs need to be better defined in the future.

DEFINING STEM CELLS INDEPENDENTLY FROM THE BEHAVIOR OF THEIR PROGENY

In this chapter, we have defined stem cells by their ability to produce offspring indefinitely while remaining in a stable physical location and cellular state. What the ultimate fate of these progeny cells is, or their manner of differentiation, has no real importance to the mechanisms that govern the stem cell itself. For example, even if each progeny cell simply moved away from its site of birth, failed to undergo any changes in its state of differentiation, and finally died, the stem cell would still be a stem cell in this sense. Although such a pointless situation is unlikely to exist normally, mutations such as *bam* and *bgcn* cause just such a change; in our view, such mutations are not stem cell mutations but mutations regulating progeny differentiation.

The term stem cell is sometimes used in a quite different sense, however, to mean the founder of a complex lineage of multiple daughter cell types. In this view, it is the complexity of its progeny cells, and in particular the regular production of at least two different types of progeny, that distinguish a cell as a stem cell. By this definition, stem cells are almost ubiquitous in embryos. More than 70% of the cell divisions during *Caenorhabditis elegans* embryogenesis are asymmetric, indicating that the progeny have different fates. All these cells would be stem cells. Most organisms lack the low cell number and invariant cell lineage of *C. elegans*; whether a cell's progeny differentiate into multiple cell types or not is only determined later, as a result of cell–cell interactions. We believe that this alternative definition of a stem cell has lost its usefulness now that the predominant role of intercellular signaling in controlling development and differentiation has been established.

FUTURE ISSUES

We have seen that GSCs, and probably SSCs, are controlled by complex signals orchestrated by surrounding somatic cells that form a niche. The structure of the niche likely gives it the ability to maintain GSCs located within it and to specify a cystoblast fate for more posteriorly located progeny cells. Ovariole tips with apparently normal morphology form in the absence of germ cells. A future goal will be to understand how the GSC niche is specified during ovarian development and how its structure is maintained. Are there commonalities in the design and specification of anatomical units that can maintain proliferative signals indefinitely in a fixed morphological framework?

Our current knowledge of the molecular regulation of stem cell behavior is imperfect but suggests that certain issues are likely to be of key importance. Hh, Wg, and Dpp signals are associated with proliferating epithelial cells at many stages of development, and they appear to be a main engine of ovarian stem cell proliferation as well. How is Hh expression maintained in the terminal filament and cap cells, and Wg expression in the cap cells? How do these potentially antagonistic signals interact to maintain a signaling center that is critical for SSC divisions and possibly for GSC activity as well? Second, what is the nature of the junction that holds GSCs to cap cells?

Finally, more needs to be learned about the requirements for a cell to become a GSC. Is a highly undifferentiated state necessary? Is it sufficient? Since GSC maintenance genes such as *nanos* and *pumilio* appear to act as repressors, one may well answer yes. This would explain why GSC daughter cells destined to become cystoblasts could be easily shifted to become GSCs. If so, converting other cells into GSCs might require that the cells' current state of differentiation be erased.

CONCLUSIONS

The *Drosophila* ovary provides excellent opportunities for studying the relationship between adult stem cells and their niches. Recent identification of intrinsic factors and signals from surrounding cells has provided significant insight into molecular mechanisms regulating the maintenance and division of ovarian stem cells, particularly germ-line stem cells. The surrounding differentiated somatic cells have been shown to function as a niche for germ-line stem cells. This will be likely true for somatic stem cells in the *Drosophila* ovary and adult stem cells in other organisms. In the future, the identification of additional signals and intrinsic factors by genetic and molecular approaches will help reveal how multiple signals from the niche are integrated to regulate the self-renewal, division, and differentiation of ovarian stem cells. Further functional and structural studies on *Drosophila* ovarian stem cell niches will reveal how niches are built during development, and how long they are maintained during the aging process. Finally, the ability of the GSC niche to reprogram other cells toward a GSC fate will be more fully assessed.

REFERENCES

Adams M.D., Celniker S.E., Holt R.A., Evans C.A., Gocayne J.D., Amanatides P.G. et al. 2000. The genome sequence of *Drosophila melanogaster*. *Science* **287**: 2185–2195.

Bopp D., Horabin I., Lersch R.A., Cline T.W., and Schedl P. 1993. Expression of the *Sex-lethal* gene is controlled at multiple levels during *Drosophila* oogenesis. *Development* **118**: 797–812.

Chenn A. and McConnell S.K. 1995. Cleavage orientation and the asymmetric inheritance of Notch1 immunoreactivity in mammalian neurogenesis. *Cell* **82**: 631–641.

Christerson L.B. and McKearin D. 1994. *orb* is required for anteroposterior and dorsoventral patterning during *Drosophila* oogenesis. *Genes Dev.* **8**: 614–628.

Clarke J.D. and Tickle C. 1999. Fate maps old and new. *Nat. Cell Biol.* **4**: E103–109.

Cox D.N., Chao A., and Lin H. 2000. *piwi* encodes a nucleoplasmic factor whose activity modulates the number and division rate of germ-line stem cells. *Development* **127**: 503–514.

Cox D.N., Chao A., Chang L., Qiao D., and Lin H. 1998. A novel class of evolutionarily conserved genes defined by *piwi* are essential for stem cell self-renewal. *Genes Dev.* **12**: 3715–3727.

de Cuevas M. and Spradling A.C. 1998. Morphogenesis of the *Drosophila* fusome and its implications for oocyte specification. *Development* **125**: 2781–2789.

de Cuevas M., Lilly M.A., and Spradling A.C. 1997. Germ-line cyst formation in *Drosophila*. *Annu. Rev. Genet.* **31**: 405–428.

Deng W. and Lin H. 1997. Spectrosomes and fusomes anchor mitotic spindles during asymmetric germ cell divisions and facilitate the formation of a polarized microtubule array for oocyte specification in *Drosophila. Dev. Biol.* **189:** 79–94.

Edgar B.A. and Lehner C.F. 1996. Developmental control of cell cycle regulators: A fly's perspective. *Science* **274:** 1646–1652.

FlyBase Consortium 1999. The FlyBase database of the *Drosophila* Genome Projects and community literature. *Nucleic Acids Res.* **27:** 85–88.

Forbes A. and Lehmann R. 1998. Nanos and Pumilio have critical roles in the development and function of *Drosophila* germ-line stem cells. *Development* **125:** 679–690.

Forbes A.J., Lin H., Ingham P.W., and Spradling A.C. 1996a. Hedgehog is required for the proliferation and specification of ovarian somatic cells prior to egg chamber formation in *Drosophila. Development* **122:** 1125.

Forbes A.J., Spradling A.C., Ingham P.W., and Lin H. 1996b. The role of segment polarity genes during early oogenesis in *Drosophila. Development* **122:** 3283–3294.

Gage F.M. 2000. Mammalian neural stem cells. *Science* **287:** 1433–1438.

Greenspan R. 1997. *Fly pushing: The theory and practice of* Drosophila *genetics.* Cold Spring Harbor Laboratory Press, Cold Spring Harbor, New York.

Harrison D. and Perrimon N. 1993. A simple and efficient generation of marked clones in *Drosophila. Curr. Biol.* **3:** 424–433.

Hake L.E. and Richter J.D. 1994. CPEB is a specificity factor that mediates cytoplasmic polyadenylation during *Xenopus* oocyte maturation. *Cell* **79:** 617–627.

Hay B., Jan L.Y., and Jan Y.N. 1988. A protein component of *Drosophila* polar granules is encoded by *vasa* and has extensive sequence similarity to ATP-dependent helicases. *Cell* **55:** 577–587.

Kelley R.L., Wang J., Bell L., and Kuroda M.I. 1997. *Sex lethal* controls dosage compensation in *Drosophila* by a non-splicing mechanism. *Nature* **387:** 195–199.

Kimble J. and Simpson P. 1997. The Lin-12/Notch signaling pathway and its regulation. *Annu. Rev. Cell Dev. Biol.* **13:** 333–361.

King R. 1970. *Ovarian development in* Drosophila melanogaster. Academic Press, New York.

King F.J. and Lin H. 1999. Somatic signaling mediated by *fs(1)Yb* is essential for germline stem cell maintenance during *Drosophila* oogenesis. *Development* **126:** 1833–1844.

Kobayashi S., Yamada M., Asaoka M., and Kitamura T. 1996. Essential role of the posterior morphogen nanos for germline development in *Drosophila. Nature* **380:** 708–711.

Lantz V., Chang J.S., Horabin J.I., Bopp D., and Schedl P. 1994. The *Drosophila* orb RNA-binding protein is required for the formation of the egg chamber and establishment of polarity. *Genes Dev.* **8:** 598–613.

Larkin M.K., Holder K., Yost C., Giniger E., and Ruohola-Baker H. 1996. Expression of constitutively active *Notch* arrests follicle cells at a precursor stage during *Drosophila* oogenesis and disrupts the anterior-posterior axis of the oocyte. *Development* **122:** 3639–3650.

Lasko P.F. and Ashburner M. 1988. The product of the *Drosophila* gene *vasa* is very similar to eukaryotic initiation factor-4A. *Nature* **335:** 611–617.

Lavoie C.A., Ohlstein B., and McKearin D.M. 1999. Localization and function of Bam protein require the *benign gonial cell neoplasm* gene product. *Dev. Biol.* **212:** 405–413.

Lawrence P. and Struhl G. 1996. Morphogens, compartments, and pattern: Lessons from *Drosophila? Cell* **85:** 951–961.

Lawson K.A., Dunn N.R., Roelen B.A.J., Zeinstra L.M., Davis A.M., Wright V.A.E., Korving J.P., and Hogan B.L.M. 1999. *Bmp4* is required for the generation of primordial germ cells in the mouse embryo. *Genes Dev.* **13:** 424–436.

Leon A. and McKearin D. 1999. Identification of TER94, an AAA ATPase protein, as a Bam-dependent component of the *Drosophila* fusome. *Mol. Biol. Cell* **10:** 3825.

Lin H. 1998. The self-renewing mechanism of stem cells in the germline. *Curr. Opin. Cell Biol.* **10:** 687–693.

Lin H. and Spradling A.C. 1993. Germline stem cell division and egg chamber development in transplanted *Drosophila* germaria. *Dev. Biol.* **159:** 140–152.

————. 1997. A novel group of *pumilio* mutations affects the asymmetric division of germline stem cells in the *Drosophila* ovary. *Development* **124:** 2463–2476.

Lin H., Yue L., and Spradling A.C. 1994. The *Drosophila* fusome, a germ-line-specific organelle, contains membrane skeletal proteins and functions in cyst formation. *Development* **120:** 947–956.

Margolis J. and Spradling A. 1995. Identification and behaviour of epithelial stem cells in the *Drosophila* ovary. *Development* **121:** 3797–3804.

Matsuzaki F. 2000. Asymmetric division of *Drosophila* neural stem cells: A basis for neural diversity. *Curr. Opin. Neurobiol.* **10:** 38–44.

Mayer K., Schoof H., Haecker A., Lenhard M., Jürgens G., and Laux T. 1998. Role of *WUSCHEL* in regulating stem cell fate in the *Arabidopsis* shoot meristem. *Cell* **95:** 805–815.

McKearin D. 1997. The *Drosophila* fusome, organelle biogenesis and germ cell differentiation: If you build it... *BioEssays* **19:** 147–152.

McKearin D. and Ohlstein B. 1995. A role for the *Drosophila* Bag-of-marbles protein in the differentiation of cystoblasts from germline stem cells. *Development* **121:** 2937–2947.

McKearin D. and Spradling A.C. 1990. *bag-of-marbles*: A *Drosophila* gene required to initiate both male and female gametogenesis. *Genes Dev.* **4:** 2242–2251.

Morrison S.J., Shah N.M., and Anderson D.J. 1997. Regulatory mechanisms in stem cell biology. *Cell* **88:** 287–298.

Murata Y. and Wharton R.P. 1995. Binding of *pumilio* to maternal *hunchback* mRNA is required for posterior patterning in *Drosophila* embryos. *Cell* **80:** 747–756.

Ohlstein B. and McKearin D. 1997. Ectopic expression of the *Drosophila* Bam protein eliminates oogenic germline stem cells. *Development* **124:** 3651–3662.

Padgett R.W. 1999. Intracellular signalling: Fleshing out the TGFβ pathway. *Curr. Biol.* **9:** R408–411.

Padgett R.W., Das P., and Krishna S. 1998. TGF-β signaling, Smads, and tumor suppressors. *BioEssays* **20:** 382–390.

Potten C.S. and Loeffler M. 1990. Stem cells: Attributes, spirals, pitfalls and uncertainties. Lessons for and from the crypt. *Development* **110:** 1001–1020.

Rørth P., Szabo K., Bailey A., Laverty T., Rehm J., Rubin G.M., Weigmann K., Milan M., Benes V., Ansorge W., and Cohen S.M. 1998. Systematic gain-of-function genetics in *Drosophila*. *Development* **125:** 1049–1057.

Schoof H., Lenhard M., Haecker A., Mayer K.F.X., Jürgens G., and Laux T. 2000. The stem cell population of *Arabidopsis* shoot meristems is maintained by a regulatory loop between the *CLAVATA* and *WUSCHEL* genes. *Cell* **100:** 635–644.

Slack J.M.W. 2000. Stem cells in epithelial tissues. *Science* **287:** 1431–1433.

Spradling A.C. 1993. Developmental genetics of oogenesis. In *The development of*

Drosophila melanogaster (eds. M. Bate and A. Martinez-Aris, pp. 1–70. Cold Spring Harbor Laboratory Press, Cold Spring Harbor, New York.

Spradling A.C., de Cuevas M., Drummond-Barbosa D., Keyes L., Lilly M., Pepling M., Xie T. 1997. The *Drosophila* germarium: Stem cells, germ line cysts, and oocytes. *Cold Spring Harbor Symp. Quant. Biol.* **62:** 25–34.

Styhler S., Nakamura A., Swan A., Suter B., and Lasko P. 1998. *vasa* is required for GURKEN accumulation in the oocyte, and is involved in oocyte differentiation and germ-line cyst development. *Development* **125:**1569–1578.

Telfer W. 1975. Development and physiology of the nurse cell-oocyte syncytium. *Adv. Insect Physiol.* **11:** 223–319.

Weissman I.L. 2000. Translating stem and progenitor cell biology to the clinic: Barriers and opportunities. *Science* **287:** 1442–1446.

Watt F.M. and Hogan B.L.M. 2000. Out of Eden: Stem cells and their niches. *Science* **287:** 1427–1430.

Xie T. and Spradling A.C. 1998. *decapentaplegic* is essential for the maintenance and division of germ line stem cells in the *Drosophila* ovary. *Cell* 1998 **94:**251–260.

———. 2000. A niche maintaining germ line stem cells in the *Drosophila* ovary. *Science* **290:** 328–330.

Xu T., Caron L.A., Fehon R.G., and Artavanis-Tsakonas S. 1992. The involvement of the *Notch* locus in *Drosophila* oogenesis. *Development* **115:** 913–922.

8

Male Germ-line Stem Cells

Amy A. Kiger[1] and Margaret T. Fuller[1,2]
[1]Department of Developmental Biology and [2] Department of Genetics
Stanford University School of Medicine
Stanford, California 94305-5329

Spermatogenesis is a classic stem cell system. Continuous production of highly differentiated, short-lived sperm is maintained throughout reproductive life by a small, dedicated population of male germ-line stem cells (GSCs). Male GSCs are unipotent, devoted solely to the generation of sperm, much like epidermal stem cells that give rise only to keratinocytes (see Chapter 19). As precursors of the spermatogonial lineage, male GSCs must maintain a balance between the production of mature sperm and the self-renewal of stem cell potential.

Male germ-line stem cells are defined by their function as persistent, clonogenic founders of differentiating germ cells. They can be identified by multiple criteria, including anatomical position within a niche in the testis and distinct behavioral and molecular phenotypes. Male GSCs exhibit many similarities to other stem cell systems. Spermatogonial stem cells are a rare, relatively quiescent population that lies in a protected region in the testis among support cells, which may regulate their behavior. Like all stem cells, male GSCs are the most resistant cells to irradiation or chemical damage. As with hematopoietic stem cells, spermatogonial stem cells in mammals are transplantable, with an ability to both expand the stem cell pool and to regenerate an entire depleted spermatogenic lineage. Spermatogonial stem cells also exhibit signature molecular features, such as high expression of β-1 integrin, much like epidermal and hematopoietic stem cells.

The function of male GSCs has broad implications for development, disease, and evolution. Spermatogenesis is fundamental for the propagation of species. Spermatogenic defects can result in infertility or disease, such as testicular germ cell cancer. The ability to identify, isolate, culture, and alter adult male GSCs will allow powerful new approaches in animal transgenics and human gene therapy relating to infertility and disease. The male germ line also offers a powerful experimental system to study fundamental questions in stem cell biology. Spermatogenesis is a well-studied and defined process with many useful tools that can be applied to stem cell research. Current advances such as functional identification of male GSCs, identification of somatic support cells, and tools to characterize their respective roles have established an important foundation for future work.

Spermatogenesis and male fertility, as dependent on the continual production of sperm, have been studied in many organisms ranging from invertebrates to vertebrates (Hannah-Alava 1965). The early germ cell stages of spermatogenesis have been investigated in arthropods (Lindsley and Tokuyasu 1980), moths (King and Akai 1971), teleosts (Upadhyay and Guraya 1973), sharks (Callard et al. 1989), reptiles and amphibians (Pudney 1995), birds (Lin and Jones 1992; Jones and Lin 1993), rodents (Leblond and Clermont 1952a; Oakberg 1956), and primates (Roussel et al. 1969; Clermont 1972; Fouquet and Dadoune 1986). Interesting parallels and contrasts in male GSC behavior have emerged from observations on different organisms. For example, the anatomical location of male GSCs and their intimate association with somatic cells are conserved in many species. One striking difference is variation in the spermatogenic cycle, such as seasonal regulation in species that undergo seasonal breeding compared to continual spermatogenesis throughout reproductive life of non-seasonal breeders.

This chapter focuses on male germ-line stem cell biology in the fruit fly *Drosophila melanogaster* and in mammals (primarily rodents). Much of the information on male GSC identification and function has resulted from the helpful tools and methods available in these systems. There are striking similarities in male GSC location, behavior, and function between *Drosophila* and mammals, suggesting that complementary approaches in the two systems will help illuminate the mechanisms of male GSC regulation.

Drosophila provides a genetic system for rapid identification of genes required for normal male GSC behavior based on unbiased mutagenesis screens (for review, see Fuller 1993). In addition, tools for mitotic recombination and genetic marking (Xu and Rubin 1993; Lee and Luo 1999) can be used in lineage analysis experiments to identify and follow the behavior of male GSCs, either in the wild type or in mutants (Gönczy and DiNardo 1996). Similar mitotic recombination tools allow tests of whether a gene required for normal stem cell behavior functions cell-autonomously (in the germ line) or non-autonomously (in the soma) (Gönczy et al. 1997; Matunis et al. 1997; Kiger et al. 2000; Tran et al. 2000). Finally, the transparency and simple organization of the *Drosophila* testis allow in vivo identification of spermatogonial stem cells and phenotypic demonstration of mutational effects without disrupting the local stem cell microenvironment.

In mammals, early spermatogonial cells, including the GSC population, can be physically manipulated. Donor male GSCs can be transplanted into recipient host testes to assay stem cell function (Brinster and Avarbock 1994; Brinster and Zimmermann 1994). The transplant assay can be used for lineage analysis or to test whether requirement for a gene function is cell-autonomous or non-cell-autonomous (Ogawa et al. 2000). As in the fly, the ability to dissect and section the mammalian testis allows phenotypic analysis of spermatogonial cells in situ. In addition, the ability to make targeted gene disruptions in mice can be used to test the genetic requirements for male GSC function.

Many of the questions that arise about male GSC biology could be asked of stem cells in any system. What regulates male GSC specification from precursor populations in the embryo? What regulates initiation of the spermatogonial stem cell divisions? How are male GSCs defined and identified? Where are GSCs located in the testis, and what cells make up their microenvironment? Do somatic cells form a niche that regulates GSC behavior? Are stem cell divisions asymmetric or symmetric? What are the molecular mechanisms that maintain a balance between self-renewal of stem cell identity and initiation of differentiation when stem cells divide? Are these critical mechanisms under intrinsic or extrinsic control?

We review these questions below, each with an introductory discussion on male GSCs in general, followed by more detailed information that specifically relates to *Drosophila* or mammalian male GSCs. For more information, see earlier reviews on germ-line stem cells (Cooper 1950; Hannah-Alava 1965; Lindsley and Tokuyasu 1980; Fuller 1993; Meistrich and van Beek 1993a; de Rooij and Grootegoed 1998; Lin 1998).

SPECIFICATION OF MALE GERM LINE AND INITIATION OF STEM CELL DIVISIONS

The male germ line proceeds through several developmental steps prior to establishment and initiation of spermatogonial stem cell divisions in the testis (Fig. 1) (for detailed description, see Pringle and Page 1997; Saffman and Lasko 1999; Wylie 1999). Primordial germ cells (PGCs) are specified as distinct from somatic cell lineages at one of the earliest stages in embryogenesis (Fig. 1a). The PGCs proliferate and migrate from their site of origin to the future position of the gonad (Fig. 1b), where they associate with somatic gonadal precursor cells to form the gonad (Fig. 1c). Once within the gonad, the PGCs differentiate in a sex-specific manner, including a distinct program of proliferation and quiescence (Fig. 1d,e).

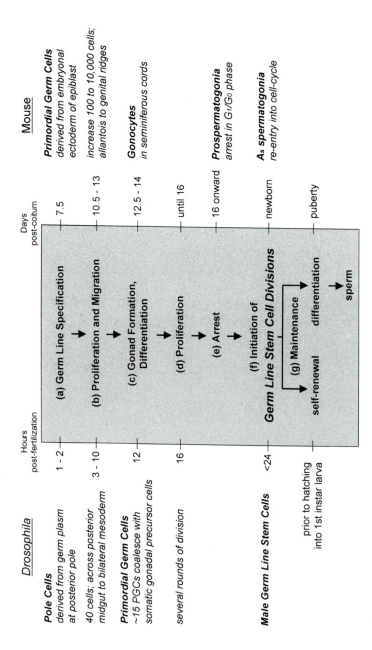

Figure 1 Specification and initiation of male germ-line stem cell divisions.

PGCs in the testis become male germ-line stem cells and initiate the first round of spermatogenesis that will produce sperm at the onset of reproductive age (Fig. 1f). Finally, male germ-line stem cell divisions are regulated so that appropriate numbers of stem cells are maintained (Fig. 1g).

When does the germ line first acquire stem cell potential? Evidence in mammals suggests that the earliest PGCs derived in the embryo already exhibit aspects of stem cell potential under certain experimental conditions. Unlike spermatogonial stem cells, however, PGCs are pluripotent, giving rise to highly differentiated cells of multiple somatic and germ cell lineages (Matsui et al. 1992; Resnick et al. 1992; Shamblott et al. 1998). In both flies and mammals, PGCs display additional characteristic differences from germ-line stem cells established in the adult male. PGCs can proliferate expansively with no differentiation. In contrast, under normal conditions, germ-line stem cells maintain their numbers and give rise to differentiating gametes. PGCs migrate throughout the embryo, whereas germ-line stem cells normally stay within a well-defined niche. Finally, PGCs are similar in appearance and behavior in both sexes, whereas germ-line stem cells are normally restricted to either male or female gametogenesis, the products of which exhibit extreme sexual dimorphism.

Environmental cues may direct the transition from PGC to male germ-line stem cell after populating the embryonic gonad. Somatic gonadal cells are required for proper development of male germ cells, including expression of sex- and stage-specific genes (Staab et al. 1996). The somatic gonad also appears to direct the sex-specific program and the timing of onset of gametogenesis (for review, see Pringle and Page 1997). However, the somatic gonadal cells do not require the presence of germ cells for testis formation (Geigy 1931; Aboim 1945; Mintz and Russell 1957).

The establishment and long-term maintenance of male germ-line stem cell divisions appear to be regulated independently. Only a subpopulation of the PGCs is maintained as male germ-line stem cells through adulthood (Hardy et al. 1979; de Rooij 1998). One hypothesis is that only some PGCs acquire and/or retain stem cell capacity, whereas other PGCs directly differentiate without self-renewing divisions. Although the mechanisms are not understood, it is thought that signals from the somatic gonad direct which cells from an initially uniform PGC population are retained and which cells differentiate.

Fly

Germ-line specification and migration in the early *Drosophila* embryo have been studied extensively (for recent reiews, see Rongo et al. 1997;

Saffman and Lasko 1999). Germ cells are the first cells formed when pole cells bud off at the posterior end of the syncytial embryo (Fig. 1a). The pole cells proliferate to yield a final population of up to 40 germ cells (Sonnenblick 1941). To reach the developing gonad, the pole cells are first passively moved with the posterior midgut invagination, then actively migrate across the midgut to contact the mesoderm (Fig. 1b). The pole cells split into two groups, migrate into bilateral clusters, and interact with a well-characterized population of somatic gonadal precursor cells (Boyle and DiNardo 1995; Boyle et al. 1997; Moore et al. 1998). Approximately 15 PGCs and 30 somatic gonadal precursor cells coalesce to form the embryonic male gonad (Sonnenblick 1941; Poirie et al. 1995). After gonad formation, the pole cells are called primordial germ cells in *Drosophila* (Fig. 1c) (Sonnenblick 1941), whereas in mammals germ cells are usually referred to as gonocytes at this stage.

Much less is known about the transition from primordial germ cell fate into male germ-line stem cell identity in *Drosophila*. Early germ cells exhibit sex-specific differences once inside the embryonic gonad. For example, a certain germ cell marker expressed in the male embryonic gonad is not expressed in females (Staab et al. 1996). Gametogenesis is also initiated at distinct times in males versus females. Male germ cell proliferation and initiation of spermatogenesis must take place prior to hatching of the embryo, because differentiating spermatogonia are found in first-instar larval testes (Fig. 1d,f) (Kerkis 1933; Sonnenblick 1941). In contrast, female germ cells do not initiate oogenesis until days later, at the time of the larval–pupal transition (King 1970). Since male GSCs are active throughout larval and adult life, stem cell activity can be assayed in larval testes, independent of adult male viability or fertility. This is helpful when studying genes required for both adult viability and stem cell behavior (see last section). From the initial ~15 PGCs in the embryonic testis, only 5–9 male germ-line stem cells are maintained in the adult testis (Fig. 1g) (Hardy et al. 1979).

Mammals

Primordial germ cells are induced in the embryonic ectoderm of the mammalian epiblast (Fig. 1a) (Everett 1943; Lawson et al. 1999; Chapter 9). In the mouse embryo at 7 days, approximately 100 PGCs are detected in the extraembryonic mesoderm based on alkaline phosphatase activity, a marker of germ cell identity (Ginsburg et al. 1990). The PGCs then migrate from the allantois along the hindgut to the genital ridges

(Saffman and Lasko 1999). PGCs proliferate during their migration (Fig. 1b), with more than 10,000 PGCs eventually populating the genital ridges (Tam and Snow 1981).

In males, PGCs are enclosed in seminiferous cords to form the gonads. The somatic environment in the seminiferous tubules triggers the male-specific differentiation of PGCs into gonocytes (Clermont and Perey 1957; Pringle and Page 1997). Gonocytes are morphologically distinct from either the PGCs or differentiating female germ cells. Gonocyte identity is marked by transition into a nonmitotic state, growth in cell size, and the onset of distinct gene expression (Huckins 1963; Li and Gudas 1997). It is hypothesized that somatic Sertoli cells in the seminiferous tubules produce an inhibitory signal that prevents differentiation of PGCs into female germ cells and allows progression along the male pathway (for review, see Pringle and Page 1997). Cessation of PGC proliferation and gonocyte survival are also dependent on the somatic cells. Whereas PGCs survived in vitro when cocultured with one of any multiple somatic cell types, gonocytes survived only when cocultured in the presence of Sertoli cells (Resnick et al. 1992; van Dissel-Emiliani et al. 1993).

Gonocytes relocate to the basal lamina during morphogenesis of seminiferous somatic cells (Orth 1993). Gonocytes undergo subsequent proliferative expansion, producing up to 50,000 cells in the mouse, then mitotically arrest in the G_1/G_0 phase until after birth (Saffman and Lasko 1999). Stem cells may develop directly from gonocytes (Clermont and Perey 1957) or may arise indirectly via prospermatogonia that differentiate at the time of the gonocyte mitotic arrest (Hilscher et al. 1974). In the newborn mouse, spermatogonial stem cells are likely to arise when proliferation resumes. Finally, onset of puberty triggers initiation of differentiation along the spermatogenic lineage. In mammals, as in the fly, it is difficult to conclude precisely when male germ-line stem cell identity is established. Some interconnected gonocytes have been found in the embryonic gonad, which may reflect initiation of spermatogenesis as early as in the gonocyte stage (Zamboni and Merchant 1973). In rat and hamster, kinetic studies indicate that some gonocytes may differentiate directly into spermatogonia (van Haaster and de Rooij 1994), suggesting that only a subpopulation of gonocytes retain stem cell status.

ROLE OF GERM-LINE STEM CELLS IN SPERMATOGENESIS

Male germ-line stem cells must self-renew as well as produce progeny that initiate differentiation. To study this crucial aspect of stem cell behavior and to unambiguously identify GSCs, we need to understand the relationship of spermatogonial stem cells to the more differentiated germ cells that comprise the spermatogenic lineage.

As in other stem cell systems, differentiation along the spermatogenic lineage progresses through three distinct compartments (Fig. 2) (Loeffler and Potten 1997; Fuchs and Segre 2000). Male GSCs maintain the lineage throughout reproductive age by balancing stem cell self-renewal with differentiation (Fig. 2, I). This balance can be obtained either by asymmetric or symmetric stem cell divisions (discussed in detail below). Stem cell daughter cells that initiate differentiation undergo several rounds of mitotic amplification divisions (Fig. 2, II). These mitotic divisions are specialized in that cytokinesis is incomplete, resulting in cysts of synchronously dividing, interconnected germ cells (Phillips 1970; Dym and Fawcett 1971). Due to the amplification divisions, a single daughter cell commit-

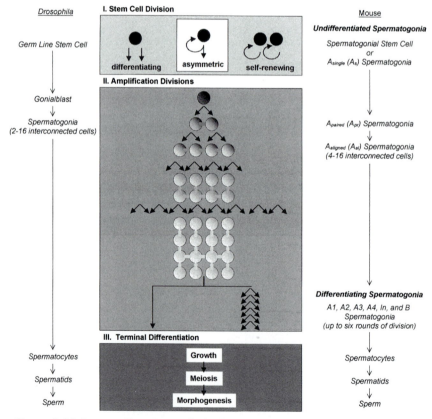

Figure 2 Male germ-line stem cells in the spermatogenic lineage.

ted to differentiation eventually gives rise to large numbers of sperm. In this regard, germ cells in the amplification divisions are comparable to progenitor cells in the hematopoietic lineage, which maintain a limited proliferative capacity (Weissman 2000). Finally, the germ cells exit from mitotic division and initiate terminal differentiation (Fig. 2, III), including progression through the stages of spermatocyte growth, the meiotic program, and morphogenesis into spermatozoa. The entire process of spermatogenesis takes approximately 10 days in *D. melanogaster*, 35 days in mice, and 61 days in rats (Clermont and Trott 1969; Lindsley and Tokuyasu 1980; Meistrich and van Beek 1993b).

Spermatogenesis is a complex process that is regulated at multiple stages. Thus, infertility is not necessarily due to a defect in the stem cell compartment. However, it has been suggested for mammals that perturbations in later stages may affect or alter stem cell behavior, indicating feedback control on the GSC population (Huckins and Oakberg 1978).

Fly

In *Drosophila*, male GSC divisions normally have an asymmetric outcome (Gönczy and DiNardo 1996). One daughter cell self-renews stem cell identity and one daughter cell initiates differentiation as a gonialblast (Fig. 2). The gonialblast is the founder spermatogonial cell that initiates the spermatogonial amplification divisions, much as the cystoblast in the *Drosophila* female germ line initiates the amplification divisions that produce interconnected germ cells of the developing egg chamber (Lin 1997). In *D. melanogaster*, precisely four rounds of synchronous amplification division invariably result in 16 interconnected spermatogonia (Tihen 1946). The number of amplification divisions varies among different *Drosophila* species, suggesting that germ cell proliferation is restricted at a distinct regulatory point that is under genetic control (Fuller 1993).

Stem cells divide asynchronously and continuously throughout larval and adult life (Cooper 1950; Hardy et al. 1979; Lindsley and Tokuyasu 1980; Gönczy and DiNardo 1996). Continuous stem cell activity ensures ongoing replenishment of gonialblasts to initiate differentiation, with the effect that all stages of spermatogenesis are present in the testis at any one time.

Mammals

In mammals, all premeiotic male germ cells, including stem cells, are called spermatogonia. The different stages of spermatogonia are roughly classified by temporal order as either undifferentiated A-type spermatogonia or differentiating spermatogonia (Leblond and Clermont 1952b; Oakberg 1956; Huckins 1971b). GSCs are among the single undifferentiated A spermatogonia, termed A$_{single}$ (A$_s$) spermatogonia. A$_s$ spermatogonia self-renew stem cell identity and give rise to other undifferentiated A-type spermatogonia that eventually differentiate. The successive stages of undifferentiated spermatogonia proliferate synchronously as A$_{paired}$ (A$_{pr}$) spermatogonia in clusters of 2 germ cells and A$_{aligned}$ (A$_{al}$) spermatogonia in clusters of 4, 8, or 16 germ cells (Fig. 2). Undifferentiated A spermatogonia develop into differentiating spermatogonia, which continue through six additional rounds of synchronous interconnected division as A$_1$, A$_2$, A$_3$, A$_4$, Intermediate, and finally, B spermatogonia (Fig. 2). Within a given region of the seminiferous tubules, mammalian spermatogenesis is cyclic, with synchronous bursts in stem cell activity alternating with periods of relative inactivity (Leblond and Clermont 1952b; Oakberg 1956) (see below).

LOCATION OF MALE GERM-LINE STEM CELLS IN THE TESTIS

Male germ-line stem cells are localized anatomically to a defined compartment within the testis. The ability to identify stem cells in situ is at present relatively unique to the male germ line, in contrast to the difficulty of unambiguously identifying most other stem cell types in vivo (e.g., hematopoietic stem cells within the bone marrow). Spermatogenesis proceeds in a spatial gradient within the testis (Figs. 3 and 4), allowing GSC activity to be easily visualized as the continual production of differentiating germ cells.

Fly

The *Drosophila* adult testis is a coiled tube closed at the apical end and opening at the base into the seminal vesicle (Fig. 3a). The progression of spermatogenesis transits the length of the tube. The GSCs reside in the germinal proliferation center at the apical testis tip (Fig. 3b,c; S) (Hardy et al. 1979). Just distal to the stem cells lie the gonialblasts and interconnected spermatogonia. Cysts of 16 growing primary spermatocytes are displaced down the testis tube, completing meiosis approximately one-third of the way toward the base. Elongating spermatids extend back up the length of the testis lumen (Fig. 3a, arrowheads) then exit the basal

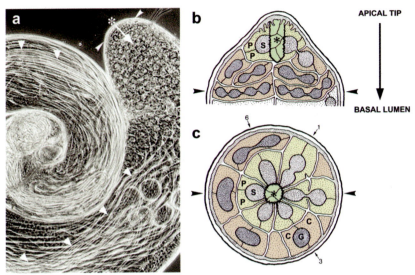

Figure 3 Location of male germ-line stem cells in the *Drosophila* testis. (*a*) The *Drosophila* adult testis is a coiled tube closed at the apical end (*asterisk*). All germ cell stages of spermatogenesis are visible through the transparent testis wall when viewed by phase microscopy. GSCs reside at the apical testis tip within the germinal proliferation center (*asterisk*). Successive stages of germ cell differentiation are displaced basally (*arrow*), with elongated sperm extending back up the testis (*arrowheads*). Schematic illustrations of (*b*) a transverse section and (*c*) a cross section through the germinal proliferation center of the testis apical tip. Asterisks and shaped arrowheads correspond approximately to those in *a*. Arrows labeled *1, 3,* and *6* denote successive stages in early spermatogenesis: (1) stem cell division, (3) formation of a differentiating germ-line cyst, and (6) initiation of spermatogonial divisions. Spermatogenesis proceeds from the apical tip to the base of the lumenal tube (*vertical arrow*). Both the GSCs (*light blue, S*) and the somatic cyst progenitor cells (*yellow, P*) divide radially and asymmetrically (*arrow 1*) around the hub (*green, asterisk*). Note that the GSCs and cyst progenitor cells normally do not divide in synchrony as drawn. The GSC daughter cell adjacent to the hub self-renews stem cell identity, whereas the daughter farthest from the hub initiates differentiation as a gonialblast (*dark blue, G*). Similarly, the cyst progenitor cells divide to give rise to one cyst progenitor cell and one cyst cell committed to differentiation (*orange, C*). One gonialblast is enclosed in two cyst cells to form a germ-line cyst (*arrow 3*), which proceeds through spermatogonial divisions (*arrow 6*). A basement membrane overlays the hub and stem cells (*gray stippled*). The testis is enclosed in a bilayer sheath made up of muscle and pigment cells (*white*). (*b, c,* Modified, with permission, from Lindsley and Tokuyasu 1980 [© Academic Press].)

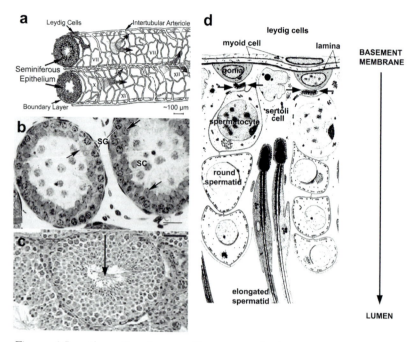

Figure 4 Location of male germ-line stem cells in the mammalian testis. (*a*) Schematic of just two seminiferous tubules from a mammalian testis. Spermatogenesis takes place in the seminiferous epithelium of the tubule lumens. Somatic boundary cells surround the seminiferous epithelium. The vasculature and somatic Leydig cells reside in the interstitial space that surrounds each tubule. Successive stages of the epithelial cycle are found along the length of the tubules, which are defined by the representative germ cell contents (Roman numerals). (Modified, with permission, from Hinton and Turner 1993 [© Oxford University Press].) (*b*) Autoradiograph of a cross-section containing two seminiferous tubules from a 21-day-old rat testis. The spermatogonia (SG) are mitotically active and incorporate ^{3}H[thymidine] at the lumen periphery. Spermatocytes (SC) are postmitotic and localize further within the lumen. Somatic Sertoli cells (*arrows*) neighbor the spermatogonia. (Modified, with permission, from Orth 1982 [©Wiley].) (*c*) Cross-section of one seminiferous tubule from an adult mouse testis stained with hematoxylin and eosin. Spermatogenesis proceeds radially inward (*arrow*), from spermatogonia at the lumenal edge to sperm in the central lumen. (Modified, with permission, from Ogawa et al. 2000.) (*d*) Schematic of a seminiferous epithelium. Spermatogenesis proceeds radially from the basement membrane to the inner lumenal space (*vertical arrow*). Spermatogonia reside adjacent to the basement membrane surrounded by somatic myoid cells. Differentiating germ cells move inward, progressing through the spermatocyte and spermatid stages. Somatic Sertoli cells flank germ cells of all stages, and form a special junction enclosing spermatogonia into an exterior, basal compartment (*small arrows*). (Modified, with permission, from Hecht 1993. [© Kluwer Academic/Plenum].)

opening (Lindsley and Tokuyasu 1980; Fuller 1993). A similar spatial gradient is observed in larval testes, with the difference that the larval testis is ovoid and normally contains only premeiotic germ cells and spermatocytes (Kerkis 1933; Sonnenblick 1941). The germ cells at the apical testis tip can be visualized by phase microscopy of live dissected testes, although the stem cells and spermatogonia are difficult to distinguish without the aid of molecular markers.

Mammals

Mammalian spermatogenesis takes place in the seminiferous epithelium, inside the multiple seminiferous tubules that compose the testis (Fig. 4a). Male GSCs lie at the tubule periphery next to the basement membrane (Hadley and Dym 1987). Germ cells move radially inward as spermatogenesis proceeds until the sperm are released into the central lumen (Fig. 4b,c). Spermatogenesis occurs in successive waves along the length of the tubules (Fig. 4a). Each wave contains a discrete cohort of germ cell stages, categorized as either 12 epithelial stages in the mouse (I–XII) or 14 stages in the rat (I–XIV) (Leblond and Clermont 1952b; Oakberg 1956). In the mouse, for example, undifferentiated spermatogonia normally divide during stages X–III, but rarely divide during the other stages (Oakberg 1971). The dynamics of the epithelial cycle imply that stem cell activity is selectively reinitiated and/or inhibited within groups of staged spermatogonia.

THE STEM CELL NICHE: THE RELATIONSHIP BETWEEN GERM-LINE STEM CELLS AND THE SOMA

Male germ-line stem cells are closely associated with somatic cells. Throughout the testis, the local microenvironment varies along with the different spermatogenic stages. Male GSCs lie within a protected region of the testis, surrounded by somatic cells that isolate them from differentiating germ cells. The close association between GSCs and specific somatic cell types or stages suggests a role for somatic support cells in regulating GSC behavior.

Fly

Drosophila male germ-line stem cells are associated with two somatic cell types within the germinal proliferation center (Figs. 3b,c and 5a,d) (Aboim 1945; Smith and Dougherty 1976; Hardy et al. 1979). GSCs lie in a ring closely apposed to a cluster of somatic apical cells (Fig. 5c) that

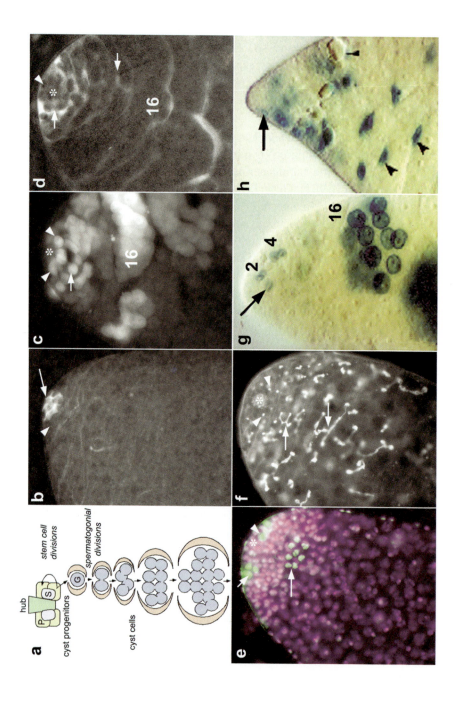

Figure 5 Identification of *Drosophila* male germ-line stem cells in the niche. (*a*) Schematic of the *Drosophila* germinal proliferation center. The GSCs (*light blue*) and somatic cyst progenitor cells (*yellow*) form a ring around the somatic hub (*green*). The germ-line gonialblast (*blue*) is encysted by two cyst cells (*orange*), then initiates the spermatogonial divisions. (*b*) The hub at the apical tip can be detected by immunofluorescence using antibodies against epithelial cell markers such as *Drosophila* E-cadherin (*arrow*). Background staining of testis was shown to help visualize the testis and is not specific to E-cadherin. The ring of GSCs that surround the hub are not visible (*arrowhead*). (*c*) The germ cells in the germinal proliferation center as detected by tissue-specific expression of the green fluorescent protein (GFP). A ring of GFP-positive, single, GSCs (*arrowheads*) surrounds the unlabeled hub (*asterisk*). Single germ cells displaced from the apex are presumptive gonialblasts formed from radial stem cell divisions (*arrow*). Interconnected germ cells in the spermatogonial stages are distinguished as clusters of 2, 4, 8, and 16 cells with GFP throughout a shared cytoplasm. (*d*) GFP expression under control of the *nanos-GAL4, UAS-GFP* transgenes is down-regulated during the spermatocyte growth phase. The somatic cyst cells in the germinal proliferation center as detected by tissue-specific expression of GFP. The cyst cell cytoplasm is thin and lacy, stretching around the germ cells. The cyst progenitor cells (*arrow at tip*) contact the hub (*asterisk*) and enclose the round, unlabeled GSCs (*arrowhead*). Cyst cells (*arrow*) continue to grow and enclose the differentiating germ cells that increase in size and number. GFP expression is via the transgenes *ptc-GAL4, UAS-GFP*. (*e*) Division patterns distinguish stem cells and gonial-blasts from spermatogonia by detection of the mitotic indicator, phosphorylated Histone 3 (*green*), and DNA (*purple*). The GSCs and gonialblasts divide asynchronously as single cells (*arrowhead*), and are normally only found near the hub (*asterisk*). Further from the hub but still within the apical tip, the interconnected spermatogonia undergo synchronous amplification divisions as groups of 2, 4 (*short arrow*), or 8 (*long arrow*) cells. At the 16-cell stage, spermatogonia exit mitosis. (*f*) Fusome structure distinguishes stem cells and gonialblasts from spermatogonia by immunofluorescence detection of components such as α-Spectrin. A ball-shaped fusome, or spectrosome (*arrowheads*), is only found adjacent to the hub (*asterisk*) in GSCs and gonialblasts. Branched fusome passes through the ring canals of interconnected clusters of 2-, 4-, 8-, and 16-cell spermatogonia and spermatocytes (*arrows*). (*g, h*) Testes analyzed 5 days after heat-shock-induced mitotic recombination and activation of the *lacZ* nuclear lineage marker. (Modified, with permission, from Gönczy and DiNardo 1996) [© Company of Biologists Ltd.].) (*g*) Lineage tracing of a persistent GSC clone using a nuclear marker. A GSC is marked as a single, dividing cell (*arrow*) adjacent to the hub (*unlabeled*). Successive progeny derived from the marked GSC are seen as more mature spermatogonial (2, 4) and spermatocyte (16) clusters. (*h*) Lineage tracing of a persistent somat-ic cyst cell clone using a nuclear marker. A cyst progenitor cell is marked as a single cell (*arrow*) near the testis apex. Progeny derived from the marked cyst progenitor cell are detected as marked cyst cell nuclei (*arrowheads*) associated with packets of developing germ cells.

form a compact structure called the hub (Hardy et al. 1979). The apical cells of the hub exhibit epithelial-like characteristics, such as localization of fasciclin III (Brower et al. 1981) and E-cadherin at the cell membrane (Fig. 5b). A pair of somatic stem cells, the cyst progenitor cells, flanks each germ-line stem cell. The cyst progenitor cells contact the hub with cytoplasmic extensions, thus enclosing the GSCs (Figs. 3b,c, and 5d) (Hardy et al. 1979). The development of hub and cyst cells does not require the presence of the germ line (Geigy 1931; Aboim 1945), supporting their somatic origin. Like the GSCs, cyst progenitor cells divide asymmetrically to self-renew a cyst progenitor cell and to produce a cyst cell that initiates differentiation (Hardy et al. 1979; Gönczy and DiNardo 1996). Two somatic cyst cells enclose one germ-line-derived gonialblast to form a unit called a germ-line cyst (Stern 1941). The two cyst cells do not divide again, but continue to enclose the growing clone of differentiating germ cells (Figs. 3b,c, and 5d). Germ cells and somatic cyst cells are easily distinguished from one another on the basis of cell morphology and marker expression.

The testis is enclosed in a sheath made up of an inner layer of muscle cells and an outer layer of squamous, pigmented cells (Geigy 1931; Stern 1941). The muscle layer of the sheath is open only over the apical cells of the hub (Hardy et al. 1979). The germinal proliferation center, however, is firmly attached to the testis apex by a thick, convoluted layer of basal lamina that overlays the hub (Fig. 3b) (Hardy et al. 1979). If the sheath is torn open from a dissected testis, cysts of differentiating germ cells spill freely away from the testis wall, while the germ cells in the germinal proliferation center remain tightly associated with the testis apex.

The number of GSCs appears to be developmentally regulated. Morphological studies by reconstruction from serial electron micrographs indicated that the number of GSCs decreases from 16–18 cells in third-instar larval testes to 5–9 cells in 3-day-old adult testes (Hardy et al. 1979). Similarly, cyst progenitor cell numbers also decrease from 19–20 cells in larval stages to 9–17 cells in the adult, with two cyst progenitor cells associated with every GSC. Concomitantly, the size and shape of the hub is compacted from a sheet of 16–18 cells into a densely packed, dome-shaped structure of 8–16 cells in the adult. It is possible that only the germ cells that maintain contact with the developing somatic hub retain GSC identity.

Mammals

Mammalian spermatogonial stem cells are neighbors to several somatic cell types along the basement membrane of the seminiferous tubule (Fig. 4d). The most closely apposed somatic cells are the large Sertoli cells.

Sertoli cells contact all stages of developing germ cells, extending processes from the basement membrane to within the central lumen of the epithelium (Russell et al. 1983). The Sertoli cells create distinct microenvironments along their length via directional secretion of multiple regulatory factors (Bardin et al. 1993). Sertoli cells form a tight junction barrier that isolates the spermatogonia into an exterior or basal compartment of the epithelium, separating them from the more differentiated germ cell stages within the interior or lumenal compartment (Fig. 4d, small arrows) (Dym and Fawcett 1970; Gilula et al. 1976). This barrier may serve to expose and/or shield stem cells from specific regulatory signals (Bardin et al. 1993). GSCs may also form junctions directly with the Sertoli cells. Desmosomes formed between spermatogonia and Sertoli cells have been described in vivo (Russell et al. 1983).

Peritubular myoid cells and the lymphatic endothelium together form a somatic boundary layer that encloses the basement membrane surrounding the spermatogonial stem cells. The myoid cells, along with Sertoli cells, secrete the underlying basement membrane as well as regulatory factors that affect Sertoli cell behavior (Skinner et al. 1985). Although the somatic Leydig cells in the intertubular spaces do not directly contact the spermatogonial stem cells, they do secrete steroids and peptides with potential regulatory roles in spermatogenesis (Ewing and Keeney 1993).

IDENTIFICATION OF MALE GERM-LINE STEM CELLS BY PHENOTYPE AND FUNCTION

Male germ-line stem cells can be distinguished from other early germ cells by distinct behavioral and molecular phenotypes. Generally, male GSCs exhibit an asynchronous pattern of mitotic division and a slower cell cycle time, making them more resistant to damage from low doses of radiation than the later undifferentiated or differentiated spermatogonia (Dym and Clermont 1970). Since the location of male germ-line stem cells within the testis is known, specific gene products can be assayed for expression in either the GSCs or their differentiated progeny. Investigation of the function of genes that are expressed in stem cells but not in more differentiated spermatogonia, or vice versa, may help uncover intrinsic mechanisms that specify stem cell self-renewal versus differentiation. In addition, such cell-type-specific expression markers greatly facilitate the analysis and interpretation of mutant phenotypes.

Stem cells are most stringently defined by their functional capacity. To be classified as a stem cell by this definition, a single, adult, male germ cell must demonstrate the ability to self-renew stem cell identity and continually produce cells that differentiate into sperm. Methods to identify male GSCs functionally have been developed for both the fly and mammalian systems.

Fly

In *Drosophila*, a combination of expression markers, characteristic subcellular structures, and division behavior are used to distinguish stem cells from later germ cell stages. In the wild-type testis, all cells undergoing mitotic division are restricted to the region of the apical tip (Figs. 3 and 5e). Stem cells and gonialblasts are distinguished from spermatogonia as the single cells that divide asynchronously close to the hub (Tihen 1946; Hardy et al. 1979; Gönczy and DiNardo 1996). In contrast, interconnected spermatogonia divide in synchrony and normally lie at a greater distance from the hub (Fig. 5e, arrows). A stem cell division was calculated to take place once every 10 hours at the apical tip of an adult testis (Lindsley and Tokuyasu 1980). Only one GSC in mitosis was observed in 50 GSCs examined morphologically (Hardy et al. 1979).

Drosophila germ cells have a characteristic subcellular structure called the fusome, which is composed of multiple membranous and cytoskeletal components, including α-spectrin (Lin et al. 1994). The fusome takes on a different shape in single germ cells and in interconnected germ cells. In GSCs and gonialblasts, this subcellular structure forms a ball-shaped spectrosome (Fig. 5f, arrowheads). Spectrosomes are normally found in a rosette of cells only one or two cells deep from the apical hub. In contrast, the fusome is extended and branched, running through the ring canals that connect mitotically related spermatogonia or spermatocytes within a cyst (Fig. 5f, arrows).

Distinct gene expression profiles can further define stem cell versus spermatogonial identities. A collection of enhancer trap lines was isolated based on distinct expression patterns of the *lacZ* marker gene in testes (Gönczy et al. 1992; Gönczy 1995). For example, the enhancer trap markers *M34a* and *S1-33* drive expression of β-galactosidase activity in the GSCs and gonialblasts at the most apical tip, but not in later stages (Gönczy 1995). Other lines mark different stages of differentiating germ cells or the accompanying somatic cyst cells. Antibodies to specific proteins also detect subpopulations of germ cells. The cytoplasmic *bag-of-marbles* protein (Bam-C) is detected in spermatogonia from the 2- to 16-cell stages, but not in the ring of germ-line stem cells around the hub (McKearin and Ohlstein 1995; Gönczy et al. 1997).

Clonal Analysis as a Test of Drosophila *Male Germ-line Stem Cell Function*

Male germ-line stem cells are genetically identified in the *Drosophila* testis by clonal analysis. The existence of GSCs was first proposed in 1929 to explain the size and distribution of clusters of identical mutations in brooding studies (Harris 1929). Analysis of the progeny from irradiated males demonstrated that large groups of identical mutant progeny must have derived from the division of one original, mutagenized germ cell. On the basis of these studies, it was proposed that a few indefinitely reproducing germ cells at each division produced one germ cell like themselves and one cell with a limited potential, allowing one germ cell to generate many sperm over an extended time (Harris 1929; Tihen 1946). Similar genetic analysis of brood patterns using a sex-linked mutable trait extended the observation, notably, that cluster size was larger when the mutation occurred in a GSC rather than at a later spermatogenic stage (Hartl and Green 1970). The results from this study accurately predicted the existence of 7–10 GSCs per adult testis and indicated that the number of germ-line stem cells stays relatively constant regardless of the number of sperm produced (consistent with earlier predictions, as reviewed in Hannah-Alava 1965). The distribution of brood clusters also suggested that the GSCs divide asynchronously, with quiescent periods of 24–48 hours.

Lineage-tracing experiments using the FLP/FRT site-specific recombination system conclusively verified both the function and location of GSCs in wild-type testes (Fig. 5g) (Gönczy and DiNardo 1996). The FLP recombinase of yeast can be used to induce site-specific recombination at *cis*-acting FRT sites incorporated into *Drosophila* chromosomes (Harrison and Perrimon 1993). The FLP/FRT system can be used to permanently mark cells by inducing mitotic recombination between differently marked homologous chromosomes or by inducing excision of a marker gene from within a single chromosome. Both germ-line stem cells and spermatogonia can be marked in this system. However, spermatogonia are present only transiently, as they eventually clear from the proliferation center within 2 days and differentiate. In contrast, stem cells persist by self-renewal of stem cell identity, continually producing waves of marked progeny undergoing spermatogenesis (Fig. 5g). Such clonal marking studies produced single, persistent, marked germ cells adjacent to the hub at the apical tip in ~50% of the induced testes examined, confirming the identity and location of germ-line stem cells deduced from ultrastructural studies (Gönczy and DiNardo 1996). The function and location of the somatic cyst progenitor stem cells were demonstrated by the same method (Fig. 5h).

The FLP/FRT lineage-tracing system can also be used in mutant genetic backgrounds to identify and follow stem cell behavior in males carrying mutations that cause stem cell defects. In addition, to test whether a gene required for stem cell function acts cell-autonomously or non-cell-autonomously, the same technology can be used to make mosaic animals in which the induced clones are homozygous for a mutation in an otherwise heterozygous background.

Mammals

In mammals, several phenotypic markers are used to distinguish the A_s spermatogonial cells from later spermatogonial stages. GSCs undergoing asynchronous mitosis or apoptosis can be detected as single cells interspersed along the periphery of the seminiferous tubule. In contrast, clusters of interconnected spermatogonia undergo mitosis and enter apoptosis synchronously within each epithelial stage (Huckins 1971b; Oakberg 1971; de Rooij and Grootegoed 1998). Due to the characteristic wavelike distribution of spermatogenic stages along the length of the seminiferous tubule, certain regions show a higher frequency of A_s stem cell proliferation, whereas other epithelial stages contain relatively inactive A_s spermatogonia. The number of A_s spermatogonia, however, remains constant throughout the epithelial cycle (Huckins 1971a). In rat and hamster, male GSCs and undifferentiated spermatogonia generally have a longer cell cycle time than do differentiating spermatogonia (Huckins 1971a; Lok et al. 1983). In rat testes, A_s stem cells are estimated to divide every 60 hours, the A_{pr} and A_{al} undifferentiated spermatogonia every 55 hours, and the differentiating spermatogonia every 42 hours (Huckins 1971a).

A-type spermatogonia, including spermatogonial stem cells, exhibit higher levels of telomerase activity (Ravindranath et al. 1997) and expression of the EE2 protein (Koshimizu et al. 1995) than later germ cell stages. Undifferentiated A spermatogonia can be further distinguished from differentiating spermatogonia on the basis of low nuclear heterochromatin (Huckins 1971b) and low levels of c-Kit expression (Schrans-Stassen et al. 1999).

Transplantation as a Test of Mammalian Germ-line Stem Cell Function

Mammalian germ-line stem cells are able to maintain stem cell function upon transplantation to a host testis. Methods for germ cell transplants have been established in the mouse testis (Brinster and Avarbock 1994;

Brinster and Zimmermann 1994). Although a mixed population of testicular cells is used for the transplant injections, only the spermatogonial stem cells are thought to establish donor-derived spermatogenesis in the host. Donor spermatogonial stem cells can provide long-term reconstitution to produce functional sperm and restore fertility in a sterile host testis, with colonization rates of >80% repopulated tubules in at least 71% of the recipient mice (Brinster and Avarbock 1994). The best colonization occurred when donor cells were injected into hosts depleted of germ cells, obtained either by cytotoxic treatment with busulfan or by genetic mutation with alleles of the *Dominant white spotting* (*W*) or *Steel* (*Sl*) loci (Brinster and Zimmermann 1994; Ohta et al. 2000; Shinohara et al. 2000). These results suggest competition between transplanted and endogenous germ-line stem cells for access to limited sites capable of supporting stem cell function, in support of the niche hypothesis.

The frequency of colonization upon transplantation indicates that germ-line stem cells are rare within the testis, consistent with the estimated two GSCs per every 10^4 germ cells (Meistrich and van Beek 1993a; Tegelenbosch and de Rooij 1993). This frequency compares with the measured frequency of approximately 1 hematopoietic stem cell in every 10^4 bone marrow cells (Spangrude et al. 1988). Individual colonization events upon transplantation can be distinct, allowing the activity of a single stem cell to be followed (Nagano et al. 1999). The ability to visualize individual stem cells verified stem cell localization at the periphery of the tubule lumen (Nagano et al. 1999). Newly transplanted spermatogonia were shown to migrate to the basement membrane, where Sertoli cells extended processes to surround the germ cells (Parreira et al. 1998, 1999).

The transplantation assay has been used to identify purification methods that enrich for male GSCs within populations of spermatogonia. Positive selection for germ cells with high expression of the specific β-1 and α-6 integrins provided a 3- to 5-fold enrichment in transplantable GSCs from mouse testes (Shinohara et al. 1999). β-1 integrin expression also cosegregates with both epidermal and hematopoietic stem cell populations (Jones and Watt 1993; Potocnik et al. 2000). Similarly, selection for binding to laminin also enriched for germ cells capable of stem cell transplantation (Shinohara et al. 1999). A negative selection method utilizing cryptorchid mice, which have a high concentration of undifferentiated spermatogonia, as the transplant donors resulted in a dramatic 50-fold enrichment of transplantable stem cells over controls (Shinohara et al. 2000). Cryptorchidism induced by retention of the testis in the body cavity leads to reversible depletion of differentiating germ cells, apparently without detriment to the stem cell population. The ability to transplant mammalian germ-line stem cells coupled with the ability to persistently transfect GSCs with retroviral constructs raises the possibility of introducing genetic modifications into the male germ line for either animal transgenics or human gene therapy (Nagano et al. 2000).

MAINTAINING A BALANCE BETWEEN TWO STEM CELL FATES: ASYMMETRIC VERSUS SYMMETRIC DIVISION

Stem cell function is twofold: Stem cells must both maintain the stem cell population and give rise to differentiating cells. The mechanisms that maintain the balance between these two daughter cell fates are the crucial question in stem cell biology. Two prevailing models have been advanced to explain how stem cells give rise to progeny with two different cell fates (Watt and Hogan 2000). The first model proposes that stem cell divisions are asymmetric, ensuring that both cell populations are evenly maintained at every division. An asymmetric outcome upon stem cell division results in one daughter cell that self-renews stem cell identity and another cell that commits to differentiation. This model was first advanced nearly 100 years ago on the basis of cytomorphological evidence in grasshopper spermatogenesis (Davis 1908), then developed by further studies in the fruit fly (Harris 1929). The second model suggests that stem cells normally undergo symmetric divisions (Wilson 1925; Huckins 1971b). Symmetric stem cell divisions must alternate between proliferative divisions, producing two stem cells, and differentiating divisions, resulting in two cells that initiate differentiation (Fig. 2). For this discussion, these models focus on the *outcome* of stem cell division and do not specify whether the mechanisms for stem cell fate decisions are intrinsically determined or extrinsically controlled.

At present, the consensus on male germ-line stem cell division pattern is split between the fly and mammalian systems (de Rooij and Grootegoed 1998; Lin 1998). However, there is not enough evidence to rule out the possibility in either system that male germ-line stem cells normally undergo both asymmetric and/or symmetric divisions.

Fly

Male germ-line stem cells in *Drosophila* usually divide with an asymmetric outcome. As described above, asymmetric stem cell divisions were first proposed to explain the appearance of large, clonal populations obtained from male brood experiments (Harris 1929; Tihen 1946). More recently, the asymmetric outcome of GSC divisions was confirmed by lineage tracing: Single, marked germ cells persisted at the testis apical tip and continually gave rise to differentiated progeny (Fig. 5g,h) (Gönczy and DiNardo 1996). By this criterion, the somatic stem cells also undergo asymmetric divisions. Although it has not yet been analyzed in the male, symmetric proliferative divisions may be possible under conditions that induce stem cell expansion to replace lost stem cells, as was described in the *Drosophila* female germ line (Xie and Spradling 1998, 2000 and Chapter 7).

Both the germ-line stem cells and cyst progenitor cells divide radially within an inherently asymmetric microenvironment (Fig. 3b,c) (Smith and Dougherty 1976; Hardy et al. 1979; Lindsley and Tokuyasu 1980). The cell fates adopted by the two stem cell daughters correlate with their physical location with respect to the hub. Upon germ-line stem cell division, the daughter cell directly adjacent to the hub and enclosed by the cyst progenitor cells retains stem cell identity and self-renewal capacity. The daughter cell displaced away from the hub becomes enclosed in cyst cells and initiates differentiation. A similar spatial relationship between the germ cells and somatic apical cells has been described for the germinal proliferation center in other insects (for review, see Hannah-Alava 1965). The conserved organization and the correlation between physical position and fate suggest that extrinsic cues from surrounding support cells may be important for the asymmetric cell fate decisions made by the two daughters of each stem cell division (see below).

Mammals

It is not yet clear whether mammalian stem cell divisions are normally asymmetric. Historically, three different models have been advanced to explain how mammalian male germ line stem cells maintain steady state (for review, see Meistrich and van Beek 1993a). All models agree that the germ-line stem cells are rare, only 0.03% of the total germ cells. In addition, all models assume that stem cells maintain a steady state so that, despite continual cell division, stem cell numbers do not increase. The A_s model is currently the most widely accepted. According to this model, A_s spermatogonial stem cells usually undergo symmetric divisions (Wilson 1925; Huckins 1971b), resulting in either two self-renewing A_s spermatogonia or two interconnected A_{pr} spermatogonia that initiate differentiation. It is possible that the cell which gives rise to A_{pr} spermatogonia is analogous to the gonialblast in *Drosophila* rather than a true stem cell. The observed delays in spermatogenesis both after irradiation (Meistrich et al. 1978) and after transplantation (Parreira et al. 1998, 1999) indicate that stem cell expansion precedes initiation of differentiation, suggesting that male GSCs can divide symmetrically to produce two stem cells under these conditions.

MOLECULAR MECHANISMS OF STEM CELL REGULATION: ROLES FOR INTRINSIC VERSUS EXTRINSIC CONTROL

Mutational analysis can be used to identify genes that mediate normal stem cell behavior. Genes required for stem cell specification can be identified in screens for mutations that disrupt stem cell formation. Genes required for the cell fate decisions that specify stem cell self-renewal can be identified in screens for mutations that lead to premature stem cell loss (Fig. 6b). Likewise, genes required for the initiation of differentiation instead of stem cell self-renewal can be identified in screens for mutations that lead to unrestricted proliferation of stem cells (Fig. 6b).

According to the stem cell niche hypothesis, the microenvironment plays a crucial role in regulating stem cell behavior. If so, then genes that are expressed in surrounding somatic support cells that extrinsically regulate germ-line stem cell behavior and genes that act intrinsically within the GSCs are both likely to be required for normal stem cell function. A somatic role in germ-line maintenance was elegantly demonstrated by ablation experiments in the nematode (Kimble and White 1981). Subsequent genetic analysis revealed the underlying molecular mechanism (Henderson et al. 1994). Maintenance of gametogenesis in the nematode syncytial gonad requires expression of the Delta-related ligand *lag-2* in the somatic distal tip cell, which signals via the Notch-like receptor *glp-1* expressed in the germ line to maintain mitotic proliferation of germ cell nuclei (Austin and Kimble 1987). Without the signal from the distal tip cell, the germ cell nuclei cease proliferation and enter meiosis and terminal differentiation.

In both flies and mammals, somatic gonadal cells have been shown to provide important signals for post-stem-cell stages of spermatogenesis. Recent evidence demonstrates that signals from somatic cells also regulate the choice of GSC fates. The best current examples from each system suggest that counteracting signals are likely to balance the choice between stem cell self-renewal and differentiation.

Fly

In *Drosophila*, specification of somatic gonadal precursor cells under control of a genetic hierarchy of pattern formation genes is necessary for gonad coalescence and subsequent PGC development into germ-line stem cells (Boyle and DiNardo 1995; Boyle et al. 1997). Screens for zygotic genes required for germ cell migration and gonad formation have also identified additional genes that act in the soma (Moore et al. 1998). Although the somatic gonad can form in the absence of germ-line cells (Aboim 1945), the behavior of somatic cells is altered in agametic testes (Gönczy and DiNardo 1996). In testis lacking germ line, cyst cells continue to proliferate and can take on an altered identity. This suggests that cross-regulation between germ cells and somatic cells may coordinate normal germinal proliferation center function. Little is known about the mechanisms that regulate the transition from primordial germ cell to stem cell identity once the germ line is established in the gonad.

A small number of genes specifically required for function of *Drosophila* male germ-line stem cells have been identified from screens for viable, male-sterile mutants. However, since spermatogenic stem cell activity initiates at the end of embryogenesis, genes essential for embryonic viability cannot readily be assessed for effects on male GSC regulation if loss-of-function mutations are homozygous lethal. Chemical mutagenesis can produce specific alleles that affect only the male germ line, weak alleles, or conditional alleles (such as temperature-sensitive alleles) of essential genes to address their roles in spermatogonial stem cell regulation. In addition, production of homozygous mutant clones in otherwise heterozygous males by mitotic recombination (described above) can be used to make gonadal mosaics to test the role of essential genes. Furthermore, the ability to make marked mutant clones in the testis can be used to test whether genes required for GSC regulation act cell-autonomously in the germ line or non-cell-autonomously in surrounding somatic support cells.

Mutations in genes required for survival or maintenance of GSCs cause loss of germ-line renewal. This phenotype can be easily identified by phase microscopy of whole testes. Typically, mutations in which germ-line stem cells are initially active but are not maintained or become quiescent lead to testes with some differentiating spermatids but loss of the developmental gradient of early germ cells at the apical tip (Fig. 7a,b). Phenotypes can range from few to many sperm, depending on whether a mutation affects establishment of stem cell identity or continual stem cell self-renewal upon division. Additional phenotypic analysis using molecular markers (as in Fig. 5) can then distinguish whether loss of early germ cell differentiation is due to loss of germ-line stem cells, stem cell quiescence, or cell death. Mutants representing all of these classes have been isolated in mutagenesis screens and are currently being characterized.

Mutations in the *Drosophila* gene *piwi* cause loss of renewing germ line in both male and female flies (Lin and Spradling 1997). Males homozygous for *piwi* mutations exhibit tiny testes with a nearly complete absence of spermatogenesis. Piwi protein is normally expressed in the early male germ cells as well as somatic hub and cyst cells (Cox et al.

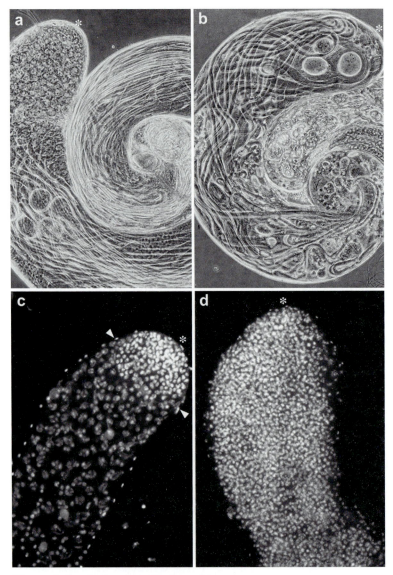

Figure 6 (See facing page for legend.)

2000). Although the male phenotype has not been examined in detail, *piwi* has been shown to be required for both the maintenance and division kinetics of *Drosophila* female GSCs. Wild-type *piwi* function appears to be required both in somatic cells and in the germ line for normal female germ-line stem cell behavior (Cox et al. 1998, 2000). Proteins homologous to Piwi have been found in a wide range of organisms from plants to humans (Cox et al. 1998). The plant homologs, *zwille* and *argonaute*, both play similar roles in maintenance of the plant meristem (Bohmert et al. 1998; Moussian et al. 1998). Mutations in the *Drosophila* gene *escargot* also disrupt maintenance of spermatogenesis; however, a substantial number of sperm are produced before male germ-line stem cells are lost (G. Hime and M. Fuller, unpubl.). Expression of *escargot* mRNA in the testis is restricted to early germ cells and the somatic hub, consistent with either an intrinsic or extrinsic role in male germ-line stem cell maintenance.

An opposite phenotype results from mutation of genes required to specify the gonialblast fate instead of germ-line stem cell self-renewal or to specify further steps of differentiation instead of spermatogonial proliferation. Unrestricted GSC self-renewal or spermatogonial mitotic amplification at the expense of differentiation can be detected by staining for DNA, which reveals expansion of compact, brightly staining mitotic cells at the apical tip (Fig. 6c,d). Overproliferation of stem cells or gonialblasts can be easily distinguished from overproliferation of interconnected spermatogonia using the gene expression, subcellular structure, and cell division behavior markers described above (Fig. 5).

Figure 6 Mutational analysis of *Drosophila* male germ-line stem cell behavior. (*a*) Phase microscopy image of a testis from a wild-type adult containing all stages of spermatogenesis, evidence of continual regeneration due to stem cell activity. Apical tip (*asterisk*). (*b*) Phase microscopy image of a testis from an adult homozygous for a mutation in a gene required for normal stem cell self-renewal, resulting in differentiation and eventual loss of the GSCs. The gradient of round early germ cells including the stem cells is no longer present at the apical tip (*asterisk*), with only sperm bundles remaining. (*c*) Testis from a wild-type adult stained with a fluorescent DNA dye. Testis shows the normal gradient of more compact, brightly staining mitotic germ cells at the apical tip (*asterisk* to *arrowheads*) followed by the more diffusely staining differentiating germ cells. (*d*) Testis from an adult mutant for *Egfr* function and stained for DNA. The testis is filled with mitotic germ cells at the expense of differentiation, seen as the expansion of brightly staining cells throughout the testis.

Genetic analysis has identified several *Drosophila* genes (*bam, bgcn, punt, schnurri*) that control the decision to exit the spermatogonial divisions at the 16-cell stage (Gönczy et al. 1997; Matunis et al. 1997). Function of two genes (*punt* and *schnurri*) is required in the somatic cyst cells to restrict spermatogonial proliferation, indicating extrinsic regulation of germ cell amplification divisions (Matunis et al. 1997). Similar extrinsic mechanisms may limit the proliferative capacity of amplifying progenitors in other lineages, such as the amplifying keratinocytes in the skin or the myeloid progenitors in the bone marrow (Fuchs and Segre 2000; Weissman 2000; Chapter 19).

Recent evidence suggests that a signal(s) from somatic cyst cells also restricts GSC self-renewal and allows differentiation of the gonialblast, thus ensuring that male germ-line stem cell divisions have an asymmetric outcome. Mutations in two different genes suggest that wild-type function of the epidermal growth factor receptor pathway is required in somatic cyst cells for the normal choice of GSC fates (Kiger et al. 2000; Tran et al. 2000). Conditional loss of function of either the *Egfr* or *raf* genes results in a massive increase in the number of early germ cells, including the GSCs and spermatogonia (Fig. 6c,d). In both mutants, many of the accumulated GSCs maintain expression of GSC markers outside of their normal niche alongside the hub or cyst progenitor cells. Accumulation of GSCs and spermatogonia is associated with a block in their differentiation, as no new spermatocytes are observed. Germ-line clones of either *Egfr* or *raf* null alleles demonstrated that wild-type function of these genes was not required in the germ line itself to allow germ-line differentiation. Cyst cell clones homozygous for mutant *raf* resulted in unrestricted proliferation of the encysted germ cells, which still contained a wild-type copy of the *raf* gene (Tran et al. 2000). These results suggest that cyst cells play a guardian role to ensure that upon GSC division, one daughter cell down-regulates the ability to self-renew stem cell identity and adopts a gonialblast fate.

Mammals

In mammals, mutations that cause germ cell depletion or early arrest of spermatogenesis are characterized initially by a "Sertoli-cell only" phenotype—atrophic tubules with few germ cells. The absence of renewing germ line can indicate a failure in germ cell specification, migration, gonad formation, or maintenance of the stem cells. Several genes are known to act extrinsically for primordial germ cell survival; for example, the growth factors LIF and OncM (Hara et al. 1998). The *Dominant white spotting* (W) and Steel (Sl) receptor–ligand pair are both needed for proper primordial germ cell proliferation and migration. Mutations in either gene result in reduced numbers of primordial germ cells in the embryonic gonad (Russell 1979; Yoshinaga et al. 1991). Interestingly, the *W* and *Sl* mutations also affect the proliferation and migration of erythropoietic and melanocytic precursors (Russell 1979). Chimera experiments testing where c-Kit and Sl function for normal germ cell development demonstrated that the receptor is only required to act in germ cells, whereas the ligand functions in the soma (Nakayama et al. 1988). Although their molecular identity or mechanism of action is not yet known, the Hertwig's anemia (*an*) and atrichosis (*at*) genes are also required for primordial germ cell survival and gonocyte development. Mice mutant for either the *an* or *at* genes have few germ cells due to germ cell death in the embryonic gonad (Chubb and Desjardins 1984; Russell et al. 1985). Finally, disruption of the growth factor BMP8b gene, which is normally expressed in early germ cells, results in a reduction in the number of spermatogonial stem cells established in the embryonic gonad, causing a delay in initiation of spermatogenesis (Zhao et al. 1996).

In other examples, loss of renewing germ line follows relatively normal germ cell specification, gonad formation, and occasionally an initial wave of spermatogenesis. However, the presently known mouse mutations that cause depletion of early germ cells all appear to affect a similar stage just downstream of the stem cells, and not stem cell self-renewal directly (de Rooij et al. 1999). Five distinct situations appear to cause developmental arrest at the switch from undifferentiated A-type spermatogonia (A_{al}) into differentiating-type spermatogonia, resulting in proliferation but not accumulation of undifferentiated A-type spermatogonia in mouse or rat testes (de Rooij et al. 1999; Meistrich et al. 2000). These situations include (1) mutations in the mouse genes *Steel* or *W* (Sl^{17H}, Sl^d, and W^f alleles) (Koshimizu et al. 1992; de Rooij et al. 1999; Ohta et al. 2000); (2) mutation of the mouse gene *juvenile spermatogonial depletion (jsd)* (Beamer et al. 1988; Mizunuma et al. 1992; de Rooij et al. 1999); (3) conditions of vitamin A deficiency (Huang and Hembree 1979; van Pelt et al. 1995; de Rooij et al. 1999); (4) cryptorchidism (Nishimune and Haneji 1981; de Rooij et al. 1999); and (5) inhibition by intratesticular testosterone after radiation or other toxicant exposures (Meistrich et al. 2000). Colonization of recipient testes with donor GSCs transplanted from *Sl* mutant or cryptorchid mice demonstrated that functional spermatogonial stem cells are in fact retained in these conditions where later stages of differentiating germ cells are depleted (Ohta et al. 2000; Shinohara et al. 2000).

Somatic cells in the testis play an important regulatory role in spermatogenesis, although most hormones and cytokines tested exhibit either pre- or post-spermatogonial effects (Desjardins and Ewing 1993). Less is known about the possible role of somatic cells in regulating spermatogonial stem cell behavior. Recently, the level of glial-cell-line-derived neurotrophic factor (GDNF) produced in Sertoli cells was implicated in regulation of spermatogonial stem cell fate decisions (Meng et al. 2000). Reduction in GDNF function disrupted stem cell maintenance, causing stem cell loss due to differentiation. Conversely, overexpression of GDNF from a transgene construct blocked early germ cell differentiation, resulting in unrestricted proliferation of stem cells and spermatogonia.

Transplantation experiments can be used in mammals to address whether genes that regulate germ-line stem cell behavior are required in the germ line or the somatic lineages. Transplantation of male germ cells between sterile W/W^v and Sl/Sl^d mutant mice demonstrated W is required in germ cells and Sl is required in the soma (Ogawa et al. 2000), in agreement with previous evidence from chimeric mice. Sl/Sl^d mutant germ cells lacking functional ligand were successfully transplanted into sterile W/W^v mutant recipient testes lacking functional receptor (Fig. 7c,d), giving rise to Sl/Sl^d-derived fertile sperm.

The cyclic nature of mammalian spermatogenesis in a given region of seminiferous tubules suggests that reentry into or exit from GSC proliferation must be regulated at distinct stages of the epithelial cycle. An inhibitory activity in testicular extracts capable of blocking the stem cell proliferation that normally reinitiates during mouse epithelial stages II and III has been reported (Clermont and Mauger 1974), possibly derived from the differentiating spermatogonia. Interestingly, the inhibitory factor was tissue- but not species-specific, suggesting that a conserved, testis-specific factor may regulate the timing of GSC divisions. More dramatic regulation of spermatogonial proliferation is seen in certain other seasonally breeding vertebrates, such as the shark (Callard et al. 1989).

Aberrations leading to germ cell neoplasia reveal important points of normal germ-line regulation in humans. Gonadoblastomas occur when PGCs fail to populate the embryonic gonad, such as in XY females, demonstrating the importance of somatic–germ cell interactions in restricting proliferation of GSC precursors (for review, see Pringle and Page 1997). Adult male germ cell tumors may derive from latent gonocytes that transformed into carcinomas in situ (CIS) (de Rooij 1998), suggesting that the developmental transition from a gonocyte to an established male GSC is a critical regulatory step.

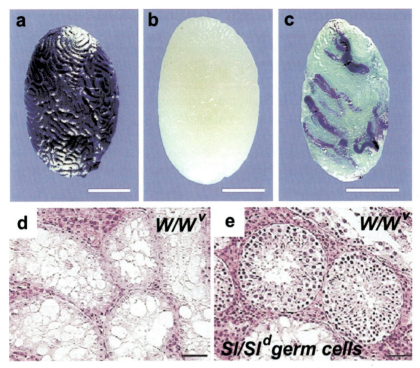

Figure 7 Transplantation of mouse male germ-line stem cells. (*a*) Whole testis from adult ROSA26 transgenic mouse with ubiquitous *lacZ* activity (*blue*) used as donor cells. (*b*) Whole testis from adult mouse without the *lacZ* transgene used as recipient host, demonstrating host cells do not stain. (*c*) Recipient testis 2 months after colonization of transplanted GSCs expressing *lacZ*. Donor-derived colonies of spermatogenesis appear as blue regions within the otherwise white seminiferous tubules of the host. (*d*) Cross-section of a tubule from an adult, sterile *W/W^v* mouse testis used as recipient host. Tubules lack spermatogenesis and contain mostly Sertoli cells. (*e*) Spermatogenesis is now evident in most tubules from an adult *W/W^v* mouse testis 1 year after transplantation of GSCs from a sterile *Sl/Sl^d* donor mouse. The *Sl/Sl^d* germ cells, although originally unable to undergo spermatogenesis in the *Sl/Sl^d* donor strain, are able to produce fertile sperm in the *W/W^v* somatic host environment. (*a*, *b*, *c*, Reprinted, with permission, from Shinohara et al. 1999 [© National Academy of Sciences]; *d*, *e* modified, with permission, from Ogawa et al. 2000.)

SUMMARY AND OUTLOOK

The male germ line offers a powerful system in which to study central questions in stem cell biology. Male germ-line stem cells have been identified in situ, allowing analysis of the role of surrounding somatic support cells in regulation of stem cell behavior. Analysis of male germ-line stem cell behavior in *Drosophila* and mammals has revealed striking parallels. The ability to combine genetic screens with well-developed descriptive analysis in both these organisms promises functional identification of genes and regulatory pathways that regulate critical aspects of stem cell biology. The ability to construct mosaic animals by germ cell transplantation in mammals or mosaic analysis in *Drosophila* allows tests of whether crucial genes control stem cell behavior by intrinsic or extrinsic mechanisms. In *Drosophila*, powerful genetic tools and the availability of the full genome sequence allow rapid identification of molecules controlling stem cell behavior. In mice, the ability to construct knockout and conditional knockout mutations allows tests of the role of candidate genes in stem cell function. These tools, and the possibility that genes identified by forward genetics in *Drosophila* may have functional homologs that can be tested in mammals, promise to reveal fundamental principles and underlying molecular pathways that may govern stem cell specification, self-renewal, and differentiation in a variety of stem cell systems.

ACKNOWLEDGMENTS

The authors acknowledge work from the laboratories whose data are included in the chapter figures, and we appreciate information provided by Ralph Brinster at the time of writing. We greatly appreciate comments on the manuscript from Marvin Meistrich, Cordula Schulz, and David Traver.

REFERENCES

Aboim A.N. 1945. Dévelopment embryonnaire et postembryonnaire des gonades normales et agamétique de *Drosophila melanogaster. Rev. Suisse Zool.* **52:** 53–154.

Austin J. and Kimble J. 1987. glp-1 is required in the germ line for regulation of the decision between mitosis and meiosis in *C. elegans. Cell* **51:** 589–599.

Bardin W.C., Gunsalus G.L., and Cheng C.Y. 1993. The cell biology of the Sertoli cell. In *Cell and molecular biology of the testis* (ed. C. Desjardins and L.L. Ewing), pp. 189–219. Oxford University Press, Oxford, United Kingdom.

Beamer W.G., Cunliffe-Beamer T.L., Shultz K.L., Langley S.H., and Roderick T.H. 1988. Juvenile spermatogonial depletion (jsd): A genetic defect of germ cell proliferation of male mice. *Biol. Reprod.* **38:** 899–908.

Bohmert K., Camus I., Bellini C., Bouchez D., Caboche M., and Benning C. 1998. AGO1 defines a novel locus of *Arabidopsis* controlling leaf development. *EMBO J.* **17:** 170–180.

Boyle M. and DiNardo S. 1995. Specification, migration and assembly of the somatic cells of the *Drosophila* gonad. *Development* **121:** 1815–1825.

Boyle M., Bonini N., and DiNardo S. 1997. Expression and function of clift in the devel-

opment of somatic gonadal precursors within the *Drosophila* mesoderm. *Development*
124: 971–982.

Brinster R.L. and Avarbock M.R. 1994. Germline transmission of donor haplotype following spermatogonial transplantation. *Proc. Natl. Acad. Sci.* **91:** 11303–11307.

Brinster R.L. and Zimmermann J.W. 1994. Spermatogenesis following male germ-cell
transplantation (comments). *Proc. Natl. Acad. Sci.* **91:** 11298–11302.

Brower D.L., Smith R.J., and Wilcox M. 1981. Differentiation within the gonads of
Drosophila revealed by immunofluorescence. *J. Embryol. Exp. Morphol.* **63:** 233–242.

Callard G., Mak P., DuBois W., and Cuevas M.E. 1989. Regulation of spermatogenesis:
The shark testis model. *J. Exp. Zool. Suppl.* **2:** 23–34.

Chubb C. and Desjardins C. 1984. Testicular function and sexual activity in senescent
mice. *Am. J. Physiol.* **247:** E569–573.

Clermont Y. 1972. Kinetics of spermatogenesis in mammals: Seminiferous epithelium
cycle and spermatogonial renewal. *Physiol. Rev.* **52:** 198–236.

Clermont Y. and Mauger A. 1974. Existence of a spermatogonial chalone in the rat testis.
Cell Tissue Kinet. **7:** 165–172.

Clermont Y. and Perey B. 1957. Quantitative study of the cell population of the seminiferous tubules of immature rats. *Am. J. Anat.* **100:** 241–268.

Clermont Y. and Trott M. 1969. Duration of the cycle of the seminiferous epithelium in
the mouse and hamster determined by means of 3H-thymidine and radioautography.
Fertil. Steril. **20:** 805–817.

Cooper K.W. 1950. Normal spermatogenesis in *Drosophila*. In *Biology of* Drosophila (ed.
M. Demerec), pp. 1–61. Wiley, New York.

Cox D.N., Chao A., and Lin H. 2000. *piwi* encodes a nucleoplasmic factor whose activity
modulates the number and division rate of germline stem cells. *Development* **127:**
503–514.

Cox D.N., Chao A., Baker J., Chang L., Qiao D., and Lin H. 1998. A novel class of evolutionarily conserved genes defined by *piwi* are essential for stem cell self-renewal.
Genes Dev. **12:** 3715–3727.

Davis H.P. 1908. Spermatogenesis in the *Acrididae* and *Locustidae*. *Bull. Mus. Comp.
Zool. (Harv. Univ.)* **53:** 59–158.

de Rooij D.G. 1998. Stem cells in the testis. *Int. J. Exp. Pathol.* **79:** 67–80.

de Rooij D.G. and Grootegoed J.A. 1998. Spermatogonial stem cells. *Curr. Opin. Cell.
Biol.* **10:** 694–701.

de Rooij D.G., Okabe M., and Nishimune Y. 1999. Arrest of spermatogonial differentiation in jsd/jsd, Sl17H/Sl17H, and cryptorchid mice. *Biol. Reprod.* **61:** 842–847.

Desjardins C. and Ewing L.L. 1993. *Cell and molecular biology of the testis.* Oxford
University Press, Oxford, United Kingdom.

Dym M. and Clermont Y. 1970. Role of spermatogonia in the repair of the seminiferous
epithelium following x-irradiation of the rat testis. *Am. J. Anat.* **128:** 265–282.

Dym M. and Fawcett D.W. 1970. The blood-testis barrier in the rat and the physiological
compartmentation of the seminiferous epithelium. *Biol. Reprod.* **3:** 308–326.

———. 1971. Further observations on the numbers of spermatogonia, spermatocytes, and
spermatids connected by intercellular bridges in the mammalian testis. *Biol. Reprod.*
4: 195–215.

Everett N.B. 1943. Observational and experimental evidences relating to the origin and
differentiation of the definitive germ cells in mice. *J. Exp. Zool.* **92:** 49–91.

Ewing L.L. and Keeney D.S. 1993. Leydig cell: Structure and function. In *Cell and molecular biology of the testis* (ed. C. Desjardins and L.L. Ewing), pp. 137–165. Oxford

University Press, Oxford, United Kingdom.

Fouquet J.P. and Dadoune J.P. 1986. Renewal of spermatogonia in the monkey (*Macaca fascicularis*). *Biol. Reprod.* **35:** 199–207.

Fuchs E. and Segre J.A. 2000. Stem cells: A new lease on life. *Cell* **100:** 143–155.

Fuller M.T. 1993. Spermatogenesis. In *The development of* Drosophila melanogaster (ed. M. Bate and A. Martinez Arias), vol. 1, pp. 71–147. Cold Spring Harbor Laboratory Press, Cold Spring Harbor, New York.

Geigy R. 1931. Action de l'ultraviolet sur le pôle germinal dans l'oeuf de *Drosophila melanogaster*. *Rev. Suisse Zool.* **38:** 187–288.

Gilula N.B., Fawcett D.W., and Aoki A. 1976. The Sertoli cell occluding junctions and gap junctions in mature and developing mammalian testis. *Dev. Biol.* **50:** 142–168.

Ginsburg M., Snow M.H., and McLaren A. 1990. Primordial germ cells in the mouse embryo during gastrulation. *Development* **110:** 521–528.

Gönczy P. 1995. "Towards a molecular genetic analysis of spermatogenesis in *Drosophila.*" Ph.D. thesis. The Rockefeller University, New York.

Gönczy P. and DiNardo S. 1996. The germ line regulates somatic cyst cell proliferation and fate during *Drosophila* spermatogenesis. *Development* **122:** 2437–2447.

Gönczy P., Matunis E., and DiNardo S. 1997. *bag-of-marbles* and *benign gonial cell neoplasm* act in the germline to restrict proliferation during *Drosophila* spermatogenesis. *Development* **124:** 4361–4371.

Gonczy P., Viswanathan S., and DiNardo S. 1992. Probing spermatogenesis in *Drosophila* with P-element enhancer detectors. *Development* **114:** 89–98.

Hadley M.A. and Dym M. 1987. Immunocytochemistry of extracellular matrix in the lamina propria of the rat testis: Electron microscopic localization. *Biol. Reprod.* **37:** 1283–1289.

Hannah-Alava A. 1965. The premeiotic stages of spermatogenesis. Adv. Genet. **13:** 157–226.

Hara T., Tamura K., de Miguel M.P., Mukouyama Y., Kim H., Kogo H., Donovan P.J., and Miyajima A. 1998. Distinct roles of oncostatin M and leukemia inhibitory factor in the development of primordial germ cells and sertoli cells in mice. *Dev. Biol.* **201:** 144–153.

Hardy R.W., Tokuyasu K.T., Lindsley D.L., and Garavito M. 1979. The germinal proliferation center in the testis of *Drosophila melanogaster*. *J. Ultrastruct. Res.* **69:** 180–190.

Harris B.B. 1929. The effects of aging of X-rayed males upon mutation frequency in *Drosophila*. *J. Hered.* **20:** 299–302.

Harrison D.A. and Perrimon N. 1993. Simple and efficient generation of marked clones in *Drosophila*. *Curr. Biol.* **3:** 424–433.

Hartl D.L. and Green M.M. 1970. Genetic studies of germinal mosaicism in *Drosophila melanogaster* using the mutable wc gene. *Genetics* **65:** 449–456.

Hecht N.B. 1993. Gene expression during male germ cell development. In *Cell and molecular biology of the testis* (ed. C. Desjardins and L.L. Ewing), pp. 400–432. Oxford University Press, Oxford, United Kingdom.

Henderson S.T., Gao D., Lambie E.J., and Kimble J. 1994. *lag-2* may encode a signaling ligand for the GLP-1 and LIN-12 receptors of *C. elegans*. *Development* **120:** 2913–2924.

Hilscher B., Hilscher W., Bulthoff-Ohnolz B., Kramer U., Birke A., Pelzer H., and Gauss G. 1974. Kinetics of gametogenesis. I. Comparative histological and autoradiographic studies of oocytes and transitional prospermatogonia during oogenesis and prespermatogenesis. *Cell Tissue Res.* **154:** 443–470.

Hinton B.T. and Turner T.T. 1993. The seminiferous tubular microenvironment. In *Cell and molecular biology of the testis* (ed. C. Desjardins and L.L. Ewing), pp. 238–265. Oxford University Press, Oxford, United Kingdom.

Huang H.F. and Hembree W.C. 1979. Spermatogenic response to vitamin A in vitamin A deficient rats. *Biol. Reprod.* **21:** 891–904.

Huckins C. 1963. Changes in gonocytes at the time of initiation of spermatogenesis in the rat. *Anat. Rec.* **145:** 243.

———. 1971a. The spermatogonial stem cell population in adult rats. II. A radioautographic analysis of their cell cycle properties. *Cell Tissue Kinet.* **4:** 313–334.

———. 1971b. The spermatogonial stem cell population in adult rats. III. Evidence for a long-cycling population. *Cell Tissue Kinet.* **4:** 335–349.

Huckins C. and Oakberg E.F. 1978. Morphological and quantitative analysis of spermatogonia in mouse testes using whole mounted seminiferous tubules. II. The irradiated testes. *Anat. Rec.* **192:** 529–542.

Jones P.H. and Watt F.M. 1993. Separation of human epidermal stem cells from transit amplifying cells on the basis of differences in integrin function and expression. *Cell* **73:** 713–724.

Jones R.C. and Lin M. 1993. Spermatogenesis in birds. *Oxf. Rev. Reprod. Biol.* **15:** 233–264.

Kerkis J. 1933. Development of gonads in hybrids between *Drosophila melanogaster* and *D. simulans*. *J. Exp. Zool.* **66:** 477–509.

Kiger A.A., White-Cooper H., and Fuller M.T. 2000. Somatic support cells restrict germ line stem cell self-renewal and promote differentiation. *Nature* **407:** 750–754.

Kimble J.E. and White J.G. 1981. On the control of germ cell development in *Caenorhabditis elegans*. *Dev. Biol.* **81:** 208–219.

King R.C. 1970. *Ovarian development in* Drosophila melanogaster. Academic Press, New York.

King R.C. and Akai H. 1971. Spermatogenesis in *Bombyx mori*. I. The canal system joining sister spermatocytes. *J. Morphol.* **124:** 143–166.

Koshimizu U., Watanabe D., Tajima Y., and Nishimune Y. 1992. Effects of W (c-kit) gene mutation on gametogenesis in male mice: Agametic tubular segments in Wf/Wf testes. *Development* **114:** 861–867.

Koshimizu U., Nishioka H., Watanabe D., Dohmae K., and Nishimune Y. 1995. Characterization of a novel spermatogenic cell antigen specific for early stages of germ cells in mouse testis. *Mol. Reprod. Dev.* **40:** 221–227.

Lawson K.A., Dunn N.R., Roelen B.A., Zeinstra L.M., Davis A.M., Wright C.V., Korving J.P., and Hogan B.L. 1999. Bmp4 is required for the generation of primordial germ cells in the mouse embryo. *Genes Dev.* **13:** 424–436.

Leblond C.P. and Clermont Y. 1952a. Definition of the stages of the cycle of the seminiferous epithelium in the rat. *Ann. N.Y. Acad. Sci.* **55:** 548–573.

———. 1952b. Spermiogenesis of rat, mouse, hamster and guinea pig as revealed by the "periodic acid-fuchsin sulfurous acid" technique. *Am. J. Anat.* **90:** 167–215.

Lee T. and Luo L.1999. Mosaic analysis with a repressible cell marker for studies of gene function in neuronal morphogenesis. *Neuron* **22:** 451–461.

Li C. and Gudas L.J. 1997. Sequences 5′ of the basement membrane laminin beta 1 chain gene (LAMB1) direct the expression of beta-galactosidase during development of the mouse testis and ovary. *Differentiation* **62:** 129–137.

Lin H. 1997. The tao of stem cells in the germline. *Annu. Rev. Genet.* **31:** 455–491.

———. 1998. The self-renewing mechanism of stem cells in the germline. *Curr. Opin. Cell. Biol.* **10:** 687–693.

Lin H. and Spradling A.C. 1997. A novel group of *pumilio* mutations affects the asymmetric division of germline stem cells in the *Drosophila* ovary. *Development* **124:** 2463–2476.

Lin H., Yue L., and Spradling A.C. 1994. The *Drosophila* fusome, a germline-specific organelle, contains membrane skeletal proteins and functions in cyst formation. *Development* **120:** 947–956.

Lin M. and Jones R.C. 1992. Renewal and proliferation of spermatogonia during spermatogenesis in the Japanese quail, *Coturnix coturnix japonica. Cell Tissue Res.* **267:** 591–601.

Lindsley D.T. and Tokuyasu K.T. 1980. Spermatogenesis. In *The genetics and biology of Drosophila* (ed. M. Ashburner and T.R.F. Wright), vol. 20, pp. 225–294. Academic Press, London.

Loeffler M. and Potten C.S. 1997. Stem cells and cellular pedigrees—A conceptual introduction. In *Stem cells* (ed. C.S. Potten), pp. 1–27. Academic Press, London.

Lok D., Jansen M.T., and D.G. de Rooij. 1983. Spermatogonial multiplication in the Chinese hamster. II. Cell cycle properties of undifferentiated spermatogonia. *Cell Tissue Kinet.* **16:** 19–29.

Matsui Y., Zsebo K., and Hogan B.L. 1992. Derivation of pluripotential embryonic stem cells from murine primordial germ cells in culture. *Cell* **70:** 841–847.

Matunis E., Tran J., Gönczy P., Caldwell K., and DiNardo S. 1997. *punt* and *schnurri* regulate a somatically derived signal that restricts proliferation of committed progenitors in the germline. *Development* **124:** 4383–4391.

McKearin D. and Ohlstein B. 1995. A role for the *Drosophila* Bag-of-marbles protein in the differentiation of cystoblasts from germline stem cells. *Development* **121:** 2937–2947.

Meistrich M.L. and van Beek M.E.A.B. 1993. Spermatogonial stem cells. In *Cell and molecular biology of the testis* (ed. C. Desjardins and L.L. Ewing), pp. 266–295. Oxford University Press, Oxford, United Kingdom.

———. 1993b. Spermatogonial stem cells: Assessing their survival and ability to produce differentiated cells. In *Methods in toxicology* (ed. R.E. Chapin and J. Heindel), vol. 3A, pp. 106–123. Academic Press, New York.

Meistrich M.L., Wilson G., Kangasniemi M., and Huhtaniemi I. 2000. Mechanism of protection of rat spermatogenesis by hormonal pretreatment: Stimulation of spermatogonial differentiation after irradiation. *J. Androl.* **21:** 464–469.

Meistrich M.L., Hunter N.R., Suzuki N., Trostle P.K., and Withers H.R. 1978. Gradual regeneration of mouse testicular stem cells after exposure to ionizing radiation. *Radiat. Res.* **74:** 349–362.

Meng X., Lindahl M., Hyvonen M.E., Parvinen M., de Rooij D.G., Hess M.W., Raatikainen-Ahokas A., Sainio K., Rauvala H., Lakso M., Pichel J.G., Westphal H., Saarma M., and Sariola H. 2000. Regulation of cell fate decision of undifferentiated spermatogonia by GDNF. *Science* **287:** 1489–1493.

Mintz B. and Russell E.S. 1957. Gene-induced embryological modifications of primordial germ cells in the mouse. *J. Exp. Zool.* **134:** 207–237.

Mizunuma M., Dohmae K., Tajima Y., Koshimizu U., Watanabe D., and Nishimune Y. 1992. Loss of sperm in juvenile spermatogonial depletion (jsd) mutant mice is ascribed to a defect of intratubular environment to support germ cell differentiation. *J. Cell Physiol.* **150:** 188–193.

Moore L.A., Broihier H.T., Van Doren M., Lunsford L.B., and Lehmann R. 1998. Identification of genes controlling germ cell migration and embryonic gonad formation in *Drosophila. Development* **125:** 667–678.

Moussian B., Schoof H., Haecker A., Jurgens G., and Laux T. 1998. Role of the ZWILLE gene in the regulation of central shoot meristem cell fate during *Arabidopsis* embryogenesis. *EMBO J.* **17:** 1799–1809.

Nagano M., Avarbock M.R., and Brinster R.L. 1999. Pattern and kinetics of mouse donor spermatogonial stem cell colonization in recipient testes. *Biol. Reprod.* **60:** 1429–1436.

Nagano M., Shinohara T., Avarbock M.R., and Brinster R.L. 2000. Retrovirus-mediated gene delivery into male germ line stem cells. *FEBS Lett.* **475:** 7–10.

Nakayama H., Kuroda H., Onoue H., Fujita J., Nishimune Y., Matsumoto K., Nagano T., Suzuki F., and Kitamura Y. 1988. Studies of Sl/Sld in equilibrium with +/+ mouse aggregation chimaeras. II. Effect of the steel locus on spermatogenesis. *Development* **102:** 117–126.

Nishimune Y. and Haneji T. 1981. Testicular DNA synthesis in vivo: Comparison between unilaterally cryptorchid testis and contralateral intact testis in mouse. *Arch. Androl.* **6:** 61–65.

Oakberg E.F. 1956. A description of spermiogenesis in the mouse and its use in analysis of the cycle of the seminiferous epithelium and germ cell renewal. *Am. J. Anat.* **99:** 391–414.

———. 1971. Spermatogonial stem-cell renewal in the mouse. *Anat. Rec.* **169:** 515–531.

Ogawa T., Dobrinski I., Avarbock M.R, and Brinster R.L. 2000. Transplantation of male germ line stem cells restores fertility in infertile mice. *Nat. Med.* **6:** 29–34.

Ohta H., Yomogida K., Dohmae K., and Nishimune Y. 2000. Regulation of proliferation and differentiation in spermatogonial stem cells: The role of c-kit and its ligand SCF. *Development* **127:** 2125–2131.

Orth J.M. 1982. Proliferation of Sertoli cells in fetal and postnatal rats: A quantitive autoradiographic study. *Anat. Rec.* **203:** 485–492.

Orth J.M. 1993. Cell biology of testicular development in the fetus and neonate. In *Cell and molecular biology of the testis* (ed. C. Desjardins and L.L. Ewing), pp. 3–57. Oxford University Press, Oxford, United Kingdom.

Parreira G.G., Ogawa T., Avarbock M.R., Franca L.R., Brinster R.L., and Russell L.D. 1998. Development of germ cell transplants in mice. *Biol. Reprod.* **59:** 1360–1370.

Parreira G.G., Ogawa T., Avarbock M.R., Franca L.R., Hausler C.L., Brinster R.L., and Russell L.D. 1999. Development of germ cell transplants: Morphometric and ultrastructural studies. *Tissue Cell* **31:** 242–254.

Phillips D.M. 1970. Insect sperm: Their structure and morphogenesis. *J. Cell. Biol.* **44:** 243–277.

Poirie M., Niederer E., and Steinmann-Zwicky M. 1995. A sex-specific number of germ cells in embryonic gonads of *Drosophila. Development* **121:** 1867–1873.

Potocnik A.J., Brakebusch C., and Fässler R. 2000. Fetal and adult hematopoietic stem cells require 1 integrin function for colonizing fetal liver, spleen, and bone marrow. *Immunity* **12:** 653–663.

Pringle M.J. and Page D.C. 1997. Somatic and germ cell sex determination in the developing gonad. In *Infertility in the male* (ed. L.I. Lipshultz and S.S. Howards), pp. 3–22.

Mosby, St. Louis, Missouri.

Pudney J. 1995. Spermatogenesis in nonmammalian vertebrates. *Microsc. Res. Tech.* **32:** 459–497.

Ravindranath N., Dalal R., Solomon B., Djakiew D., and Dym M. 1997. Loss of telomerase activity during male germ cell differentiation. *Endocrinology* **138:** 4026–4029.

Resnick J.L., Bixler L.S., Cheng L., and Donovan P.J. 1992. Long-term proliferation of mouse primordial germ cells in culture. *Nature* **359:** 550–551.

Rongo C., Broihier H.T., Moore L., Van Doren M., Forbes A., and Lehmann R. 1997. Germ plasm assembly and germ cell migration in *Drosophila. Cold Spring Harbor Symp. Quant. Biol.* **62:** 1–11.

Roussel J.D., Parrott M.W., and Tuttle L.W. 1969. A preliminary study of injury and recovery of the male germinal epithelium and spermatogenesis in *Macaca mulatta* following whole body cobalt-60 gamma irradiation. *J. Reprod. Fertil.* **18:** 177–178.

Russell E.S. 1979. Hereditary anemias of the mouse: A review for genetics. *Adv. Genet.* **20:** 357–459.

Russell E.S., McFarland E.C., and Peters H. 1985. Gametic and pleiotropic defects in mouse fetuses with Hertwig's macrocytic anemia. *Dev. Biol.* **110:** 331–337.

Russell L.D., Tallon-Doran M., Weber J.E., Wong V., and Peterson R.N. 1983. Three-dimensional reconstruction of a rat stage V Sertoli cell: III. A study of specific cellular relationships. *Am. J. Anat.* **167:** 181–192.

Saffman E.E. and Lasko P. 1999. Germline development in vertebrates and invertebrates. *Cell Mol. Life Sci.* **55:** 1141–1163.

Schrans-Stassen B.H., van de Kant H.J., de Rooij D.G., and van Pelt A.M. 1999. Differential expression of c-kit in mouse undifferentiated and differentiating type A spermatogonia. *Endocrinology* **140:** 5894–5900.

Shamblott M.J., Axelman J., Wang S., Bugg E.M., Littlefield J.W., Donovan P.J., Blumenthal P.D., Huggins G.R., and Gearhart J.D. 1998. Derivation of pluripotent stem cells from cultured human primordial germ cells (erratum *Proc. Natl. Acad. Sci.* [1999] **96:**1162). *Proc. Natl. Acad. Sci.* **95:** 13726–13731.

Shinohara T., Avarbock M.R., and Brinster R.L. 1999. β_1- and α_6-integrin are surface markers on mouse spermatogonial stem cells. *Proc Natl. Acad. Sci.* **96:** 5504–5509.

———. 2000. Functional analysis of spermatogonial stem cells in Steel and cryptorchid infertile mouse models. *Dev. Biol.* **220:** 401–411.

Skinner M.K., Tung P.S., and Fritz I.B. 1985. Cooperativity between Sertoli cells and testicular peritubular cells in the production and deposition of extracellular matrix components. *J. Cell. Biol.* **100:** 1941–1947.

Smith P.A. and Dougherty J.F. 1976. The premeiotic stages of spermatogenesis in *Drosophila melanogaster. Amer. Zool.* **16:** 189.

Sonnenblick B.P. 1941. Germ cell movements and sex determination of the gonads in the *Drosophila* embryo. *Proc. Natl. Acad. Sci.* **26:** 373–381.

Spangrude G.J., Heimfeld S., and Weissman I.L. 1988. Purification and characterization of mouse hematopoietic stem cells (erratum *Science* [1989] **244:**1030). *Science* **241:** 58–62.

Staab S., Heller A., and Steinmann-Zwicky M. 1996. Somatic sex-determining signals act on XX germ cells in *Drosophila* embryos. *Development* **122:** 4065–4071.

Stern C. 1941. The growth of the testes in *Drosophila*: I. The relation between vas deferens and testis within various species. *J. Exp. Zool.* **87:** 113–158.

Tam P.P. and Snow M.H. 1981. Proliferation and migration of primordial germ cells during compensatory growth in mouse embryos. *J. Embryol. Exp. Morphol.* **64:** 133–147.

Tegelenbosch R.A. and de Rooij D.G. 1993. A quantitative study of spermatogonial multiplication and stem cell renewal in the C3H/101 F1 hybrid mouse. *Mutat. Res.* **290:** 193–200.

Tihen J.A. 1946. An estimate of the number of cell generations preceding sperm formation in *Drosophila melanogaster. Am. Nat.* **80:** 389–393.

Tran J., Brenner T.J., and DiNardo S. 2000. Somatic control over the germline stem cell lineage during *Drosophila* spermatogenesis. *Nature* **407:** 764–757.

Upadhyay S.N. and Guraya S.S. 1973. Histochemical studies on the spermatogenesis of some telecost fishes. *Acta. Anat.* **86:** 484–514.

van Dissel-Emiliani F.M., de Boer-Brouwer M., Spek E.R., van der Donk J.A., and de Rooij D.G. 1993. Survival and proliferation of rat gonocytes in vitro. *Cell Tissue Res.* **273:** 141–147.

van Haaster L.H. and de Rooij D.G. 1994. Partial synchronization of spermatogenesis in the immature Djungarian hamster, but not in the immature Wistar rat. *J. Reprod. Fertil.* **101:** 321–326.

van Pelt A.M., van Dissel-Emiliani F.M., Gaemers I.C., van der Burg M.J., Tanke H.J., and de Rooij D.G. 1995. Characteristics of A spermatogonia and preleptotene spermatocytes in the vitamin A-deficient rat testis. *Biol. Reprod.* **53:** 570–578.

Watt F.M. and Hogan B.L. 2000. Out of Eden: Stem cells and their niches. *Science* **287:** 1427–1430.

Weissman I.L. 2000. Stem cells: Units of development, units of regeneration, and units in evolution. *Cell* **100:** 157–168.

Wilson E.B. 1925. *The cell in development and heredity.* Macmillan, New York.

Wylie C. 1999. Germ cells. *Cell* **96:** 165–174.

Xie T. and Spradling A.C. 1998. decapentaplegic is essential for the maintenance and division of germline stem cells in the *Drosophila* ovary. *Cell* **94:** 251–260.

Xie T. and Spradling A.C. 2000. A niche maintaining germline stem cells in the *Drosophila* ovary. *Science* **290:** 328–330.

Xu T. and Rubin G.M. 1993. Analysis of genetic mosaics in developing and adult *Drosophila* tissues. *Development* **117:** 1223–1237.

Yoshinaga K., Nishikawa S., Ogawa M., Hayashi S., Kunisada T., and Fujimoto T. 1991. Role of *c-kit* in mouse spermatogenesis: Identification of spermatogonia as a specific site of *c-kit* expression and function. *Development* **113:** 689–699.

Zamboni L. and Merchant H. 1973. The fine morphology of mouse primordial germ cells in extragonadal locations. *Am. J. Anat.* **137:** 299–335.

Zhao G.Q., Deng K., Labosky P.A., Liaw L., and Hogan B.L. 1996. The gene encoding bone morphogenetic protein 8B is required for the initiation and maintenance of spermatogenesis in the mouse. *Genes Dev.* **10:** 1657–1669.

9
Primordial Germ Cells as Stem Cells

Brigid Hogan
Department of Cell Biology
Vanderbilt University School of Medicine
Nashville, Tennessee 37232

Germ cells are the precursors of the mature gametes, making their status as stem cells apparently unassailable. The fusion of the gametes to produce a totipotent zygote initiates the whole program of embryonic development, leading to the formation of the stem cells of all adult tissues as well as the next generation of germ cells. Focusing on mammals, in this review, I examine how germ cells arise and whether their precursors are stem cells in their own right. I also discuss how the study of germ cells and their precursors sheds light on the important questions of what controls pluripotency and how genomes are reprogrammed. For the purposes of this review, I define stem cells as a cell population that has the capacity both to self-renew and to give rise to at least one kind of nondividing, fully differentiated descendant.

The germ cell lineage usually originates as a very small founding population that is segregated from somatic cells early in development, at least in organisms where the overall body plan is also established early (Dixon 1994). Perhaps the physical separation of germ cells from organizing centers helps to protect them from the influence of potent signaling factors and morphogenetic movements. In vertebrates and *Drosophila,* there is considerable proliferation of the founding population as it moves from its site of origin to the gonads. The term primordial germ cells (PGCs) is strictly applied to the diploid germ cell precursors that transiently exist in the embryo before they enter into close association with the somatic cells of the gonad and become irreversibly committed as germ cells. Male and female PGCs are indistinguishable, and in mammals both will finally stop dividing and enter into meiosis when associated with the somatic cells of the ovary, or even with tissues such as the adrenal gland outside the gonads. However, in the testis, PGCs behave differently, since they come under the influence of the XY gonadal cells that produce a short-range, diffusible, meiosis-inhibiting factor. Male PGCs therefore normally undergo mitotic arrest in G_1 as prospermatogonial stem cells that do not divide again until puberty (for review, see McLaren 1994; Sassone-Corsi 1997). Some limited proliferation of spermatogonial stem cells can be obtained in culture (Nagano et al. 1998). Therefore, the mammalian germ line consists of two distinct stem cell populations, the transient population of PGCs outside the gonad and the spermatogonial stem cells within, that self-renew and differentiate into sperm throughout the fertile life of the adult male (Fig. 1).

THE ORIGIN OF PRIMORDIAL GERM CELLS: INHERITANCE OF CYTOPLASMIC DETERMINANTS VERSUS INDUCTION BY EXTRINSIC FACTORS

In most organisms studied, but with several exceptions including mammals and birds (Dixon 1994), the segregation of pluripotent germ cells from somatic cells involves maternal factors or determinants. These are deposited in the cytoplasm of the egg and during cleavage are asymmetrically segregated into a small number of blastomeres that subsequently differentiate into PGCs. Germ cell determinants are complexes of RNA

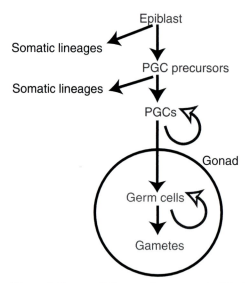

Figure 1 Germ cell lineage in mammals. Pluripotent cells (that express *Oct4*) are shown. Stem cell self-renewal is shown as a curved arrow. In the gonad only the male germ cells constitute a stem cell population; oocytes do not proliferate.

and protein that have been best characterized in *Caenorhabditis elegans* (where they associate into organelles called P granules) and in *Drosophila* (where they constitute the polar granules or pole plasm). For example, in *Drosophila*, components include oskar, nanos, vasa, and tudor. Ectopic expression of oskar in the *Drosophila* blastula is sufficient to initiate the formation of ectopic germ cells. However, in *C. elegans*, P granule components are necessary but not sufficient for the specification of germ cells (for review, see Ephrussi and Lehmann 1992; Hubbard and Greenstein 2000). Very little is known about the way in which germ plasm components regulate gene expression and cell behavior in germ cell precursors (for review, see Wylie 1999). In *C.elegans*, zygotic gene expression and possibly mRNA stability are repressed in germ-line blastomeres by at least one P granule component (the protein PIE-1) (for review, see Seydoux and Strome 1999). Other gene products, for example, the polycomb group MES proteins, are involved in transcriptional silencing at the level of chromatin structure. One hypothesis, therefore, is that a number of independent repression mechanisms protect germ cells in *C. elegans* from responding to signals that normally restrict the developmental options of somatic cell lineages. By shutting down gene expression, the germ cell lineage is kept pluripotential (for discussion, see Dixon 1994).

The properties and behavior of germ plasm in *Xenopus*, and similarities with *Drosophila* polar granules, have been thoroughly discussed previously (Wylie 1999). Homologs of vasa, a component of *Drosophila* polar granules, have recently been identified in zebrafish primordial germ cells (Braat et al. 1999; Weidinger et al. 1999).

Mammals and chick (Ginsberg 1994) apparently do not have maternally derived germ cell determinants. Mouse genes that encode homologs of *Drosophila* polar granule components, for example, vasa (*Mvh*) and germ cell-less (*Gcl*), are not expressed in PGCs but in adult male germ cells (Fujiwara et al. 1994; Leatherman et al. 2000). If maternally encoded germ plasm is absent from mammals, what regulates PGC formation? The current idea is that PGC precursors are induced in the embryo by secreted signaling factors produced by adjacent extraembryonic cells. It is still possible that the localized production of these inducing factors is under the control of maternal determinants segregated to extraembryonic cells, but this hypothesis has not yet been tested.

To enable critical evaluation of the induction of PGCs, a brief description of early mouse development is in order (Fig. 2). At around the time of implantation (~4.0–4.5 days post coitum, dpc) the blastocyst consists of two populations of cells; an outer epithelial layer of trophoblast

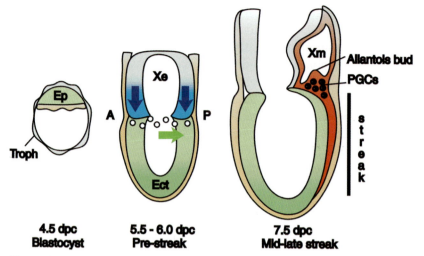

Figure 2 Model for the development of PGCs in the mouse embryo. At 4.5 dpc the blastocyst consists of an outer layer of trophoblast (Troph) surrounding the epiblast (Ep; *green*) and the primitive or visceral endoderm (*orange*). By 5.5–6.0 dpc, the epiblast has given rise to the embryonic ectoderm (Ect) and the trophoblast has formed the extraembryonic ectoderm (Xe). Signals from the Xe, for example BMP4 and probably BMP8b (*blue arrows*), are thought to induce PGC precursors (*open circles*) in the proximal epiblast. These move from anterior to posterior (A–P; *green arrow*). By 7.5 dpc, mesoderm has been generated (*red*) in the primitive streak and extraembryonic region (Xm). Descendants of the PGC precursors are allocated to either the extraembryonic mesoderm or PGC (*filled circles*) lineages.

cells that surrounds a tightly packed cluster of undifferentiated inner cell mass (ICM) cells. The ICM subsequently differentiates into an inner epiblast or embryonic ectoderm population and an outer primitive or extraembryonic visceral endoderm. After implantation, all cell types proliferate rapidly and the trophoblast forms a knob-like mass of cells known as the extraembryonic ectoderm, and the epiblast cells become organized into a cup-shaped epithelium. There is a clear morphological demarcation or junction between the epiblast and the extraembryonic ectoderm, and lineage analysis strongly suggests there is no mixing of cells between the two tissues after about 4.0 dpc. Around 6.0 dpc, the embryo begins to undergo gastrulation. Proximal epiblast cells move posteriorly, lose their epithelial organization, and give rise to unpolarized mesodermal cells. The first cells to delaminate from the epiblast give rise to extraembryonic mesoderm, whereas cells that drop out later give rise to embryonic mesoderm in the primitive streak. As described in detail below, the first time PGCs can be clearly distinguished from somatic cells in the mouse embryo is around 7.5 dpc. A cluster of about 45–50 cells that express high levels of the genes encoding tissue nonspecific alkaline phosphatase (TNAP) and the OCT4 transcription factor can be identified posterior to the primitive streak at the base of the allantois. They are surrounded by somatic mesoderm cells that express much lower levels of these markers (see Anderson et al. 2000).

Several lines of evidence show that PGCs arise from cells in the epiblast, although the precise time at which the PGC progenitors are committed to their fate has not been determined. The first evidence comes from the elegant lineage analysis experiments of Kirstie Lawson (Lawson and Hage 1994). She injected single cells in the epiblast at the prestreak (pregastrulation) and early streak stages with a fluorescent lineage marker and then cultured the embryos for 40 hours and determined the location of labeled descendants. Analysis showed that PGCs (as judged by alkaline phosphatase staining) were derived from cells originally located in the proximal region of the prestreak epiblast, dispersed within about three cell diameters of the junction with the extraembryonic ectoderm. A crucial finding was that no injected epiblast cells gave rise to PGCs alone. Cells that generated labeled PGCs also gave rise to labeled cells in the extraembryonic mesoderm (most frequently allantois, but also amnion and extraembryonic mesoderm of the yolk sac). This finding showed that the so-called PGC precursor cell population must generate descendants committed to either the extraembryonic mesoderm or the germ cell lineages. It is thought that this allocation takes place when the precursors are posterior to the primitive streak at around 7.5 dpc, but nothing is known about the mechanisms involved. For example, the process may be stochastic and cell-autonomous or influenced by extrinsic factors. It may involve lateral inhibition, or asymmetric cell division and the localization of zygotic (rather than maternal) gene products to the PGC lineage. One limitation of the cell lineage analysis described above is that it does not say anything about the time at which the PGC precursors are first set aside. It only tells us that they already exist at 6.0 dpc in the prestreak epiblast. The process leading to the generation of the precursors could have been initiated significantly earlier.

The fact that PGC precursors are located in the epiblast close to the junction with the extraembryonic ectoderm suggests that this environment contains factors inducing PGC precursor fate. To test this hypothesis, Tam and Zhou (1996) carried out an embryonic grafting experiment. They isolated clumps of 5–20 distal epiblast cells from early streak stage embryos of a reporter transgenic line that expresses β-galactosidase constitutively in all cells. The pieces were then grafted close to the junction with the extraembryonic ectoderm of wild-type, early streak stage (6.5 dpc) embryos, and the chimeric embryos were cultured in vitro. Analysis of these embryos showed many lacZ-positive cells in the extraembryonic and posterior mesoderm. In a very small number of embryos a few PGCs could be found that coexpressed alkaline phosphatase and β-galactosidase. This important experiment indicated that distal embryonic ectoderm cells, which would normally have developed into anterior ectoderm or neurectoderm, can change in response to exogenous signals and acquire more ventral posterior cell fates, including that of PGCs. However, it does not reveal the whole window of time when induction of PGC precursors normally takes place; it only tells us that the inducing activity is still available at the early streak stage. In fact, it may be that induction occurs over an extended period of time, with some epiblast cells receiving sufficient inducing signal early, even at the blastocyst stage, and others not until 6.5 dpc.

If mouse or human blastocysts are grown in vitro, the ICM can give rise to pluripotential embryonic stem (ES) cell lines that can both self-renew indefinitely and give rise to multiple cell types in culture. When mouse ES cells are injected into a blastocyst, they mix with the ICM cells and contribute to all the tissues of the embryo except for the trophoblast and extraembryonic ectoderm or extraembryonic visceral endoderm. Some of the ES cells are able to differentiate along the germ cell lineage. Since the ES cells have undergone extensive proliferation in culture, this finding argues strongly against maternally inherited factors in the epiblast or ICM playing a role in germ cell determination in mammals. However, the results again shed no light on when or how the induction of the germ cell precursors first takes place.

EVIDENCE THAT FACTORS PRODUCED BY THE TROPHOBLAST OR EXTRAEMBRYONIC ECTODERM PLAY A ROLE IN MAMMALIAN GERM-LINE DEVELOPMENT

The experiments described above suggest that germ-line-inducing factors are present near the junction between the trophoblast and ICM or extraembryonic ectoderm and epiblast. The first evidence for the nature of the factors came from the observation that embryos homozygous null for the gene encoding the transforming growth factor β (TGFβ)-related growth factor, bone morphogenetic protein 4 (BMP4), completely lack both an allantois (assessed morphologically) and PGCs (assessed by staining for either alkaline phosphatase or the carbohydrate antigen,

SSEA-1 [Lawson et al. 1999; N.R. Dunn and B.L.M. Hogan, unpubl.]).
Bmp4 is first expressed at high levels in the extraembryonic ectoderm and
only later in the extraembryonic mesoderm cells in the allantois and posterior primitive streak surrounding the PGCs (Lawson et al. 1999). *Bmp4*
is not expressed in the founding population of PGCs. The early expression pattern of *Bmp4* suggests that the protein secreted by the extraembryonic ectoderm induces cells in the proximal epiblast to assume the fate
of PGC/allantois precursors. The finding that wild-type ES cells cannot
rescue the mutant phenotype, even when they contribute more than 90%
of the cells in chimeric embryos, supports this hypothesis. Finally, *Bmp4*
heterozygous embryos have a significantly smaller founding population
of PGCs than normal, even though, once formed, the cells proliferate at
the same rate as wild-type PGCs. This is consistent with a model in which
BMP4 produced by the extraembryonic ectoderm acts in a dose-dependent manner to control the fate of the pluripotent proximal epiblast cells.
According to this model, epiblast cells that receive the highest dose of
BMP4 over the longest period have a high probability of becoming PGC
precursors, whereas cells receiving a lower dose are more likely to give
rise to extraembryonic or lateral mesoderm.

Further experiments are needed to distinguish between this model
and alternatives. For example, rather than acting instructively, BMP4 may
function simply as a permissive factor, maintaining the survival of PGC
precursors segregated by a different mechanism. One prediction of the
instructive or morphogen model is that in *Bmp4* homozygous mutants
(and in mutants of genes encoding receptors or components of downstream signaling pathways), the fate of cells in the proximal epiblast,
including those that normally give rise to PGC precursors, is changed to
more dorsal/anterior cell types. Another prediction is that BMP protein
should induce PGC precursors in isolated epiblasts. However, it is possible that BMP4 is necessary but not sufficient for inducing PGC precursors, and that additional factors, including ones made by the visceral
endoderm, are required. Recent data suggest that at least one factor
secreted by the extraembryonic ectoderm functions in collaboration with
BMP4 to control PGC development. This is the related protein, BMP8b,
made exclusively by the extraembryonic ectoderm at this stage of development (Ying et al. 2000). BMP8b may act independently as a homo-
dimer or possibly form biologically active heterodimers with BMP4,
although the data do not support the hypothesis that such heterodimers are
obligatory for PGC precursor formation. Finally, it is not yet known
whether BMP4 and BMP8b act directly on the epiblast, or indirectly
through the extraembryonic endoderm.

Further analysis of the role of cell–cell interactions in early PGC development would be greatly facilitated by the development of specific molecular markers both for PGC precursors before they have moved into the posterior primitive streak and for the descendants of these precursors that have differentiated along the PGC lineage.

CHARACTERISTICS OF MAMMALIAN PGCs BEFORE THEY REACH THE GONAD AND MAINTENANCE OF THE PLURIPOTENT STATE

The founding population of PGCs of the 7.5-dpc mouse embryo under-goes two important processes en route to their final resting place in the gonads. The cells proliferate, and they migrate along the endoderm of the hind gut, through the mesentery and into the genital ridges. Most PGCs have reached the ridges at 11.5 dpc, and proliferation ceases by about 13.5 dpc. Migration is common to germ cells of several organisms; e.g., *Drosophila*, *Xenopus*, zebrafish, and chick. However, since it is not obvi-ously relevant to the stem cell status of PGCs, it will not be considered further here, and readers are referred to other reviews and papers (Wylie 1999; Anderson et al. 2000; Bendel-Stenzel et al. 2000). It should be noted, however, that chick PGCs migrate to the gonads via the blood-stream (Ginsberg 1994), but no intravascular PGCs have been seen in mammals, even though their migration route carries them near major blood vessels.

Proliferation increases the number of PGCs in the embryo from around 150 at 8.5 dpc to about 25,000 by 13.5 dpc (Tam and Snow 1981), giving a population doubling time of about 16 hours. It is not known whether the number of cell divisions undergone by each PGC in vivo is invariant.

Unlike hematopoietic stem cells, there are still very few molecular markers characteristic of mammalian PGCs. Indeed, no gene is yet known that is exclusively expressed in PGCs and PGC precursors. The markers that are most frequently used to distinguish PGCs after about 7.5–8.5 dpc are TNAP (MacGregor et al. 1995), stage-specific embryonic antigen-1 (SSEA1, a complex surface carbohydrate), and OCT4 (a POU-domain transcription factor).

OCT4 (encoded by the *Pou5f1* gene in mice and also known as OCT3/4) is of particular interest because it appears to be a key regulator of the pluripotential phenotype. It is expressed in all the cells of the cleav-age-stage embryo and late-stage morula, but switched off in the tro-phoblast, and remains active in the embryonic ectoderm and primitive endoderm until gastrulation. It is then gradually down-regulated in the derivatives of the embryonic ectoderm and endoderm, and by 8.5 dpc is only expressed in the PGCs. It is finally extinguished in the germ line when the PGCs begin to differentiate in the gonad, only to be reactivated as the gametes reach maturity (Pesce et al. 1998). This pattern of expression led to the hypothesis that OCT4 is a guardian of the pluripotential phenotype and prevents cells from becoming restricted in their developmental potential. This idea is supported by the observation that *Pou5f1* null embryos lack an inner cell mass and consist entirely of trophoblast cells (Nichols et al. 1998). More recent studies have suggested that the precise level of *Pou5f1* expression in undifferentiated ES cells regulates their differentiation in vitro (Niwa et al. 2000). Intermediate levels of OCT4 protein appear to favor the pluripotential, undifferentiated phenotype, whereas low levels promote the differentiation of ES cells into trophoblast, and high levels into endoderm and mesoderm. It is thought that OCT4 maintains the undifferentiated state by regulating gene transcription in collaboration with coactivators such as SOX2 or ROX-1. High levels of these cofactors may be maintained by signaling through the IL-6/LIF (leukemia inhibitory factor) receptor subunit, gp130, mediated by STAT-3 activation. As described in the next section, LIF is a cytokine that was recognized for its ability to maintain the undifferentiated state of ES cells in vitro. However, homozygous null *Lif* mutant embryos develop normally, so that if gp130 signaling plays a role in vivo, it must be activated by LIF-related cytokines. Obviously, an important goal is to identify genes up- or down-regulated by OCT4 in pluripotential epiblast cells and PGCs in vivo. One candidate is *Fgf4* (Ambrosetti et al. 1997); another is *Kit* (see below). It is noteworthy that OCT4 appears to regulate gene expression in mammalian PGCs rather differently from pole plasm determinants in *C.elegans*, which apparently function by generally repressing gene expression in the PGCs.

   Mammalian PGCs are distinguished from somatic cells by a number of genome-wide modifications. Normally, during preimplantation development, zygotic DNA is demethylated, except at sites associated with allele-specific parental imprinting (Monk et al. 1987). Remethylation occurs in somatic cells before gastrulation, but the PGCs (and presumably their precursors) do not undergo this epigenetic modification. In addition, PGCs go one step further and remove the methylation of parentally imprinted loci that persists in somatic cells (Kato et al. 1999). This reprogramming appears to occur gradually, as the PGCs migrate to the genital ridges, and is completed by 13.5 dpc. New imprints are subsequently added during germ cell maturation. Erasure of parental imprinting in PGCs has two consequences. First, PGCs that have not yet begun their differentiation into mature germ cells are unique in having no modification of their genome at all, at least at the level of DNA methylation (Kato et al. 1999). This may be necessary to erase the epigenetic influences or modifications of the parents and to restore the totipotency of the germ line. Second, PGCs late in the migratory pathway or just arrived in the gonad have a different phenotype from PGCs at 13.5 dpc. It could therefore be argued that the proliferation phase of PGCs does not strictly speaking involve a self-renewal, but rather the rapid amplification of a transitional precursor population.

Another difference in genomic modification between PGCs and somatic cells is the fact that female PGCs avoid random inactivation of their X chromosomes, at least during the early stages of their existence (Tam et al. 1994). Both X chromosomes are active in the epiblast until shortly before gastrulation, when a wave of random X inactivation goes through the population (Tan et al. 1993). However, at the earliest time they can be recognized, which is posterior to the primitive streak and in the hindgut endoderm, most PGCs still have two active X chromosomes. By the time they have reached the gonad, however, most have asynchronously undergone X inactivation. The X chromosomes are then reactivated before the onset of meiosis. Understanding how the PGCs initially avoid X inactivation will provide important information about the mechanism of germ-line specification at the genomic level.

PROLIFERATION OF PGCs

At least three different extracellular ligand/receptor signaling systems have been identified that promote the survival and proliferation of PGCs. These are (1) stem cell factor and its tyrosine kinase receptor, (2) bFGF and FGF receptors, and (3) cytokines of the interleukin/LIF family and their receptors that signal through a common gp130 subunit.

Stem cell factor (SCF, also known as Steel factor and mast cell growth factor) encoded by the *Mgf* (formerly *Steel*) locus, and its transmembrane tyrosine kinase receptor, c-KIT, encoded by the *Kit* (formerly *W*) gene, were first identified as growth factors for PGCs from genetic analysis in the mouse. *Mgf* is expressed in the somatic cells through which the PGCs migrate, whereas *Kit* is expressed by the PGCs themselves, at least until a few days after arrival in the genital ridge when it is down-regulated (Bendel-Stenzel et al. 2000; Manova and Bachvarova 1991).

A role for FGFs and receptors (e.g., FGFR1 and 2) in promoting PGC proliferation was first suggested from experiments in which purified bFGF was added to cells in culture (Matsui et al. 1992; Resnick et al. 1998). Whether FGFs play a role in vivo is not known, but *Fgf 3,4, 5,* and

8 genes are variously expressed in the epiblast, posterior primitive streak, and mesoderm along the migration route of the PGCs.

Other factors that promote the survival and proliferation of PGCs in vitro are leukemia inhibitory factor (LIF), oncostatin M (OSM), interleukin-6 (IL-6), and ciliary neurotrophic factor (CNTF), all members of the IL-6/LIF cytokine family (Cheng et al. 1994; Koshimizu et al. 1996; Hara et al. 1998 and references therein). These factors function through a dimeric transmembrane receptor expressed in PGCs. One subunit of the receptor (e.g., LIF receptor-β) binds specific ligands. The other is a common, non-ligand-binding subunit called glycoprotein 130 (gp130) that acts as a signal transducer by activating STAT-3. Antibodies to gp130 block the activity of LIF on PGCs (Koshimizu et al. 1996). LIF was first tested for its effect on PGCs in vitro because it promotes the undifferentiated, pluripotent phenotype of mouse ES cells in culture; in the absence of LIF and feeder cells, ES cells rapidly differentiate. As described in the previous section, recent studies suggest that LIF functions in combination with a specific level of OCT4 to maintain the undifferentiated phenotype. Signaling through gp130 is therefore likely to play a key role in maintaining the pluripotency and self-renewal ability of PGCs. However, despite the key role apparently played by LIF/gp130 in controlling the PGC phenotype, it is still unclear which member(s) of the ligand family functions in vivo, since mice lacking LIF, LIFRβ, and IL-6 all have normal numbers of PGCs (Koshimizu et al. 1996; Wylie 1999). Likewise, mutation of genes encoding IL-4 and IL-2R has no effect on PGC number even though IL-4 promotes the survival of PGCs in vitro (Cooke et al. 1996). The most likely explanation is that several interleukins regulate PGC proliferation and survival and can compensate for each other in vivo.

Finally, it is very likely that as-yet-unidentified growth factors influence PGC proliferation because optimal growth of the cells in vitro requires fibroblast cell feeder layers. The possible identity of some of these factors has been discussed previously (Bendel-Stenzel et al. 1998).

Although SCF, LIF, and FGF alone have some activity on PGC survival and proliferation in vitro, in combination they have a dramatic effect on the behavior of cells isolated before about 13.5 dpc. Rather than showing a finite number of cell doublings in vitro, the PGCs continue to proliferate indefinitely (Matsui et al. 1992; Resnick et al. 1992; Labosky et al. 1994a). Moreover, the PGCs change their phenotype to resemble pluripotent ES cells that are derived from the inner cell mass cells of the blastocyst. Precisely how this "transdifferentiation" from a PGC to ES cell phenotype is brought about is not known. Like ES cells, embryonic germ-cell-derived cell lines (known as EG cells) can differentiate extensively in culture and can contribute to all the tissues of the embryo, including the germ line, when injected into a host blastocyst (Labosky et al. 1994b; Stewart et al. 1994). However, many undifferentiated EG cells have differences in the methylation of imprinted loci compared with ES cells (Labosky et al. 1994b; Tada et al. 1997). This reflects the fact, discussed in the previous section, that PGCs remove allele-specific parental imprints as they migrate toward, and enter, the gonads. This phenotype is dominant, because if EG cells are fused with somatic cells (thymic lymphocyte), there is demethylation of several imprinted and non-imprinted genes in the somatic nuclei (Tada et al. 1997). It is not yet known whether human EG cell lines show differences in the methylation of imprinted loci (Shamblott et al. 1998).

A process similar to the transdifferentiation of PGCs to EG cells in vitro may occur during the rare in vivo development of teratocarcinomas in the testis of some strains of mice, e.g., 129/Sv. The frequency of testicular teratomas can be increased from about 1% to 95% in the 129/Sv strain by the introduction of the homozygous *Ter* mutation, but the identity of this modifier is not yet known (Asada et al. 1994). Teratomas can also be induced experimentally in vivo in mice by transplanting genital ridges to ectopic sites, or in some rodents from extraembryonic endoderm cells of the early yolk sac (Sobis and Vandeputte 1982). Evidence suggests that this reflects the transdifferentiation of endoderm cells, rather than proliferation of yolk sac cells that have remained undifferentiated.

WHAT CHANGES WHEN PGCs ENTER THE GONAD AND COME INTO CLOSE ASSOCIATION WITH SOMATIC CELLS? THE END OF THE ROAD FOR PGCs

When PGCs enter the genital ridge, they come into close association with somatic gonadal cells derived from the intermediate mesoderm, and after continuing proliferation for a few days, they differentiate into germ cells. By about 13.5 dpc, female PGCs are entering into the prophase of meiosis, while male germ cells go into mitotic arrest and do not resume mitosis until the onset of puberty.

In the mouse, there is a down-regulation of c-KIT receptors in germ cells in the gonad (Manova and Bachvarova 1991). This presumably plays a role in making the germ cells unresponsive to stem cell factor after they have entered the gonad. Since the formation of teratomas is rare, a whole variety of additional mechanisms probably operate normally to protect intragonadal PGCs from the influence of other mitogenic factors. These mechanisms also appear to operate in PGCs that fail to reach the gonad, since extragonadal teratomas, which are presumed without any direct evidence to be derived from PGCs, are also rare. As discussed earlier, PGCs that come to lie in the fetal adrenal gland cease proliferating and enter meiosis in the mouse (Francavilla and Zamboni 1985). However, experiments in which *Xenopus* PGCs were isolated from the mesentery, labeled in vitro, and then transplanted into the blastoceol cavity of host embryos provided evidence that under these conditions the cells could become incorporated into various tissues and differentiate into somatic cells such as muscle and notochord (Wylie et al. 1985). Analogous experiments in which in-vitro-labeled PGCs from 10.5-dpc mouse embryos were injected into blastocysts failed to show incorporation into either somatic tissues or the germ line (P. Donovan et al., pers. comm.). The ability of individual PGCs to change their fate in ectopic sites in vivo needs to be explored in more detail using robust genetic lineage markers.

In conclusion, PGCs constitute a stem cell population that plays important, evolutionarily conserved roles in germ-line development. The advantages of this population for the organism are that it expands the initially very small pool of germ cell precursors, moves them from extraembryonic regions to the gonads, and helps to ensure that the cells are protected from influences driving them down somatic lineages. The PGCs thus remain pluripotential until they come to the end of the road and differentiate into germ cells.

ACKNOWLEDGMENTS

I thank colleagues in my lab who have worked with such enthusiasm on PGCs, in particular Drs. Yasuhisa Matsui, Trish Labosky, N. Ray Dunn, and Takeshi Fujiwara. Thanks also to Molly Weaver for critical comments on the manuscript. I am an Investigator of the Howard Hughes Medical Institute.

REFERENCES

Ambrosetti D.-C., Basilico C., and Dailey L. 1997. Synergistic activation of the fibroblast growth factor 4 enhancer by Sox2 and Oct-3 depends on protein-protein interactions facilitated by a specific spatial arrangement of factor binding site. *Mol. Cell. Biol.* **17:** 6321–6329.

Anderson R., Copeland T.K., Scholer H., Heasman J., and Wylie C. 2000. The onset of germ cell migration in the mouse embryo. *Mech. Dev.* **91:** 61–68.

Asada Y., Varnum D.S., Frankel W.N., and Nadeau J.H. 1994. A mutation in the Ter gene causing increased susceptibility to testicular teratomas maps to mouse chromosome 18. *Nat. Genet.* **6:** 363–368.

Bendel-Stenzel M., Anderson R., Heasman J., and Wylie C. 1998. The origin and migration of primordial germ cells in the mouse. *Semin. Cell Dev. Biol.* **9:** 393–400.

Bendel-Stenzel M.R., Gomperts M., Anderson R., Heasman J., and Wylie C. 2000. The role of cadherins during primordial germ cell migration and early gonad formation in the mouse. *Mech. Dev.* **91:** 143–152.

Braat A.K., Zandbergen T., van de Water S., Goos H.J., and Zivkovic D. 1999. Characterization of zebrafish primordial germ cells: Morphology and early distribution of vasa RNA. *Dev. Dyn.* **216:** 153–167.

Cheng L., Gearing D.P., White L.S., Compton D.L., Schooley K., and Donovan P.J. 1994. Role of leukemia inhibitory factor and its receptor in mouse primordial germ cell growth. *Development* **120:** 3145–3153.

Cooke J.E., Heasman J., and Wylie C.C. 1996. The role of interleukin-4 in the regulation of mouse primordial germ cell numbers. *Dev. Biol.* **174:** 14–21.

Dixon K.E. 1994. Evolutionary aspects of primordial germ cell formation. *Ciba Found. Symp.* **182:** 92–119.

Ephrussi A. and Lehmann R. 1992. Induction of germ cell formation by oskar. *Nature* **358:** 387–392.

Francavilla S. and Zamboni L. 1985. Differentiation of mouse ectopic germinal cells in intra- and perigonadal locations. *J. Exp. Zool.* **233:** 101–109.

Fujiwara Y., Komiya T., Kawabata H., Sato M., Fujimoto H. Furusawa M., and Noce T. 1994. Isolation of a DEAD-family protein gene that encodes a murine homolog of *Drosophila* vasa and its specific expression in germ cell lineage. *Proc. Natl. Acad. Sci.* **91:** 12258–12262.

Ginsberg M. 1994. Primordial germ cell formation in birds. *Ciba Found. Symp.* **182:** 52–67.

Hara T., Tamura K., de Miguel M.P., Mukouyama Y., Kim H., Kogo H., Donovan P.J., and Miyajima A. 1998. Distinct roles of oncostatin M and leukemia inhibitory factor in the development of primordial germ cells and sertoli cells in mice. *Dev. Biol.* **201:** 144–153.

Hubbard E.J. and Greenstein D. 2000. The *Caenorhabditis elegans* gonad: A test tube for cell and developmental biology. *Dev. Dyn.* **218:** 2–22.

Kato Y., Rideout W.M., III, Hilton K., Barton S.C., Tsunoda Y., and Surani M.A. 1999. Developmental potential of mouse primordial germ cells. *Development* **126:** 1823–1832.

Koshimizu U., Taga T., Watanabe M., Saito M., Shirayoshi Y., Kishimoto T., and Nakatsuji N. 1996. Functional requirement of gp130-mediated signaling for growth and survival of mouse primordial germ cells in vitro and derivation of embryonic germ (EG) cells. *Development* **122:** 1235–1242.

Labosky P.A., Barlow D.P., and Hogan B.L.M. 1994a. Embryonic germ cell lines and their derivation from mouse primordial germ cells. *Ciba Found. Symp.* **182:** 157–178.

———. 1994b. Mouse embryonic germ (EG) cell lines: Transmission through the germline and differences in the methylation imprint of insulin-growth factor 2 receptor (Igf2r) gene compared with embryonic stem (ES) cell lines. *Development* **120:** 3197–3204.

Lawson K.A. and Hage W.J. 1994. Clonal analysis of the origin of primordial germ cells in the mouse. *Ciba Found. Symp.* **182:** 68–91.

Lawson K.A., Dunn N.R., Roelen B.A., Zeinstra L.M., Davis A.M., Wright C.V., Korving J.P., and Hogan B.L. 1999. Bmp4 is required for the generation of primordial germ cells in the mouse embryo. *Genes Dev.* **13:** 424–436.

Leatherman J.L., Kaestner K.H., and Jongens T.A. 2000. Identification of a mouse germ cell-less homologue with conserved activity in *Drosophila*. *Mech. Dev.* **92:** 145–153.

MacGregor G.R., Zambrowicz B.P., and Soriano P. 1995. Tissue non-specific alkaline phosphatase is expressed in both embryonic and extraembryonic lineages during mouse embryogenesis but is not required for migration of primordial germ cells. *Development* **121:** 1487–1496.

Manova K. and Bachvarova R.F. 1991. Expression of c-kit encoded at the W locus of mice in developing embryonic germ cells and presumptive melanoblasts. *Dev. Biol.* **146:** 312–324.

Matsui Y., Zsebo K., and Hogan B.L.M. 1992. Derivation of pluripotential embryonic stem cells from murine promordial germ cells in culture. *Cell* **70:** 841–847.

McLaren A. 1994. Germline and soma: Interactions during early mouse development. *Sem. Dev. Biol.* **5:** 43–49.

Monk M., Boubelik M., and Lehnert S. 1987. Temporal and regional changes in DNA methylation in the embryonic, extraembryonic and germ cell lineages during mouse embryo development. *Development* **99:** 371–382.

Nagano M., Avarbock M.R., Leonida E.B., Brinster C.J., and Brinster R.L. 1998. Culture of mouse spermatogonial stem cells. *Tissue Cell* **30:** 389–397.

Nichols J., Zevnik B., Anastassiadis K., Niwa H., Klewe-Nebenius D., Chambers I., Scholer H., and Smith A. 1998. Formation of pluripotent stem cells in the mammalian embryo depends on the POU transcription factor Oct4. *Cell* **95:** 379–391.

Niwa H., Miyazaki J., and Smith A.G. 2000. Quantitative expression of oct-3/4 defines differentiation, dedifferentiation or self-renewal of ES cells. *Nat. Genet.* **24:** 372–376.

Pesce M., Wang X., Wolgemuth D.J., and Schöler H. 1998. Differential expression of Oct-4 transcription factor during mouse germ cell differentiation. *Mech. Dev.* **71:** 89–98.

Resnick J.L., Bixler L.S., Cheng L., and Donovan P.J. 1992. Long-term proliferation of mouse primordial germ cells in culture. *Nature* **359:** 550–551.

Resnick J.L., Ortiz M., Keller J.R., and Donovan P.J. 1998. Role of fibroblast growth factors and their receptors in mouse primordial gem cell growth. *Biol. Reprod.* **59:** 1224–1229.

Sassone-Corsi P. 1997. Transcriptional checkpoints determining the fate of male germ cells. *Cell* **88:** 163–166.

Seydoux G. and Strome S. 1999. Launching the germline in *Caenorhabditis elegans:* Regulation of gene expression in early germ cells. *Development* **126:** 3275–3283.

Shamblott M.J., Axelman J., Wang S., Bugg S., Littlefield J.W., Donovan P.J., Blumenthal P.D., Huggins G.R., and Gearhart J.D. 1998. Derivation of pluripotent stem cells from cultured human primordial germ cells. *Proc. Natl. Acad. Sci.* **95:** 13726–13731.

Sobis H. and Vandeputte M. 1982. Development of teratomas from yolk sac of genetically sterile embryos. *Dev. Biol.* **92:** 553–556.

Stewart C.L., Gadi I., and Bhatt H. 1994. Stem cells from primordial germ cells can reenter the germ line. *Dev. Biol.* **161:** 626–628.

Tada M., Tada T., Lefebvre L., Barton S., and Surani M. 1997. Embryonic germ cells induce epigenetic reprogramming of somatic nucleus in hybrid cells. *EMBO J.* **16:** 6510–6520.

Tam P.P.L. and Snow M.H.L. 1981. Proliferation and migration of primordial germ cells during compensatory growth in mouse embryos. *J. Embryol. Exp. Morphol.* **64:** 133–147.

Tam P.P.L. and S.X. Zhou 1996. The allocation of epiblast cells to ectodermal and germ-line lineages is influenced by the position of the cells in the gastrulating mouse embryo. *Dev. Biol.* **178:** 124–132.

Tam P.P.L., Zhou S.X., and Tan S.-S. 1994. X-chromosome activity of the mouse primordial germ cells revealed by the expression of an X-linked *lac-Z* transgene. *Development* **120:** 2925–2932.

Tan S.-S., Williams E.A., and Tam P.P.L. 1993. X-chromosome inactivation occurs at different times in different tissues of the post-implantation mouse embryo. *Nat. Genet.* **3:** 170–174.

Weidinger G., Wolke U., Koprunner M., Klinger M., and Raz E. 1999. Identification of tissues and patterning events required for distinct steps in early migration of zebrafish primordial germ cells. *Development* **126:** 5295–5307.

Wylie C. 1999. Germ cells. *Cell* **96:** 165–174.

Wylie C.C., Heasman J., Snape A., O'Driscoll M., and Holwill S. 1985. Primordial germ cells of *Xenopus laevis* are not irreversibly determined early in development. *Dev. Biol.* **112:** 66–72.

Ying Y., Liu X.-M., Marble A., Lawson K.A., and Zhao G.-Q. 2000. Requirement of Bmp8b for the generation of primordial germ cells in the mouse. *Mol. Endocrinol.* **14:** 1053–1063.

10
Embryonic Stem Cells

Austin Smith
Centre for Genome Research
University of Edinburgh
Scotland, United Kingdom

Embryonic stem (ES) cells are pluripotent stem cell lines derived directly from early mouse embryos without use of immortalizing or transforming agents. They can be propagated as homogeneous stem cell cultures
and expanded without apparent limit. Unusually among established cell
lines, ES cells maintain a stable euploid karyotype. Yet more remarkably,
ES cells retain the character of embryo founder cells, even after prolonged culture and extensive manipulation. Thus, they are able to reinte-
grate fully into embryogenesis when returned to the early embryo.
Chimeric mice can be produced in which ES cell descendants are represented among all cell types, including functional gametes. ES cells are
also readily amenable to sophisticated genome engineering, in particular
via homologous recombination. These properties are widely exploited to
introduce gene knock-outs and other precise genetic modifications into
the mouse germ line.

The ability to propagate pluripotent ES cells presents unique opportunities for experimental analysis of gene regulation and function during
self-renewal, cell commitment, and differentiation. The combination of
intrinsic and extrinsic factors that maintain developmental identity and
potency is beginning to be defined. Progress is also being made toward
understanding and controlling lineage- and/or cell-type-specific differentiation of ES cells in vitro. When harnessed effectively, ES cell differentiation can provide defined cell populations for pharmacological testing
and cellular transplantation. Generation of ES cell equivalents from other
species, most particularly human, is now anticipated for realization of the
full power of ES cell technologies both as research tools and, ultimately,
as cell therapy reagents.

ORIGINS OF MOUSE EMBRYONIC STEM CELLS

Pluripotent Stem Cells in the Early Embryo

The mammalian fetus develops from a founder population of cells that are present before and shortly after implantation (Hogan et al. 1994). These cells are pluripotent, meaning that they are individually capable of giving rise to derivatives of each of the three primary germ layers and to germ cells. Initially defined as the entire internal cell component of the blastocyst, the inner cell mass (ICM), pluripotent cells are segregated to a subcompartment, the epiblast, prior to implantation. After implantation the epiblast expands rapidly to generate the cellular substrate for gastrulation and formation of the embyro proper. Once gastrulation commences, the epiblast cells (often termed primitive or embryonic ectoderm at this stage) progressively differentiate into definitive mesoderm, endoderm, and ectoderm. Pluripotent cells are thus succeeded by lineage-committed precursors in the fetus.

Although the possibility that rare pluripotent cells may persist cryptically within differentiated tissues has not been definitively excluded (Weissman 2000), the epiblast per se is clearly transient and does not appear to meet one of the conventional criteria for a stem cell population, persistence throughout the lifetime of the organism. However, a range of experimental interventions in mouse embryos have revealed that epiblast cells are highly plastic and that their self-renewal and differentiation are regulated according to the embryonic context. Thus, the ICM and epiblast can adjust to either the removal or addition of significant numbers of cells and still give rise to a normal fetus (Hogan et al. 1994). Indeed, this capacity to accommodate extra cells provides the foundation on which chimeric fetuses are produced (Gardner 1998). The destined tissue contribution of epiblast cells is dictated by their position in the egg cylinder at the onset of gastrulation (Beddington 1983; Lawson et al. 1991), but they can adopt new fates if grafted heterotopically (Beddington 1983; Tam and Zhou 1996). Most strikingly, if the early mouse embryo is removed from the uterus and the epiblast cells are grafted to a permissive ectopic site, such as the testis or kidney capsule of a syngeneic or immunocompromised mouse, they will generate large multidifferentiated tumors known as teratocarcinomas (Solter et al. 1970). Teratocarcinomas contain differentiated cell types of all germ layers and, in addition, an undifferentiated, proliferative component that can be maintained on serial transplantation. Teratocarcinomas can be produced at a high frequency from single epiblasts (Diwan and Stevens 1976), but not at all from postgastrulation embryos. The persistence and expansion of undifferentiated stem cells in embryo-derived teratocarcinomas indicates that mouse epiblast cells do in fact have an intrinsic potential for prolonged self-renewal.

Embryonal Carcinoma Cells

The undifferentiated component of teratocarcinoma is described as embryonal carcinoma due to its resemblance to early embryonic tissue. The propagation of this population can be maintained in explant culture, and continuous embryonal carcinoma, or EC, cell lines may be derived (Evans 1972). EC cells have several distinctive features (for review, see Martin 1980). In particular, they are often capable of multilineage differentiation. Crucially, this capacity is retained by clonal isolates (Kleinsmith and Pierce 1964; Martin and Evans 1975), formally establishing the presence of pluripotent stem cells. Along with evidence of similarities in immunophenotype and protein expression profile to the ICM/epiblast, this gave rise to the concept that EC cells are counterparts of normal pluripotent embryo cells. The finding that EC cells could participate in embryonic development and contribute to chimeric fetuses and, in some cases, even live offspring (Brinster 1974; Papaioannou et al. 1975; 1978), substantiated this notion. This ability demonstrates that the capacity of EC cells for extended self-renewal in teratocarcinomas or in culture does not represent an oncogenic transformation (Martin 1980). In this regard, it is noteworthy that the epiblast does not express G_1 cyclins (Wianny et al. 1998) and is therefore unlikely to be subject to normal cell cycle control mechanisms. The corollary of extrauterine teratocarcinoma development is that extended self-renewal of epiblast within the embryo is actively suppressed.

However, the derivation of EC cells via expansion in tumors, usually involving serial transfers, compromises their genetic constitution. Almost all have an aneuploid karyotype, and more subtle changes are also likely due to the pressure for selective growth advantage. Indeed, most EC cells show some restrictions in differentiation potential and in their ability to integrate normally into embryogenesis (Martin 1980). Consequently, their value as a developmental model is undermined, and they do not provide a suitable system for germ-line transgenesis.

Derivation of Embryonic Stem Cells

Studies with EC cells laid the intellectual and experimental groundwork for the establishment of "true" embryo stem cell cultures. A seminal point was the realization that pluripotency was best sustained in a coculture system. Martin and Evans observed that in primary cultures of teratocarcinoma, EC cells tended to thrive in proximity to differentiated cell types but to expand poorly in isolation. This prompted investigation of the potential of established cell lines to support EC cell propagation. Coculture with mitotically inactivated embryonic fibroblasts was found not only to allow the efficient establishment of EC cultures, but also to result in stem cells with high differentiation capacity (Martin and Evans 1975; Martin et al. 1977). It was reasoned that the fibroblasts were providing some critical nutrient or trophic factor support, hence they were described as "feeder" cells.

Feeders were employed in renewed efforts to establish cell cultures directly from cultured embryos (Hogan and Tilly 1977). In 1981, the derivation of pluripotent cell lines from mouse blastocysts was reported (Evans and Kaufman 1981; Martin 1981). The protocols for ES cell derivation are relatively simple (Robertson 1987). Embryros at the expanded blastocyst stage are plated, either intact or following immunosurgical isolation of the ICM, onto a feeder layer. Conventional tissue culture medium is supplemented with 2-mercaptoethanol and 10–20% fetal calf serum. After several days of culture, epiblast outgrowths are disaggregated and replated onto fresh feeders. Various types of differentiated colonies arise along with colonies of undifferentiated morphology (Robertson 1987). The latter are individually dissociated and replated. If secondary colonies of undifferentiated cells arise, these can generally be expanded further, and continuous ES cell lines can be established.

Factors Influencing ES Cell Derivation

Establishing an ES cell culture entails the liberation of pluripotent epiblast cells from their fated differentiation. Prior induction of diapause (implantation delay) appears to enhance the efficiency of ES cell generation (Robertson 1987). This may be attributable to an increase in epiblast cell numbers during diapause (Evans and Kaufman 1983), although this is relatively modest. Perhaps more likely is that the arrest of normal development pre-configures the epiblast cells for continued self-renewal by activating dependency on cytokine signaling for maintenance of pluripotency (J. Nichols and A.G. Smith, in prep.). The process by which a state of continuous self-renewal is arrived at is not automatic, however, and is poorly understood. The standard protocol can reproducibly yield ES cell lines from inbred 129 strains and somewhat less efficiently from C57BL/6 strains. However, usually only a minority of embryos give rise to ES cells, suggesting that some epigenetic event is rate-limiting.

Furthermore, the isolation of ES cell lines from other strains of mice has generally proven very problematic. Thus, there is a strong genetic component to ES cell derivation. Interestingly, this is not reflected in the propensity of embryos to give rise to teratocarcinomas, which does not exhibit significant strain dependency (Damjanov et al. 1983).

Isolation of epiblast cells from inductive influences of adjacent hypoblast (Beddington and Robertson 1999) is reported to enhance the efficiency of ES cell derivation (Brook and Gardner 1997). Brook and Gardner even demonstrate the derivation of multiple ES cell lines from separate cells of the same epiblast by this approach, although it remains to be shown formally that all cells of the epiblast are equally competent to produce ES cells. Removal of differentiated lineages has been applied to circumvent nonpermissiveness in CBA mice (McWhir et al. 1996; Brook and Gardner 1997), but whether this will hold for other strains has not been reported.

It is evident that ES cells originate from the epiblast (Evans and Kaufman 1983; Gardner and Brook 1997), that is, after differentiation of the hypoblast, but the point of embryo development at which capacity to generate ES cells is lost is not clear. To date no success has been reported with egg cylinder stages, even though these give rise to teratocarcinomas very efficiently. Possibly the epithelial organization of the egg cylinder imposes constraints on epiblast cells that may be disrupted on ectopic grafting but are not readily erased in primary culture.

Embryonic Germ Cells

In addition to experimental induction from explanted embryos, teratocarcinomas can originate spontaneously from germ cells. Testicular teratocarcinoma is particularly prevalent in strain 129 mice. The evidence that undifferentiated germ cells can give rise to embryonal carcinoma remained something of a curiosity in the absence of methods for propagating germ cells in vitro. Following molecular cloning of the *Steel* growth factor and the cytokine leukemia inhibitory factor (LIF; see below), limited expansion of germ cells became possible (Matsui et al. 1991). Building on this, it was found that on additional inclusion of basic fibroblast growth factor (FGF-2) in the cultures, mouse primordial germ cells converted after several days in culture into cells resembling ES cells that could then be maintained indefinitely (Matsui et al. 1992; Resnick et al. 1992). These are termed embryonic germ (EG) cells to denote their origin. In most respects, they are indistinguishable from blastocyst-derived ES cells, including pluripotency and even germ-line competence

(Labosky et al. 1994; Stewart et al. 1994). However, irregularities in imprinting arising from their germ cell origin can compromise full developmental potential so that EG cells may colonize chimeras less effectively than ES cells. Evidence has also been presented that EG cells retain the unique capacity of germ cells to erase imprints (Tada et al. 1997), a property that has not been shown in ES cells.

PLURIPOTENCY OF EMBRYONIC STEM CELLS

Teratocarcinoma Formation

ES cells closely resemble EC cells in morphology, growth behavior, and marker expression. This relationship extends to the capacity to give rise to multidifferentiated teratomas and teratocarcinomas. ES cells readily produce tumors containing well-differentiated mesodermal, ectodermal, and endodermal tissue and cell types (Evans and Kaufman 1983). The representation of undifferentiated stem cells in the tumors tends to be less than in EC cell-generated teratocarcinomas, most likely reflecting the latter's history of tumor selection. The ability clonally to give rise to teratocarcinomas is a defining feature of pluripotent embryo cells, shared by ES, EG, and EC cells.

Integration into the Developing Embryo

The most extraordinary feature of ES cells is that, even after extended propagation on tissue culture plastic in synthetic media, they remain capable of participating in normal embryogenesis. Several techniques can be used to introduce ES cells into the preimplantation mouse embryo, but regardless of method of delivery, the ES cells can colonize all fetal lineages plus yolk sac mesoderm (Bradley et al. 1984). Consistent with their epiblast origin, ES cells contribute poorly to extraembryonic endoderm and rarely, if ever, to trophoblast (Beddington and Robertson 1989). In contrast to EC cells, ES cells behave relatively consistently in their ability to integrate into the embryo and produce viable chimeras. ES cells produce functional differentiated progeny in all tissues and organs. Genetic coat-color markers therefore provide a simple and fairly reliable means of monitoring overall chimeric contribution.

Incorporation into embryogenesis not only confirms that ES cells are pluripotent, but also demonstrates that they can respond appropriately to developmental cues for proliferation, differentiation, migration, and patterning. ES cells thus retain in full the identity and capacity of resident epiblast cells.

Germ-line Transmission

A key property of ES cells is that they maintain a euploid karyotype. This is crucial because a balanced diploid chromosome complement is permissive for meoisis. Thus, unlike EC cells, if ES cells colonize the germ-cell lineage in a chimera, they are capable of progression to functional gametes. The landmark of deriving mice from cultured stem cells was reported by the Evans laboratory in 1984 (Bradley et al. 1984). In the early days of ES cell culture, germ-line transmission was often elusive. This became more frequent as the skills required for maintaining the diploid pluripotent phenotype were disseminated. Retention of germ-line competence depends absolutely on adherence to a rigorous tissue culture regime, with avoidance of any untoward selective pressures such as overgrowth or nutrient deprivation. Of course, random mutational events will always occur in the culture and epigenetic modifications may also arise; for example, alterations in imprinting status (Dean et al. 1998), so it is advisable to use low-passage stocks and/or to isolate new subclones periodically for transgenic work.

The great majority of ES cell lines are 40XY. The implication that two active X chromosomes may somehow be disadvantageous for ES cell propagation is consistent with the high incidence of spontaneous X chromosome deletions found in established XX ES lines (Rastan and Robertson 1985). In any case, the XY genotype confers particular advantages for establishing germ-line transmission. Not only can male chimeras produce more offspring than females, but XY cells can convert the undifferentiated genital ridge of an XX recipient into testicular development. Since XX germ cells do not survive in a male gonad, this phenomenon of sex conversion results in chimeric males in which all the mature germ cells are of ES cell origin (Bradley et al. 1984). In addition, it has been observed that the extent of contribution of strain 129 ES cells to chimeras is strongly influenced by the genotype of the recipient embryo. In particular, microinjection into C57BL/6 blastocysts results in very high ES cell contributions and a greatly increased frequency of germ-line transmission (Schwartzberg et al. 1989).

ES Cell-derived Fetuses

ES cells are not in themselves capable of generating a blastocyst and should therefore not be described as totipotent. The issue of whether ES cells are self-sufficient for generation of the fetal component of the conceptus has been addressed by Nagy et al. (1991, 1993), who introduced ES cells into tetraploid recipient embryos. In tetraploid embryos, extraembryonic lineages are produced normally but fetal lineages develop poorly. Consequently, in chimeras between tetraploid and diploid embryos, the fetus becomes almost exclusively colonized by the diploid cells. ES cells show a similar propensity to dominate the tetraploid contribution to the fetus, and such fetuses can develop to term. Thus, it can be argued that ES cells alone are competent to generate the entire fetus. However, although there may be few or possibly no tetraploid cells persisting in the animal at birth, a resident tetraploid ICM compartment is present initially.

To date, fetal development has not been reported following microsurgical replacement of the ICM with ES cells. Therefore, requirement for a "normalizing" signal from the host ICM to induce ES cells to reenter into an embryonic differentiation program cannot be discounted. Furthermore, although liveborn offspring may be obtained from ES cell–tetraploid chimeras, many embryos die in utero, and those that do persist usually die shortly after birth, in contrast to the situation with ICM chimeras. This is likely attributable to cryptic epigenetic or possibly mutational changes that have arisen during derivation or propagation of the ES cells. Such changes may be masked in diploid chimeras. Consequently, ES cells that give good somatic and germ-line colonization in diploid chimeras vary greatly in performance in the tetraploid setting (Nagy et al. 1993). Thus, a note of caution is required in any assertion that an ES cell is unaltered from an epiblast cell in situ.

GENOME MANIPULATION IN ES CELLS

Insertional Mutagenesis and Gene Trapping

DNA can be introduced into ES cells by conventional infection or transfection protocols. Their capacity for clonogenic expansion then allows independent integrants to be expanded and transgenic mice to be generated (Robertson 1986). Random insertion of viral vectors into the ES cell genome has been employed to mutate and tag genes in phenotype-driven screens (Robertson et al. 1986). Gene trapping is a refinement of this approach that facilitates isolation of a disrupted gene and can allow a degree of preselection for desired categories of target gene based on expression pattern or subcellular localization of the gene product (Gossler et al. 1989; Friedrich and Soriano 1991; Skarnes et al. 1995; Forrester et al. 1996). This technique has been widely used as a gene discovery tool in mice and further pursued as a method for annotated mutagenesis of the entire mouse genome (Hicks et al. 1997; Zambrowicz et al. 1998).

Targeted Gene Modification

The major use of ES cell genetic modification to date, however, has been for the directed modification of nominated genes, known as gene targeting. Pioneering work in the mid-1980s established that transfected DNA could be integrated into designated loci in the ES cell genome via homologous recombination (Thomas and Capecchi 1987). In 1989 the first incidence of germ-line transmission of a targeted allele was reported (Thompson et al. 1989), demonstrating that the manipulations and drug selections involved in isolating homologous recombinant clones did not in themselves compromise ES cell pluripotency.

There are now well-established procedures for introducing a range of different types of modifications, such as deletion, point mutation, reporter insertion, or coding sequence replacement, into the mouse genome. Conditional mutations can be created by incorporation of site-specific recombinase technology. In such cases, short recognition sequences for a recombinase such as Cre or Flp are targeted by homologous recombination to flank the gene segment of interest. This interval can then be deleted in a stage- or tissue-specific fashion by appropriate transgenic expression of the recombinase (Gu et al. 1994; Schwenk et al. 1998).

Chromosome Engineering

The use of site-specific recombination can be extended to the engineering of long-range modifications in the ES cell and thence the mouse genome (Smith et al. 1995; Su et al. 2000; Zheng et al. 2000). Deletions, inversions, duplications, or translocations can be generated according to the respective orientation and *cis* or *trans* localization of the recombinase recognition sequences. This is a powerful method for interrogating the genome, increasingly so with the amassing of sequence information and gene localization data.

Autonomous chromosomal elements have also been introduced into ES cells via cell fusion (Shen et al. 1997, 2000; Tomizuka et al. 1997; Hernandez et al. 1999). These minichromosomes can be maintained stably in ES cells and chimeras, and in some cases, can be transmitted through the germ line. This creates the foundations of a system for genetic dissection of centromere function in mammalian mitosis and meiosis. Minichromosome vectors may also find applications in biotechnology; for example, the creation of humanized antibodies.

MAINTENANCE OF ES CELL PLURIPOTENCY

Symmetrical Self-renewal

ES cells multiply by symmetrical cell division. They can routinely be expanded to give relatively homogeneous and undifferentiated populations (Fig. 1), judged by morphology, marker expression, efficient generation of equipotent subclones, and reproducibly broad colonization of chimeras from a few cells. This expansion can be continued over several weeks, and very large (10^9–10^{10}) populations of substantially pure stem cells can be generated. In fact, ES cells appear to be immortal (Suda et al. 1987) and show no evidence of either crisis or senescence, in contrast to other primary cultures (see Chapter 5).

The symmetric amplification of ES cells contrasts with most other stem cells ex vivo and, in conjunction with the facility for genetic manipulation, provides a tractable system for experimental characterization of self-renewal.

Oct-3/4: Governor of Transcription and Fate in Pluripotent Cells

Oct-3/4 is a POU family transcriptional regulator restricted to early embryos, germ-line cells, and undifferentiated EC, EG, and ES cells (Pesce et al. 1998). In vivo, zygotic expression of Oct-3/4 is essential for

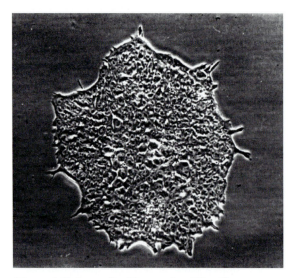

Figure 1 Colony of self-renewing ES cells.

the initial development of pluripotential capacity in the ICM (Nichols et al. 1998b). In ES cells, continuous function of Oct-3/4 is necessary to maintain pluripotency (Niwa et al. 2000). If Oct-3/4 expression is acutely eliminated in ES cells, self-renewal ceases and an unorthodox differentiation process is triggered. Instead of forming the normal ES cell derivatives, endoderm and mesoderm, the cells differentiate into trophoblast (Fig. 2). In the presence of FGF-4 and feeders, it is even possible to isolate trophoblast stem (TS) cells (see Chapter 12). The interest of this observation is that the differentiation of trophectoderm and ICM in the mouse blastocyst is considered to be associated with a segregation of developmental capacity such that the former can generate only trophoblast lineages and the latter only yolk sac and fetal tissues. Consistent with this, ES cells do not normally form trophoblast either in vitro, in teratomas, or in chimeras. It appears that this developmental restriction may be necessary for manifestation of pluripotency and is imposed directly by

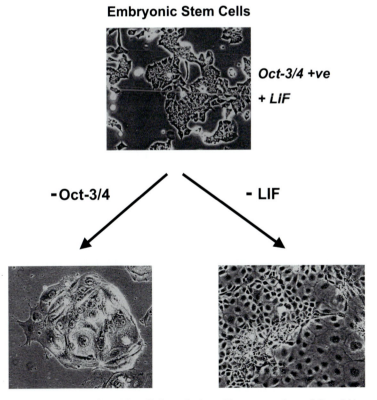

Figure 2 Alternative ES cell fates induced by repression of Oct-3/4 or withdrawal of LIF.

Oct-3/4. In other words, Oct-3/4 acts in part as a lock that prevents default differentiation into trophoblast (Niwa et al. 2000).

Oct-3/4 also contributes positively to pluripotency by directing expression of multiple target genes (Saijoh et al. 1996). This is achieved via interaction with several coactivators (Scholer et al. 1991; Ambrosetti et al. 1997; Ben-Shushan et al. 1998), and probably also corepressors. The complexity of Oct-3/4 function is indicated by the finding that marginally increased expression in ES cells provokes differentiation, but in this case into endoderm and mesoderm (Niwa et al. 2000). Although Oct-3/4 is normally down-regulated during pluripotent cell differentiation, this is a consequence rather than a cause of germ-layer commitment. Indeed, in the ICM, Oct-3/4 levels transiently increase in nascent hypoblast (Palmieri et al. 1994). One hypothesis is that differential lineage commitment may be determined by altered interaction of Oct-3/4 with specific partners, expression or activity of which may be regulated by inductive signals.

Finally, although Oct-3/4 seems to be a pivotal player in the determination of pluripotent cell fate, maintenance of Oct-3/4 expression is not in itself sufficient to sustain the pluripotent phenotype (Niwa et al. 2000). Significantly, an extrinsic signal is also needed.

Cytokine Stimulation of Self-renewal

In monoculture using media supplemented with serum alone, ES cells can neither be derived nor maintained. As discussed above, ES cells were originally isolated by coculture with a feeder layer. Subsequently it was discovered that the feeders can be substituted by conditioned medium preparations (Smith and Hooper 1983; Smith and Hooper 1987), indicating that their key function is to provide trophic stimulation. In fact, a purified cytokine, leukemia inhibitory factor (LIF), is sufficient to sustain ES cell self-renewal (Smith et al. 1988; Williams et al. 1988). This effect is exclusive to LIF and a small group of related cytokines that act via the gp130 receptor (Yoshida et al. 1994). LIF is expressed by feeder cells, and this expression is elevated in the presence of ES cells (Rathjen et al. 1990). LIF does not act via inducing expression of Oct-3/4 because transgenic expression of Oct-3/4 does not remove the requirement for LIF (Niwa et al. 2000).

On withdrawal of LIF (or feeders), proliferation continues, but differentiation is induced and ES cells do not persist beyond a few days. It has been suggested that self-renewal equates to the inhibition of differentiation (Weissman 2000). However, this is only true provided survival and division are constitutive. In the case of ES cells, replication does indeed appear to be autonomous. The cell cycle is uncoupled from cdk/cyclin checkpoints in G_1 (Savatier et al. 1995; Wianny et al. 1998), and no method has been reported for producing quiescence in ES cells. Apoptosis can be induced in ES cells (Sabapathy et al. 1997; Koyanagi-Katsuta et al. 2000), however, which implies that an anti-apoptotic pathway could be a crucial element of the self-renewal signal. Although ES cells remain viable in defined media lacking LIF, serum, or added growth factors, this is heavily dependent on cell density, suggesting a requirement for autocrine survival signaling.

Two major signal transduction pathways are recruited downstream of ligand-induced dimerization of gp130 receptors. The latent transcription factor STAT3 is activated by tyrosine phosphorylation mediated by JAK kinases (Lutticken et al. 1994), and engagement of the adapters SHP2 and Gab1 lead to stimulation of the Ras-Erk mitogen-activated protein kinase cascade (Takahashi-Tezuka et al. 1998). Analysis of modified receptors indicated that recruitment of STAT3 is essential for ES cell propagation (Niwa et al. 1998). This conclusion was substantiated by demonstration that expression of the dominant interfering STAT3F molecule induced differentiation in the presence of LIF. In contrast, suppression of the SHP2/Erk signaling arm actually enhanced ES cell self-renewal (Burdon et al. 1999b). Finally, studies with directly activatable or constitutively activated variants of STAT3 have provided strong evidence that this transcription factor alone can provide the self-renewal signal in serum-supplemented medium (Matsuda et al. 1999; C. Stracey et al., in prep.).

Cytokines of the LIF family are not dedicated to stem cell regulation, but have diverse effects on a variety of cell types (Kishimoto et al. 1994). Interestingly, most of these actions are to promote differentiation, for example of myeloid cells or astrocyte precursors, or to induce expression of differentiated functions, such as acute phase protein synthesis by hepatocytes. STAT3 is the major mediator of these responses. Therefore, ES cell self-renewal is stimulated by a conventional signal transduction pathway, but the output of this signal, inhibition of differentiation, is peculiar to the stem cell context. A key task is to define the level of interaction, direct or indirect, with Oct-3/4 and to identify the important target genes in ES cells. These are likely to include repressed genes, expression of which could direct commitment and differentiation.

Intracellular Signaling Network in ES Cells

The antagonistic effect of SHP2 and Erk activation on self-renewal (Burdon et al. 1994b) can partly be explained by a negative regulation of

JAK-STAT signaling by SHP2 tyrosine phosphatase activity (Symes et al. 1997). In addition, blockade of the Erk activating enzyme MEK1 with the inhibitor PD05809 reduces ES cell differentiation both in monolayer and aggregate culture. Continued cell proliferation without stimulation of Erk activation is unusual but may be accounted for by the lack of restriction on entry into S phase in ES cells (Savatier et al. 1995; Burdon et al. 1999a). Promotion of self-renewal by PD05809 further implies that there is likely to be a direct pro-differentiative effect of Erk activation. This relates not only to coupling downstream of gp130, but to growth factors and other inductive stimuli that signal through the Ras-Raf-MEK-Erk cascade, and probably also to aspects of integrin signaling that involve Erk activation.

As discussed above, self-renewal may require suppression of apoptosis. It remains to be determined whether the anti-apoptotic function that has been ascribed to STAT3 in other cell systems is operative in ES cells, or whether activation of the PI3-kinase/Akt pathway may fulfill such a role.

The requirement to achieve and maintain a high level of STAT3 activation and low level of Erk activity may underlie some of the difficulty experienced in ES cell derivation. It is significant, therefore, that application of PD05809 can increase the efficiency of ES cell establishment by promoting expansion of primary stem cell colonies (T. Burdon et al., in prep.). It is also noteworthy that, although ES cells established on feeders can be adapted to grow on gelatin in the presence of LIF, this is generally preceded by extensive differentiation, and the stem cells that persist and regenerate the cultures are often compromised and show reduced contribution to chimeras. This may indicate that the signaling network is tuned slightly differently during culture on feeders and must be readjusted for growth in LIF alone.

Although ES cells employ classical signal transduction mechanisms, the likely existence of stem-cell-specific signaling adapters should not be overlooked. For example, Erk activation in response to various stimuli appears attenuated in ES cells relative to other cell types, despite the presence of comparable levels of Erk proteins (T. Burdon et al., in prep.). This probably results in part from expression of an altered form of the Gab1 adapter protein in ES cells that suppresses linkage of certain receptors to the Ras-Erk cascade. Such redirection of primary signal transduction so as to minimize pro-differentiative outputs may turn out to be a cardinal aspect of stem cell propagation in general.

Alternative Pathways of Self-renewal

The dependency of ES cells on gp130 signaling presents a paradox, however. In vivo, a critical role for the gp130 pathway in the epiblast is evident only on induction of embryonic diapause (J. Nichols et al., in prep.). In uninterrupted embryogenesis, there is no apparent requirement for LIF, gp130, or STAT3 prior to gastrulation. This implies that normal expansion of the epiblast is either autonomous or under the direction of a separate signaling pathway. The regulative properties of the epiblast (Hogan et al. 1994) argue against the former. For example, giant blastocysts made by aggregation of two or more cleavage embryos produce normal-sized egg cylinders after implantation on the same time schedule as ordinary blastocysts. Conversely, small blastocysts created by splitting 2-cell embryos "catch up" after implantation and produce full-sized egg cylinders. Regulation of the epiblast population occurs within 36 hours of implantation. This adaptive response may be governed via juxtacrine signaling within the epiblast compartment or by paracrine stimulation from neighboring tissue.

ES cells provide both an assay for, and a potential source of, epiblast regulatory signals (Heath and Smith 1988). Like epiblast, ES cells can be sustained independently of gp130 and STAT3, at least transiently (Dani et al. 1998). Such a process operates in addition to LIF signaling during culture of ES cells on mouse embryo fibroblast feeders (I. Chambers and A.G. Smith, unpubl.). The factor(s) and signaling mechanisms that mediate this effect have yet to be characterized at the molecular level, however. Evidence has also been presented that pluripotent cells may be maintained in a slightly altered state using conditioned medium from the HepG2 human hepatocyte cell line. Under such conditions, cell morphology, expression of certain genes, differentiation behavior, and ability to colonize the embryo are altered. Significantly, this transition appears reversible with regard to all these features. Therefore, it either reflects an inherent plasticity of the ES cell phenotype (Smith 1992) or marks two distinct but continuous stages of normal epiblast progression (Rathjen et al. 1999; Lake et al. 2000). It will be of interest to resolve whether integrin signaling may contribute to ES cell regulation, given its significance for hematopoietic, keratinocyte, and other stem cell populations, and requirement for egg cylinder development (Fassler and Meyer 1995; Fassler et al. 1995; Fuchs and Segre 2000).

IN VITRO DIFFERENTIATION OF ES CELLS

A major aspiration at the outset of EC and ES cell research was to elucidate the decision-making processes in lineage commitment and cell type differentiation of pluripotent cells. This issue is now reemerging to the fore with increasing interest in the application of ES cell systems for efficient in vitro analysis of gene function and pharmacological screening, and for the potential development of cell therapy. From their differentiation in teratomas and chimeras, ES cells clearly have the capacity to produce every type of fetal and adult cell. Understanding and controlling cell fate determination remains a major challenge, however.

Differentiation in Embryoid Bodies

Our abilities to direct pluripotent cells into specific pathways and then to support the viability and maturation of individual differentiated phenotypes in vitro are currently limited, and the approaches are rather unsophisticated. The principal method used to trigger differentiation of ES cells into defined cell types is cell aggregation in suspension culture. This technique, originally developed with EC cells (Martin and Evans 1975; Martin et al. 1977), leads to formation of multidifferentiated structures called embryoid bodies. In these structures, the developmental program of ICM/epiblast cells is reactivated in the ES cells. Cellular differentiation proceeds in a similar fashion to that which occurs in the embryo, albeit in the absence of proper axial organization or elaboration of a body plan (Doetschman et al. 1985). Each embryoid body develops multiple different cell types. A range of differentiated products can readily be obtained, including yolk sac endoderm, cardiomyocytes, embryonic and definitive hematopoietic cells, endothelial cells, skeletal myocytes, adipocytes, neurons, and glia (Weiss and Orkin 1996). It is possible to bias the differentiation for or against certain cell types by addition of retinoic acid (Rohwedel et al. 1999). However, the final cultures are always a heterogeneous mixture of various cell types.

In the absence of knowledge of how to instruct ES cells into a lineage of choice, which in any case may never be completely effective in the context of complex multicellular interactions that occur in an embryoid body, an alternative approach is to isolate cells of interest from the mixture of differentiation products. For hematopoietic cells, this can readily be done by selective culture in semi-solid media in the presence of hematopoietic growth factors (Wiles and Keller 1991). A complementary strategy is to purify lineage-specific precursors or terminal differentiated phenotypes based on marker gene expression. This can be achieved by immunopurification where suitable cell-surface markers are available, or more generally by introduction of a transgene marker conferring drug resistance and/or cell-sorting capacity (Klug et al. 1996; Li et al. 1998).

Differentiation in Monolayer Culture

ES cells differentiate readily in monolayer culture when deprived of LIF or feeder support. Various differentiated morphologies emerge, and markers of mesoderm and endoderm become expressed. However, the identities of the major cell types produced under such conditions have not been carefully defined. It is possible that many of the cells may not represent bona fide embryonic or fetal phenotypes but rather could be aberrant products arising from misregulated or scrambled differentiation programs. Nonetheless, in a very elegant study, Nishikawa has shown that distinct mesodermal subsets can be produced during monolayer differentiation, and in particular that clonogenic endothelial and hematopoietic progenitors can be isolated by fluorescence-activated cell sorting (FACS) (Nishikawa et al. 1998). These progenitors can even proceed to form vasculature (Yamashita et al. 2000). This is a very significant result because it establishes that "true" differentiation can be uncoupled from morphogenesis and does not require complex multicellular interactions. Furthermore, the development of some lineages is actually suppressed by such interactions and is therefore enhanced by purifying the precursors. This finding also has implications on a practical level because monolayer culture is much more amenable than aggregation for experimental dissection and manipulation. For example, the application of candidate inductive signaling molecules such as Wnts and BMPs is likely to have more profound and interpretable consequences in homogeneous monolayer cultures than on embryoid bodies. Use of defined media will likely be required to realize the full potential of this approach (Wiles and Johansson 1999).

Mechanism of Differentiation

Do ES cells undergo asymmetric division during differentiation? In the absence of LIF, undifferentiated ES cells are rapidly depleted from the cultures. This must occur either by symmetrical division leading to differentiation of both daughter cells, or by a limited number of asymmetric divisions followed by selective death of the stem cells. The absence of any overt polarity in ES cells in monolayer culture might suggest that there is no foundation for development of asymmetry. However, this issue should be investigated directly by time lapse recordings. It would also be instructive to determine whether in embryoid bodies the initial differentiation of an outer layer of extraembryonic endoderm is an asymmetric event or is directed solely by external position.

Although there is also selective activation of a small number of specialized genes, lineage commitment is in essence a restriction of global gene expression potential. This entails the heritable repression of the majority of non-housekeeping genes. How such epigenetic mechanisms operate and how they may be erased during nuclear transfer or dedifferentiation has yet to be determined. Important insights could be obtained, however, by studying how chromatin architecture is modified during ES cell differentiation.

The chromatin organization in a pluripotent cell nucleus must be permissive for activation of lineage-specific gene transcription. A noteworthy observation from gene trapping studies is that many developmentally regulated genes are already transcriptionally active at low levels in undifferentiated ES cells. It is also possible to detect allegedly tissue-restricted transcripts in ES cells by reverse transcription PCR. This is reminiscent of the "lineage priming" concept proposed for hematopoietic stem cells (Hu et al. 1997); but if stem cells express lineage-specific genes, how is the undifferentiated pluripotent state maintained? There are at least three possible and nonexclusive explanations:

1. The level of expression of differentiation genes may not be functionally significant, but may simply reflect random transcription occurring through open chromatin.
2. Commitment may require coordinated expression of a battery of genes, individual expression of which has no consequence.
3. Stem-cell-specific transcriptional determinants may specifically antagonize the action of lineage commitment genes.

Self-renewal of ES cells appears to rely on an interplay of conflicting intracellular signals and transcriptional determinants. This is so finely balanced that the alternative outcome of differentiation can readily be triggered (Fig. 3). Thus, some level of "spontaneous" differentiation is usually evident in ES cell cultures. It will be interesting to discover whether other types of stem cells are regulated in a similar manner such that they are constantly "poised" to differentiate.

PLURIPOTENT EMBRYO CELLS FROM OTHER SPECIES

Derivation of permanent stem cell lines that fulfill the criteria of epiblast origin, sustained symmetrical self-renewal, pluripotency, integration into fetal development, and germ-line colonization has to date only been validated in mice. Germ-line colonization from cultured cells has been reported in chickens and medaka fish, but only after short-term culture (Pain et al. 1996; Hong et al. 1998). Chimeras have been reported in rabbits, pigs, and cattle, but in no case has germ-line colonization been corroborated. These data may suggest that the situation in the mouse is the exception rather than the rule. The ES cell phenotype represents a ground state for mouse epiblast or primordial germ cells in teratocarcinomas or

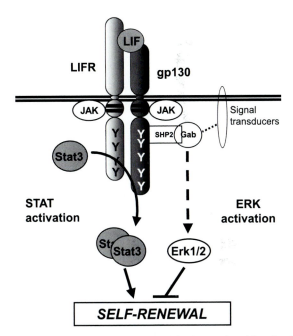

Figure 3 ES cell self-renewal is determined by the balance between conflicting signals.

ex vivo. However, although diploid stem cell cultures can readily be derived from rat ICMs, rather than exhibiting multilineage differentiation, these cells appear restricted to extraembryonic development (M. Buehr and A.G. Smith, unpubl.). It may be significant in this regard that ectopically grafted rat embryos do not produce teratocarcinomas (Skreb et al. 1971) and that rat epiblast appears to retain the ability to produce hypoblast even into egg cylinder stages (Nichols et al. 1998a). Therefore, the possibility should be considered that the ES cell phenomenon is specific to inbred laboratory mice and that the ground state in other species may differ and perhaps even be a more primitive "pre-pluripotent" cell.

Stem cell cultures have also been established from human blastocysts (Thomson et al. 1998). These cells can generate teratomas in immuno-compromised mice and show some capacity for multilineage differentiation in vitro (Reubinoff et al. 2000). Therefore, they could represent human equivalents of ES cells. However, the critical functional tests of chimera contribution and gamete production obviously should not be undertaken for ethical reasons. It is noteworthy that these human cells differentiate into trophoblast, indicating that they may not represent exactly the same developmental stage as mouse ES cells. Furthermore, they are difficult to expand and seemingly do not respond to LIF (Reubinoff et al.

2000). Intriguingly, human EG-like cells derived from fetal primordial germ cells, in contrast, appear to be dependent on LIF for continued propagation (Shamblott et al. 1998). The molecular characterization of these human cells and comparison against mouse ES and EG cells is now a pressing issue, particularly in light of the desire to develop human pluripotent cells for regenerative therapies (Gearhart 1998; Smith 1998).

ACKNOWLEDGMENTS

I thank all past and present members of the laboratory for their intellectual and practical contributions toward the goal of understanding embryonic stem cells. Our research is supported by the UK Biotechnology and Biological Sciences Research Council and Medical Research Council, and by the International Human Frontiers in Science Program.

REFERENCES

Ambrosetti D.-C., Basilico C., and Dailey L. 1997. Synergistic activation of the fibroblast growth factor 4 enhancer by sox2 and oct-3 depends on protein-protein interactions facilitated by a specific spatial arrangement of factor binding sites. *Mol. Cell. Biol.* **17:** 6321–6329.

Beddington R. 1983. The origin of the fetal tissues during gastrulation in the rodent. In *Development in mammals* (ed. M.H. Johnson), vol. 5, pp. 1–32. Elsevier, Amsterdam, The Netherlands.

Beddington R.S.P. and Robertson E.J. 1989. An assessment of the developmental potential of embryonic stem cells in the midgestation mouse embryo. *Development* **105:** 733–737.

———. 1999. Axis development and early asymmetry in mammals. *Cell* **96:** 195–209.

Ben-Shushan E., Thompson J.R., Gudas L.J., and Bergman Y. 1998. *Rex-1*, a gene encoding a transcription factor expressed in the early embryo, is regulated via Oct-3/4 and Oct-6 binding to an octamer site and a novel protein, Rox-1, binding to an adjacent site. *Mol. Cell. Biol.* **18:** 1666–1878.

Bradley A., Evans M.J., Kaufman M.H., and Robertson E. 1984. Formation of germ-line chimeras from embryo-derived teratocarcinoma cell lines. *Nature* **309:** 255–256.

Brinster R.L. 1974. The effect of cells transferred into the mouse blastocyst on subsequent development. *J. Exp. Med.* **140:** 1049–1056.

Brook F.A. and Gardner R.L. 1997. The origin and efficient derivation of embryonic stem cells in the mouse. *Proc. Natl. Acad. Sci.* **94:** 5709–5712.

Burdon T., Chambers I., Niwa H., Stracey C., and Smith A.G. 1999a. Signaling mechanisms regulating self-renewal and differentiation of pluripotent embryonic stem cells. *Cells Tiss. Organs* **165:** 131–143.

Burdon T., Stracey C., Chambers I., Nichols J., and Smith A. 1999b. Suppression of SHP-2 and ERK signalling promotes self-renewal of mouse embryonic stem cells. *Dev. Biol.* **210:** 30–43.

Damjanov I., Bagasra O., and Solter D. 1983. Genetic and epigenetic factors regulate the evolving malignancy of embryo-derived teratomas. *Cold Spring Harb. Conf. Cell Proliferation* **10:** 501–517.

Dani C., Chambers I., Johnstone S., Robertson M., Ebrahimi B., Saito M., Taga T., Li M., Burdon T., Nichols J., and Smith A.G. 1998. Paracrine induction of stem cell renewal by LIF-deficient cells: A new ES cell regulatory pathway. *Dev. Biol.* **203:** 149–162.

Dean W., Bowden L., Aitchison A., Klose J., Moore T., Meneses J.J., Reik W., and Feil R. 1998. Altered imprinted gene methylation and expression in completely ES cell-derived mouse fetuses: Association with aberrant phenotypes. *Development* **125:** 2273–2282.

Diwan S.B. and Stevens L.C. 1976. Development of teratomas from ectoderm of mouse egg cylinders. *J. Natl. Cancer Inst.* **57:** 937–942.

Doetschman T.C., Eistetter H., Katz M., Schmidt W., and Kemler R. 1985. The in vitro development of blastocyst-derived embryonic stem cell lines: Formation of visceral yolk sac, blood islands and myocardium. *J. Embryol. Exp. Morphol.* **87:** 27–45.

Evans M.J. 1972. The isolation and properties of a clonal tissue culture strain of pluripotent mouse teratoma cells. *J. Embryol. Exp. Morphol.* **28:** 163–176.

Evans M.J. and Kaufman M. 1981. Establishment in culture of pluripotential cells from mouse embryos. *Nature* **292:** 154–156.

———. 1983. Pluripotential cells grown directly from normal mouse embryos. *Cancer Surv.* **2:** 185–208.

Fassler R. and Meyer M. 1995. Consequences of lack of $\beta1$ integrin gene expression in mice. *Genes Dev.* **9:** 1896–1908.

Fassler R., Pfaff M. Murphy J., Noegel A.N., Johannson S., Timpi R., and Albrecht A. 1995. The lack of $\beta1$ integrin gene in embryonic stem cells affects cell morphology, migration and adhesion, but not integration into the inner cell mass of blastocysts. *J. Cell Biol.* **128:** 979–988.

Forrester L.M., Nagy A., Sam M., Watt A., Stevenson L., Bernstein A., Joyner A.L., and Wurst W. 1996. An induction gene trap screen in embryonic stem cells: Identification of genes that respond to retinoic acid in vitro. *Proc. Natl. Acad. Sci.* **93:** 1677–1682.

Friedrich G. and Soriano P. 1991. Promoter traps in embryonic stem cells: A genetic screen to identify and mutate developmental genes in mice. *Genes Dev.* **5:** 1513–1523.

Fuchs E. and Segre J.A. 2000. Stern cells: A new lease on life. *Cell* **100:** 143–155.

Gardner R.L. 1998. Contributions of blastocyst micromanipulation to the study of mammalian development. *BioEssays* **20:** 168–180.

Gardner R.L. and Brook F.A. 1997. Reflections on the biology of embryonic stem cells. *Int. J. Dev. Biol.* **41:** 235–243.

Gearhart J. 1998. New potential for human embryonic stem cells. *Science* **282:** 1061–1062.

Gossler A., Joyner A.L., Rossant J., and Skarnes W.C. 1989. Mouse embryonic stem cells and reporter constructs to detect developmentally regulated genes. *Science* **244:** 463–465.

Gu H., Marth J.D., Orban P.C., Mossmann H., and Rajewsky K. 1994. Deletion of a DNA polymerase β gene segment in T cells using cell type-specific gene targeting. *Science* **265:** 103–106.

Heath J.K. and Smith A.G. 1988. Regulatory factors of embryonic stem cells. *J. Cell. Sci. (Suppl.)* **10:** 257–266.

Hernandez D., Mee P.J., Martin J.E., Tybulewicz V.L., and Fisher E.M. 1999. Transchromosomal mouse embryonic stem cell lines and chimeric mice that contain freely segregating segments of human chromosome 21. *Hum. Mol. Genet.* **8:** 923–933.

Hicks G.G., Shi E.G., Li X.M., Li C.H., Pawlak M., and Ruley H.E. 1997. Functional genomics in mice by tagged sequence mutagenesis. *Nat Genet* **16:** 338–344.

Hogan B.L.M. and Tilly R. 1977. In vitro culture and differentiation of normal mouse blastocysts. *Nature* **265:** 626–629.

Hogan B., Beddington R., Costantini F., and Lacy E. 1994. *Manipulating the mouse embryo: A laboratory manual.* Cold Spring Harbor Laboratory Press, Cold Spring Harbor, New York.

Hong Y., Winkler C., and Schartl M. 1998. Efficiency of cell culture derivation from blastula embryos and of chimera formation in the medaka (*Oryzias latipes*) depends on donor genotype and passage number. *Dev. Genes Evol.* **208:** 595–602.

Hu M., Krause D., Greaves M., Sharkis S., Dexter M., Heyworth C., and Enver T. 1997. Multilineage gene expression precedes commitment in the hemopoietic system. *Genes Dev.* **11:** 774–785.

Kishimoto T., Taga T., and Akira S. 1994. Cytokine signal transduction. *Cell* **76:** 253–262.

Kleinsmith L.J. and Pierce G.B. 1964. Multipotentiality of single embryonal carcinoma cells. *Cancer Res.* **24:** 1544–1552.

Klug M.G., Soonpaa M.H., Koh G.Y., and Field L.J. 1996. Genetically selected cardiomyocytes from differentiating embryonic stem cells form stable intracardiac grafts. *J. Clin. Invest.* **98:** 216–224.

Koyanagi-Katsuta R., Akimitsu N., Arimitsu N., Hatano T., and Sekimizu K. 2000. Apoptosis of mouse embryonic stem cells induced by single cell suspension. *Tissue Cell* **32:** 66–70.

Labosky P.A., Barlow D.P., and Hogan B.L. 1994. Mouse embryonic germ (EG) cell lines: Transmission through the germline and differences in the methylation imprint of insulin-like growth factor 2 receptor (Igf2r) gene compared with embryonic stem (ES) cell lines. *Development* **120:** 3197–3204.

Lake J., Rathjen J., Remiszewski J., and Rathjen P.D. 2000. Reversible programming of pluripotent cell differentiation. *J. Cell Sci.* **113:** 555–566.

Lawson K.A., Meneses J.J., and Pedersen R.A. 1991. Clonal analysis of epiblast fate during germ layer formation in the mouse embryo. *Development* **113:** 891–911.

Li M., Pevny L., Lovell-Badge R., and Smith A. 1998. Generation of purified neural precursors from embryonic stem cells by lineage selection. *Curr. Biol.* **8:** 971–974.

Lutticken C., Wegenka U.M., Yuan J., Buschmann J., Schindler C., Ziemiecki A., Harpur A.G., Wilks A.F., Yasukawa K., Taga T., Kishimoto T., Barbieri G., Pellegrini S., Sendtner M., Heinrich P.C., and Horn F. 1994. Association of transcription factor APRF and protein kinase Jak1 with the interleukin-6 signal transducer gp130. *Science* **263:** 89–92.

Martin G.R. 1980. Teratocarcinomas and mammalian embryogenesis. *Science* **209:** 768–776.

———. 1981. Isolation of a pluripotent cell line from early mouse embryos cultured in medium conditioned by teratocarcinoma stem cells. *Proc. Natl. Acad. Sci.* **78:** 7634–7638.

Martin G.R. and Evans M.J. 1975. The formation of embryoid bodies in vitro by homogeneous embryonal carcinoma cell cultures derived from isolated single cells. In *Teratomas and differentiation* (eds. M.I. Sherman and D. Solter), pp. 169–187. Academic Press, New York.

Martin G.R., Wiley L.M., and Damjanov I. 1977. The development of cystic embryoid bodies in vitro from clonal teratocarcinoma stem cells. *Dev. Biol.* **61:** 230–244.

Matsuda T., Nakamura T., Nakao K., Arai T., Katsuki M., Heike T., and Yokota T. 1999. STAT3 activation is sufficient to maintain an undifferentiated state of mouse embryonic stem cells. *Embo J.* **18:** 4261–4269.

Matsui Y., Zsebo K., and Hogan B.L.M. 1992. Derivation of pluripotential embryonic stem cells from murine primordial germ cells in culture. *Cell* **70:** 841–847.

Matsui Y., Toksoz D., Nishikawa S., Nishikawa S.-I., Williams D., Zsebo K., and Hogan B.L.M. 1991. Effect of Steel factor and leukaemia inhibitory factor on murine primordial germ cells in culture. *Nature* **353:** 750–752.

McWhir J., Schnieke A.E., Ansell R., Wallace H., Colman A., Scott A.R., and Kind A.J. 1996. Selective ablation of differentiated cells permits isolation of embryonic stem cell lines from murine embryos with a non-permissive genetic background. *Nat. Genet.* **14:** 223–226.

Nagy A., Rossant J., Nagy R., Abramow-Newerly W., and Roder J.C. 1993. Derivation of completely cell culture-derived mice from early-passage embryonic stem cells. *Proc. Natl. Acad. Sci.* **90:** 8424–8428.

Nagy A., Gocza E., Merentes Diaz E., Prideaux V.R., Ivanyi E., Markkula M., and Rossant J. 1991. Embryonic stem cells alone are able to support fetal development in the mouse. *Development* **110:** 815–821.

Nichols J., Smith A., and Buehr M. 1998a. Rat and mouse epiblasts differ in their capacity to generate extraembryonic endoderm. *Reprod. Fertil. Dev.* **10:** 517–525.

Nichols J., Zevnik B., Anastassiadis K., Niwa H., Klewe-Nebenius D., Chambers I., Scholer H., and Smith A. 1998. Formation of pluripotent stem cells in the mammalian embryo depends on the POU transcription factor Oct-4. *Cell* **95:** 379–391.

Nishikawa S.I., Nishikawa S., Hirashima M., Matsuyoshi N., and Kodama H. 1998. Progressive lineage analysis by cell sorting and culture identifies FLK1[+]VE-cadherin[+] cells at a diverging point of endothelial and hemopoietic lineages. *Development* **125:** 1747–1757.

Niwa H., Miyazaki J., and Smith A.G. 2000. Quantitative expression of Oct-3/4 defines differentiation, dedifferentiation or self-renewal of ES cells. *Nat. Genet.* **24:** 372–376.

Niwa H., Burdon T., Chambers I., and Smith A.G. 1998. Self-renewal of pluripotent embryonic stem cells is mediated via activation of STAT3. *Genes Dev.* **12:** 2048–2060.

Pain B., Clark M.E., Shen M., Nakazawa H., Sakurai M., Samarut J., and Etches R.J. 1996. Long-term in vitro culture and characterisation of avian embryonic stem cells with multiple morphogenetic potentialities. *Development* **122:** 2339–2348.

Palmieri S.L., Peter W., Hess H., and Scholer H.R. 1994. Oct-4 transcription factor is differentially expressed in the mouse embryo during establishment of the first two extraembryonic cell lineages involved in implantation. *Dev. Biol.* **166:** 259–267.

Papaioannou V.E., McBurney M.W., Gardner R.L., and Evans M.J. 1975. Fate of teratocarcinoma cells injected into early mouse embryos. *Nature* **258:** 70–73.

Papaioannou V.E., Gardner R.L., McBurney M.W., Babinet C., and Evans M.J. 1978. Participation of cultured teratocarcinoma cells in mouse embryogenesis. *J. Embryol. Exp. Morphol.* **44:** 93–104.

Pesce M., Gross M.K., and Scholer H. 1998. In line with our ancestors: *Oct-4* and the mammalian germ. *BioEssays* **20:** 722–732.

Rastan S. and Robertson E.J. 1985. X-chromosome deletions in embryo-derived (EK) cell lines associated with lack of X-chromosome inactivation. *J. Embryol. Exp. Morphol.* **90:** 379–388.

Rathjen P.D., Toth S., Willis A., Heath J.K., and Smith A.G. 1990. Differentiation inhibiting activity is produced in matrix-associated and diffusible forms that are generated by alternate promoter usage. *Cell* **62:** 1105–1114.

Rathjen J., Lake J.A., Bettess M.D., Washington J.M., Chapman G., and Rathjen P.D. 1999. Formation of a primitive ectoderm like cell population, EPL cells, from ES cells in response to biologically derived factors. *J. Cell. Sci.* **112:** 601–612.

Resnick J.L., Bixler L.S., Cheng L., and Donovan P.J. 1992. Long-term proliferation of mouse primordial germ cells in culture. *Nature* **359:** 550–551.

Reubinoff B.E., Pera M.F., Fong C.Y., Trounson A., and Bongso A. 2000. Embryonic stem cell lines from human blastocysts: Somatic differentiation in vitro (see comments) (erratum *Nat. Biotechnol.* [2000] **18:** 559). *Nat. Biotechnol.* **18:** 399–404.

Robertson E.J. 1986. Pluripotential stem cell lines as a route into the mouse germ line. *Trends.Genet.* **2:** 9–13.

———. 1987. Embryo-derived stem cell lines. In *Teratocarcinomas and embryonic stem cells: A practical approach* (ed. E.J. Robertson), pp. 71–112. IRL Press, Oxford, United Kingdom.

Robertson E., Bradley A., Kuehn M., and Evans M. 1986. Germ-line transmission of genes introduced into cultured pluripotential cells by retroviral vector. *Nature* **323:** 445–448.

Rohwedel J., Guan K., and Wobus A.M. 1999. Induction of cellular differentiation by retinoic acid in vitro. *Cells Tiss. Organs* **165:** 190–202.

Sabapathy K., Klemm M., Jaenisch R., and Wagner E.F. 1997. Regulation of ES cell differentiation by functional and conformational modulation of p53. *EMBO J.* **16:** 6217–6229.

Saijoh Y., Fukii H., Meno C., Sato M., Hirota Y., Nagamatsu S., Ikeda M., and Hamada H. 1996. Identification of putative downstream genes of Oct-3, a pluripotent cell-specific transcription factor. *Genes Cells* **1:** 239–252.

Savatier P., Lapillonne H., van Grunsven L.A., Rudkin B.B., and Samarut J. 1995. Withdrawal of differentiation inhibitory activity/leukaemia inhibitory factor up-regulates D-type cyclins and cyclin-dependent kinase inhibitors in mouse embryonic stem cells. *Oncogene* **12:** 309–322.

Scholer H.R., Ciesiolka T., and Gruss P. 1991. A nexus between Oct-4 and E1A: Implications for gene regulation in embryonic stem cells. *Cell* **66:** 291–304.

Schwartzberg P.L., Goff S.P., and Robertson E.J. 1989. Germ-line transmission of a c-abl mutation produced by targeted gene disruption in ES cells. *Science* **246:** 799–803.

Schwenk F., Kuhn R., Angrand P.O., Rajewsky K., and Stewart A.F. 1998. Temporally and spatially regulated somatic mutagenesis in mice. *Nucleic Acids Res.* **26:** 1427–1432.

Shamblott M.J., Axelman J., Wang S., Bugg E.M., Littlefield J.W., Donovan P.J., Blumenthal P.D., Huggins G.R., and Gearhart J.D. 1998. Derivation of pluripotent stem cells from cultured human primordial germ cells. *Proc. Natl. Acad. Sci.* **95:** 13726–13731.

Shen M.H., Yang J., Loupart M.L., Smith A., and Brown W. 1997. Human mini-chromosomes in mouse embryonal stem cells. *Hum. Mol. Genet.* **6:** 1375–1382.

Shen M.H., Mee P.J., Nichols J., Yang J., Brook F., Gardner R.L., Smith A.G., and Brown W.R. 2000. A structurally defined mini-chromosome vector for the mouse germ line. *Curr. Biol.* **10:** 31–34.

Skarnes W.C., Moss J.E., Hurtley S.M., and Beddington R.S. 1995. Capturing genes encoding membrane and secreted proteins important for mouse development. *Proc.*

Natl. Acad. Sci. **92:** 6592–6596.

Skreb N., Svajger A., and Levak-Svajger B. 1971. Growth and differentiation of rat egg cylinders under the kidney capsule. *J. Embryol. Exp. Morphol.* **25:** 47–55.

Smith A.G. 1992. Mouse embryo stem cells: Their identification, propagation and manipulation. *Semin. Cell Biol.* **3:** 385–399.

———. 1998. Cell therapy: In search of pluripotency. *Curr. Biol.* **8:** 802–804.

Smith A.G. and Hooper M.L. 1987. Buffalo rat liver cells produce a diffusible activity which inhibits the differentiation of murine embryonal carcinoma and embryonic stem cells. *Dev. Biol.* **121:** 1–9.

Smith A.G., Heath J.K., Donaldson D.D., Wong G.G., Moreau J., Stahl M., and Rogers D. 1988. Inhibition of pluripotential embryonic stem cell differentiation by purified polypeptides. *Nature* **336:** 688–690.

Smith A.J.H., De Sousa M.A., Kwabi-Addo B., Heppell-Parton A., Impey H., and Rabbitts P. 1995. A site-directed chromosomal translocation induced in embryonic stem cells by Cre/*loxP* recombination. *Nat. Genet.* **9:** 376–385.

Smith T.A. and Hooper M.L. 1983. Medium conditioned by feeder cells inhibits the differentiation of embryonal carcinoma cultures. *Exp. Cell Res.* **145:** 458–462.

Solter D., Skreb N., and Damjanov I. 1970. Extrauterine growth of mouse egg cylinders results in malignant teratoma. *Nature* **227:** 503–504.

Stewart C.L., Gadi I., and Bhatt H. 1994. Stem cells from primordial germ cells can reenter the germ line. *Dev. Biol.* **161:** 626–628.

Su H., Wang X., and Bradley A. 2000. Nested chromosomal deletions induced with retroviral vectors in mice. *Nat. Genet.* **24:** 92–95.

Suda Y., Suzuki M., Ikawa Y., and Aizawa S. 1987. Mouse embryonic stem cells exhibit indefinite proliferative potential. *J. Cell. Physiol.* **133:** 197–201.

Symes A., Stahl N., Reeves S.A., Farruggella T., Servidei T., Gearan T., Yancopoulos G., and Fink J.S. 1997. The protein tyrosine phosphatase SHP-2 negatively regulates ciliary neurotrophic factor induction of gene expression. *Curr. Biol.* **7:** 697–700.

Tada M., Tada T., Lefebvre L., Barton S.C., and Surani M.A. 1997. Embryonic germ cells induce epigenetic reprogramming of somatic nucleus in hybrid cells. *EMBO J.* **16:** 6510–6520.

Takahashi-Tezuka M., Yoshida Y., Fukada T., Ohtani T., Yamanaka Y., Nishida K., Nakajima K., Hibi M., and Hirano T. 1998. Gab1 acts as an adapter molecule linking the cytokine receptor gp130 to ERK mitogen-activated protein kinase. *Mol. Cell. Biol.* **18:** 4109–4117.

Tam P. and Zhou S.X. 1996. The allocation of epiblast cells to ectodermal and germ-line lineages is influenced by the position of the cells in the gastrulating mouse embryo. *Dev. Biol.* **178:** 124–132.

Thomas K.R. and Capecchi M.R. 1987. Site directed mutagenesis by gene targeting in mouse embryo-derived stem cells. *Cell* **51:** 503–512.

Thompson S., Clarke A.R., Pow A.M., Hooper M.L., and Melton D.W. 1989. Germ line transmission and expression of a corrected gene produced by gene targetting in embryonic stem cells. *Cell* **56:** 313–321.

Thomson J.A., Itskovitz-Eldor J., Shapiro S.S., Waknitz M.A., Swiergiel J.J., Marshall V.S., and Jones J.M. 1998. Embryonic stem cell lines derived from human blastocysts. *Science* **282:** 1145–1147.

Tomizuka K., Yoshida H., Uejima H., Kugoh H., Sato K., Ohguma A., Hayasaka M., Hanaoka K., Oshimura M., and Ishida I. 1997. Functional expression and germline transmission of a human chromosome fragment in chimaeric mice (see comments). *Nat. Genet.* **16:** 133–143.

Weiss M.J. and Orkin S.H. 1996. In vitro differentiation of murine embryonic stem cells. *J. Clin. Invest.* **97:** 591–595.

Weissman I.L. 2000. Stem cells: Units of development, units of regeneration, and units in evolution. *Cell* **100:** 157–168.

Wianny F., Real F.X., Mummery C.L., Van Rooijen M., Lahti J., Samarut J., and Savatier P. 1998. G1-phase regulators, cyclin D1, cyclin D2, and cyclin D3: Up-regulation at gastrulation and dynamic expression during neurulation. *Dev. Dyn.* **212:** 49–62.

Wiles M.V., and Johansson B.M. 1999. Embryonic stem cell development in a chemically defined medium. *Exp. Cell. Res.* **247:** 241–248.

Wiles M.V. and Keller G. 1991. Multiple hematopoietic lineages develop from embryonic stem (ES) cells in culture. *Development* **111:** 259–267.

Williams R.L., Hilton D.J., Pease S., Willson T.A., Stewart C.L., Gearing D.P., Wagner E.F., Metcalf D., Nicola N.A., and Gough N.M. 1988. Myeloid leukaemia inhibitory factor maintains the developmental potential of embryonic stem cells. *Nature* **336:** 684–687.

Yamashita J., Itoh H., Hirashima M., Ogawa M., Nishikawa S., Yurugi T., Naito M., Nakao K., and Nishikawa S. 2000. Flk-1-positive cells derived from embryonic stem cells serve as vascular progenitors. *Nature* **408:** 92–96.

Yoshida K., Chambers I., Nichols J., Smith A., Saito M., Yasukawa K., Shoyab M., Taga T., and Kishimoto T. 1994. Maintenance of the pluripotential phenotype of embryonic stem cells through direct activation of gp130 signaling pathways. *Mech. Dev.* **45:** 163–171.

Zambrowicz B.P., Friedrich G.A., Buxton E.C., Lilleberg S.L., Person C., and Sands A.T. 1998. Disruption and sequence identification of 2000 genes in mouse embryonic stem cells. *Nature* **392:** 608–611.

Zheng B., Sage M., Sheppeard E.A., Jurecic V., and Bradley A. 2000. Engineering mouse chromosomes with Cre-loxP: Range, efficiency, and somatic applications. *Mol. Cell. Biol.* **20:** 648–655.

11

Embryonal Carcinoma Cells as Embryonic Stem Cells

Peter W. Andrews and Stefan A. Przyborski
Department of Biomedical Science
University of Sheffield
Sheffield S10 2TN, United Kingdom

James A. Thomson
Wisconsin Regional Primate Research Center
and The Department of Anatomy
University of Wisconsin School of Medicine
Madison, Wisconsin 53715-1299

Embryonal carcinoma (EC) cells are the stem cells of teratocarcinomas. These tumors, which present a caricature of embryogenesis, have fascinated pathologists for many hundreds of years. Indeed, Wheeler (1983), in his excellent review of the history of these tumors, mentions that the earliest reference to what is evidently a teratoma, a benign form, is found on clay tablets from the Chaldean Royal Library of Nineveh dating from 600 to 900 B.C. Among these tablets, devoted to methods of predicting the future, one sign is described, *"When a woman gives birth to an infant that has three feet, two in their normal position (attached to the body), and the third between them, there will be great prosperity in the land"* (Ballantyne 1894). Such an optimistic forecast perhaps foretells the value that modern biologists have found in EC cells as tools for the study of cell differentiation in embryonic development and cancer.

Teratomas and teratocarcinomas occur in a range of manifestations (Table 1). The most common are ovarian dermoid cysts. These form from oocytes that are parthogenetically activated and begin development but eventually become disorganized, giving rise to a teratoma containing a haphazard array of embryonic tissues (Fig. 1). Such tumors are generally benign, but they can grow to very large sizes. Teratomas also occur, although more rarely, in other sites, including the base of the spine in newborn infants, and it is a tumor of this type that is evidently the subject of the Chaldean writer.

Stem Cell Biology © 2001 Cold Spring Harbor Laboratory Press 0-87969-575-7/01 $5 +. 00

Table 1 Simplified classification of germ cell tumors

Histological type	Description	Comments
Teratoma	A tumor containing an array of differentiated somatic cell types.	The differentiated cells may be organized into well recognizable anatomical structures (e.g., teeth) or be haphazardly arranged. These tumors are often benign, but their malignant potential is well known. The most common form is the benign "dermoid cyst" of the ovary.
Embryonal carcinoma	"Undifferentiated" epithelial cells resembling embryonic cells of the ICM and the primitive ectoderm.	Highly malignant tumors; the cells are generally regarded as stem cells able to differentiate into a range of histological cell types.
Teratocarcinoma	A tumor contain both teratoma and embryonal carcinoma.	The malignancy of these tumors is generally ascribed to their embryonal carcinoma component.
Yolk sac carcinoma	Cells resemble those of the extraembryonic "yolk sac."	In the mouse these cells may resemble parietal or visceral yolk sac; in humans no such clear distinction is evident. Human yolk sac carcinoma typically produces α-fetoprotein.
Choriocarcinoma	Cells resemble cyto- and syncytiotrophoblast of the placenta.	These do not occur in GCTs of the laboratory mouse.
Seminoma	Relatively uniform cells resembling "primordial germ cells."	A malignancy tumor that does not occur in the laboratory mouse; known as Dysgerminoma in females.
Spermatocytic seminoma	Heterogeneous cells resembling a caricature of spermatogenesis.	A low malignancy tumor occurring in older men, and generally regarded as distinct from all other GCTs.

The histopathology and classification of germ cell tumors is complex and controversial. The descriptions above may be regarded as oversimplified by experienced pathologists, but they represent common usage among developmental and cell biologists. More detailed descriptions and discussion may be found in histopathology texts (see, e.g., Mostofi and Price 1973).

Of greater clinical significance to cancer biologists are the teratocarcinomas of the testis (Dixon and Moore 1952; Mostofi and Price 1973). These tumors are a subgroup of cancers that, because of their histological complexity, site of origin, and apparent caricature of embryogenesis, have

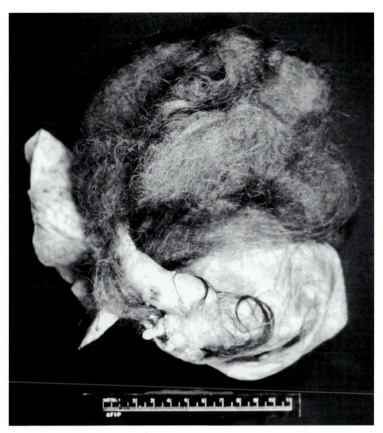

Figure 1 Human ovarian teratoma, or dermoid cyst. Although a wide range of more or less well organized tissues may be found in these tumors, masses of hair and teeth (*bottom left*) are especially common. (Courtesy, Department of Pathology, University of Sheffield.)

generally been thought to arise from germ cells (Fig. 2). Germ cell tumors (GCT) account for almost all testicular cancers and are always malignant. They occur typically in young post-pubertal men, with a peak incidence in the third decade of life (Møller 1993). Although they are rare, their incidence has increased markedly over the past 50 years, and their medical significance also reflects the young age of the patients. On the other hand, GCT are among the most treatable cancers since the advent of *cis*-platinum-based therapy in the 1970s (Einhorn 1987; Stoter 1987).

Testicular GCT are usually divided into seminomas and non-seminomas (Damjanov 1990, 1993). Seminomas are, histologically, relatively homogeneous tumors consisting of cells that resemble primordial germ cells, in contrast to the non-seminomas, which are histologically hetero-

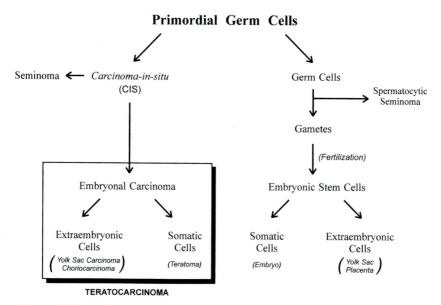

Figure 2 Schematic representation of a common view of germ cell tumor histogenesis and its parallel with embryogenesis.

geneous and may, confusingly, also contain elements of seminoma. More striking, however, is the frequent occurrence of somatic tissues such as nerve, bone, or muscle in non-seminomatous GCT as well as a histologically undifferentiated cell type known as embryonal carcinoma (EC). EC cells are now known to be the key malignant stem cells of these tumors, capable of differentiating into the wide range of somatic cells that comprise the teratomatous elements. The term teratocarcinoma is used to refer to GCT containing both embryonal carcinoma and teratoma components. Other elements of non-seminomatous GCT include highly malignant cells corresponding to the yolk sac (yolk sac carcinoma) and trophoblast (choriocarcinoma). Embryonal carcinoma, yolk sac carcinoma, and, rarely, choriocarcinoma may all occur alone, or combined with one another, as well as with teratoma elements.

TERATOCARCINOMAS IN THE LABORATORY MOUSE

Pathologists have long held the notion that the formation of teratocarcinomas in some way reflects the processes of embryonic development, and that EC cells perhaps resemble undifferentiated stem cells from the early embryo (Dixon and Moore 1952; Damjanov and Solter 1974). However, the rarity of the human tumors and the sporadic nature of similar tumors in animals limited their study until Stevens and Little (1954) discovered that about 1% of male mice of strain 129 develop testicular teratomas (Stevens and Hummel 1957; Stevens 1967a). This provided the starting point for a detailed study that led through the characterization of murine EC cells to the eventual development of embryonic stem (ES) cell lines from mouse embryos in 1981 (Evans and Kaufman 1981; Martin 1981).

The teratomas of 129 male mice can be observed by 15 days of embryonic development, as structures described as embryoid bodies within the seminiferous tubules of the fetal gonad. Stevens (1964) estimated that such teratomas originated between 11 and 12 days of development. He also showed that the incidence of these tumors can be increased by transplanting the genital ridges of early embryos to the testis capsule of adult mice. Furthermore, although no other strain of mouse regularly produces testicular teratomas spontaneously, transplantation of the genital ridges from embryos of the A/He strain also resulted in the formation of teratomas (Stevens 1970a). There is a very narrow window in development when the genital ridges are susceptible to such manipulation. Primordial germ cells, which are first identifiable in the extraembryonic yolk sac, migrate through the hindgut to the genital ridges, arriving at about 11 days of development (Bendel-Stenzel et al. 1998). The greatest incidence of induced teratomas occurred after transplanting genital ridges from 12 to 12.5 day embryos, and fell dramatically when genital ridges from older embryos were transplanted. An upper limit of about 13.5 days implies some changes in the germ cells after arriving in the genital ridge rendering them resistant to transformation. This could be associated with their entering mitotic arrest soon after their arrival in the genital ridge.

Confirmation of the germ cell origin of the spontaneous and experimental testicular teratomas came from studies of mice homozygous for mutations at the *Steel (Sl)* locus (Stevens 1967b). The *Sl* locus encodes stem cell factor (SCF), a growth factor required for survival of the various stem cells including melanocytes, hematopoietic stem cells, and primordial germ cells (Besmer 1991). Viable *Sl/Sl* homozygotes are infertile since the primordial germ cells do not survive migration. After crossing *Sl* on to the 129 background, Stevens found that the genital ridges from *Sl/Sl* mice did not yield teratomas, confirming the origin of those tumors from primordial germ cells. Curiously, however, males heterozygous for *Steel (Sl/+)* exhibit an increased incidence of teratomas (Stevens 1964). The reason for this has never been elucidated. However, the receptor for SCF is encoded by the *W* locus, which encodes the c-*kit* oncogene. One wonders whether, in the presence of suboptimal SCF levels that might occur in *Sl/+* mice, expression of *W/c-kit* might be up-regulated, with subsequent effects on germ cell proliferation.

Subsequently, Stevens identified another strain of laboratory mouse, the LT strain, that exhibits ovarian teratomas at high frequency (Stevens and Varnum 1974). In this case, it is evident that oocytes within the ovary frequently undergo parthogenetic activation and initiate embryonic development that becomes progressively disorganized, forming tumors that appear to be the counterparts of benign ovarian cysts in humans.

Despite its long history, the genetic basis for the susceptibility of 129 mice to teratoma development remains unclear. A mutation, *Ter,* occurring in a subline 129/terSv, causes teratomas to develop with a much higher frequency than in the original 129/Sv line (Stevens 1973). Backcross analysis of 129/ter mice has shown that the *Ter* gene is located on chromosome 18 within 0.6 cM of *Grl1* (Asada et al. 1994; Sakurai et al. 1994), but its molecular identity is currently unknown. Strangely, *Ter/Ter* mice exhibit a reduced number of germ cells (Noguchi and Noguchi 1985). Thus, counterintuitively, the mutations at two loci (*Sl* and *Ter*) known to increase susceptibility to germ cell tumors also appear to reduce germ cell viability and/or proliferation. To date, no mutations causing hyperproliferation of mouse germ cells are known (Noguchi et al. 1996). *Ter* is a modifying gene that is neither sufficient nor necessary for GCT formation and does not cause tumors on backgrounds other than 129 (Sakurai et al. 1994). Evidently, susceptibility to teratomas is polygenic and is presumably influenced by environmental or stochastic factors, since penetrance is low.

The testicular tumors formed spontaneously in 129 mice or following genital ridge transplantation can be divided into those that can be retransplanted into other syngeneic mice, and those that cannot (Stevens and Hummel 1957). The retransplantable tumors, termed teratocarcinomas, contain groups of cells identified as EC cells by comparison with the EC cells recognized in human teratocarcinomas. Kleinsmith and Pierce (1964) provided the first evidence that these EC cells are the malignant stem cells of teratocarcinomas: Transplantation of single EC cells from one tumor to a new host proved sufficient to result in the formation of a new teratocarcinoma containing the full range of differentiated elements seen in the parental tumor. Thus, not only are the EC cells the malignant stem cells of the tumor, they are also the repository of the pluripotent nature of these tumors. Non-retransplantable teratomas did not contain EC cells.

Although testicular teratomas can only be induced in a limited number of strains, teratomas can also be formed from many other strains of mice if rather earlier embryos, notably at about 7 days of development at the egg cylinder stage, are transplanted to ectopic sites (Stevens 1970b; Solter et al. 1970, 1979). As in the ovarian parthogenetic tumors, these embryos continue to grow, become disorganized, and form teratomas or, in some cases, retransplantable teratocarcinomas containing EC cells. Whether retransplantable teratocarcinomas are formed depends on the host strain into which the embryo is transplanted, and not on the genotype of the embryo itself (Solter et al. 1981). Solter and Damjanov (1979) also showed that the outcome of these experiments is dependent on the immune status of the host. Thus, whereas C3H embryos transplanted to C3H hosts typically form teratocarcinomas, teratomas were mostly formed if the C3H host had been rendered immunodeficient by neonatal thymectomy and sublethal irradiation. This phenomenon remains unexplained. One possibility is that the persistence of EC cells is fostered by a factor produced by the immune system; alternatively, it was suggested that higher levels of natural killer cells in mice deficient for T-lymphocytes might be detrimental to EC cell survival.

Murine Embryonal Carcinoma Cell Lines

Cell cultures of EC cells derived from murine teratocarcinomas were first reported by Kahn and Ephrussi in 1970. Subsequently, several groups established murine EC cell lines, although with some difference in emphasis and techniques (Fig. 3a). Many of these lines can be maintained as undifferentiated EC cells in vitro but are able to form teratocarcinomas when transplanted back to an appropriate mouse host (Evans 1972; Jakob et al. 1973; Martin and Evans 1974; Nicolas et al. 1975). They are said to

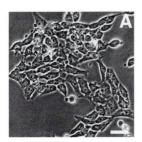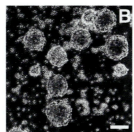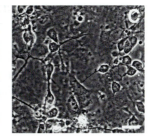

Figure 3 The murine pluripotent EC cell line, PCC7 (Pfeiffer et al. 1981). (*A*) Undifferentiated EC cells. (*B*) Embryoid bodies formed by culture in suspension. (*C*) Differentiation into neurons and other cell types after induction with retinoic acid. Bars: (*A*) 20 μm; (*B*) 100 μm; (*C*) 15 μm.

be "pluripotent"; however, some EC cell lines evidently lose this ability to differentiate and are termed "nullipotent" (Bernstine et al. 1973).

Some of the pluripotent lines also differentiate in culture, but the circumstances vary between lines and between laboratories. For example, among EC lines derived by Jakob and her colleagues, PCC3 EC cells remain undifferentiated if kept proliferating in subconfluent cultures (Nicolas et al. 1975). However, if allowed to reach confluence and maintained in that condition for several days, these cells differentiate spontaneously, yielding a variety of cell types, including nerve and muscle. Maintenance of other pluripotent EC lines in an undifferentiated state, however, was found to depend on culture on feeder layers of transformed mouse fibroblasts (Martin and Evans 1975). The STO line of transformed mouse fibroblasts rapidly became the standard feeder widely used for such cells. In this case, differentiation can be induced by removing the EC cells from the feeder cells. It was found particularly advantageous to force the cells to grow in suspension without attachment to a substrate by culture in bacteriological petri dishes. Under these conditions, the cells aggregate and form structures known as embryoid bodies, in which an inner core of EC cells is surrounded by a layer of cells resembling the visceral endoderm of an early mouse conceptus. Gradually these embryoid bodies become histologically complex and cystic, and a wide variety of differentiated cells grow out when the embryoid bodies are plated on a substrate that permits attachment.

Relationship to the Early Embryo

It had long been hypothesized from studies of human teratocarcinomas that EC cells might resemble stem cells from the early embryo. During the 1960s and early 1970s, research in a different sphere, in the biology of the immune system and the genetics of transplantation, focused attention on the role of the cell surface in regulating cell behavior. The area of immunogenetics that led to the development of techniques for producing antisera to specific cell-surface antigens had also led to the notion that these antigens might play a role in the regulation of cell differentiation (Boyse and Old 1969). The coincidence of these ideas with the availability of cultured EC cells quickly led to experiments to identify specific *embryonic* cell-surface antigens. One approach, adopted by Artzt et al. (1973), was to immunize adult 129 mice with EC cells (they chose the F9 line) that were also of 129 origin. Prevailing concepts of immunology suggested that, because of tolerance, the only antigens to which the adult 129 mice would form antibodies would be those expressed only on the "embryonic" EC cells and not on any adult cells. Anti-F9 sera produced in 129 mice did indeed detect, in cytotoxicity and immunofluorescence assays, an antigen expressed by EC cells but not by a range of other more differentiated cells. This same antigen was also expressed by cells of the inner cell mass (ICM) of the embryonic blastocyst. This relationship, as well as similar expression of other markers like alkaline phosphatase, taken together with a comparable capacity for differentiation, led to the notion that EC cells are a malignant counterpart of ICM embryonic cells (Jacob 1978).

The nature of the F9 antigen became controversial because of suggestions that it was related to key cell-surface molecules encoded by the *T-locus*, the complex genetics of which was then poorly understood (Kemler et al. 1976). The difficulties of working with polyclonal antisera meant that the precise nature of this anti-F9 activity was never resolved, although a link to the *T-locus* became progressively unlikely (Gachelin et al. 1982). Nevertheless, the hypothesis provided a strong stimulus to mouse developmental biology both in ideas and technology, just as approaches based on molecular genetics and monoclonal antibodies became available. The advent of monoclonal antibodies led to the production of reagents that identify antigens with similar characteristics to the F9 antigen. Perhaps the most notable of these monoclonal antibody-defined EC cell antigens is stage-specific embryonic antigen-1 (SSEA1), which was subsequently shown to involve an oligosaccharide epitope known as the Lewis-X (Le^x) antigen (Solter and Knowles 1978; Gooi et al. 1981). SSEA1 is commonly expressed by murine EC cells and embryonic ICM cells, and it seems likely that the polyclonal 129 anti-F9 serum contained significant levels of antibodies recognizing this epitope.

The proposition that EC cells are indeed the counterpart of ICM cells was soon tested directly by transferring small numbers of EC cells to blastocysts, which were subsequently re-implanted into pseudopregnant females. In the first experiments, reported by Brinster (1974), EC cells derived from an agouti mouse were injected into a blastocyst from an albino strain: A mouse was born that had patches of agouti fur as well as albino fur, indicating that some of its fur derived from the implanted EC cells. Others subsequently made more detailed experiments and demonstrated that the implanted EC cells in some cases contributed to almost all tissues of the host embryo (Papaioannou et al. 1975), and in rare cases it was reported that the germ line of the resultant chimeras was derived from the EC component (Mintz and Illmensee 1975). Not only did the experiments serve to demonstrate the close relationship of EC cells to the ICM, but they also suggested that their malignant character, seen in their ability to form retransplantable teratocarcinomas, was suppressed in the embryo. Indeed, as long suggested from the human studies, their differentiated derivatives were themselves generally not malignant, supporting the ideas of Pierce that the formation of cancers, and not only of teratocarcinomas, is associated with defects in the normal mechanisms of stem cell differentiation (Pierce 1974). In fact, it became evident that suppression of malignancy is not always complete, perhaps reflecting subtle genetic abnormalities in some of the EC cell lines (Papaioannou and Rossant 1983). Nevertheless, the concept of suppression of malignancy survives even though there are many exceptions, and oncologists treating human GCT are generally wary of persistent teratoma lesions in successfully treated patients, because of their potential for regaining malignancy.

Although murine teratocarcinomas were initially described as being euploid, it gradually became evident that small karyotypic changes frequently occurred. It seems likely that continued growth as a tumor, or extended growth in culture, leads to the accumulation of mutations that promote a transformed phenotype. That some EC cells lose their ability to differentiate could well reflect selection for mutations that interfere with differentiation. Indeed, cell hybrids formed between EC cells and somatic cells, notably thymocytes, often continue to exhibit an EC phenotype with a greater capacity for differentiation than the parental EC cells (Andrews and Goodfellow 1980). This suggests that wild-type alleles derived from the somatic cell parent complement "anti-differentiation" mutations derived from the parental EC cells.

Differentiation of EC Cells in Culture

Initial studies of EC cell differentiation focused on their ability to differentiate spontaneously under a variety of circumstances, most notably after producing embryoid bodies when cultured in suspension (Fig. 3b) (Martin and Evans 1975). However, although this differentiation to a wide range of cell types is intriguing, the range of cell types produced and the uncontrolled nature of the differentiation make study of the underlying processes difficult. A significant advance was the discovery that an apparently nullipotent EC cell line, F9, can be induced to differentiate by exposure to retinoic acid (Strickland and Mahdhavi 1978). After exposure to both retinoic acid and cAMP, F9 generated cells that closely resemble parietal endoderm (Strickland et al. 1980). Although retinoic acid had been known for many years to play a key role in epidermal cell differentiation, the results with F9 cells focused the attention of developmental biologists on the role of this important derivative of vitamin A in regulating embryonic development. Subsequently, if F9 cells are cultured in suspension in the presence of retinoic acid, they form embryoid bodies in which the outer layer of cells resembles visceral endoderm, while the inner cells retain the EC phenotype (Hogan et al. 1983). Thus, apparently, F9 cells can be switched between differentiating into visceral or parietal endoderm by altering the conditions of induction. It was later shown that retinoic acid is able to induce the differentiation of a number of mouse EC cell lines such as PCC7 (Fig. 3) (Pfeiffer et al. 1981). Perhaps the most well known of such EC lines is P19, which differentiates in a predominantly neural direction when exposed to retinoic acid (Jones-Villeneuve et al. 1982), but in a mesodermal direction, with the formation of muscle cells, when exposed to another agent, dimethylsulfoxide (DMSO) (McBurney et al. 1982). EC cell differentiation can also be induced by other agents such as hexamethylene bisacetamide (HMBA) (Jakob et al. 1978).

There is no doubt that studies of mouse EC cells in culture provided insights into molecules that play a role in embryonic development and regulate differentiation of embryonic cells. Moreover, the experience with EC cells provided the foundations for the development of ES cell lines (Evans and Kaufman 1981; Martin 1981). However, with the rapid advances in molecular genetics that have allowed access to the early mouse embryo, the availability of ES cells has reduced the necessity for studying EC cells. On the other hand, although their capacity for differentiation is substantially less than that of ES cells, EC cell lines may be more robust and simpler for some experimental purposes.

HUMAN EC CELLS

While embryogenesis in the laboratory mouse became progressively more accessible to experimental study, analysis of human development remained, and indeed still remains, severely restricted, not only by ethical considerations but also by the logistical problems of working with human embryos. Nevertheless, although recent developments in biology indicate a strong conservation of regulatory mechanisms throughout phylogeny, stretching from the nematode worm all the way to mammalian development, there is no doubt that each species presents unique features and that human development differs in significant ways from that of other mammals. Human EC cell lines provide an opportunity to investigate mechanisms that regulate embryonic cell differentiation in a way that is pertinent to early human development, while also shedding light on a medically significant form of cancer.

Cell lines were first derived from human germ cell tumors and maintained as xenografts in the 1950s (Pierce et al. 1957). Later, several lines were established in culture, notably TERA1, TERA2, and SuSa, described during the 1970s (Fogh and Trempe 1975; Hogan et al. 1977). Initial studies of these cell lines highlighted similarities with the mouse EC cells. In particular, some of the human GCT-derived cell lines were reported to express the F9 antigen and, later, SSEA1 (Hogan et al. 1977; Holden et al. 1977; Solter and Knowles 1978). It was first assumed that this was consistent with human EC cells expressing the F9 antigen, like murine EC cells. However, a comparative study by Andrews et al. (1980) of a range of cell lines derived from GCT, and a more detailed analysis of one of these, 2102Ep (Andrews et al. 1982), led to the conclusion that human EC cells differ in a number of respects from their murine counterparts. In particular, SSEA1, which had become a hallmark of murine EC cells, appeared *not* to be expressed by human EC cells, in contradiction to the earlier studies, although it is expressed by some derivative cells following differentiation. On the other hand, two new antigens, SSEA3 and SSEA4, which are expressed by cleavage-stage murine embryos but not ICM or EC cells, are present on human EC cells (Andrews et al. 1982; Damjanov et al. 1982; Shevinsky et al. 1982; Kannagai et al. 1983a).

SSEA3 and -4 are epitopes associated with globoseries glycolipids expressed on the cell surface (Table 2) (Kannagi et al. 1983a,b). In contrast, SSEA1 is an epitope associated with a lactoseries glycolipid that contains a different core structure, although it is synthesized from the same precursor, lactosylceramide (Gooi et al. 1981; Kannagi et al. 1982). Murine EC cells and early embryos express the Forssman antigen, which also possesses a globoseries core structure (Willison et al. 1982). However, the terminal disaccharide, galactosaminyl galactosamine, which forms the Forssman epitope, occurs in the mouse but not in humans. One possibility is that the terminal structures forming the SSEA3 and -4 epitopes in humans might not occur in mouse EC cells because of competition by the enzyme forming the terminal Forssman epitope. Perhaps the more significant issue is the similarity between human and murine EC cells in their expression of globoseries glycolipid core structures, rather than differences in the terminal modifications of these oligosaccharides (Fenderson et al. 1987).

The SSEA3 and -4 epitopes are members of the P blood group system, and the red blood cells of most people express both epitopes. However, a very small number of individuals lack the ability to synthesize the P blood group substance, which has been identified with globoside,

Table 2 Glycolipid antigens identified in human EC cells and their differentiated derivatives

Antigen	Terminal carbohydrate structures forming the epitope	Lactosyl ceramide core
SSEA3	Galβ1→3GalNAcβ1→3Galα1→	
SSEA3, SSEA4	NeuNAcα→3Galβ1→3GalNAcβ1→3Galα1→	
Globo H	Fucα1→2Galβ1→3GalNAcβ1→3Galα1→	
Globo A	GalNAcα1→3Galβ1→3GalNAcβ1→3Galα1→	
	2	
	↑	
	Fucα1	

Galβ1→4Glcβ1→Cer

SSEA1	Galβ1→4GlcNAcβ1→ ——————	
	3	
	↑	
	Fucα1	

| ME311 | (9-0-acetyl)NeuNAcα2→8NeuNAcα2→ | |
| A2B5 | NeuNAcα2→8NeuNAcα2→8NeuNAcα2→ | |

The globoseries antigens SSEA3, SSEA4, globo A, and globo H (Kannagi et al 1983a,b; Fenderson et al 1987), the lactoseries antigen SSEA1 (Kannagi et al. 1982; Gooi et al. 1981), and the ganglioseries antigens, ME311 and A2B5 (Thurin et al. 1985; Fenderson et al. 1987) are all synthesized by extension from a common precursor, lactosyl ceramide. The enzymes responsible for addition of the third sugar residues (galactosyl, glucosaminyl, and sialyl transferase, respectively) appear to regulate the rate-limiting step that controls which synthetic pathway predominates (Chen et al. 1989).

and these individuals are also unable to produce the SSEA3 or -4 antigens (Tippett et al. 1986). Interestingly, women lacking the P blood group antigens have a high rate of spontaneous abortions (Race and Sanger 1975), perhaps because of their ability to mount an immune reaction to antigens such as SSEA3 and –4, which studies of EC cells suggested are expressed on the very early embryo (Tippett et al. 1986). It also transpires that red blood cells of about 1% of Caucasians do not express SSEA4, which has been equated to a previously identified blood group antigen called Luke. It is not known whether Luke (–)/SSEA4(–) individuals also have high rates of spontaneous abortions, or what other consequences might flow from this polymorphism.

Another set of antigens that have been identified in human EC cells are epitopes associated with keratan sulfate, notably TRA-1-60 and TRA-1-81 (Andrews et al. 1984a; Badcock et al. 1999), as well as GCTM2, K21, and K4 (Rettig et al. 1985; Pera et al. 1988). It appears that these epitopes are commonly expressed by human EC cells, and indeed some, notably TRA-1-60, have been shown to be useful serum markers in germ cell tumor patients as they are shed by EC cells (Marrink et al. 1991; Mason et al. 1991; Gels et al. 1997). A workshop to compare expression of a variety of antigens by a large panel of human GCT cells confirmed that SSEA3, SSEA4, TRA-1-60, TRA-1-81, and GCTM2 are all characteristic markers of human EC cells (Andrews et al. 1996).

Differentiation of Human EC Cells

A striking feature of many established human EC cell lines is their lack of ability to differentiate into well-recognizable cell types. This might, in part, reflect their evolution in tumors, since an ability to differentiate would tend to limit tumor growth and so provide a selective disadvantage for stem cells, whereas acquisition of an inability to differentiate would provide a strong selective advantage. Unlike murine EC cells, human EC cells are highly aneuploid, and it is easy to envisage that genetic changes which inhibit their differentiation might occur readily during their development. This facet of human GCT biology makes difficult the definition of EC cells, since an ability to differentiate is generally taken as a key diagnostic feature of an EC phenotype, and of course, the particular interest of EC cells to developmental biologists lies in their ability to differentiate. Recently, we observed that hybrids formed between 2102Ep, a relatively nullipotent EC line, and NTERA2 pluripotent EC cells appeared to retain an ability to differentiate (C. Duran and P.W. Andrews, unpubl.). Therefore, we concluded that 2102Ep cells fail to differentiate because of a loss of some function rather than acquisition of an active inhibitor of differentiation.

Nevertheless, a number of human EC cell lines do show morphological changes, accompanied by changes in expression of various markers, when cultured under different conditions. In particular, many undergo a transition to a "large flat" phenotype when cultured at low cell densities. This has been examined in closest detail in the 2102Ep EC cell line (Andrews et al. 1982). Low-density culture of these cells results in down-regulation of SSEA3, and the appearance of SSEA1. The low-density, SSEA1 (+) cells also activate expression of fibronectin (Andrews 1982), and some produce human chorionic gonadotropin (HCG) and resemble trophoblastic giant cells (Damjanov and Andrews 1983). The mechanism of low-density-induced differentiation is unclear. It is evidently not due to low levels of an autocrine factor produced by the EC cells themselves, as conditioned medium from high-density cultures does not inhibit the phenomenon. Additionally, inhibition of cadherin-mediated cell:cell adhesion by culture in medium with low levels of Ca^{++} does not induce this type of differentiation (Giesberts et al. 1999). Nevertheless, some short-range signal between cells must be involved.

The apparent trophoblast differentiation seen in low-density cultures of 2102Ep, and some other human EC cell lines, reflects a notable difference between murine and human GCT; namely, the frequent occurrence of trophoblastic elements in human but not mouse teratocarcinomas (Damjanov and Solter 1974). The observation that murine EC cells appear to make trophoblastic elements only rarely, if at all, correlates with the notion that murine EC cells are equivalent to late ICM, or primitive ectoderm cells which have lost the capacity for trophoblastic differentiation. A corollary of these observations is that human EC cells correspond to an earlier stage of embryonic development than mouse EC cells (e.g., cleavage-stage embryos), or that the embryonic cells to which the human cells are related possess a wider range of potency than the corresponding mouse cells at the same stage of embryonic development.

Although many human EC cells do not appear to differentiate in response to retinoic acid, a number of lines that do differentiate extensively have been described. For example, GCT27 is an EC cell line that requires maintenance on feeder layers to prevent differentiation (Pera et al. 1989). When removed from feeders, the cells undergo differentiation into a variety of cell types that include extraembryonic endodermal cells and cells with neural properties. They respond to retinoic acid, yielding cells resembling extraembryonic endoderm (Roach et al. 1993), and also differentiate in response to BMP2 (Pera and Herzfeld 1998). Other EC lines that differentiate extensively include NCR-G3 (Hata et al. 1989; Umezawa et al. 1996), NCC IT (Teshima et al. 1988; Damjanov et al. 1993), and NEC14 (Hasegawa et al. 1991). However, perhaps the most extensively studied is the TERA2 line.

The TERA2 Pluripotent EC Line

The TERA2 teratocarcinoma cell line is one of the oldest extant human GCT lines (Fogh and Trempe 1975), but it was several years before it was recognized as a pluripotent EC cell because cultures of these cells frequently contain multiple cell types and may, depending on culture conditions, contain very few EC cells. A more robust subline, NTERA2, was derived by Andrews et al. (1984b) after passage of TERA2 through an athymic (nu/nu) (nude) mouse in which it formed a xenograft tumor with marked teratoma features. TERA2 and NTERA2 xenografts contain multiple cell types, most notably glandular structures and neural elements (Fig. 4). Single-cell clones of NTERA2 were isolated, and NTERA2 clone D1 (often abbreviated NT2/D1) became the standard line that is now widely used. NTERA2 cells express characteristics in common with other human EC cells such as 2102Ep, for example, SSEA3 and SSEA4, as well as TRA-1-60 and high levels of the liver isozyme of alkaline phosphatase. Interestingly, unlike many other human EC lines, the TERA2-derived lines do not express any placental-like ALP activity and show no evidence of trophoblastic differentiation when cultured at low cell density, although induction of both SSEA1 and fibronectin occurs.

Not only do NTERA2 EC cells form well-differentiated teratomas when grown as xenografts in nude mice, they also respond to retinoic acid and other agents in culture (Fig. 5) (Andrews 1984). After exposure to 10^{-5} or 10^{-6} M retinoic acid, NTERA2 cells rapidly lose their EC phenotype, acquiring a substantially different growth pattern and cellular morphology. Cultures exposed to retinoic acid typically lose expression of EC markers such as SSEA3, SSEA4, or TRA-1-60 over a 1- to 2-week period (Fig. 6). At the same time, a variety of other antigens, notably ganglioseries glycolipids, appear on the surface of the cells (Fenderson et al. 1987). Generally, a 2- to 3-day exposure to retinoic acid is sufficient to commit almost all the cells to differentiate, and within 2–3 weeks, EC cells are not detectable in the cultures.

Differentiation of NTERA2 EC cells is characterized not only by changes in surface antigen expression, but also by changes in susceptibility to infection with certain viruses, notably human cytomegalovirus (HCMV) and human immunodeficiency virus (HIV). For example,

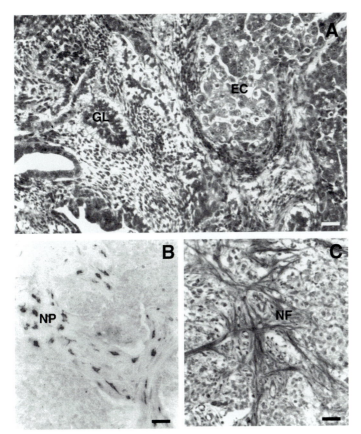

Figure 4 Xenograft tumor of NTERA2 human EC cells grown in a SCID mouse. (*A*) Staining with hematoxylin and eosin, showing glandular structures (GL) and patches of embryonal carcinoma (EC); (*B*) staining for Nissl substance indicating neural perikarya (NP); (*C*) silver staining of neural fibers (NF). Bars: (*A*) 60 μm; (*B, C*) 40 μm.

NTERA2 stem cells are resistant to infection with HCMV and HIV, whereas the differentiated cells are permissive for the replication of both viruses (Gönczöl et al. 1984; Hirka et al. 1991). In the case of HCMV, resistance results from inactivity of the major immediate early promoter of the virus in the EC cells (Lafemina and Hayward 1988; Nelson and Groudine 1986).

Many genes also show a marked regulation during NTERA2 differentiation. For example, *Oct4*, which is characteristically expressed by EC cells and ES cells, is down-regulated following retinoic acid induction of NTERA2 cells (S.A. Przyborski and P.W. Andrews, unpubl.). At the same

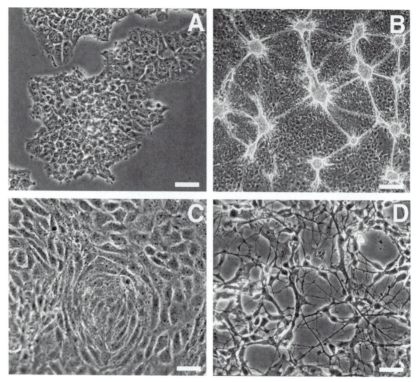

Figure 5 Cultures of NTERA2 human EC cells. Phase contrast micrographs of NTERA2 cultures showing: (*A*) undifferentiated NTERA2 human EC stem cells; (*B, C*) differentiated derivatives after 3–4 weeks' exposure to 10 μM retinoic acid and 3 mM HMBA, respectively; (*D*) cultures enriched for NTERA2-derived neurons as previously described (Pleasure et al. 1992). Bars: (*A, B, C*) 50 μm; (*D*) 500 μm.

time, a number of other genes are induced. Among these is a member of the *Wnt* family, *Wnt13*, that is not expressed by NTERA2 or other human EC cells, but is induced strongly upon retinoic acid induction (Wakeman et al. 1998). Curiously, we have not detected expression of other members of the *Wnt* family during NTERA2 differentiation whereas, for example, *Wnt1* has been noted to be induced during differentiation of the mouse EC line P19 (Papkoff 1994). Members of the *Frizzled* family of genes that encode putative receptors for *Wnt* are also expressed in various patterns during NTERA2 differentiation, and we have speculated that this may indicate a possible role for *Wnt* signaling in controlling the types of cells that are generated during differentiation (Wakeman et al. 1998 and unpubl.). Lithium, an inhibitor of GSK3β, which is a component of the Wnt signaling pathway, is also able to induce NTERA2 differentiation,

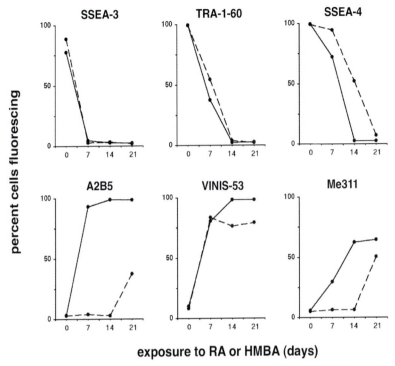

exposure to RA or HMBA (days)

Figure 6 Changes in cell-surface antigen expression by NTERA2 cells during differentiation induced by either 10 μM retinoic acid (*solid line*) or 3 mM HMBA (*broken line*), analyzed by immunofluorescence and flow cytofluorimetry. SSEA3, SSEA4, and TRA-1-60 are EC-cell-specific antigens (Andrews et al. 1996), whereas A2B5, VINIS53, and ME311 are antigens induced upon differentiation (Fenderson et al. 1987; Andrews et al. 1990). SSEA3, SSEA4, A2B5, and ME311 are associated with glycolipids (see Table 1), whereas TRA-1-60 is a keratan sulfate-associated antigen (Badcock et al. 1999) and VINIS53 recognizes NCAM (P.W. Andrews, unpubl.).

and we have speculated that this might indicate a potential for EC cell differentiation to be modulated by Wnt signaling (Giesberts et al. 1999).

One gene family that is subject to marked up-regulation following retinoic acid treatment is the *Hox* family. Mammalian *Hox* genes are encoded by four separate clusters located throughout the mammalian genome (Wright 1991). These clusters are related in organization to those that occur in lower vertebrates and invertebrates such as *Drosophila*, and the temporal and spatial pattern of expression of the genes along the anterior–posterior axis of the developing embryo is related to their positions in the clusters. *Hox* genes located at the 3′ ends of the clusters have a more anterior pattern of expression than those found in the 5′ ends of the clusters. Mavilio and his colleagues observed that many *Hox* genes are induced during differentiation of NTERA2 cells (Mavilio et al. 1988) and, moreover, their expression is induced in a retinoic acid-dosage-dependent manner that relates to the position of *Hox* genes within the gene clusters (Simeone et al. 1990). Thus, *Hox* genes located at the 3′ ends of the *Hox* clusters are inducible to maximum level by low concentrations of retinoic acid (less than 10^{-7}M) whereas genes located at the 5′ ends of the clusters require much higher concentrations of 10^{-5} and 10^{-6} M retinoic acid for maximum induction. It was suggested that this feature reflects a possible role of retinoic acid in patterning the anterior–posterior axis of the developing embryo. The temporal sequence of *Hox* gene activation is also related to their position in the gene clusters, 3′-end genes appearing substantially before 5′-end genes.

As retinoic-acid-induced differentiation of NTERA2 EC cells progresses, neural markers become evident and neurons expressing neurofilament proteins and a typically neuronal morphology appear, most usually during the second week after first exposure to retinoic acid (Fig. 5B) (Andrews 1984; Lee and Andrews 1986). Neurons derived from NTERA2 after retinoic acid treatment probably comprise only 2–5% of all the differentiated cells, but they are the most obvious and prominent ones. These neurons express tetrodotoxin-sensitive sodium channels (Rendt et al. 1989) and exhibit regenerative membrane potentials, as well as a wide variety of other neural characteristics, such as glutamate receptors and voltage-gated calcium channels (Pleasure and Lee 1993; Younkin et al. 1993; Squires et al. 1996). Neurons may be purified from the cultures by techniques involving differential trypsinization and treatment with mitotic inhibitors (Fig. 5D) (Pleasure et al. 1992). Recently, it has been suggested that these NTERA2-derived neurons could be implanted into the central nervous system to correct neural deficits resulting from various diseases. Thus, in rats, such neurons will apparently survive and integrate functionally to correct partial defects resulting from experimentally induced stroke (Borlongan et al. 1998; Hurlbert et al. 1999; Muir et al. 1999; Philips et al. 1999).

The differentiation of NTERA2 cells into neurons appears in many ways to recapitulate the steps that occur during embryonic development of the nervous system (Figs. 7 and 8) (Przyborski et al. 2000). For example, *nestin,* a gene that encodes an intermediate neurofilament protein characteristic of proliferating neuroprogenitors, is rapidly up-regulated soon after NTERA2 EC cells are exposed to retinoic acid. This transient rise of *nestin* expression is immediately followed by increases in expres-

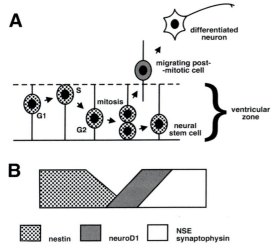

Figure 7 Gene expression in developing CNS neurons of the vertebrate embryo. (*A*) Neuronal precursors proliferate in the ventricular zone of the neural tube. As these cells repeatedly divide and pass through the cell cycle, the position of their perikarya oscillates within this germinal epithelium as indicated (G_1, S, G_2, mitosis). Cells leave the mitotic cycle, migrate out of the ventricular zone, and commence differentiation. The levels of previously characterized neural genes change markedly during this process and can be used as indicators of neuronal development. (*B*) Schematic illustrating the regulated expression of *nestin, neuroD1, neuron-specific enolase (NSE),* and *synaptophysin* in proliferating, postmitotic, and terminally differentiating embryonic neurons, respectively, during the formation of the vertebrate CNS.

sion of *neuroD1,* a bHLH transcription factor localized in postmitotic neuroblasts of the developing nervous system. Subsequently, genes typical of terminally differentiated neurons become expressed; for example, neuron-specific enolase and synaptophysin.

NTERA2 EC cells are susceptible to induction not only with retinoic acid but also with a number of other agents, most notably hexamethylene bisacetamide (HMBA) (Andrews et al. 1990) and members of the BMP family (Andrews et al. 1994). NTERA2 cells induced with 3 mM HMBA are distinct from those induced with retinoic acid, and neural elements are mostly not evident (Fig. 5C), although one good marker of differentiation induced by HMBA is NCAM. BMPs, notably BMP7, also induce NTERA2 differentiation, yielding again a distinct set of cells. On the other hand, there are some overlaps in the nature of the cells induced by these agents. For example, we have found the induction of smooth muscle actin following exposure to BMP7, but also, at rather lower levels, fol-

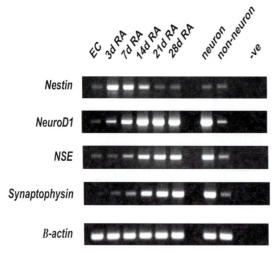

Figure 8 Expression of neurogenic genes during NTERA2 development. RT-PCR analysis of molecular markers for proliferating (*nestin*), postmitotic (*neuroD1*), and maturing (*NSE, synaptophysin*) neurons during retinoic-acid-induced differentiation of NTERA2 human EC cells. Purified neurons and nonneuron samples were prepared from 28-day retinoic-acid-induced NTERA2 cultures using the method of Pleasure et al. (1992). Expression of β-actin was used to assess RT DNA levels as shown.

lowing retinoic acid induction (Qualtrough 1998). Although many of the markers typical of retinoic acid induction are not expressed soon after treatment with HMBA, the HMBA-induced cultures eventually often express some of the markers that are typical of retinoic-acid-treated cultures, and a few neurons are occasionally observed. Thus, although the pathways of differentiation induced by these three agents, retinoic acid, HMBA, and BMP7, are predominantly different, they nevertheless seem to overlap with one another and the pathways are not mutually exclusive.

The nature of the nonneural cells seen in differentiating cultures of NTERA2, whether induced by retinoic acid, HMBA, or BMP7, are not fully characterized. Although the appearance of smooth muscle actin suggests the appearance of smooth muscle cells, we have never noted expression of *MyoD*, or the induction of cells corresponding to skeletal or cardiac muscle, which would indicate mesodermal differentiation; nor has endodermal differentiation been observed. It appears that NTERA2 EC cells are committed to ectoderm but that the nature of the ectodermal pathways induced depends on the culture conditions applied. Under some conditions, for example after retinoic acid induction, the cells adopt a fate more akin to dorsal ectoderm and give rise to neural derivatives, whereas in other circumstances they may give rise to more ventral types of ectoderm. Smooth muscle induction may be indicative of differentiation corresponding to neural crest derivatives. However, not only the NTERA2 EC cells, but also a number of other human EC lines express *Brachyury* even though mesodermal differentiation has not been observed (Gokhale et al. 2000). Whether this expression of *Brachyury* indicates a competence for mesodermal differentiation that is not realized under the available culture conditions, or whether *Brachyury* is not an indicator of competence for mesodermal differentiation in humans, remains to be ascertained. On the other hand, the gross aneuploidy of NTERA2 cells, in common with other human EC cells, may be indicative of genetic changes that interfere with their developmental potential.

PRIMATE ES CELL LINES

Although human EC cells resemble mouse EC cells in some respects, they differ from them in a number of important areas. Thus, the relationship of human EC cells to human embryonic stem (ES) cells was, to some extent, in question not least because of the extensive chromosomal changes seen in EC cells. However, recently, primate ES cell lines have been isolated from rhesus monkeys, common marmosets, and humans, and they have proved to share many of the characteristics previously defined for human EC cells.

The primate ES cells were derived by plating an isolated ICM on fibroblasts in the presence of serum, but in the absence of other exogenous growth factors (Thomson et al. 1995, 1996, 1998; Thomson and Marshall 1998; Reubinoff et al. 2000). These conditions are similar to those used for the derivation of some human EC cell lines, and for the derivation of mouse ES cells prior to the identification of leukemia inhibitory factor (LIF) as a critical mediator of mouse ES cell self-renewal (Smith et al. 1988; Williams et al. 1988). Human embryonic germ (EG) cell lines have also been isolated from fetal germ cells plated on fibroblasts in the presence of serum, but their derivation required supplementation of the medium with LIF, basic fibroblast growth factor, and forskolin (Shamblott et al. 1998).

The factors produced by fibroblasts that are required for human ES and EG cell self-renewal are unknown. Mouse ES cells remain undifferentiated and proliferate in the absence of fibroblasts if LIF, or other LIF cytokine family members such as ciliary neurotropic factor (CNF) or oncostatin M, are present (Smith et al. 1988; Williams et al. 1988;

Conover et al. 1993; Rose et al. 1994). Each of these factors acts through the LIF receptor complex, a heterodimer of the LIF receptor and the IL-6 signal transducer, gp130 (Yoshida et al. 1994). However, primate ES cells cultured in the presence of LIF and in the absence of fibroblasts uniformly differentiate or die within about 7–10 days (Thomson and Marshall 1998; Thomson et al. 1995, 1996, 1998; Reubinoff et al. 2000). Rhesus ES cells grown on primary fibroblasts derived from homozygous LIF-knockout mice continue undifferentiated proliferation for at least three passages (Thomson and Marshall 1998). Some human EC cell lines are feeder-dependent, and LIF, oncostatin M, and CNF also fail to prevent their differentiation (Roach et al. 1993). Given the reported importance of LIF in the culture of human EG cells, further work is warranted to clarify whether the gp130 signaling pathway is active at all in primate ES cells, or whether an entirely different signaling pathway mediates undifferentiated proliferation.

Human, rhesus monkey, and common marmoset ES cells all express a shared repertoire of cell-surface antigens that is similar to that of undifferentiated human EC cells, including SSEA3, SSEA4, TRA-1-60, TRA-1-81, and alkaline phosphatase (Thomson et al. 1995, 1996, 1998; Thomson and Marshall 1998; Reubinoff et al. 2000). Human EG cells similarly express these markers, but they also express the lactoseries glycolipids, SSEA1 (Shamblott et al. 1998), which is not expressed by human EC and primate ES cells. The pattern of markers expressed by both primate ES cells and human EG cells differs from those expressed by mouse ES cells, underscoring basic differences in early mouse and human embryology.

The morphologies of primate ES cells and human EC cells are very similar (Fig. 9), but are distinct from the reported morphology of human EG cells. Primate ES cells form relatively flat, compact colonies that dissociate into single cells easily in trypsin or in Ca^{++}/Mg^{++}-free medium, whereas human EG cells form tight, more spherical colonies that are refractory to routine dissociation methods. In general, undifferentiated growth of human EC cells is promoted at high cell densities. In contrast, primate ES cells differentiate rapidly if they are allowed to pile up after the cultures grow to confluence. It is not yet clear whether the cell-surface marker and morphological differences between human ES cells and human EG cells reflect fundamental biological differences, or merely differences in culture conditions.

Primate ES cells share with human EC cells the ability to differentiate to extraembryonic lineages, including yolk sac and trophoblast (Thomson et al. 1995, 1996, 1998; Thomson and Marshall 1998;

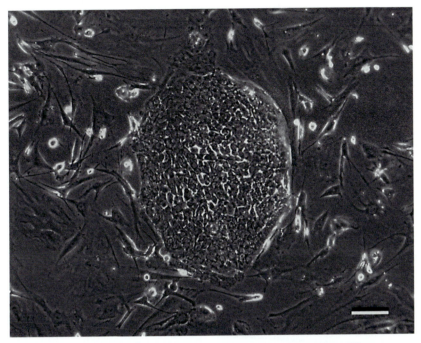

Figure 9 Human ES cell colony on fibroblast feeder layers. Bar, 75 μm.

Reubinoff et al. 2000). Mouse ES cells rarely contribute to trophoblast in chimeras, and it is unclear whether the rare ES-cell-derived cells that integrate into the trophoblast are functional trophoblast cells (Beddington et al. 1989). Primate ES cell lines will spontaneously differentiate in vitro to endoderm (probable extraembryonic endoderm) and trophoblast, evidenced by the secretion of α-fetoprotein and chorionic gonadotropin into the culture medium (Thomson et al. 1995, 1996, 1998; Thomson and Marshall 1998; Reubinoff et al. 2000). In the mouse embryo, the last cells capable of contributing to derivatives of both trophectoderm and all three embryonic germ layers are early ICM cells of the expanding blastocyst (Winkel and Pederson 1988). The timing of commitment to ICM or trophectoderm has not been established for any primate species, but because human EC/ES cells can differentiate to trophoblast and to derivatives of all three germ layers, and because they express SSEA3 and SSEA4, human EC/ES cells may resemble an earlier stage of embryogenesis than mouse EC/ES cells (Andrews et al. 1980). However, the fact that mouse ES cells will contribute to the trophoblast even rarely in chimeras suggests that they may have the developmental potential to form trophoblast, but that the environmental conditions in chimeras simply do not allow efficient differentiation to trophoblast by ES cells. Indeed, it has recently been demonstrated that repression of Oct4 in mouse ES cells induced trophectoderm differentiation (Niwa et al. 2000).

Like their mouse ES/EC counterparts, primate ES cell lines have both more advanced and more consistent developmental potentials than human EC cell lines, possibly reflecting the malignant origin and the severe karyotypic abnormalities of the EC cells (Roach et al. 1993). Human and rhesus ES cells injected into SCID mice consistently form teratomas with advanced differentiated structures of all three embryonic germ layers, including smooth and striated muscle, bone, cartilage, gut and respiratory epithelium, keratinizing squamous epithelium, neurons, and ganglia (Fig. 10). What is remarkable about the primate ES cell teratomas is not only the range of individual cell types, but also the formation of complex structures requiring coordinated interactions between different cell types. For example, the development of neural tube-like structures, gut-like

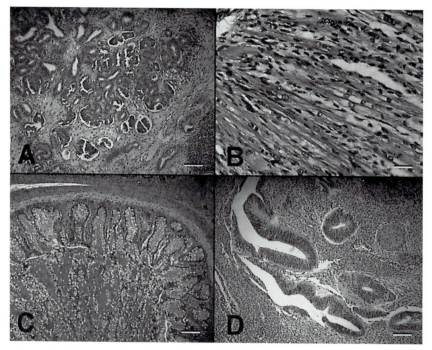

Figure 10 Teratoma from human ES cells injected into SCID beige mice: (*A*) Fetal glomeruli; (*B*) striated muscle; (*C*) gut; (*D*) neural epithelium. Bars: (*A, D*) 100 μm; (*B*) 50 μm; (*C*) 167 μm.

structures, and hair follicles requires highly coordinated interactions between different cell types. Finally, perhaps the most impressive example of organized epithelial–mesenchymal interactions in these primate ES cell tumors is the formation of well-organized tooth buds, complete with ameloblasts, odontoblasts, and intervening dentin. The formation of teratomas by human EG cells has not been described, but differentiation of derivatives of all three embryonic germ layers in vitro has been reported (Shamblott et al. 1998).

CONCLUSION

The past 20 years have been marked by a dramatic increase in our understanding of mammalian development, most notably in the laboratory mouse. In part, this has been a consequence of the revolution in molecular genetics, and the finding that many regulatory mechanisms have been highly conserved throughout phylogeny. It has also had its roots in the study of teratocarcinomas and their EC stem cells. Those studies provided a stimulus to thought and approaches to embryonic development at a time when other tools were limited. They provided access to key molecules and genes that play a role in development, and they continue to provide a convenient experimental system for addressing some questions about the mechanisms that regulate embryonic cell differentiation. The culmination of that work was the development of techniques for culturing ES cells, which now provide the key route to genetic manipulation of the laboratory mouse.

Although human embryogenesis undoubtedly resembles that of other mammalian species, there are certainly differences at the morphological as well as at the cellular and molecular levels. Given the logistical as well as ethical and legal difficulties surrounding work with human embryos, teratocarcinomas and their EC stem cells derived from human germ cell tumors provide a useful tool for helping to translate findings in species more tractable to experimental study to the human situation. For example, we have investigated the pattern of expression of various glycolipid antigens, and there are certainly aspects of their expression that are distinct between human and mouse EC cells and, evidently, embryos. The recent characterization of human and monkey ES cells has validated the presumption that human EC cells do relate to pluripotent cells of the very early embryo, as in the mouse model, so that results from EC cell lines will continue to provide important pointers for future study. In some ways, the capacity of EC cell differentiation is limited, and the availability of human ES cell lines will extend the range of questions that can be addressed in vitro. On the other hand, the limitations of EC cells can sometimes be put to advantage, as EC cells provide a simpler and more robust experimental system. Human EC and ES lines are likely to remain complementary tools.

Apart from their value as experimental tools, pluripotent stem cells are likely sources of specific differentiated cell types for tissue replacement therapies for a whole host of diseases. Some have already made a start in this direction using EC-cell-derived neurons. Eventually, ES cells may provide the source of choice for such treatments because of their evident "normality" and the lesser likelihood of reversion to a malignant phenotype. Nevertheless, our current ability to culture human ES cells, and our understanding of their biology, rests on many decades of work with their tumor-derived counterparts, the EC cells of murine and human teratocarcinomas.

REFERENCES

Andrews P.W. 1982. Human embryonal carcinoma cells in culture do not synthesize fibronectin until they differentiate. *Int. J. Cancer.* **30:** 567–571.

———. 1984. Retinoic acid induces neuronal differentiation of a cloned human embryonal carcinoma cell line *in vitro.* Dev. Biol. **103:** 285–293.

Andrews P.W., Banting G.S., Damjanov I., Arnaud D., and Avner P. 1984a. Three monoclonal antibodies defining distinct differentiation antigens associated with different high molecular weight polypeptides on the surface of human embryonal carcinoma cells. *Hybridoma* **3:** 347–361.

Andrews P.W., Bronson D.L., Benham F., Strickland S., and Knowles B.B. 1980. A comparative study of eight cell lines derived from human testicular teratocarcinoma. *Int. J. Cancer* **26:** 269–280.

Andrews P.W., Goodfellow P.N., Shevinsky L., Bronson D.L., and Knowles B.B. 1982. Cell surface antigens of a clonal human embryonal carcinoma cell line: Morphological and antigenic differentiation in culture. *Int. J. Cancer* **29:** 523–531.

Andrews P.W. and Goodfellow P.N. 1980. Antigen expression by somatic cell hybrids of a murine embryonal carcinoma cell with thymocytes and L cells. *Somat. Cell Genet.* **6:** 271–284.

Andrews P.W., Nudelman E., Hakomori S.-I., and Fenderson B.A. 1990. Different patterns of glycolipid antigens are expressed following differentiation of TERA-2 human embryonal carcinoma cells induced by retinoic acid, hexamethylene bisacetamide (HMBA) or bromodeoxyuridine (BUdR). *Differentiation* **43:** 131–138.

Andrews P.W., Damjanov I., Berends J., Kumpf S., Zappavingna V., Mavilio F., and Sampath K. 1994. Inhibition of proliferation and induction of differentiation of pluripotent human embryonal carcinoma cells by osteogenic protein-1 (or bone morphogenetic protein-7). *Lab. Invest.* **71:** 243–251.

Andrews P.W., Damjanov I., Simon D., Banting G., Carlin C., Dracopoli N.C., and Fogh J. 1984b. Pluripotent embryonal carcinoma clones derived from the human teratocarcinoma cell line Tera-2: Differentiation *in vivo* and *in vitro.* Lab. Invest. **50:** 147–162.

Andrews P.W., Casper J., Damjanov I., Duggan-Keen M., Giwercman A., Hata J.I., von Keitz, A., Looijenga L.H.J., Millán J.L., Oosterhuis J.W., Pera M., Sawada M., Schmoll H.J., Skakkaebaek N.E., van Putten W., and Stern P. 1996. Comparative analysis of cell surface antigens expressed by cell lines derived from human germ cell tumors. *Int. J. Cancer* **66:** 806–816.

Artzt K., Dubois P., Bennett D., Condamine H., Babinet C., and Jacob F. 1973. Surface antigens common to mouse cleavage embryos and primitive teratocarcinoma cells in culture. *Proc. Natl. Acad. Sci.* **70:** 2988–2992.

Asada Y., Varnum D.S., Frankel W.N., and Nadeau J.H. 1994. A mutation in the *ter* gene causing increased susceptibility to testicular teratomas maps to mouse chromosome 18. *Nat. Genet.* **6:** 363–368.

Badcock G., Pigott C., Goepel J., and Andrews P.W. 1999. The human embryonal carcinoma marker antigen TRA-1-60 is a sialylated keratan sulphate proteoglycan. *Cancer Res.* **59:** 4715–4719.

Ballantyne J.W. 1894. The teratological records of Chaldea. *Teratologia* **1:** 127–142.

Beddington R.S.P. and Robertson E.J. 1989. An assessment of the developmental potential of embryonic stem cells in the midgestation mouse embryo. *Development* **105:** 733–737.

Bendel-Stenzel M., Anderson R., Heasman J., and Wylie C. 1998. The origin and migration of primordial germ cells in the mouse. *Semin. Cell Dev. Biol.* **9:** 393–400.

Bernstine E.G., Hooper M.L., Grandchamp S., and Ephrussi B. 1973. Alkaline phosphatase activity in mouse teratoma. *Proc. Natl. Acad. Sci.* **70:** 3899–3903.

Besmer P. 1991. The kit ligand encoded at the murine Steel locus: A pleiotropic growth and differentiation factor. *Curr. Opin. Cell Biol.* **3:** 939–946.

Borlongan C.V., Tajima Y., Trojanowski J., Lee V.M.Y., and Sanberg P.R. 1998. Cerebral ischemia and CNS transplantation: Differential effects of grafted fetal rat striatal cells and human neurons derived from a clonal cell line. *NeuroReport* **9:** 3703–3709.

Boyse E.A. and Old L.J. 1969. Some aspects of normal and abnormal cell surface genetics. *Annu. Rev. Genet.* **3:** 269–290.

Brinster R.L. 1974. The effect of cells transferred into the mouse blastocyst on subsequent development. *J. Exp. Med.* **140:** 1049–1056.

Chen C., Fenderson B.A., Andrews P.W., and Hakomori S.-I. 1989. Glycolipid-glycosyltransferases in human embryonal carcinoma cells during retinoic acid-induced differentiation. *Biochemistry* **28:** 2229–2238.

Conover J.C., Ip N.Y., Poueymirou W.T., Bates B., Goldfarb M.P., DeChiara T.M., and Yancopoulos G.D. 1993. Ciliary neutotrophic factor maintains the pluripotentiality of embryonic stem cells. *Development* **119:** 559–565.

Damjanov I. 1990. Teratocarcinoma stem cells. *Cancer Surv.* **9:** 303–319.

———. 1993. Pathogenesis of testicular germ cell tumors. *Eur. Urol.* **23:** 2–7.

Damjanov I. and Andrews P.W. 1983. Ultrastructural differentiation of a clonal human embryonal carcinoma cell line in vitro. *Cancer Res.* **43:** 2190–2198.

Damjanov I. and Solter D. 1974. Experimental teratoma. *Current Top. Pathol.* **59:** 69–130.

Damjanov I., Horvat B., and Gibas Z. 1993. Retinoic acid-induced differentiation of the developmentally pluripotent human germ cell tumor-derived cell line, NCCIT. *Lab Invest.* **68:** 220–232.

Damjanov I., Fox N., Knowles B.B., Solter D., Lange P.H., and Fraley E.E. 1982. Immunohistochemical localisation of murine stage specific embryonic antigens in human testicular germ cell tumors. *Am. J. Pathol.* **108:** 225–230.

Dixon F.S. and Moore R.A. 1952. Tumors of the male sex organs. In *Atlas of tumor pathology*, vol. 8. (fascicles 31b and 32). Armed Forces Institute of Pathology, Washington, D.C.

Einhorn L.H. 1987. Treatment strategies of testicular cancer in the United States. *Int. J. Androl.* **10:** 399–405.

Evans M.J. 1972. The isolation and properties of a clonal tissue culture strain of pluripotent mouse teratoma cells. *J. Embryol. Exp. Morphol.* **28:** 163–176.

Evans M.J. and Kaufman M.H. 1981. Establishment in culture of pluripotential cells from mouse embryos. *Nature* **292:** 154–156.

Fenderson B.A., Andrews P.W., Nudelman E., Clausen H., and Hakomori S.-I. 1987. Glycolipid core structure switching from globo- to lacto- and ganglio-series during retinoic acid-induced differentiation of TERA-2-derived human embryonal carcinoma cells. *Dev. Biol.* **122:** 21–34.

Fogh J. and Trempe G. 1975. New human tumor cel lines. In *Human tumor cells in vitro* (ed. J. Fogh), pp. 115–159. Plenum Press, New York.

Gachelin G., Delarbre C., Coulon-Morelec M.J., Keil-Dlouha V., and Muramatsu T. 1982. F9 antigens: A re-evaluation. In *Teratocarcinoma and embryonic cell interactions* (eds. T. Muramatsu et al.), pp. 121–140. Japan Scientific Societies Press, Tokyo.

Gels M.E., Marrink J., Visser P., Sleijfer D.T., Droste J.H.J., Hoekstra H.J., Andrews P.W., and Koops H.S. 1997. Importance of a new tumor marker TRA-1-60 in the follow-up of patients with clinical state I nonseminomatous testicular germ cell tumors. *Ann. Surg. Oncol.* **4:** 321–327.

Giesberts A.N., Duran C., Morton I.E., Piggot C., and Andrews P.W. 1999. Role of cadherin-mediated cell-cell adhesion in differentiation of human embryonal carcinoma cell lines. *Mech. Dev.* **83:** 115–125.

Gokhale P.J., Giesberts A.N., and Andrews P.W. 2000. *Brachyury* is expressed by human teratocarcinoma cells in the absence of mesodermal differentiation. *Cell Growth Differ.* **11:** 157–162.

Gönczöl E., Andrews P.W., and Plotkin S.A. 1984. Cytomegalovirus replicates in differentiated but not undifferentiated human embryonal carcinoma cells. *Science* **224:** 159–161.

Gooi H.C., Feizi T., Kapadia A., Knowles B.B., Solter D., and Evans M.J. 1981. Stage specific embryonic antigen involves $\alpha 1 \rightarrow 3$ fucosylated type 2 blood group chains. *Nature* **292:** 156–158.

Hasegawa T., Hara E., Takehana K., Nakada S., Oda K., Kawata M., Kimura H., and Sekiya S. 1991. A transient decrease in N-myc expression and its biological role during differentiation of human embryonal carcinoma cells. *Differentiation* **47:** 107–117.

Hata J., Fujita H., Ikeda E., Matsubayashi Y., Kokai Y., and Fujimoto J. 1989. Differentiation of human germ cell tumor cells. *Hum. Cell* **2:** 382–387.

Hirka G., Prakesh K., Kawashima H., Plotkin S.A., Andrews P.W., and Gönczöl E. 1991. Differentiation of human embryonal carcinoma cells induces human immunodeficiency virus permissiveness which is stimulated by human cytomegalovirus coinfection. *J. Virol.* **65:** 2732–2735.

Hogan B.L.M., Barlow D.P., and Tilly R. 1983. F9 teratocarcinoma cells as a model for the differentiation of parietal and visceral endoderm in the mouse embryo. *Cancer Surv.* **2:** 115–140.

Hogan B., Fellows M., Avner P., and Jacob F. 1977. Isolation of a human teratoma cell line which expresses F9 antigen. *Nature* **270:** 515–518.

Holden S., Bernard O., Artzt K., Whitmore W.F., and Bennett D. 1977. Human and mouse embryonal carcinoma cells in culture share an embryonic antigen (F9). *Nature* **270:** 518–520.

Hurlbert M.S., Gianani R.I., Hutt C., Freed C.R., and Kaddis F.G. 1999. Neural transplantation of hNT neurons for Huntington's disease. *Cell Transplant.* **8:** 143–151.

Jacob F. 1978. Mouse teratocarcinoma and mouse embryo. *Proc. R. Soc. Lond. B Biol. Sci.* **201:** 249–270.

Jakob H., Dubois P., Eisen H., and Jacob F. 1978. Effets de l'hexaméthylènebisacétamide sur la différenciation de cellules de carcinome embryonnaire. *C.R. Acad. Sci.* **286:** 109–111.

Jakob H., Boon T., Gaillard J., Nicolas J.-F., and Jacob F. 1973. Tératocarcinoma de la souris: Isolement, culture, et proprieties de cellules à potentialities multiples. *Ann. Microbiol. Inst. Pasteur.* **124B:** 269–282.

Jones-Villeneuve E.M., McBurney M.W., Rogers K.A., and Kalnins V.I. 1982. Retinoic acid induces embryonal carcinoma cells to differentiate into neurons and glial cells. *J. Cell Biol.* **94:** 253–262.

Kahn B.W. and Ephrussi B. 1970. Developmental potentialities of clonal in vitro cultures of mouse testicular teratoma. *J. Natl. Cancer Inst.* **44:** 1015–1029.

Kannagi R., Nudelman E., Levery S.B., and Hakomori S. 1982. A series of human erythrocyte glycosphingolipids reacting to the monoclonal antibody directed to a developmentally regulated antigen, SSEA-1. *J. Biol. Chem.* **257:** 14865–14874.

Kannagi R., Cochran N.A., Ishigami F., Hakomori S.-I., Andrews P.W., Knowles B.B., and Solter D. 1983a. Stage-specific embryonic antigens (SSEA-3 and -4) are epitopes of a unique globo-series ganglioside isolated from human teratocarcinoma cells. *EMBO J.* **2:** 2355–2361.

Kannagi R., Levery S.B., Ishigami F., Hakomori S., Shevinsky L.H., Knowles B.B., and Solter D. 1983b. New globoseries glycosphingolipids in human teratocarcinoma reactive with the monoclonal antibody directed to a developmentally regulated antigen, stage-specific embryonic antigen 3. *J. Biol. Chem.* **258:** 8934–8942.

Kemler R., Babinet C., Condamine H., Gachelin G., Guénet J.L., and Jacob F. 1976. Embryonal carcinoma antigen and the *T/t* locus of the mouse. *Proc. Natl. Acad. Sci.* **73:** 4080–4084.

Kleinsmith L.J. and Pierce G.B. 1964. Multipotentiality of single embryonal carcinoma cells. *Cancer Res.* **24:** 1544–1552.

Lafemina R.L. and Hayward G.S. 1988. Differences in cell-type-specific blocks to immediate early gene expression and DNA replication of human, simian and murine cytomegalovirus. *J. Gen. Virol.* **69:** 355–374.

Lee V.M.-Y. and Andrews P.W. 1986. Differentiation of NTERA-2 clonal human embryonal carcinoma cells into neurons involves the induction of all three neurofilament proteins. *J. Neurosci.* **6:** 514–521.

Marrink J., Andrews P.W., van Brummen P.J., de Jong H.J., Sleijfer D., Schraffordt-Koops H., and Oosterhuis J.W. 1991. TRA-1-60: A new serum marker in patients with germ cell tumors. *Int. J. Cancer* **49:** 368–372.

Martin G.R. 1981. Isolation of a pluripotent cell line from early mouse embryos cultured in medium conditioned by teratocarcinoma stem cells. *Proc. Natl. Acad. Sci.* **78:** 7634–7636.

Martin G.R. and Evans M.J. 1974. The morphology and growth of a pluripotent teratocarcinoma cell line and its derivatives in tissue culture. *Cell* **2:** 163–172.

————. 1975. Differentiation of clonal lines of teratocarcinoma cells: Formation of embryoid bodies *in vitro*. *Proc. Natl. Acad. Sci.* **72**: 1441–1445.

Mason M.D., Pera M.F., and Cooper S. 1991. Possible presence of an embryonal carcinoma-associated proteoglycan in the serum of patients with testicular germ cell tumors. *Eur. J. Cancer* **27**: 300

Mavilio F., Simeone A., Boncinelli E., and Andrews P.W. 1988. Activation of four homeobox gene clusters in human embryonal carcinoma cells induced to differentiate by retinoic acid. *Differentiation* **37**: 73–79.

McBurney M.W., Jones-Villeneuve E.M., Edwards M.K., and Anderson P.J. 1982. Control of muscle and neuronal differentiation in a cultured embryonal carcinoma cell line. *Nature.* **299**: 165–167.

Mintz B. and Illmensee K. 1975. Normal genetically mosaic mice produced from malignant teratocarcinoma cells. *Proc. Natl. Acad. Sci.* **72**: 3585–3589.

Møller H. 1993. Clues to the aetiology of testicular germ cell tumors from descriptive epidemiology. *Eur. Urol.* **23**: 8–15.

Mostofi F.K. and Price E.B. 1973. Tumours of the male genital system. In *Atlas of tumor pathology,* 2nd series, (fascicle 8). Armed Forces Institute of Pathology, Washington, D.C.

Muir J.K., Raghupathi R, Saatman K.E., Wilson C.A., Lee V.M.Y., Trojanowski J.Q., Philips M.F., and McIntosh T.K. 1999. Terminally differentiated human neurons survive and integrate following transplantation into the traumatically injured rat brain. *J. Neurotrauma* **16**: 403–411.

Nelson J.A. and Groudine M. 1986. Transcriptional regulation of the human cytomegalovirus major immediate-early gene is associated with induction of Dnase I-hypersensitive sites. *Mol. Cell. Biol.* **6**: 452–461.

Nicolas J.-F., Dubois P., Jakob H., Gaillard J., and Jacob F. 1975. Tératocarcinome de la souris: Différenciation en culture d'une lignée de cellules primitives à potentialities multiples. *Ann. Microbiol. Inst. Pasteur* **126A**: 3–22.

Niwa H., Miyazaki J., and Smith A.G. 2000. Quantitative expression of Oct-3/4 defines differentiation, dedifferentiation or self-renewal of ES cells. *Nat. Genet.* **24**: 372–376.

Noguchi M., Watanabe C., Kobayashi T., Kuwashima M., Sakurai T., Katoh H., and Moriwaki K. 1996. The *ter* mutation responsible for germ cell deficiency but not testicular nor ovarian teratocarcinogenesis in *ter/ter* congenic mice. *Dev. Growth Differ.* **38**: 59–69.

Noguchi T. and Noguchi M. 1985. A recessive mutation (*ter*) causing germ cell deficiency and a high incidence of congenital testicular teratomas in 129/Sv-ter mice. *J. Natl. Cancer. Inst.* **75**: 385–391.

Papaioannou V.E. and Rossant J. 1983. Effects of the embryonic environment on proliferation and differentiation of embryonal carcinoma cells. *Cancer Surv.* **2**: 165–183.

Papaioannou V.E., McBurney M.W. Gardner R.L., and Evans M.J. 1975. Fate of teratocarcinoma cells injected into early mouse embryos. *Nature* **258**: 70–73.

Papkoff J. 1994. Identification and biochemical characterization of secreted Wnt-1 protein from P19 embryonal carcinoma cells induced to differentiate along the neuroectodermal lineage. *Oncogene* **9**: 313–317.

Pera M.F. and Herzfeld D. 1998. Differentiation of human pluripotent teratocarcinomas stem cells induced by bone morphogenetic protein-2. *Reprod. Fertil. Dev.* **10**: 551–555.

Pera M.F., Cooper S., Mills J., and Parrington J.M. 1989. Isolation and characterization of a multipotent clone of human embryonal carcinoma cells. *Differentiation* **42**: 10–23.

Pera M.F., Blasco-Lafita M.J., Cooper S., Mason M., Mills J., and Monaghan P. 1988.

Analysis of cell-differentiation lineage in human teratomas using new monoclonal antibodies to cytostructural antigens of embryonal carcinoma cells. *Differentiation* **39:** 139–149.

Pfeiffer S.E., Jakob H. Mikoshiba K., Dubois P., Guènet J.L., Nicolas J.F., Gaillard J., Chevance G., and Jacob F. 1981. Differentiation of a teratocarcinoma line: Preferential development of cholinergic neurons. *J. Cell Biol.* **88:** 57–66.

Philips M.F., Muir J.K., Saatman K.E., Raghupathi R., Lee V.M.Y., Trojanowski J.Q., and McIntosh T.K. 1999. Survival and integration of transplanted postmitotic human neurons following experimental brain injury in immunocompetent rats. *J. Neurosurg.* **90:** 116–124.

Pierce G.B. 1974. Neoplasms, differentiations and mutations. *Am. J. Pathol.* **77:** 103–118.

Pierce G.B., Verney E.L., and Dixon F.J. 1957. The biology of testicular cancer I. Behaviour after transplantation. *Cancer Res.* **17:** 134–138.

Pleasure S.J. and Lee V.M.Y. 1993. NTERA-2 cells a human cell line which displays characteristics expected of a human committed neuronal progenitor cell. *J. Neurosci. Res.* **35:** 585–602.

Pleasure S.J., Page C., and Lee V.M.Y. 1992. Pure, postmitotic, polarized human neurons derived from NTERA-2 cells provide a system for expressing exogenous proteins in terminally differentiated neurons. *J. Neurosci.* **12:** 1802–1815.

Przyborski S., Morton I.E., Wood A., and Andrews P.W. 2000. Developmental regulation of neurogenesis in the pluripotent human embryonal carcinoma cell line NTERA-2. *Eur. J. Neurosci.* **12:** 3521–3528.

Qualtrough J.D. 1988. "Bone morphogenetic proteins in human embryonal carcinoma cells." Ph.D. thesis, University of Sheffield, Sheffield, United Kingdom.

Race R.R. and Sanger R. 1975. *Blood groups in man,* 6th edition. Blackwell Scientific, Oxford, United Kingdom.

Rendt J., Erulkar S., and Andrews P.W. 1989. Presumptive neurons derived by differentiation of a human embryonal carcinoma cell line exhibit tetrodotoxin-sensitive sodium currents and the capacity for regenerative responses. *Exp. Cell Res.* **180:** 580–584.

Rettig W.J., Cordon-Cardo C., Ng J.S. Oettgen H.F., Old L.J., and Lloyd K.O. 1985. High-molecular-weight glycoproteins of human teratocarcinomas defined by monoclonal antibodies to carbohydrate determinants. *Cancer Res.* **45:** 815–821.

Reubinoff B.E, Pera M.F., Fong C.Y., Trounson A., and Bongso A. 2000. Embryonic stem cell lines from human blastocysts: Somatic differentiation in vitro. *Nat. Biotechnol.* **18:** 399–404.

Roach S., Cooper S., Bennett W., and Pera M.F. 1993. Cultured cell lines from human teratomas—Windows into tumor growth and differentiation and early human development. *Eur. Urol.* **23:** 82–88.

Rose T.M., Weiford D.M., Gunderson N.L., and Bruce A.G. 1994. Oncostatin-M (OSM) inhibits the differentiation of pluripotent embryonic stem cells *in vitro. Cytokine* **6:** 48–54.

Sakurai T., Katoh H., Moriwaki K., Noguchi T., and Noguchi M. 1994. The *Ter* primordial germ cell deficiency mutation maps near Grl-1 on mouse chromosome 18. *Mamm. Genome* **5:** 333–336.

Shamblott M.J., Axelman J., Wang S., Bugg E.M., Littlefield J.W., Donovan P.J., Blumethal P.D., Huggins G.R., and Gearhard J.D. 1998. Derivation of pluripotent stem cells from cultured human primordial germ cells. *Proc. Natl. Acad. Sci.* **95:** 13726–13731.

Shevinsky L.H., Knowles B.B., Damjanov I., and Solter D. 1982. A stage specific embryonic antigen (SSEA-3) defined by a monoclonal antibody to murine embryos and expressed on pre-implantation embryos and human teratocarcinoma cells. *Cell* **30:** 697–705.

Simeone A., Acampora D., Arcioni L., Andrews P.W., Boncinelli E., and Mavilio F. 1990. Sequential activation of human HOX2 homeobox genes by retinoic acid in human embryonal carcinoma cells. *Nature* **346:** 763–766.

Smith A.G., Heath J.K., Donaldson D.D., Wong G.G., Moreau J., Stahl M., and Rogers D. 1988. Inhibition of pluripotential embryonic stem cell differentiation by purified polypeptides. *Nature* **336:** 688–690.

Solter D. and Damjanov I. 1979. Teratocarcinomas rarely develop from embryos transplanted into athymic mice. *Nature* **278:** 554–555.

Solter D. and Knowles B.B. 1978. Monoclonal antibody defining a stage-specific mouse embryonic antigen (SSEA-1). *Proc. Natl. Acad. Sci.* **75:** 5565–5569.

Solter D., Dominis M., and Damjanov I. 1979. Embryo-derived teratocarcinomas: I. The role of strain and gender in the control of teratocarcinogenesis. *Int. J. Cancer* **24:** 770–772.

———. 1981. Embyro-derived teratocarcinoma. III. Development of tumors from teratocarcinoma-permissive and non-permissive strain embryos transplanted to F1 hybrids. *Int. J. Cancer* **28:** 479–483.

Solter D., Skreb N., and Damjanov I. 1970. Extrauterine growth of mouse egg-cylinders results in malignant teratoma. *Nature* **227:** 503–504.

Squires P.E., Wakeman J.A., Chapman H., Kumpf S., Fiddock M.D., Andrews P.W., and Dunne M.J. 1996. Regulation of intracellular Ca^{2+} in response to muscarinic and glutamate receptor agonists during the differentiation of NTERA2 human embryonal carcinoma cells into neurons. *Eur. J. Neurosci.* **8:** 783–793.

Stevens L.C. 1964. Experimental production of testicular teratomas in mice. *Proc. Natl. Acad. Sci.* **52:** 654–661.

———. 1967a. The biology of teratomas. *Adv. Morphology* **6:** 1–31.

———. 1967b. Origin of testicular teratomas from primordial germ cells in mice. *J. Natl. Cancer Inst.* **38:** 549–552.

———. 1970a. Experimental production of testicular teratomas in mice of strains 129, A/He and their F_1 hybrids. *J. Natl. Cancer Inst.* **44:** 929–932.

———. 1970b. The development of transplantable teratocarcinomas from intratesticular grafts of pre- and post-implantation mouse embryos. *Dev. Biol.* **21:** 364–382.

———. 1973. A new inbred subline of mice (129/terSv) with a high incidence of spontaneous congenital testicular teratomas. *J. Natl. Cancer Inst.* **50:** 235–242.

Stevens L.C. and Hummel K.P. 1957. A description of spontaneous congenital testicular teratomas in strain 129 mice. *J. Natl. Cancer. Inst.* **18:** 719–747.

Stevens L.C. and Little C.C. 1954. Spontaneous testicular teratomas in an inbred strain of mice. *Proc. Natl. Acad. Sci.* **40:** 1080–1087.

Stevens L.C. and Varnum D.S. 1974. The development of teratomas from parthenogenetically activated ovarian mouse eggs. *Dev. Biol.* **37:** 369–380.

Stoter G. 1987. Treatment strategies of testicular cancer in Europe. *Int. J. Androl.* **10:** 407–415.

Strickland S. and Mahdavi V. 1978. The induction of differentiation in teratocarcinomas stem cells by retinoic acid. *Cell* **15:** 393–403.

Strickland S., Smith K.K., and Marotti K.R. 1980. Hormonal induction of differentiation in teratocarcinoma stem cells: Generation of parietal endoderm by retinoic acid and dibutyryl cAMP. *Cell* **21:** 347–355.

Teshima S., Shimosato Y., Hirohashi S., Tome Y., Hayashi I., Kanazawa H., and Kakizoe

T. 1988. Four new human germ cell tumor cell lines. *Lab. Invest.* **59**: 328–336.

Thomson J.A. and Marshall V.S. 1998. Primate embryonic stem cells. *Curr. Top. Dev. Biol.* **38**: 133–165.

Thomson J.A., Kalishman J., Golos T.G., Durning M., Harris C.P., and Hearn J.P. 1996. Pluripotent cell lines derived from common marmoset (*Callithrix jacchus*) blastocysts. *Biol. Reprod.* **55**: 688–690.

Thomson J.A., Itskovitz-Eldor J., Shapiro S.S., Waknitz M.A., Swiergiel J.J., Marshall V.S., and Jones J.M. 1998. Embryonic stem cell lines derived from human blastocysts. *Science* **282**: 1145–1147.

Thomson J.A., Kalishman J., Golos T.G., Durning M., Harris C.P., Becker R.A., and Hearn J.P. 1995. Isolation of a primate embryonic stem cell line. *Proc. Natl. Acad. Sci.* **92**: 7844–7848.

Thurin J., Herlyn M., Hindsgaul O., Stromberg, J., Karlsson K., Elder D., Steplewski Z., and Koprowski H. 1985. Proton NMR and fast atom bombardment mass spectrometry analysis of the melanoma-associated ganglioside 9-0-acetyl-GD$_3$. *J. Biol. Chem.* **260**: 14556–14563.

Tippett P., Andrews P.W., Knowles B.B., Solter D., and Goodfellow P.N. 1986. Red cell antigens P (globoside) and Luke: Identification by monoclonal antibodies defining the murine stage-specific embryonic antigens -3 and -4 (SSEA-3 and -4). *Vox Sang.* **51**: 53–56.

Umezawa A., Maruyama T., Inazawa J., Imai S., Takano T., and Hata J. 1996. Induction of mcl1/EAT, Bcl-2 related gene, by retinoic acid or heat shock in the human embryonal carcinoma cells, NCR-G3. *Cell Struct. Funct.* **21**: 143–150.

Wakeman J.A., Walsh J., and Andrews P.W. 1998. Human *Wnt-13* is developmentally regulated during the differentiation of NTERA-2 pluripotent human embryonal carcinoma cells. *Oncogene* **17**: 179–186

Wheeler J.E. 1983. History of teratomas. In *The human teratomas: Experimental and clinical biology* (eds. I. Damjanov et al.), pp. 1–22. Humana Press, Clifton, New Jersey.

Williams R., Hilton D., Pease S., Wilson T., Stewart C., Gearing D., Wagner E., Metcalf D., Nicola N., and Gough N. 1988. Myeloid-leukemia inhibitory factor maintains the developmental potential of embryonic stem cells. *Nature* **336**: 684–687.

Willison K.R., Karol R.A., Suzuki A., Kundu S.K., and Marcus D.M. 1982. Neutral glycolipid antigens as developmental markers of mouse teratocarcinomas and early embryos: An immunologic and chemical analysis. *J. Immunol.* **129**: 603–609.

Winkel G.K. and Pederson R.A. 1988. Fate of the inner cell mass in mouse embryos as studied by microinjection of lineage tracers. *Dev. Biol.* **127**: 143–156.

Wright C.V. 1991. Vertebrate homeobox genes. *Curr. Opin. Cell Biol.* **3**: 976–982.

Yoshida K., Chambers I., Nichols J., Smith A., Saito M., Yasukawa K., Shoyab M., Taga T., and Kishimoto T. 1994. Maintenance of the pluripotential phenotype of embryonic stem cells through direct activation of GP130 signalling pathways. *Mech. Dev.* **45**: 163–171.

Younkin D.P., Tang C.M., Hardy M., Reddy U.R., Shi Q.Y., Pleasure S.J., Lee V.M.Y., and Pleasure D. 1993. Inducible expression of neuronal glutamate receptor channels in the NT2 human cell line. *Proc. Natl. Acad. Sci.* **6**: 2174–2178.

12
Trophoblast Stem Cells

Tilo Kunath, Dan Strumpf, and Janet Rossant
Samuel Lunenfeld Research Institute
Mount Sinai Hospital
Toronto, Canada M5G 1X5

Satoshi Tanaka
Laboratory of Cellular Biochemistry
Vet. Med. Sci. /Animal Resource Sci.
University of Tokyo,1-1-1 Yayoi
Bunkyo-ku, Tokyo, Japan 113-8657

THE TROPHOBLAST LINEAGE AND PLACENTAL DEVELOPMENT

In the mammalian embryo, the formation of the extraembryonic lineages, the trophectoderm and primitive endoderm, precedes the differentiation of cells that will contribute to the fetus itself. The precocious differentiation of these lineages in mammals is related to their essential roles in promoting survival of the embryo in the uterine environment. Cells of the primitive endoderm give rise to the endoderm layers of the yolk sacs, whereas descendants of the trophectoderm will form the trophoblast portion of the placenta (Fig. 1). The development of both extraembryonic lineages has been reviewed previously (Rossant 1986, 1995). The scope of the following discussion is to provide an overview of trophectoderm development in the preimplantation embryo and of the trophoblast lineage and placenta in postimplantation stages, as the basis for the study of trophoblast stem cells.

The trophectoderm is the first cell type to differentiate in the mammalian embryo. In the mouse, it is morphologically distinguishable by the blastocyst stage (3.5 days post coitum [dpc]), where it forms an outer monolayer of cells surrounding the blastocoelic cavity and the inner cell mass (ICM) (Fig. 1A). The trophectoderm cells are characterized by their flattened epitheloid-like appearance, with apical tight junction complexes. In addition, trophectoderm cells harbor sodium pumps (Na^+, K^+-ATPase) whose activity leads to accumulation of fluid within the blastocoel cavity, resulting in blastocoel expansion. This process is thought to

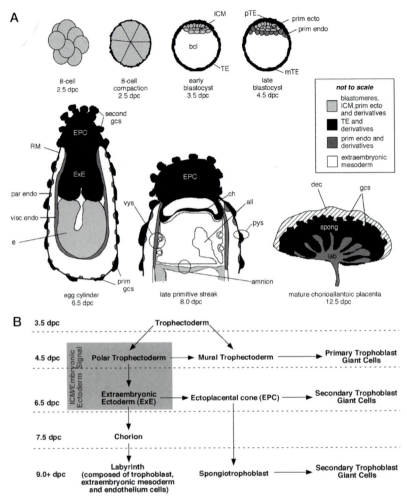

Figure 1 Development of the trophoblast lineage. (*A*) The development of the trophoblast is presented in the context of the development of the embryo proper and extraembryonic tissues. (*ICM*) Inner cell mass; (*TE*) trophectoderm; (*bcl*) blastocoel; (*pTE*) polar trophectoderm; (*mTE*) mural trophectoderm; (*prim ecto*) primitive ectoderm; (*prim endo*) primitive endoderm; (*second gcs*) secondary giant cells; (*EPC*) ectoplacental cone; (*ExE*) extraembryonic ectoderm; (*RM*) Reichert's membrane; (*par endo*) parietal endoderm; (*visc endo*) visceral endoderm; (*e*) embryonic ectoderm; (*prim gcs*) primary giant cells; (*vys*) visceral yolk sac; (*ch*) chorion; (*all*) allantois; (*pys*) parietal yolk sac; (*dec*) maternal decidua; (*spong*) spongiotrophoblast; (*lab*) labyrinthine trophoblast. (*B*) This diagram presents a model for the development of the trophoblast lineage from the blastocyst stage (3.5 dpc) through the formation of the chorioallantoic placenta, with an emphasis on stages and developmental origins of the trophoblast. Interaction with the ICM or its derivatives is crucial for the proliferation and maintenance of a trophoblast stem-cell population (*gray shading*).

facilitate hatching from the zona pellucida, a thick protein coat surrounding the embryo (Wiley et al. 1990).

The distinction of the trophectoderm from the ICM may be initiated during the events of compaction at the eight-cell stage, when cells become polarized. During successive divisions, cells that inherit an apical region will end up in the trophectoderm, while apolar cells contribute to the ICM. However, irreversible commitment of individual cells to the trophoblast lineage does not occur until the blastocyst stage (Rossant and Vijh 1980; Johnson and Ziomek 1981; Pedersen 1986).

In the blastocyst, trophectoderm cells make up approximately 75% of the total cell number (Copp 1978), underscoring the fact that most of the cells in the embryo at this stage are set aside for the role of establishing the maternal-embryonic contact. By 4.5 dpc, at the peri-implantation stage, the formation of different trophectodermal subtypes is initiated. While the cells overlying the ICM continue to divide and form the polar trophectoderm, the cells away from the ICM, the mural trophectoderm, cease dividing, but continue to replicate their DNA (Fig.1A) (Copp 1978). This process, known as endoreduplication, gives rise to cells with multiple copies of their genome (Barlow and Sherman 1972). They will form the primary trophoblast giant cells that mediate implantation of the embryo into the uterine epithelium and later take on endocrine functions (Gardner and Johnson 1972).

Following implantation, the polar trophectoderm continues to divide and grows initially toward the blastocoelic cavity, to form the extraembryonic ectoderm (ExE), and then outward to form the ectoplacental cone (EPC) (Copp 1979). This typical directional growth may occur due to mechanical constraints placed on the implanting blastocyst by the uterine wall (Gardner et al. 1973; Copp 1979). Secondary trophoblast giant cells arise at the periphery of the EPC and eventually come to surround the entire embryo and its membranes. These cells provide direct contact with the maternal environment during the early part of pregnancy. These polyploid cells appear phenotypically indistinguishable from primary giant cells of the blastocyst (Fig. 1A).

At 8.5 dpc, formation of the chorioallantoic placenta is initiated by fusion of the diploid trophoblast of the EPC and chorionic plate with the allantois, a structure derived from extraembryonic mesoderm (Fig. 1A). Subsequently, by 10.0 dpc, three distinctive trophoblast cell layers are formed, which persist for the rest of gestation. The innermost layer, the labyrinth, is formed following the attachment of the allantois to the chorion, and eventually will be the site for exchange of nutrients and gases with the maternal blood. This function is achieved via the large surface area of the labyrinthine layer, formed through extensive folding and branching that occur as it develops. The intermediate compact layer of spongiotrophoblast cells, through which the maternal blood cells pass, is formed as a consequence of the expansion and flattening of the EPC after 7.5 dpc. The third layer, the outer layer of giant cells, is formed from the postmitotic trophoblast cells lying at the periphery of the EPC, and practically covers the entire placenta. The trophoblast cells perform many other functions connected with survival in the uterus, including hormone and cytokine production and immune protection of the fetus (Cross et al. 1994; Cross 2000).

EVIDENCE FOR THE EXISTENCE OF TROPHOBLAST STEM CELLS IN VIVO

A basic requirement for cells within a specific lineage to serve as stem cells is their ability for self-renewal, and the capacity to give rise to all descendants of that lineage. The existence of such cells in the trophoblast lineage of the mouse has been implied by numerous studies, as summarized below.

Studies on the Trophoblast Lineage

As discussed earlier, following implantation the mural trophoblast cells of the blastocyst stop dividing and transform into primary giant cells, while the polar trophoblast cells continue to divide (Copp 1978). In culture, mural trophectoderm fragments were shown to form trophectoderm vesicles that induce decidual reactions when transferred to uteri of pseudopregnant recipients. Although these vesicles implanted at equal efficiencies as control blastocysts, only a limited number of giant cells were recognized at the sites of implantation of the trophectoderm (Gardner and Johnson 1972). This suggested that the mural trophectoderm by itself is limited in its ability to contribute additional giant cells due to its inability to proliferate. Indeed, a later study showed that further increase in the number of primary giant cells relies on cell division originating in the polar trophectoderm followed by cell migration to the mural trophectoderm (Copp 1979). Thus, these experiments demonstrated that trophectoderm proliferation relies on cell division to be maintained in the polar trophectoderm.

Ectopic transplantation of EPC led to the formation of trophoblast giant cells at the transplantation sites (Kirby et al. 1966; Avery and Hunt 1969). This suggested that postimplantation trophoblast still required some positive signal to maintain its proliferation. In addition, it was demonstrated that transplanting or culturing pieces of ExE isolated from mouse embryos up to 8.5 dpc also resulted in cells with the morphological characteristics of trophoblast giant cells, emphasizing the similarity between the properties of the ExE and EPC (Rossant and Ofer 1977).

The ExE and EPC are not identical, however, although they are both diploid trophectoderm derivatives. They respond differently to different culture conditions: EPC cells gave rise to giant cells under all conditions tested, whereas ExE exhibited a period of sustained proliferation in some conditions (Rossant and Tamura-Lis 1981). The two tissues also differed in their 2D protein synthetic profiles (Johnson and Rossant 1981). During in vitro culture, ExE cells pass through a brief stage of diploid maintenance and synthesis of EPC-like proteins before transforming into giant cells. Under the same conditions, EPC cells rapidly commenced giant cell transformation. In addition, when 5.5 dpc and 6.5 dpc ExE were injected into 3.5 dpc blastocysts, they contributed to ExE as well as the EPC and trophoblast giant cells in resulting chimeras (Rossant et al. 1978). Taken together, all these results suggest that the diploid ExE may act as a stem cell pool for the postimplantation trophoblast, giving rise to EPC cells as well as secondary giant cells.

ICM and Its Derivatives in Trophoblast Proliferation

Giant cell transformation is apparently the normal path of differentiation of all trophoblast cells of the blastocyst not in contact with the ICM (Gardner et al. 1973). This process begins at the abembryonic pole of the mouse blastocyst and eventually involves the whole trophectoderm except those cells in the region immediately overlaying the ICM (Dickson 1966). Reconstitution experiments involving the injection of ICM cells into mural trophoblastic vesicles resulted in the development of normal embryos (Gardner et al. 1973), thus suggesting the ICM is an active source of signals promoting trophoblast proliferation. Continued dependence of trophoblast proliferation on the ICM and its derivatives could be important in ensuring that the development of the trophoblast is coordinated with that of the embryo it supports. Indeed, it was suggested that cell division in the diploid ExE trophoblast cells may be maintained by their proximity to the embryo proper during postimplantation stages, whereas EPC cells farther away from the ICM derivatives will transform into the secondary giant cell population (Gardner et al. 1973). Maintaining postimplantation trophoblast cells in close contact with one another in the absence of ICM derivatives was insufficient to maintain them in a diploid state (Ilgren 1981; Rossant and Tamura-Lis 1981).

However, when pieces of ExE were inserted into embryonic tissue, graft-ed ectopically, and scored for the presence of trophoblast giant cells, none was observed. In control grafts, where ExE was not enclosed in embry-onic tissue, trophoblast giant cells were readily found. Thus, it appears that a signal emanating from the embryonic tissues was able to maintain the ExE cells in a diploid state. In contrast, EPC cells analyzed in similar conditions differentiated into trophoblast giant cells, further suggesting that the ExE is likely the source of stem cells for the trophoblast lineage (Rossant and Tamura-Lis 1981).

Model for the Postimplantation Trophoblast Cell Lineage

From all the studies described above, it is possible to present a model for the early trophoblast cell lineage incorporating the role of the ICM and its derivatives in the induction and maintenance of trophoblast proliferation (Fig. 1B) (Copp 1979; Rossant and Tamura-Lis 1981). The model pre-sents a pathway of differentiation in which the diploid polar trophecto-derm of the blastocyst gives rise to the ExE. A diploid cell population is maintained in the ExE, but it is also capable of producing diploid EPC cells. Self-renewal in the diploid EPC cells is limited, and some go on to form secondary giant cells. Maintenance of a diploid cell population within the polar trophectoderm or the ExE is dependent on interaction with the ICM or the embryonic ectoderm, respectively (Fig. 1B, gray shading). In the mature chorioallantoic placenta, the spongiotrophoblast, components of the labyrinth, and the giant cells are direct descendants of the trophoblast lineage.

EVIDENCE FOR FGF SIGNALING IN THE PREIMPLANTATION EMBRYO AND ITS IMPORTANCE FOR TROPHOBLAST PROLIFERATION

As described earlier, the proliferative capacity of diploid cells within the trophoblast lineage depends on their interaction with the ICM or its deriv-atives. Recent expression and genetic studies point to a critical role of fibroblast growth factor (FGF) signaling in regulation of proliferation and development in the trophoblast lineage.

The FGF family consists of at least 22 FGF ligands that function in various processes throughout embryonic development (Hoshikawa et al. 1998; Miyake et al. 1998; Ohbayashi et al. 1998; Nishimura et al. 1999; Szebenyi and Fallon 1999; N. Itoh, unpubl.). FGF4 is the only ligand known to be expressed in the preimplantation embryo. *Fgf4* transcripts can be detected at the 1-cell stage through to the blastocyst stage, where its expression becomes confined to the ICM (Niswander and Martin 1992; Rappolee et al. 1994). During peri- and postimplantation stages (4.5–6.0 dpc), it continues to be expressed solely in the epiblast in a uniform pattern (Niswander and Martin 1992). Embryos homozygous for an *Fgf4* null mutation die shortly after implantation (5.5 dpc). Their postimplantation phenotype was characterized by impaired growth of the embryonic component (Feldman et al. 1995). This defect is suggested to occur after implantation, since *Fgf4*$^{-/-}$ blastocysts appeared normal when compared to wild-type littermates. Nonetheless, the presence of maternal *Fgf4* mRNA or protein may partially compensate for the loss of zygotic transcripts. This in turn could allow additional cell divisions, resulting in extended survival of the embryos until the postimplantation stage. In vitro outgrowths from mutant blastocysts revealed the lack of ICM and endoderm, which could be partially rescued by exogenous FGF4 (Feldman et al. 1995). Exogenous administration of FGF4 to wild-type cultured ICM cells resulted in proliferation of these cells and promoted their differentiation into parietal and/or primitive endoderm (Rappolee et al. 1994). Thus, it appeared that FGF4 serves as a critical component for the survival and development of the ICM in the early postimplantation phase of mouse embryogenesis. However, *Fgf4*$^{-/-}$ embryonic stem (ES) cells can be generated, and they proliferate normally in vitro, although growth and survival of the differentiated cell types that arise from null ES cells are affected (Wilder et al. 1997). This discrepancy between the effects of loss of FGF4 in ES cells and embryos could be explained by an additional requirement for FGF4 in signaling to the trophectoderm lineage. Some data to support this were observations that administration of FGF4 to blastocyst outgrowths led to an increase in the number of outgrowing trophectoderm cells (Chai et al. 1998). Furthermore, addition of FGF4 to *Oct4*$^{-/-}$ embryos, which only make trophectoderm, also promoted its proliferation (Nichols et al. 1998).

FGF signaling is mediated through the cooperative interaction of high-affinity tyrosine kinase receptors and heparin sulfate proteoglycans. The group of high-affinity FGF receptors consists of four members, FGFR1–FGFR4 (Szebenyi and Fallon 1999). There is some cross-reactivity between the four receptors and ligands, FGF1–FGF9, and some alternatively spliced forms of FGFR1–FGFR3 have ligand specificity (Ornitz et al. 1996). Isoforms of all four FGF receptors bind FGF4, and expression of all four receptors has been detected at the blastocyst stage (Rappolee et al. 1998; Haffner-Krausz et al. 1999). Both *Fgfr3* and *Fgfr4* transcripts are detectable in all early blastocyst cells, with the latter being more pronounced in the trophectoderm (Rappolee et al. 1994). However, these receptors are unlikely to play a critical role in trophoblast development, since embryos mutant for *Fgfr3* only, or *Fgfr3* and *Fgfr4*, display late skeletal and lung defects, respectively (Colvin et al. 1996; Deng et al. 1996; Weinstein et al. 1998). A recent analysis of *Fgfr2* expression pattern in the preimplantation embryo reveals an early onset of expression of two alternatively spliced forms of this receptor (termed IIIb and IIIc) that differ in an extracellular Ig domain. The *Fgfr2 IIIc* transcript is present in the oocyte, whereas the *FgfR2 IIIb* isoform is first detected in the two-cell stage. Both alternatively spliced transcripts are detected through the compacted morula stage. Whole-mount in situ and immunohistochemistry analyses detect *Fgfr2* expression specifically in the outer cell layer of the morula. These cells later give rise to the trophectoderm, where the expression of *Fgfr2* persists in the expanded blastocyst (Haffner-Krausz et al. 1999). Postimplantation expression of *Fgfr2* in the trophoblast lineage continues in the ExE through the late-streak stage (Ciruna and Rossant 1999). The generation of two different *Fgfr2* mutations led to embryonic lethality at different stages (Arman et al. 1998; Xu et al. 1998). The more severe *Fgfr2* phenotype resulted in embryos that implanted randomly with respect to the mesometrial–antimesometrial axis of the uterus. These embryos died at 4.5–5.5 dpc. Since the trophectoderm mediates implantation, these observations suggested that the lethality of these mutants was due to trophoblast defects (Arman et al. 1999). Analysis of the other allele of *Fgfr2* revealed that mutant embryos die at 10.0–11.0 dpc due to placental failure. The lethal defects are characterized by failure in chorioallantoic fusion in about one-third of the mutant embryos, and others lack the labyrinthine portion of the placenta (Xu et al. 1998). Thus, *Fgfr2* appears to be important also for later stages of placental development. Since different regions of the *Fgfr2* locus were targeted, it is possible that only one is a null and the other is a new allele. The early, severe phenotype could be the result of a dominant-negative allele that inhibited all FGF signaling or the later, less severe phenotype could be due to a hypomorphic allele that allowed partial FGFR2 signaling to occur. The discrepancy between these two phenotypes has yet to be resolved. However, genetic background cannot account for the differences, since both mutants were analyzed on a 129 background.

Evidence for a critical role for FGF signaling in the proliferation and development of the trophectoderm was further demonstrated by the analysis of mouse embryos that express a dominant negative FGF receptor (dnFGFR) (Chai et al. 1998). In mosaic embryos, cell division ceased at the fifth cell division in all cells that expressed the mutant receptor, resulting in an overall lower number of cells in these mosaic blastocysts. Moreover, no mitotic trophoblast cells adjacent to the ICM were found to express dnFGFR, whereas expression of dnFGFR was detected in post-mitotic trophoblast cells farther away from the ICM. Thus, it seems that functional FGF signaling, probably via the FGF4 ligand and FGFR2 receptor, is essential for trophoblast proliferation in vivo, and in culture, as discussed below.

DERIVATION OF TROPHOBLAST STEM CELL LINES

Several attempts have been made to culture trophoblast cells ex vivo. Invariably, the cultures differentiated into postmitotic giant cells, and consequently, cell lines were not established (Rossant and Tamura-Lis 1981). However, the recent evidence implicating FGF signaling in trophoblast proliferation and development warranted a renewed attempt at trophoblast cultures. Initially, the ExE of 6.5 dpc embryos was isolated and disaggregated into a near-single-cell suspension with trypsin. These ExE cells were plated in the presence of FGF4 and its required cofactor, heparin. In these conditions, the ExE cells eventually differentiated into giant cells, indicating that FGF4 alone was not sufficient to maintain trophoblast cells in a proliferative state. However, when the ExE cells were plated on a feeder layer of mouse embryonic fibroblasts (MEFs) in the same conditions, the ExE cells produced epithelial colonies that could be passaged without differentiation into giant cells (Tanaka et al. 1998). Upon removal of FGF4 or the MEFs, the epithelial cells ceased to divide and differentiated into giant cells (Fig. 2A,B). As described below, gene expression studies and chimeric analysis determined these cells to be of trophoblast origin, and they retained the capacity to contribute to all trophoblast cell types in vivo. Thus, they were termed trophoblast stem (TS) cells. First, the general properties of TS cells are described, including their derivation, maintenance in culture, differentiation, and their developmental potential in chimeras. This is followed by gene expression studies of TS cells in their proliferative state and as they differentiate.

TS cell lines can be derived from several different stages of development. In addition to the ExE of 6.5 dpc embryos, TS cell lines have been derived from 3.5 dpc blastocysts and the chorionic ectoderm of 7.5 dpc embryos. However, TS cell lines could not be derived from the embryonic ectoderm or the EPC of 6.5 dpc embryos. This suggests that TS cells exist in vivo for at least a 4-day window within the trophoblast lineage. TS cell lines derived from different stages of development exhibited similar properties in culture, and their gene expression profiles and developmental

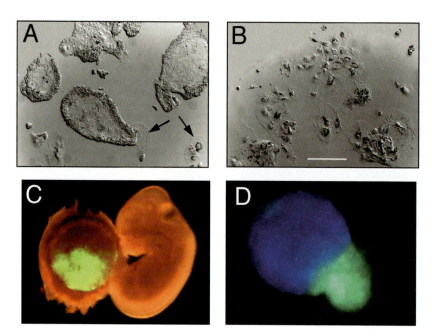

Figure 2 TS cells grown in the presence (*A*) and absence (*B*) of FGF4 and MEF-conditioned medium (MEF-CM). The stem cells grow as tight epithelial sheets with distinctly defined borders. Differentiated giant cells are indicated (*arrows*). In the absence of FGF4 and MEF-CM the cells transform into giant cells with large nuclei and dark, perinuclear deposits. *Bar*, 50 μm. (*C*) TS cell chimera at 11.5 dpc generated by blastocyst injection of EGFP-TS cells. (*D*) Cellular aggregate between ES cells and EGFP-TS cells, where the ES cells are transgenic for cyan fluorescent protein (CFP) (*cyan*).

potential were indistinguishable. The efficiency of TS cell derivation is very high, approaching 100% of explanted embryos. Furthermore, the ability to generate lines is not strain-dependent, as observed for ES cell line derivation, and male and female lines can be generated equally well.

TS cell lines are dependent on both FGF4 and MEFs. If either component is removed, or if the cofactor for FGF4, heparin, is removed, the cultures differentiate into giant cells. However, FGF4 may be replaced with either FGF1 or FGF2 without loss of stem cell maintenance. This is not surprising, since FGF1 and FGF2 can activate the same receptors as FGF4 (Zimmer et al. 1993). More interestingly, the MEFs may be replaced with MEF-conditioned medium (MEF-CM) (Tanaka et al. 1998). This CM must be present at a critical concentration to be effective, suggesting that there is a soluble factor or factors in the MEF-CM required for TS cell maintenance (Fig. 2A,B). The identification of the critical MEF-CM component(s) should shed more light on the requirements of trophoblast stem cells in vivo. The identity of the required factor in the MEF-CM has remained elusive. Several candidates, such as the ligands LIF, EGF, BMP2, and BMP7, have been unable to replace the MEF-CM in TS cell cultures. Even the nature of the stem-cell-promoting effect of the feeder cells is still unknown. Biochemical characterization of the MEF-CM, such as by protease treatments and fractionations, is under way.

As mentioned above, TS cells were observed to differentiate into cells that morphologically resembled trophoblast giant cells. Fluorescence-activated cell scan (FACS) analysis of propidium iodide-stained cells confirmed that they were indeed increasing their DNA content, as do giant cells in vivo. These FACS studies also supported the microscopy observations that TS cell lines are considerably heterogeneous. The FACS profiles of TS cells grown in stem cell conditions indicated that ~10% of the cells exhibited an increased ploidy, which is indicative of differentiation. In an attempt to reduce the heterogeneity of the cultures, TS cells were FACS-sorted on the basis of DNA content using the vital dye, Hoechst 33342. TS cells with a 2N DNA content were selectively FACS-sorted from higher ploidy cells and cultured. These 2N-sorted TS cells were considerably less heterogeneous in culture, and their FACS profiles confirmed these observations.

The most convincing results that speak to the true stem cell nature of TS cell lines were their specific and exclusive contributions to trophoblast lineages in chimera studies. When TS cell lines were injected into 3.5 dpc blastocysts, contributions were only observed in trophoblast lineages and never in embryonic lineages or extraembryonic tissues derived from mesodermal and endodermal lineages, such as the yolk sac (Tanaka et al. 1998). Chimeras were analyzed from 6.5 dpc conceptuses through to term placenta. Contributions were observed in all trophoblast subtypes, but some preferences were observed. In early chimeras, TS cells were found to contribute most frequently to the ExE and less frequently to the EPC. Contributions to the giant cell layer were rare, and when they were observed, the clones were small. At later stages of development, TS cells contributed well to the labyrinth and the spongiotrophoblast, but to a lesser extent to the secondary giant cell layer. In fact, large clones in the trophoblast were observed right up to the edge of the placenta where the secondary giant cells begin to form, but the TS cells rarely contributed to the secondary giant cell layer itself (Fig. 2C). These restrictions may reflect the mode of generation of chimeras via blastocyst injection, where much of the trophectoderm has already formed. If technical difficulties with aggregation of TS cells with morulae can be overcome, more extensive colonization of the trophoblast can be expected. Another interesting observation was the coherent nature of most of the TS cell clones (Fig. 2C). This was reminiscent of clones in the primitive endoderm lineage and in direct contrast to the very mosaic contributions observed in the embryo proper (Gardner and Cockroft 1998).

GENE EXPRESSION STUDIES

The genes expressed by TS cells cultured in stem cell conditions, and as they differentiate, closely resemble the gene expression profile of the trophoblast lineage in vivo (Table 1). The receptor, *Fgfr2*, and the transcription factors, *Cdx2*, *mEomesodermin* (*mEomes*), and *Err2* are all expressed in early diploid trophoblast cells, the ExE (Beck et al. 1995; Luo et al. 1997; Arman et al. 1999; Ciruna and Rossant 1999). In agreement with these in vivo observations, these genes are strongly expressed in TS cells and are down-regulated as they differentiate. The secreted ligand, BMP4, is expressed in the ExE of the early mouse conceptus (Lawson et al. 1999) and is expressed only in stem cells and not in differentiated TS cells (S. Tanaka, unpubl.).

The basic helix-loop-helix (bHLH) transcription factor, Mash2, and the novel gene *Tpbp* (formerly *4311*), are expressed in the EPC and spongiotrophoblast (Lescisin et al. 1988; Guillemot et al. 1994). In TS cells, *Mash2* and *Tpbp* were not expressed in stem cells, but were induced upon differentiation. A similar pattern was observed for the transcription factor, Gcm1 (Basyuk et al. 1999; S. Tanaka, unpubl.). Placental lactogen-1 (PL-1) is a hormone secreted by giant cells (Faria et al. 1991). Expression of this gene was only detected in differentiated TS cells. Hand1, a bHLH transcription factor, is also expressed in differentiated trophoblast lineages such as the EPC and the giant cells (Cross et al. 1995). However, *Hand1* was highly expressed in both stem and differentiated TS cells, which was not in agreement with the pattern in vivo.

Genes representative of other early embryo cell types were not detected in TS cells. Oct4, a transcription factor expressed in the early embryonic ectoderm (Palmieri et al. 1994), was not detected in TS cells. *Brachyury*, a mesodermal marker (Wilkinson et al. 1990), and *Hnf4*, an endodermal marker (Duncan et al. 1994), were also not expressed in TS cells.

With few exceptions, the gene expression profile of TS cells in culture is largely representative of the trophoblast in vivo. ExE-specific genes are expressed in TS cells maintained in stem cell conditions, whereas EPC and giant-cell-specific genes are induced upon differentiation.

Table 1 Comparison of gene expression between TS cells and the trophoblast in vivo

Gene	Class	Expression in TS cells		Expression in the trophoblast
		(stem)	(differentiated)	
Fgfr2	receptor tyrosine kinase	+	–	TE, ExE, ChE
Cdx2	*caudal*-related homeobox transcription factor	+	–	TE, ExE, ChE, Spong
mEomes	T-box transcription factor	+	–	TE, ExE, ChE
Err2	orphan nuclear receptor	+	–	ExE, ChE
Bmp4	TGFβ ligand	+	–	ExE, ChE
Mash2	bHLH transcription factor	–	+	EPC, Spong
Gcm1	novel transcription factor	–	+	ChE, Lab
Tpbp	novel	–	+	EPC, Lab
PL-1	lactogen	–	–	TE, GC

(TE), trophectoderm; (ExE) extraembryonic ectoderm; (ChE) chorionic ectoderm; (Spong) spongiotrophoblast; (Lab) labyrinthine trophoblast; (GC) giant cell layer.

NEW MODEL FOR TROPHOBLAST DEVELOPMENT

With the derivation of FGF4-dependent TS cell lines and recent expression and mutational data, an updated model of trophoblast development can be formulated. The most significant change from the former model is the identification of a major component of the embryo-derived signal required for the maintenance and proliferation of trophoblast stem cells in vivo. In addition, transcription factors thought to be critical for the trophoblast lineage have been added to the model (Fig. 3). It is proposed that the growth factor, FGF4, produced and secreted by the ICM (and later by the embryonic ectoderm), signals to the overlying trophoblast cells via an FGFR, of which FGFR2 is a good candidate, maintaining them in a diploid, proliferative state. As trophoblast cells are displaced distally from the embryo proper, they cease to receive the embryo-derived signals and begin to differentiate into other trophoblast subtypes, such as EPC cells and giant cells. It is not known whether the differentiated trophoblast subtypes are default states that are manifested after removal of stem-cell-maintaining signals or whether there are additional signals that promote differentiation. The ex vivo culture system of TS cells would suggest the former, but the mechanism in vivo is not likely to be that simple.

The transcriptional regulation of *Fgf4* has been well studied in cultured cells. The findings suggest that two transcription factors, Oct4 and Sox2 (an HMG-box transcription factor), synergistically activate *Fgf4* expression in the embryo proper (Yuan et al. 1995). The *Oct4* null muta-

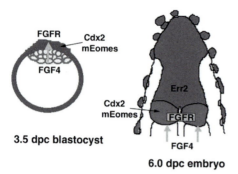

Figure 3 New model for trophoblast development. At the blastocyst stage, FGF4 is proposed to signal from the ICM to the overlying trophoblast through an FGFR turning on or maintaining such genes as *Cdx2* and *mEomes* in the TS cell pool. At postimplantation stages, a similar signaling pathway is likely occurring with additional critical transcription factors, such as *Err2*.

tion resulted in embryos with significantly reduced levels of *Fgf4* expression (Nichols et al. 1998). The major putative receptor for FGF4 in the trophoblast is FGFR2. The expression data and mutant analysis make this receptor the best candidate to functionally receive the embryo-derived FGF4 signal. In fact, the more severe *Fgfr2* mutant embryos exhibit a peri-implantation lethal phenotype. Interestingly, the embryos implanted randomly and not at the abembryonic pole, implying that the trophecto-derm of the blastocyst was equivalent and did not segregate into polar and mural regions (Arman et al. 1998). The *Fgfr2* gene is differentially spliced to encode two receptors (IIIb and IIIc) that differ in their ligand specificity. Targeted mutation of the IIIb isoform resulted in a later phenotype that differed from both of the two *Fgfr2* mutations. The pups died at birth with major limb and lung abnormalities (De Moerlooze et al. 2000). When *Fgfr2* mutant embryos had their placentas rescued by tetraploid aggregations, the embryonic phenotype was strikingly similar to the IIIb isoform mutation mentioned above (Arman et al. 1999). These results indicated that the IIIb isoform was critical for signaling in the embryo proper and that the IIIc isoform of *Fgfr2* is likely the functional receptor in the trophoblast. This would predict that a IIIc isoform-specific mutation would phenocopy the complete null mutation.

Among the transcription factors known to be expressed in TS cells, Cdx2 and mEomes are among the most interesting because they belong to gene families that are known to be regulated by FGF signaling in other vertebrates. *Cdx2* is a member of the *caudal*-related subfamily of homeobox genes. Since the discovery of the prototypic member, *caudal*, in

Drosophila melanogaster, numerous orthologs have been isolated from both invertebrates and vertebrates (He et al. 1997). Studies on *Xcad3*, a *Xenopus caudal* homolog, indicated that this gene was an immediate-early target of FGF signaling (Isaacs et al. 1998). Of the three *caudal*-related genes known to exist in the mouse (*Cdx1*, *Cdx2*, and *Cdx4*), only *Cdx2* was found to be expressed in trophoblast tissues (Beck et al. 1995). It would be of interest to determine whether *Cdx2* is a direct target of the FGF4–FGFR signal in the trophoblast. Interestingly, the *Cdx2* null phenotype is similar, if not identical, to the severe *Fgfr2* mutation (Chawengsaksophak et al. 1997), suggesting a critical role for *Cdx2* in the trophoblast and consistent with its being a putative target of FGF signaling.

The T-box gene family, of which *mEomes* is a member, defines a large group of transcription factors with a conserved DNA-binding domain known as the T-box (Papaioannou and Silver 1998). The prototypic T-box gene, *Brachyury* (*T*), was shown to be an FGF immediate-early response gene in *Xenopus* (Smith et al. 1991). Studies in zebrafish also found two T-box genes, *no tail* (*T* homolog) and *spadetail*, to be regulated by FGF signaling (Griffin et al. 1995, 1998). However, it was not determined whether this regulation was direct or indirect. *mEomes* is first expressed in the trophectoderm of the 3.5 dpc blastocyst and is later restricted to the ExE of the early postimplantation embryo (Ciruna and Rossant 1999; Hancock et al. 1999). A targeted mutation of this gene resulted in embryonic lethality shortly after implantation due to trophectoderm defects (Russ et al. 2000). This phenotype was similar to the *Cdx2* null mutation and one of the *Fgfr2* mutations, suggesting that FGF signaling may also regulate *mEomes*.

FUTURE PERSPECTIVES

The derivation and characterization of trophoblast stem cell lines has provided a new cell culture system for studying trophoblast development and placentation in the mouse. The ability of TS cells to both differentiate in culture and contribute to trophoblast tissues in vivo is unique among trophoblast or placental cell lines studied to date. When TS cell lines are compared to other rodent trophoblast cell lines, several fundamental differences can be noted. The Rcho-1 cell line from a rat choriocarcinoma has the ability to differentiate directly into giant cells in vitro, which makes it a valuable system for studying giant cell differentiation and endoreduplication (Faria and Soares 1991). However, the starting population is tetraploid, and they do not differentiate into other trophoblast subtypes, such as labyrinthine or spongiotrophoblast cells, and their ability to contribute to chimeras has not been reported. The SM cell lines (SM9-1, SM9-2, and SM-10) were derived from mouse mid- to late-gestation placentas (Sharma 1998). These cell lines exhibit differential invasiveness in culture, but their inability to differentiate restricts their usefulness as models for broad aspects of trophoblast development.

Both ES and TS cell lines express genes that are highly representative of their tissues of origin, but several exceptions can be noted. TS and ES cells can differentiate into several cell types in culture, and both exclusively contribute to their respective lineages in chimeric conceptuses. TS and ES cells behave as classic stem cells in vitro with indefinite maintenance of a stem cell pool that generates different progeny. However, in vivo they both show a limited period of stem-cell-like activity. Their existence in vivo is relatively short (3–4 days) in comparison to the length of gestation, and they are restricted to the earliest moments of development.

Numerous interactions are thought to occur between the epiblast and trophoblast in vivo. With the availability of both TS and ES cells, these interactions may be studied ex vivo. Preliminary experiments have shown that TS and ES cells do interact to form coherent aggregates in suspension cultures (D. Strumpf et al., unpubl.). Interestingly, the cells most often segregate to form a structure where a group of ES cells is interacting with a group of TS cells at a planar surface, reminiscent of the situation in vivo (Fig. 2D). Phenomena such as primordial germ cell induction and mesoderm induction may be investigated in such TS–ES cell aggregates.

The universality of the existence of TS cells in other mammalian species has yet to be determined. However, attempts to derive TS cell lines from other species are under way. It is encouraging to note that a porcine trophoblast cell line, TE1, has been derived that shares several morphological characteristics with mouse TS cell lines (Flechon et al. 1995). This cell line is dependent on feeder cells, but a requirement for FGF signaling has not been established.

Since the placenta is the most diverged organ among mammals, and there are considerable differences between human and mouse trophoblast development, the derivation of human TS cell lines would provide a significant model of the human placenta, which would not be redundant with mouse TS cell lines. Although blastocyst formation in the mouse and human appear quite similar, the events following implantation are quite different. The mouse polar trophectoderm exhibits rapid proliferation subsequent to implantation to give rise to the ExE, whereas many of the human trophectodermal cells undergo cell fusion to immediately form the multinucleated syncytiotrophoblast. There is a layer of diploid trophoblast cells between the syncytiotrophoblast and the epiblast, known as the cytotrophoblast. If TS cells exist in human, they would most likely arise from the cytotrophoblast layer. However, rapid proliferation of the cytotrophoblast layer does not occur until the early villous stage, which is about 7 days after implantation (Benirschke and Kaufmann 1995). These observations suggest that TS cells may more likely be found in later stages of human placental development rather than in the blastocyst. Human TS cell lines could be of potential therapeutic use, such as in the production of clinically useful hormones or cell-based therapies for patients with placental insufficiencies.

ACKNOWLEDGMENTS

The authors' work described here was supported by the Canadian Institutes of Health Research.

REFERENCES

Arman E., Haffner-Krausz R., Gorivodsky M., and Lonai P. 1999. Fgfr2 is required for limb outgrowth and lung-branching morphogenesis. *Proc. Natl. Acad. Sci.* **96:** 11895–11899.

Arman E., Haffner-Krausz R., Chen Y., Heath J.K., and Lonai P. 1998. Targeted disruption of fibroblast growth factor (FGF) receptor 2 suggests a role for FGF signaling in pre-gastrulation mammalian development. *Proc. Natl. Acad. Sci.* **95:** 5082–5087.

Avery G.B. and Hunt C.V. 1969. The differentiation of trophoblast giant cells in the mouse, studied in kidney capsule grafts. *Transplant. Proc.* **1:** 61–66.

Barlow P.W. and Sherman M.I. 1972. The biochemistry of differentiation of mouse trophoblast: Studies on polyploidy. *J. Embryol. Exp. Morphol.* **27:** 447–465.

Basyuk E., Cross J.C., Corbin J., Nakayama H., Hunter P., Nait-Oumesmar B., and Lazzarini R.A. 1999. Murine Gcm1 gene is expressed in a subset of placental trophoblast cells. *Dev. Dyn.* **214:** 303–311.

Beck F., Erler T., Russell A., and James R. 1995. Expression of Cdx-2 in the mouse embryo and placenta: Possible role in patterning of the extra-embryonic membranes. *Dev. Dyn.* **204:** 219–227.

Benirschke K. and Kaufmann P. 1995. *Pathology of the human placenta*, 3rd edition Springer-Verlag, New York.

Chai N., Patel Y., Jacobson K., McMahon J., McMahon A., and Rappolee D.A. 1998. FGF is an essential regulator of the fifth cell division in preimplantation mouse embryos. *Dev. Biol.* **198:** 105–115.

Chawengsaksophak K., James R., Hammond V.E., Kontgen F., and Beck F. 1997. Homeosis and intestinal tumours in Cdx2 mutant mice. *Nature* **386:** 84–87.

Ciruna B.G. and Rossant J. 1999. Expression of the T-box gene *Eomesodermin* during early mouse development. *Mech. Dev.* **81:** 199–203.

Colvin J.S., Bohne B.A., Harding G.W., McEwen D.G., and Ornitz D.M. 1996. Skeletal overgrowth and deafness in mice lacking fibroblast growth factor receptor 3. *Nat. Genet.* **12:** 390–397.

Copp A.J. 1978. Interaction between inner cell mass and trophectoderm of the mouse blastocyst. I. A study of cellular proliferation. *J. Embryol. Exp. Morphol.* **48:** 109–125.

———. 1979. Interaction between inner cell mass and trophectoderm of the mouse blastocyst. II. The fate of the polar trophectoderm. *J. Embryol. Exp. Morphol.* **51:** 109–20.

Cross J.C. 2000. Genetic insights into trophoblast differentiation and placental morphogenesis. *Semin. Cell Dev. Biol.* **11:** 105–113.

Cross J.C., Werb Z., and Fisher S.J. 1994. Implantation and the placenta: Key pieces of the development puzzle. *Science* **266:** 1508–1518.

Cross J.C., Flannery M.L., Blanar M.A., Steingrimsson E., Jenkins N.A., Copeland N.G., Rutter W.J., and Werb Z. 1995. *Hxt* encodes a basic helix-loop-helix transcription factor that regulates trophoblast cell development. *Development* **121:** 2513–2523.

De Moerlooze L., Spencer-Dene B., Revest J., Hajihosseini M., Rosewell I., and Dickson C. 2000. An important role for the IIIb isoform of fibroblast growth factor receptor 2 (FGFR2) in mesenchymal-epithelial signalling during mouse organogenesis. *Development* **127:** 483–492.

Deng C., Wynshaw-Boris A., Zhou F., Kuo A., and Leder P. 1996. Fibroblast growth factor receptor 3 is a negative regulator of bone growth. *Cell* **84:** 911–921.

Dickson A.D. 1966. The form of the mouse blastocyst. *J. Anat.* **100:** 335–348.

Duncan S.A., Manova K., Chen W.S., Hoodless P., Weinstein D.C., Bachvarova R.F., and Darnell J.E., Jr. 1994. Expression of transcription factor HNF-4 in the extraembryonic endoderm, gut, and nephrogenic tissue of the developing mouse embryo: HNF-4 is a marker for primary endoderm in the implanting blastocyst. *Proc. Natl. Acad. Sci.* **91:** 7598–7602.

Faria T.N. and Soares M.J. 1991. Trophoblast cell differentiation: Establishment, characterization, and modulation of a rat trophoblast cell line expressing members of the placental prolactin family. *Endocrinology* **129:** 2895–2906.

Faria T.N., Ogren L., Talamantes F., Linzer D.I., and Soares M.J. 1991. Localization of placental lactogen-I in trophoblast giant cells of the mouse placenta. *Biol. Reprod.* **44:** 327–331.

Feldman B., Poueymirou W., Papaioannou V.E., DeChiara T.M., and Goldfarb M. 1995. Requirement of FGF-4 for postimplantation mouse development. *Science* **267:** 246–249.

Flechon J.E., Laurie S., and Notarianni E. 1995. Isolation and characterization of a feeder-dependent, porcine trophectoderm cell line obtained from a 9-day blastocyst. *Placenta* **16:** 643–658.

Gardner R.L. and Cockroft D.L. 1998. Complete dissipation of coherent clonal growth occurs before gastrulation in mouse epiblast. *Development* **125:** 2397–2402.

Gardner R.L. and Johnson M.H. 1972. An investigation of inner cell mass and trophoblast tissues following their isolation from the mouse blastocyst. *J. Embryol. Exp. Morphol.* **28:** 279–312.

Gardner R.L., Papaioannou V.E., and Barton S.C. 1973. Origin of the ectoplacental cone and secondary giant cells in mouse blastocysts reconstituted from isolated trophoblast and inner cell mass. *J. Embryol. Exp. Morphol.* **30:** 561–572.

Griffin K., Patient R., and Holder N. 1995. Analysis of FGF function in normal and no tail zebrafish embryos reveals separate mechanisms for formation of the trunk and the tail. *Development* **121:** 2983–2994.

Griffin K.J., Amacher S.L., Kimmel C.B., and Kimelman D. 1998. Molecular identification of spadetail: Regulation of zebrafish trunk and tail mesoderm formation by T-box genes. *Development* **125:** 3379–3388.

Guillemot F., Nagy A., Auerbach A., Rossant J., and Joyner A.L. 1994. Essential role of Mash-2 in extraembryonic development. *Nature* **371:** 333–336.

Haffner-Krausz R., Gorivodsky M., Chen Y., and Lonai P. 1999. Expression of Fgfr2 in the early mouse embryo indicates its involvement in preimplantation development. *Mech. Dev.* **85:** 167–172.

Hancock S.N., Agulnik S.I., Silver L.M., and Papaioannou V.E. 1999. Mapping and expression analysis of the mouse ortholog of *Xenopus Eomesodermin. Mech. Dev.* **81:** 205–208.

He T.C., da Costa L.T., and Thiagalingam S. 1997. Homeosis and polyposis: A tale from the mouse. *Bioessays* **19:** 551–555.

Hoshikawa M., Ohbayashi N., Yonamine A., Konishi M., Ozaki K., Fukui S., and Itoh N. 1998. Structure and expression of a novel fibroblast growth factor, FGF-17, preferentially expressed in the embryonic brain. *Biochem. Biophys. Res. Commun.* **244:** 187–191.

Ilgren E.B. 1981. On the control of the trophoblastic giant-cell transformation in the mouse: Homotypic cellular interactions and polyploidy. *J. Embryol. Exp. Morphol.* **62:** 183–202.

Isaacs H.V., Pownall M.E., and Slack J.M. 1998. Regulation of Hox gene expression and posterior development by the *Xenopus* caudal homologue Xcad3. *EMBO J.* **17:** 3413–3427.

Johnson M.H. and Rossant J. 1981. Molecular studies on cells of the trophectodermal lineage of the postimplantation mouse embryo. *J. Embryol. Exp. Morphol.* **61:** 103–116.

Johnson M.H. and Ziomek C.A. 1981. The foundation of two distinct cell lineages within the mouse morula. *Cell* **24:** 71–80.

Kirby D.R. Billington W.D., and James D.A. 1966. Transplantation of eggs to the kidney and uterus of immunised mice. *Transplantation* **4:** 713–718.

Lawson K.A., Dunn N.R., Roelen B.A., Zeinstra L.M., Davis A.M., Wright C.V., Korving J.P., and Hogan B.L. 1999. Bmp4 is required for the generation of primordial germ cells in the mouse embryo. *Genes Dev.* **13:** 424–436.

Lescisin K.R., Varmuza S., and Rossant J. 1988. Isolation and characterization of a novel trophoblast-specific cDNA in the mouse. *Genes Dev.* **2:** 1639–1646.

Luo J., Sladek R., Bader J.A., Matthyssen A., Rossant J., and Giguere V. 1997. Placental abnormalities in mouse embryos lacking the orphan nuclear receptor ERR-β. *Nature* **388:** 778–782.

Miyake A., Konishi M., Martin F.H., Hernday N.A., Ozaki K., Yamamoto S., Mikami T., Arakawa T., and Itoh N. 1998. Structure and expression of a novel member, FGF-16, on the fibroblast growth factor family. *Biochem. Biophys. Res. Commun.* **243:** 148–152.

Nichols J., Zevnik B., Anastassiadis K., Niwa H., Klewe-Nebenius D., Chambers I., Scholer H., and Smith A. 1998. Formation of pluripotent stem cells in the mammalian embryo depends on the POU transcription factor Oct4. *Cell* **95:** 379–391.

Nishimura T., Utsunomiya Y., Hoshikawa M., Ohuchi H., and Itoh N. 1999. Structure and expression of a novel human FGF, FGF-19, expressed in the fetal brain. *Biochim. Biophys. Acta.* **1444:** 148–151.

Niswander L. and Martin G.R. 1992. *Fgf-4* expression during gastrulation, myogenesis, limb and tooth development in the mouse. *Development* **114:** 755–768.

Ohbayashi N., Hoshikawa M., Kimura S., Yamasaki M., Fukui S., and Itoh N. 1998.

Structure and expression of the mRNA encoding a novel fibroblast growth factor, FGF-18. *J. Biol. Chem.* **273:** 18161–18164.

Ornitz D.M., Xu J., Colvin J.S., McEwen D.G., MacArthur C.A., Coulier F., Gao G., and Goldfarb M. 1996. Receptor specificity of the fibroblast growth factor family. *J. Biol. Chem.* **271:** 15292–15297.

Palmieri S.L., Peter W., Hess H., and Scholer H.R. 1994. Oct-4 transcription factor is differentially expressed in the mouse embryo during establishment of the first two extraembryonic cell lineages involved in implantation. *Dev. Biol.* **166:** 259–267.

Papaioannou V.E. and Silver L.M. 1998. The T-box gene family. *Bioessays* **20:** 9–19.

Pedersen R.A. 1986. Potency, lineage and allocation in preimplantation mouse embryos. In *Experimental approaches to mammalian embryonic development* (ed. J. Rossant and R.A. Pederson), pp. 3–34. Cambridge University Press, London, United Kingdom.

Rappolee D.A., Patel Y., and Jacobson K. 1998. Expression of fibroblast growth factor receptors in peri-implantation mouse embryos. *Mol. Reprod. Dev.* **51:** 254–264.

Rappolee D.A., Basilico C., Patel Y., and Werb Z. 1994. Expression and function of FGF-4 in peri-implantation development in mouse embryos. *Development* **120:** 2259–2269.

Rossant, J. 1986. Development of extraembryonic cell lineages in the mouse embryo. In *Experimental approaches to mammalian embryonic development* (ed. J. Rossant and R.A. Pederson), pp. 97–120. Cambridge University Press, London, United Kingdom.

———. 1995. Developnment of the extraembryonic lineages. *Semin Dev. Biol.* **6:** 237–247.

Rossant J. and Ofer L. 1977. Properties of extra-embryonic ectoderm isolated from postimplantation mouse embryos. *J. Embryol. Exp. Morphol.* **39:** 183–194.

Rossant J. and Tamura-Lis W. 1981. Effect of culture conditions on diploid to giant-cell transformation in postimplantation mouse trophoblast. *J. Embryol. Exp. Morphol.* **62:** 217–227.

Rossant J. and Vijh K.M. 1980. Ability of outside cells from preimplantation mouse embryos to form inner cell mass derivatives. *Dev. Biol.* **76:** 475–482.

Rossant J., Gardner R.L., and Alexandre H.L. 1978. Investigation of the potency of cells from the postimplantation mouse embryo by blastocyst injection: A preliminary report. *J. Embryol. Exp. Morphol.* **48:** 239–247.

Russ A.P., Wattler S., Colledge W.H., Aparicio S.A., Carlton M.B., Pearce J.J., Barton S.C., Surani M.A., Ryan K., Nehls M.C., Wilson V., and Evans M.J. 2000. *Eomesodermin* is required for mouse trophoblast development and mesoderm formation. *Nature* **404:** 95–99.

Sharma R.K. 1998. Mouse trophoblastic cell lines. II. Relationship between invasive potential and proteases. *In Vivo* **12:** 209–217.

Smith J.C., Price B.M., Green J.B., Weigel D., and Herrmann B.G. 1991. Expression of a *Xenopus* homolog of *Brachyury (T)* is an immediate-early response to mesoderm induction. *Cell* **67:** 79–87.

Szebenyi G. and Fallon J.F. 1999. Fibroblast growth factors as multifunctional signaling factors. *Int. Rev. Cytol.* **185:** 45–106.

Tanaka S., Kunath T., Hadjantonakis A.K., Nagy A., and Rossant J. 1998. Promotion of trophoblast stem cell proliferation by FGF4. *Science* **282:** 2072–2075.

Weinstein M., Xu X., Ohyama K., and Deng C.X. 1998. FGFR-3 and FGFR-4 function cooperatively to direct alveogenesis in the murine lung. *Development* **125:** 3615–3623.

Wilder P.J., Kelly D., Brigman K., Peterson C.L., Nowling T., Gao Q.S., McComb R.D., Capecchi M.R., and Rizzino A. 1997. Inactivation of the FGF-4 gene in embryonic stem cells alters the growth and/or the survival of their early differentiated progeny. *Dev. Biol.* **192**: 614–629.

Wiley L.M., Kidder G.M., and Watson A.J. 1990. Cell polarity and development of the first epithelium. *BioEssays* **12**: 67–73.

Wilkinson D.G., Bhatt S., and Herrmann B.G. 1990. Expression pattern of the mouse T gene and its role in mesoderm formation. *Nature* **343**: 657–659.

Xu X., Weinstein M., Li C., Naski M., Cohen R.I., Ornitz D.M., Leder P., and Deng C. 1998. Fibroblast growth factor receptor 2 (FGFR2)-mediated reciprocal regulation loop between FGF8 and FGF10 is essential for limb induction. *Development* **125**: 753–765.

Yuan H., Corbi N., Basilico C., and Dailey L. 1995. Developmental-specific activity of the FGF-4 enhancer requires the synergistic action of Sox2 and Oct-3. *Genes Dev.* **9**: 2635–2645.

Zimmer Y., Givol D., and Yayon A. 1993. Multiple structural elements determine ligand binding of fibroblast growth factor receptors. Evidence that both Ig domain 2 and 3 define receptor specificity. *J. Biol. Chem.* **268**: 7899–7903.

13

Hematopoietic Stem Cells: Molecular Diversification and Developmental Interrelationships

Stuart H. Orkin
Howard Hughes Medical Institute
Harvard Medical School
Boston, Massachusetts 02115

Blood cells are continuously produced throughout our lifetime from rare pluripotent bone marrow stem cells, called hematopoietic stem cells (HSCs). HSCs are endowed with two characteristics: They give rise to additional HSCs through self-renewal and also undergo differentiation to progenitor cells that become variously committed to different hematopoietic lineages (Weissman 2000). Operationally, HSCs are best described as those cells capable of reconstituting the hematopoietic system of a recipient individual. Indeed, this defining in vivo property forms the basis of bone marrow transplantation, which was first developed as a lifesaving clinical procedure nearly a half century ago.

Despite the recognition decades ago that HSCs exist, many questions regarding their origins, regulation, and developmental potential remain unresolved. These include (1) How are HSCs formed during development? (2) How do they choose between a resting state and self-renewal/differentiation? (3) How is the remarkable diversity of blood cells (red cells, white cells [neutrophils and monocytes/macrophages], T- and B-lymphocytes, megakaryocytes, mast cells, eosinophils) established at the molecular level? (4) How can our prior views and understanding of HSCs be reconciled with recent findings of unsuspected plasticity of HSCs and other somatic cells?

DEFINITIONS AND MARKERS OF HSCS

Characterization of HSCs by their function, that is, by their capacity to sustain long-term multilineage hematopoiesis in a recipient individual, has provided an assay system for cell populations separated by cell-surface markers defined by monoclonal antibodies to surface molecules. In general, the bone marrow of adult animals, most often mice, has been used as the source of potential HSCs. In the mouse, cells of the c-kit$^+$, sca-1$^+$, thy-1^{lo}, lineage-negative phenotype are able to reconstitute recipients at limiting dilution (Weissman 2000). Extrusion of dyes such as Hoechst 33324 and Rhodamine 123 has also been successfully used to identify populations greatly enriched in HSCs. A preoccupation in the field has been phenotypic description of *the* HSC. This goal has provided lively discussion among investigators, because it appears that there are subsets of HSCs. For example, the surface marker CD34 was initially believed to be present on all HSCs. More recent evidence points to the existence of rare CD34$^-$ HSCs (Osawa et al. 1996). Indeed, the CD34$^+$ state may reflect activation of HSCs (Sato et al. 1999). Moreover, separation of cells on the basis of Hoechst fluorescence at two emission wavelengths allows the identification of both replicating and quiescent HSCs (Goodell et al. 1996). The apparent diversity of HSCs and the failure of in vitro biological assays (at least to date) to define HSCs hamper *direct* molecular characterization of HSCs. Furthermore, study of the parameters controlling activation of HSCs from a resting state and symmetric versus asymmetric divisions has also been impeded. Techniques to expand HSCs in vitro or to immortalize HSCs while retaining their multipotential properties are needed both for improved biological characterization and for clinical application.

A simplified scheme of blood cell development from the HSC to mature lineages is depicted in Figure 1 (for details, see Akashi et al. 2000).

ORIGIN(S) OF HSCs

The hematopoietic system is an embryologic derivative of mesoderm. In vertebrates, hematopoiesis takes place at successive anatomic sites. Embryonic (or primitive) hematopoiesis occurs in the blood islands of the yolk sac (YS) (~E7.5–11 in the mouse). Definitive (or adult) hematopoiesis is transient in the fetal liver (FL) (~E11–16 in the mouse) but later sustained throughout life in the bone marrow (BM). This temporal pattern is consistent with a simple model in which HSCs arise first, and perhaps uniquely, in the YS and then seed the FL and later the BM through the circulation. Indeed, experiments more than 30 years ago were described in support of this sequence (Moore and Metcalf 1970). Chick–quail chimera experiments suggested an alternative scenario, as an independent site of hematopoietic cell generation was identified within

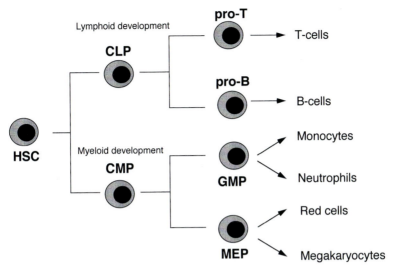

Figure 1 Schematic view of hematopoiesis. The hierarchy of blood cell development is depicted from hematopoietic stem cells (HSC) to the mature circulating blood cells shown to the right. Proposed common progenitors, defined by separation of populations and bioassays, are indicated as CLP (common lymphoid progenitor), CMP (common myeloid progenitor), pro-T (T-lymphoid progenitor), pro-B (B-cell progenitor), GMP (granulocyte/macrophage progenitor), and MEP (megakaryocyte/erythroid progenitor) (for details, see Akashi et al. 2000).

the embryo proper in the para-aortic splanchnopleura/aorta, gonad, mesonephros region (commonly called the AGM). AGM precursors of hematopoietic cells are present prior to the onset of circulation (Cumano et al. 2000). In contrast to the YS-derived progenitors, they provide multilineage differentiation upon transplantation into irradiated adult recipients. Analogous AGM-derived hematopoietic progenitors have been identified in the mouse (Medvinsky and Dzierzak 1996). These findings implicate the AGM as a region in which HSCs are born, and argue against a contribution of YS-derived progenitors to the adult hematopoietic system. This latter view has been challenged, however, by other experiments in which YS-derived progenitors are transplanted into *newborn* rather than adult recipients (Yoder et al. 1997). In this setting, definitive HSCs are observed in the YS, in fact in greater numbers than in the AGM region (at E9) (Yoder and Hiatt 1999). As investigators continue to debate the relative contribution of YS and AGM regions to adult hematopoiesis, a working model posits that multiple, probably independent, origins of HSCs exist in development. The milieu into which HSCs are introduced (e.g., newborn or adult) influences how they are scored by in vivo assays.

A common, emerging theme in the complex origin of HSCs is an intimate relationship between hematopoietic and vascular development. In the vertebrate YS the first blood cells, embryonic red blood cells, arise in close apposition to the endothelial cells of the blood islands. This proximity and the temporal development of the blood and vascular lineages suggested the existence of a common precursor, the hemangioblast (Pardanaud et al. 1989). Recent findings, as reviewed in Chapter 15, provide experimental support for this hypothesis in the mouse (Choi et al. 1998). Within the embryo proper as well, there is compelling evidence for a close interrelationship between the hematopoietic and vascular programs. Indeed, in this setting, data are more compatible with the emergence of definitive hematopoietic progenitors (presumably HSCs) from a subset of the vascular compartment (dubbed hemogenic endothelium). First, in chick–quail chimera experiments, two subsets of mesoderm have been defined: a dorsal one (the somite) that produces pure angioblasts (angioblastic potential) and a second, ventral one (the splanchnopleural mesoderm) that generates cells with dual endothelial and hematopoetic potentials (Pardanaud and Dieterlen-Lievre 1999). In agreement with these findings, $CD34^+$ hematopoietic cells have been observed in the floor of the aorta in the developing mouse and human (Tavian et al. 1996; Delassus et al. 1999). In addition, putative definitive hematopoietic cells $(CD34^+)$ are seen in the proximal umbilical and vitelline arteries, two potential sites of HSC emergence. In accord with this, intra-aortic, vitelline, and umbilical hematopoietic clusters are visualized in mice harboring a *lacZ* knock-in of the Cbfa2 (AML1) gene, which is essential for formation of definitive hematopoietic cells (see below) (North et al. 1999).

In vitro studies also argue for a role for endothelial cells in the origin of hematopoietic cells. For example, sorting of endothelial cells of E9.5 YS and embryos for a VE-cadherin$^+$, $CD34^+$, flk-1$^+$(a receptor for vascular endothelial growth factor [VEGF]), $CD31^+$, $CD45^-$, Ter 119$^-$ phenotype yields a population able to generate blood cells of all lineages, including lymphocytes (Nishikawa et al. 1998). An unresolved question is the relationship of these "hemogenic" endothelial cells to presumptive hemangioblasts.

REGULATORY GENES REQUIRED FOR FORMATION OR MAINTENANCE OF STEM CELLS

Although the anatomic origins of HSCs are not fully resolved, several transcription factors have been demonstrated to be required for either the generation or maintenance/proliferation of HSCs. As with other transcriptional components, their in vivo requirements have been revealed through gene targeting of ES cells in mice. Two factors, SCL/tal-1 and Lmo2, are essential for the generation of any hematopoietic cells, either at the YS stage or later in development (Porcher et al. 1996; Robb et al. 1996; Yamada et al. 1998). Thus, these factors are necessary for all aspects of primitive and definitive hematopoesis. Moreover, both are required for proper vascular development in the YS, consistent with their expression in the hemangioblast (Visvader et al. 1998; Yamada et al. 2000). Remarkably, each factor was first identified through chromosomal translocations in acute T-cell leukemia (T-ALL). Indeed, the SCL/tal-1 gene, which encodes a member of the basic helix-loop-helix (bHLH) family, is activated by an upstream deletion or translocation in perhaps 25% of T-ALL, and SCL/tal-1 and Lmo2 expression is more frequently seen in this entity, even without evident chromosomal alterations (Begley and Green 1999). Lmo2 protein, a LIM-only polypeptide, is specifically associated with SCL/tal-1 as well as a novel LIM-interacting polypeptide, Ldb1. Moreover, a multiprotein complex containing SCL/tal-1, Lmo2, Ldb1, the ubiquitous bHLH heterodimerization partner E12/47, and GATA-1 (see below) has been observed in erythroid and progenitor cells (Wadman et al. 1997). Whereas SCL/tal-1 (as a heterodimer with E12/47) binds to consensus E-box DNA target sites, Lmo2 does not recognize DNA by itself, but rather appears to provide a bridging function in transcription.

Precisely how SCL/tal-1 and Lmo2 function to promote hematopoietic development is as yet unresolved. The simplest interpretation of available data suggests that these factors are required for the specification of the hematopoietic fate from mesoderm. Expression of SCL/tal-1, Lmo2, and GATA-1 together in *Xenopus* embryos leads to hematopoietic specification in areas of the embryo that would normally exhibit other fates (Mead et al. 1998). In addition, injection of SCL/tal-1 RNA into wild-type zebrafish appears to promote both vascular and hematopoietic development, largely by expanding the hemangioblast population (Gering et al. 1998). Overexpression of SCL/tal-1 cDNA in zebrafish *cloche* mutant embryos also complements defects in blood and vessel development (Liao et al. 1998).

The genes acted upon by SCL-1/tal-1 and Lmo2 that act in transcription to specify hematopoiesis are largely unknown. One possible transcriptional target gene for SCL/tal-1 is that for the membrane tyrosine kinase c-kit, the receptor for stem cell factor (SCF, c-kit ligand), a growth factor for multipotential and mast cells. Defining the roles of SCL/tal-1 in transcription, however, is complicated by recent findings pointing to major DNA-binding-*independent* functions in development (Porcher et al. 1999). For example, formation of primitive erythroid cells and definitive hematopoietic progenitors takes place without site-specific DNA binding by SCL/tal-1 but requires an intact HLH domain that directs heterodimerization. By inference, therefore, protein–protein interactions of SCL/tal-1, presumably with Lmo2 in this context, are pivotal for HSC generation.

The formation of definitive hematopoietic cells (and HSCs), but not YS erythroid cells, requires AML1 (also known as Cbfa2), a transcription factor related to *Drosophila runt* (Okuda et al. 1996; Wang et al. 1996). As opposed to SCL/tal-1 and Lmo2, which are transcriptionally activated by chromosomal rearrangements, AML1 is expressed as a fusion protein with a variety of partners in diverse translocations in leukemia. In many of these instances, it is believed that the resultant fusion protein functions as a dominant-negative inhibitor of AML1 function (Okuda et al. 1998). In the absence of AML1, mouse embryos die at mid-gestation without any definitive hematopoietic cells (Okuda et al. 1996; Wang et al. 1996). No progenitors can be scored in colony assays, and homozygous mutants of a *lacZ* knock-in at the locus fail to generate hematopoietic clusters at sites of definitive hematopoietic cell formation, such as the floor of the aorta, and the vitelline and umbilical arteries (North et al. 1999). Again, the specific target genes regulated by AML1 that are required for HSC formation are unknown. From studies in myeloid cells, it has been demonstrated that growth factor receptors such as granulocyte colony-stimulating factor (G-CSF) may be controlled by AML1 in association with other myeloid-restricted transcriptional regulators (Zhang et al. 1996).

Production of a normal number of HSCs appears to depend on the expression of yet another transcription factor, GATA-2, a member of the GATA family (see below) (Tsai et al. 1994). GATA-2 is highly expressed in immature progenitors and then down-regulated in many, but not all, hematopoietic lineages. Forced expression of GATA-2 inhibits transition from a multipotential progenitor to a committed erythroid precursor (Briegel et al. 1993). Loss of GATA-2 function in mice is embryonic-lethal due to marked anemia (Tsai et al. 1994). Although the numbers of YS progenitors are modestly reduced in GATA-2$^{-/-}$ embryos, definitive progenitors are ~100-fold less than wild type. The precise level at which GATA-2 is required is uncertain. During mouse, zebrafish, and *Xenopus* development, GATA-2 expression parallels that of SCL/tal-1 and Lmo2 in regions fated for hematopoiesis (Detrich et al. 1995). It is conceivable, therefore, that GATA-2 functions within transcriptional complexes, perhaps including SCL/tal-1 and Lmo2 (Vyas et al. 1999), involved in establishing the hematopoietic program. Alternatively, GATA-2 may be required somewhat later in the pathway, perhaps to sustain the viability or proliferative capacity of immature progenitors. The presence of HSCs, albeit at a greatly reduced number in the absence of GATA-2, is consistent with this latter view.

A pivotal decision for HSCs is whether to remain in a resting G_0 state or to commit to self-renewal or production of progenitors. Relatively little is known regarding the regulation of such choices. Recent evidence, however, suggests that the cyclin-dependent kinase inhibitor, p21 (cip1/waf1), may be required to maintain HSC quiescence (Cheng et al. 2000). In p21$^{-/-}$ mice, HSC proliferation and their absolute numbers were increased under normal homeostatic conditions. However, these HSCs were more susceptible to cell-cycle-specific myelotoxic injury. Increased cell cycling also was observed to lead to stem cell exhaustion. Thus, p21 may constitute a molecular switch controlling the entry of HSC into cycle.

DIFFERENTIATION AND DIVERSIFICATION OF STEM CELLS

Although our understanding of how HSCs are induced to form is rudimentary, considerably more is known regarding the intrinsic cellular machinery for selection of lineage from a multipotential hematopoietic cell and subsequent differentiation. The growth and differentiation of hematopoietic cells are sustained by growth factors, cytokines that may act on cells of many lineages (e.g., SCF) or principally on a single one (e.g., erythropoietin). A consensus view, not held uniformly (Metcalf 1998), is that signaling pathways activated through the receptor for these growth factors foster viability and are permissive for proliferation, but are not determinative with respect to lineage choice (Goldsmith et al. 1998; Socolovsky et al. 1998; Stoffel et al. 1999). That is, critical decisions of lineage are executed by nuclear regulatory factors, acting to establish transcriptional programs characteristic of each precursor and lineage. Rather than attempting to provide a comprehensive summary of hematopoietic transcriptional factors, here I illustrate some underlying principles that derive from recent studies.

DOMINANT LINEAGE SELECTION OR REPROGRAMMING

The sine qua non for a "master" regulator is its potential to alter the differentiation phenotype of a cell into which it is introduced. For ex vivo assessment of function, investigators rely on available cell lines that are not irreversibly "frozen" in a given state. In practice, the cell lines suitable for these experiments are limited. Thus, we may underestimate at this time the extent to which some transcription factors are competent to program differentiation of specific lineages. Nonetheless, several clear-cut examples of lineage reprogramming have been reported and serve to illustrate common principles.

The zinc-finger protein GATA-1 is normally expressed at a low level in multipotential progenitors and at higher levels in erythroid precursors, megakaryocytes, mast cells, and eosinophils (Orkin 1992). Knock-out studies in mice demonstrate that GATA-1 is essential for the maturation of both erythroid and megakaryocyte precursors, but not for their initial generation (Weiss et al. 1994; Fujiwara et al. 1996; Shivadasani et al. 1997). It is hypothesized that the related GATA factor GATA-2 shares functions with GATA-1 and, in effect, substitutes for GATA-1 in lineage commitment. This view is consistent with forced expression experiments in two different systems. For example, expression of GATA-1 (or GATA-2 or GATA-3) in a myeloid cell 416B of mouse origin leads to the acquisition of megakaryocytic markers (Visvader and Adams 1993; Visvader et al. 1995). Similarly, introduction of GATA-1 into chicken progenitors transformed with a *myb-ets* retrovirus reprograms cells to three different fates—erythroid, eosinophil, and megakaryocytic (Kulessa et al. 1995). The level at which GATA-1 is expressed appears to determine the specific lineage that arises. In both systems, lineage reprogramming is accompanied by down-regulation of the myeloid markers of the host cells. Thus, in addition to activating a megakaryocytic/eosinophilic/erythroid program, GATA-1 acts to turn off the program of a "contralateral" lineage in which it is not normally expressed. Lineage antagonism, established through critical hematopoietic transcription factors, is emerging as a newly recognized and consistent theme (see below).

Another major hematopoietic transcription factor, PU.1, an ets protein, is able to induce myeloid lineage commitment in multipotential chicken progenitors, and in conjunction with GATA-1 and the basic-zipper protein C/EBP, promotes formation of eosinophils (Nerlov and Graf 1998; Nerlov et al. 1998). Again, concomitant with up-regulation of myeloid or eosinophil markers, down-regulation of multipotential markers is observed. In the absence of PU.1 in the mouse, myeloid and lymphoid development is perturbed (Scott et al. 1994, 1997; McKercher et al. 1996). In this setting, however, immature PU.1$^{-/-}$ progenitors are formed but are unable to proliferate or differentiate (DeKoter et al. 1998). Thus, as with GATA-1, gain-of-function experiments establish functions in lineage selection, whereas loss of function in vivo does not entirely ablate lineage commitment. This difference most likely rests on compensatory mechanisms available in vivo that are not operative in simpler, test cellular systems.

COMBINATORIAL POSITIVE ACTIONS OF HEMATOPOIETIC TRANSCRIPTION FACTORS

Whereas early views of mammalian differentiation highlighted the dominance of single "master" regulators, such as the bHLH factor myoD in myogenesis (Weintraub et al. 1991), a more sophisticated appreciation has emerged in recent years. Rather than acting in "isolation," key regulatory factors function within a cellular context. In experimental systems the outcome observed depends considerably on the character of the cells in which dominant regulators are expressed. Clear examples of this principle are apparent from studies of hematopoietic regulators.

In probing the mechanisms by which GATA-1 participates in transcription in the context of a GATA-1-negative erythroid precursor cell line (Weiss et al. 1997), it became apparent that the transcriptional action of GATA-1 might depend on a cell-restricted cofactor. The hypothetical cofactor was isolated by a yeast two-hybrid screen and dubbed "FOG" for *F*riend *o*f *G*ATA-1 (Tsang et al. 1997). Indeed, physical interaction of FOG, a multitype zinc-finger protein, with the N finger of GATA-1 is essential for the completion of both erythroid and megakaryocytic differentiation (Tsang et al. 1998; Crispino et al. 1999). Mutations of the N finger of GATA-1 that specifically disrupt interaction with FOG, but retain the DNA-binding contribution of the finger, lead to impaired erythropoiesis and platelet formation and function, both in test systems in culture and in human patients (Crispino et al. 1999; Nichols et al. 2000). Similarly, myeloid development relies on the combined presence and action of PU.1 and C/EBP, and eosinophil formation on C/EBP and GATA-1. Although direct experimental verification is not available, one may extrapolate these concepts to suggest that T-lymphoid cells might be GATA-3$^+$, Ikaros factor$^+$, PU.1$^-$, GATA-1$^-$, whereas B cells are PU.1$^+$, GATA-3$^-$, GATA-1$^-$, Pax-5$^+$. By extension, each lineage can be defined by its transcription factor "haplotype" (Akashi et al. 2000), just as cell-surface phenotypes have traditionally been used in immunology.

SUPPRESSION OF OTHER LINEAGES AS A MECHANISM OF LINEAGE SELECTION

Whereas lineage choice has traditionally been viewed as strictly a positive event, the concomitant down-regulation of markers of one or multiple lineages upon activation of a program, such as that described above for GATA-1 (Visvader et al. 1992; Kulessa et al. 1995), suggests that the manner in which multipotential cells choose a differentiation pathway may be more complex than heretofore imagined. Indeed, experiments that define the role of Pax-5 in B-lymphoid development illustrate how central suppression of alternative fates may be in lineage selection (Nutt et al. 1998, 1999). Prior experiments had shown that Pax-5 is essential for B-cell development (Urbanek et al. 1994). More recently, it has become evident that pro-B cells lacking Pax-5 are not restricted in their lineage fate (Nutt et al. 1999). Under stimulation with suitable cytokines, these pro-B cells are able to differentiate into macrophages, osteoclasts, dendritic cells, granulocytes, and natural killer cells. Remarkably, Pax-5$^{-/-}$ progenitors reconstitute the T-lymphoid system upon introduction into host mice (Rolink et al. 1999). Thus, commitment to B-cell development through Pax-5 involves suppression of alternative lineages. Investing complementary actions (activation and suppression) in individual transcription factors provides a parsimonious means of coordinating developmental decisions, particularly where multiple potential fates are available.

ANTAGONISM OF KEY HEMATOPOIETIC FACTORS AND REINFORCEMENT OF LINEAGE CHOICES

Mechanisms mediating antagonism between lineages are becoming clarified. Recent findings suggest that cross-regulation between lineage-restricted transcription factors is exerted at the level of protein–protein interaction as well as in transcription. GATA-1 and PU.1 serve as the dominant factors for erythroid/megakaryocytic and myeloid development, respectively. Expression of PU.1 in erythroid precursors arrests differentiation and leads to erythroleukemia (Moreau-Gachelin et al. 1990, 1996). Indeed, GATA-1 and PU.1 proteins interact. Association of the amino terminus and ets-domain of PU.1 with the C-finger of GATA-1 (or other GATA factors) blocks DNA binding by GATA-1 (Rekhtman et al. 1999; Zhang et al. 2000). Although DNA binding by PU.1 remains unaffected, *trans*-activation by PU.1 is impaired upon interaction with GATA-1, possibly due to displacement of a transcriptional cofactor, proposed to be c-jun (Zhang et al. 1999; Nerlov et al. 2000). Thus, cross-interactions between these factors serve to favor one lineage (erythroid/megakaryocytic or myeloid) at the expense of the "contralateral" option. Unknown mechanisms, either direct or indirect, then serve to down-regulate transcription of GATA-1 in myeloid lineages and PU.1 in erythroid/megakaryocytic cells.

Another example of cross-regulation in lineage choice is provided by recent observations of the roles of C/EBP and FOG in eosinophil selection (Querfurth et al. 2000). Chicken eosinophils generated in the myb-ets system by GATA-1 and C/EBP do not express appreciable FOG. Expression of FOG in these cells leads to down-regulation of eosinophil markers and acquisition of multipotential cell markers. Expression of a regulated C/EBP transgene in multipotential cells leads to rapid transcriptional shutoff of FOG, which acts in this setting as a repressor of the action of GATA-1 at transcriptional targets, such as the gene Eos47. Therefore, induction of eosinophil-specific genes is proposed to require repression of FOG expression, and consequently, relief of FOG repression of GATA-1. In the presence of enforced FOG expression, multipotential cells fail to differentiate into eosinophils. Differentiation reflects a "collapse" of the multipotential state, a finding reminiscent of that seen in the absence of Pax-5.

Antagonism established through cross-regulation of critical factors serves not only to execute a lineage choice, but also to reinforce this decision. Although irreversible differentiation might result, the option of reversing these regulatory loops remains, as long as chromatin events do not silence transcription of these factors.

Combined positive and negative regulatory influences on lineage choice are summarized in general terms in Figure 2.

CONCENTRATION-DEPENDENT ACTIONS OF HEMATOPOIETIC TRANSCRIPTION FACTORS

In reprogramming of chicken progenitors to eosinophil, erythroid, and thromboblast lineages by GATA-1, Kulessa and colleagues (1995) observed that the level at which GATA-1 was expressed correlated with the lineage outcome. Intermediate levels were observed in eosinophils and erythroid cells, and high levels in thromboblasts. Of interest, levels of expression differed by only a few fold between lineages. Although these findings might be explained by titration of DNA targets at different GATA-1 concentrations, it seems more likely that assembly (or disassembly) of protein complexes is influenced by subtle concentration changes, particularly given the nature of generally weaker protein–protein interactions. Reducing the expression of GATA-1 in vivo by approximately threefold due to a targeted mutation of *cis*-regulatory elements results in markedly impaired erythroid cell maturation (McDevitt et al. 1997). Thus, high concentrations of GATA-1 protein are needed to drive cell maturation.

Concentration-dependent influences of PU.1 on differentiation have recently been noted (DeKoter and Singh 2000). In particular, reintroduc-

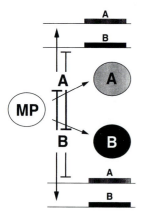

Figure 2 Positive and antagonistic regulatory interactions. A model of the simplest lineage choice is depicted here. A multipotential progenitor (MP) is able to generate two lineages, A and B (all shown in circles). Transcription factor A is expressed specifically within precursors of lineage A and is required for their maturation; conversely, factor B is required for lineage B. The factors are shown above and below to feed back in positive fashion to regulate their own respective transcription, whereas factor A represses transcription of the factor B gene, and B represses transcription of the A gene. Moreover, as shown in the center, factors A and B interfere with each other's function through direct protein–protein interactions. According to this model, a choice between fates A and B is reinforced by antagonism exerted both at the protein–protein and transcriptional levels.

tion of PU.1 into PU.1$^{-/-}$ progenitors rescues both macrophage and B-cell differentiation. However, high-level expression favors macrophage development and blocks B-cell development. It is hypothesized that PU.1 in this instance may antagonize the action of Pax-5 via protein interactions.

COEXPRESSION OF LINEAGE FACTORS IN MULTIPOTENTIAL PROGENITORS

Among the lineage-restricted transcription factors, the majority are expressed, at least at low level, in hematopoietic progenitors that have yet to choose a lineage (Jimenez et al. 1992). After lineage commitment, markers of other lineages are extinguished. Furthermore, additional markers of specific lineages, such as DNase I hypersensitivity of immunoglobulin loci, are present in multipotential cells but absent in selected lineages (erythroid, myeloid). Multilineage gene expression has also been documented at the single-cell level by PCR (Hu et al. 1997). These findings have led to the hypothesis that multipotential progenitors are "testing" various options or poised in a molecular sense to pursue any one of multiple paths. This notion of multipotential cell plasticity is readily reconciled with findings reviewed above regarding cross-regulatory interactions of transcription factors and the assembly of complexes that may be highly dependent on protein concentrations (if not modifications). We envision that immature progenitors may express regulatory factors generally ascribed to specific lineages, perhaps at low level, in bursts, or in a cell-cycle-dependent fashion. Lineage commitment is then associated with increased expression (or activity) of such factors, coupled with antagonistic mechanisms that serve to reinforce an initial, and rather tentative, decision.

UNEXPECTED PLASTICITY OF HSCs AND STEM CELLS FOR OTHER TISSUES

Cell biologic and molecular findings have provided a working conceptual framework in which to consider the events from HSC to individual hematopoietic lineages. Recent evidence, however, suggests unprecedented plasticity of HSCs. For example, populations of presumptive muscle stem cells (satellite cells) contribute to hematopoiesis upon transplantation into mice (Gussoni et al. 1999; Jackson et al. 1999). Conversely, purified HSC populations contribute to muscle (Gussoni et al. 1999). Prior evidence also suggested that peripheral blood contains $CD34^+$, presumptive endothelial progenitors, whose relationship to traditional $CD34^+$ hematopoietic progenitors is unknown (Asahara et al. 1997). The most extreme example of stem cell plasticity thus far described is the generation of hematopoietic cells in the mouse from cultured clonal neural stem cells (Bjornson et al. 1999). Although it has yet to be proven formally in these instances that isolated single cells are endowed with inherent plasticity of the magnitude revealed in these recent studies, it is highly unlikely that low-level contamination of one population with another can account for the results. Rather, it seems that cells are reeducated in some unknown manner by the local microenvironment to adopt new fates, or dedifferentiate into multipotent somatic cells that then redifferentiate along a new path. Although the signals mediating these phenomena are unknown, the suggestion that cell culture conditions may prime muscle stem cells for hematopoietic contribution in vivo (Jackson et al. 1999) hints at experimental approaches to dissecting the relevant components. Determining the environment cues responsible for stem cell plasticity and relating these to the control of critical transcription factors are challenges for the future.

REFERENCES

Akashi K., Traver D., Miyamoto T., and Weissman I.L. 2000. A clonogenic common myeloid progenitor that gives rise to all myeloid lineages. *Nature* **404:** 193–197.

Asahara T., Murohara T., Sullivan A., Silver M., van der Zee R., Li T., Witzenbichler B., Schatteman G., and Isner J.M. 1997. Isolation of putative progenitor endothelial cells for angiogenesis. *Science* **275:** 964–966.

Begley C.G. and Green A.R. 1999. The SCL gene: from case report to critical hematopoietic regulator. *Blood* **93:** 2760–2770.

Bjornson C.R., Rietze R.L., Reynolds B.A., Magli M.C., and Vescovi A.L. 1999. Turning brain into blood: A hematopoietic fate adopted by adult neural stem cells in vivo. *Science* **283:** 534–537.

Briegel K., Lim K.-C., Plank C., Beug H., Engel J., and Zenke M. 1993. Ectopic expression of a conditional GATA-2/estrogen receptor chimera arrests erythroid differentiation in a hormone-dependent manner. *Genes Dev.* **7:** 1097–1109.

Cheng T., Rodrigues N., Shen H., Yang Y., Dombkowski D., Sykes M., and Scadden D.T. 2000. Hematopoietic stem cell quiescence maintained by p21. *Science* **287:** 1804–1808.

Choi K., Kennedy M., Kazarov A., Papadimitriou J.C., and Keller G. 1998. A common precursor for hematopoietic and endothelial cells. *Development* **125:** 725–732.

Crispino J.D., Lodish M.B., MacKay J.P., and Orkin S.H. 1999. Use of altered specificity mutants to a specific protein-protein interaction in differentiation: The GATA-1:FOG complex. *Mol. Cell* **3:** 219–228.

Cumano A., Dieterlen-Lievre F., and Godin I. 2000. The splanchnopleura/AGM region is the prime site for the generation of multipotent hemopoietic precursors, in the mouse embryo. *Vaccine* **18:** 1621–1623.

DeKoter R.P. and Singh H. 2000. Regulation of B lymphocyte and macrophage development by graded expression of PU.1. *Science* **288:** 1439–1441.

DeKoter R.P., Walsh J.C., and Singh H. 1998. PU.1 regulates both cytokine dependent proliferation and differentiation of granulocyte/macrophage progenitors. *EMBO J.* **17:** 4456–4468.

Delassus S., Titley I., and Enver T. 1999. Fucntional and molecular analysis of hematopoietic progenitors derived from the aorta-gonad-mesonephros region of the mouse embryo. *Blood* **94:** 1495–1503.

Detrich H.W., Kieran M.W., Chan F.W., Barone L.M., Yee K., Rundstadler J.A., Pratt S., Ransom D., and Zon L.I. 1995. Intra-embryonic hematopoietic cell migration during vertebrate development. *Proc. Natl. Acad. Sci.* **92:** 10713–10717.

Fujiwara Y., Browne C.P., Cunniff K., Goff S.C., and Orkin S.H. 1996. Arrested development of embryonic red cell precursors in mouse embryos lacking transcription factor GATA-1. Proc. Natl. Acad. Sci. **93:** 12355–12358.

Gering M., Rodaway A.R.F., Gottgens B., Patient R.K., and Green A.R. 1998. The SCL gene specifies haemangioblast development from early mesoderm. *EMBO J.* **17:** 4029–4045.

Goldsmith M.A., Mikami A., You Y., Liu K.D., Thomas L., Pharr P., and Longmore G.D. 1998. Absence of cytokine receptor-dependent specificity in red blood cell differentiation in vivo. *Proc. Natl. Acad. Sci.* **95:** 7006–7011.

Goodell M.A., Brose K., Paradis G., Conner A.S., and Mulligan R.C. 1996. Isolation and functional properties of murine hematopoietic stem cells that are replicating in vivo. *J. Exp. Med.* **183:** 1797–1806.

Gussoni E., Soneoka Y., Strickland C.D., Buzney E.A., Khan M.K., Flint A.F., Kunkel L.M., and Mulligan R.C. 1999. Dystrophin expression in the mdx mouse restored by stem cell transplantation. *Nature* **401**: 390–394.

Hu M., Kruase D., Greaves M., Sharkis S., Dexter M., Heyworth C., and Enver T. 1997. Multilineage gene expression precedes commitment in the hemopoietic system. *Genes Dev.* **11**: 774–785.

Jackson K.A., Mi T., and Goodell M.A. 1999. Hematopoietic potential of stem cells isolated from murine skeletal muscle. *Proc. Natl. Acad. Sci.* **96**: 14482–14486.

Jimenez G., Griffiths S.D., Ford A.M., Greaves M.F., and Enver T. 1992. Activation of the β-globin locus control region precedes commitment to the erythroid lineage. *Proc. Natl. Acad. Sci.* **89**: 10618–10622.

Kulessa H., Frampton J., and Graf T. 1995. GATA-1 reprograms avian myelomonocytic cells into eosinophils, thromboblasts and erythroblasts. *Genes Dev.* **9**: 1250–1262.

Liao E.C., Paw B.H., Oates A.C., Pratt S.J., Postlethwait J.H., and Zon L.I. 1998. SCL/Tal-1 transcription factor acts downstream of *cloche* to specify hematopoietic and vascular progenitors in zebrafish. *Genes Dev.* **12**: 621–626.

McDevitt M.A., Shivdasani R.A., Fujiwara Y., Yang H., and Orkin S.H. 1997. A "knock-down" mutation created by *cis*-element gene targeting reveals the dependence of red blood cell maturation on the level of transcription factor GATA-1. *Proc. Natl. Acad. Sci.* **94**: 6781–6785.

McKercher S.R., Torbett B.E., Anderson K.L., Henkel G.W., Vestal D.J., Baribault H., Klemnsz M., Feeney A.J., Wu G.E., Paige C.J., and Maki R.A. 1996. Targeted disruption of the PU.1 gene results in multiple hematopoietic abnormalities. *EMBO J.* **15**: 5647–5658.

Mead P.E., Kelley C.M., Hahn P.S., Piedad O., and Zon L.I. 1998. SCL specifies hematopoietic mesoderm in *Xenopus* embryos. *Development* **125**: 2611–2620.

Medvinsky A. and Dzierzak E. 1996. Definitive hematopoiesis is autonomously initiated by the AGM region. *Cell* **86**: 897–906.

Metcalf D. 1998. Lineage commitment and maturation in hematopoietic cells: The case for extrinsic regulation. *Blood* **92**: 345–347.

Moore M.S.A. and Metcalf D. 1970. Ontogeny of the haemopoietic system: Yolk sac origin of in vivo and in vitro colony forming cells in the developing mouse embryo. *Br. J. Haematol.* **18**: 279–296.

Moreau-Gachelin F., Ray D., Tambourin P., Tavitian A., Klemsz M.J., McKercher S.R., Celada A., Van Beveren C., and Maki R.A. 1990. The Pu.1 transcription factor is the product of the putative oncogene Spi-1. *Cell* **61**: 1166.

Moreau-Gachelin F., Wendling F., Molina T., Denis N., Titeux M., Grimber G., Briand P., Vainchenker W., and Tavitian A. 1996. Spi-1/PU.1 transgenic mice develop multistep erythroleukemias. *Mol. Cell. Biol.* **16**: 2453–2463.

Nerlov C. and Graf T. 1998. PU.1 induces myeloid lineage commitment in multipotent hematopoietic progenitors. *Genes Dev.* **12**: 2403–2412.

Nerlov C., Querfurth E., Kulessa H., and Graf T. 2000. GATA-1 interacts with the myeloid PU.1 transcription factor and represses PU.1-dependent transcription. *Blood* **95**: 2543–2551.

Nerlov C., McNagny K.M., Doderlein G., Kowenz-Leutz E., and Graf T. 1998. Distinct C/EBP functions are required for eosinophil lineage commitment and maturation. *Genes Dev.* **12**: 2413–2423.

Nichols K.E., Crispino J.D., Poncz M., White J.G., Orkin S.H., Maris J.M., and Weiss M.J.

2000. Familial dyserythropoietic anaemia and thrombocytopenia due to an inherited mutation in GATA1. *Nat. Genet.* **24:** 266–270.

Nishikawa S.-I., Nishikawa S., Kawamoto H., Yoshida H., Kizumoto M., Kataoka H., and Katsura Y. 1998. In vitro generation of lymphohematopoietic cells from endothelial cells purified from murine embryos. *Immunity* **8:** 761–769.

North T., Gu T.-L., Stacy T., Wang Q., Howard L., Binder M., Marin-Padilla M., and Speck N.A. 1999. *Cbfa2* is required for the formation of intra-aortic hematopoietic clusters. *Development* **126:** 2563–2575.

Nutt S.L., Heavey B., Rolink A.G., and Busslinger M. 1999. Commitment to the B-lymphoid lineage depends on the transcription factor Pax5. *Nature* **401:** 556–562.

Nutt S.L., Morrison A.M., Dorfler P., Rolink A., and Busslinger M. 1998. Identification of BSAP (Pax-5) target genes in early B-cell development by loss- and gain-of-function experiments. *EMBO J.* **17:** 2319–2333.

Okuda T., Deursen J.V., Hiebert S.W., Grosveld G., and Downing J.R. 1996. AML1, the target of multiple chromosomal translocations in human leukemia, is essential for normal fetal liver hematopoiesis. *Cell* **84:** 321–330.

Okuda T., Cai Z., Yang S., Lenny N., Lyu C.J., van Deursen J.M., Harada H., and Downing J.R. 1998. Expression of a knocked-in AML1-ETO leukemia gene inhibits the establishment of normal definitive hematopoiesis and directly generates dysplastic hematopoietic progenitors. *Blood* **91:** 3134–3143.

Orkin S.H. 1992. GATA-binding transcription factors in hematopoietic cells. *Blood* **80:** 575–581.

Osawa M., Hanada K., Hamada H., and Nakauchi H. 1996. Long-term lymphohematopoietic reconstitution by a single CD34-low/negative hematopoietic stem cell. *Science* **273:** 242–245.

Pardanaud L. and Dieterlen-Lievre F. 1999. Manipulation of the angiopoietic/hemangiopoietic commitment in the avian embryo. *Development* **126:** 617–627.

Pardanaud L., Yassine F., and Dieterlen-Lievre F. 1989. Relationship between vasculogenesis, angiogenesis, and haemopoiesis during avian ontogeny. *Development* **105:** 473–485.

Porcher C., Liao E.C., Fujiwara Y., Zon L.I., and Orkin S.H. 1999. Specification of hematopoietic and vascular development by the bHLH transcription factor SCL without direct DNA binding. *Development* **126:** 4603–4615.

Porcher C., Swat W., Rockwell K., Fujiwara Y., Alt F. W., and Orkin S.H. 1996. The T-cell leukemia oncoprotein SCL/tal-1 is essential for development of all hematopoietic lineages. *Cell* **86:** 47–57.

Querfurth E., Schuster M., Kulessa H., Crispino J.D., Doderlein G., Orkun S.H., Graf T., and Nerlov C. 2000. Antagonism between C/EBPb and FOG in eosinophil lineage commitment of multipotent hematopoietic progenitors. *Genes Dev.* **14:** 2515–2525.

Rekhtman N., Radparvar F., Evans T., and Skoultchi A.I. 1999. Direction interaction of hematopoietic transcription factors PU.1 and GATA-1: Functional antagonism in erythroid cells. *Genes Dev.* **13:** 1398–1411.

Robb L., Elwood N.J., Elefanty A.G., Kontgen F., Li R., Barnett L.D., and Begley C.G. 1996. The scl gene product is required for the generation of all hematopoietic lineages in the adult mouse. *EMBO J.* **15:** 4123–4129.

Rolink A.G., Nutt S.L., Melchers F., and Busslinger M. 1999. Long-term in vivo reconstitution of T-cell development by Pax5- deficient B-cell progenitors (see comments). *Nature* **401:** 603–606.

Sato T., Laver J.H., and Ogawa M. 1999. Reversible expression of CD34 by murine hematopoietic stem cells. *Blood* **94:** 2548–2554.

Scott E.W., Simon M.C., Anastasi J., and Singh H. 1994. Requirement of transcription factor PU.1 in the development of multiple hematopoietic lineages. *Science* **265:** 1573–1577.

Scott E.W., Fisher R.C., Olson M.C., Kehrli E.W., Simon M.C., and Singh H. 1997. PU.1 functions in a cell-autonomous manner to control the differentiation of multipotential lymphoid-myeloid progenitors. *Immunity* **6:** 437–447.

Shivadasani R.A., Fujiwara Y., McDevitt M.A., and Orkin S.H. 1997. A lineage-selective knockout establishes the critical role of transcription factor GATA-1 in megakaryocyte growth and platelet development. *EMBO J.* **16:** 3965–3973.

Socolovsky M., Lodish H.F., and Daley G.Q. 1998. Control of hematopoietic differentiation: Lack of specificity in signaling by cytokine receptors. *Proc. Natl. Acad. Sci.* **95:** 6573–6575.

Stoffel R., Ziegler S., Ghilardi N., Ledermann B., de Sauvage F.J., and Skoda R.C. 1999. Permissive role of thrombopoietin and granulocyte colony-stimulating factor receptors in hematopoietic cell fate decisions in vivo. *Proc. Natl. Acad. Sci.* **96:** 698–702.

Tavian M., Coulombel L., Luton D., Clemente H.S., Dieterlen-Lievre F., and Peault B. 1996. Aorta-associated CD34$^+$ hematopoietic cells in the early human embryo. *Blood* **87:** 67–72.

Tsai F.-Y., Keller G., Kuo F.C., Weiss M.J., Chen J.-Z., Rosenblatt M., Alt F., and Orkin S.H. 1994. An early haematopoietic defect in mice lacking the transcription factor GATA-2. *Nature* **371:** 221–226.

Tsang A.C., Visvader J.E., Turner C.A., Fujiwara Y., Yu C., Weiss M.J., Crossley M., and Orkin S.H. 1997. FOG, a multitype zinc finger protein, acts as a cofactor for transcription factor GATA-1 in erythroid and megakaryocytic differentiation. *Cell* **90:** 109–119.

Tsang A.P., Fujiwara Y., Hom D.B., and Orkin S.H. 1998. Failure of megakaryopoiesis and arrested erythropoiesis in mice lacking the GATA-1 transcriptional cofactor FOG. *Genes Dev.* **12:** 1176–1188.

Urbanek P., Wang Z.-Q., Fetka I., Wagner E.R., and Busslinger M. 1994. Complete block of early B cell differentiation and altered patterning of the posterior midbrain in mice lacking Pax5/BSAP. *Cell* **79:** 901–912.

Visvader J. and Adams J.M. 1993. Megakaryocytic differentiation induced in 416B myeloid cells by GATA-2 and GATA-3 transgenes or 5-azacytidine is tightly coupled to GATA-1 expression. *Blood* **82:** 1493–1501.

Visvader J.E., Fujiwara Y., and Orkin S.H. 1998. Unsuspected role for the T-cell leukemia protein SCL/tal-1 in vascular development. *Genes Dev.* **12:** 473–479.

Visvader J.E., Elefanty A.G., Strasser A., and Adams J.M. 1992. GATA-1 but not SCL induces megakaryocytic differentiation in an early myeloid line. *EMBO J.* **11:** 4557–4564.

Visvader J.E., Crossley M., Hill J., Orkin S.H., and Adams J.M. 1995. The C-terminal zinc finger of GATA-1 or GATA-2 is sufficient to induce megakaryocytic differentiation of an early myeloid cell line. *Mol. Cell. Biol.* **15:** 634–641.

Vyas P., McDevitt M.A., Cantor A.B., Katz S., Fujiwara Y., and Orkin S.H. 1999. Different sequence requirements for expression in erythroid and megakaryocytic cells within a regulatory element upstream of the GATA-1 gene. *Development* **126:** 2799–2811.

Wadman I.S., Osada H., Grutz G.G., Agulnick A.D., Westphal H., Forster A., and Rabbitts T.H. 1997. The LIM-only protein Lmo2 is a bridging molecule assembling an erythroid, DNA-binding complex which include TAL1, E47, GATA-1, and Ldb1/NL1 proteins. *EMBO J.* **16:** 3145–3157.

Wang Q., Stacy T., Binder M., Marin-Padilla M., Sharpe A.H., and Speck N.A. 1996. Disruption of the *Cbfa2* gene causes necrosis and hemorrhaging in the central nervous system and blocks definitive hematopoiesis. *Proc. Natl. Acad. Sci.* **93:** 3444–3449.

Weintraub H., Davis R., Tapscott S., Thayer M., Krause M., Benezra R., Blackwell T.K., Turner D., Rupp R., Hollenberg S., Zhuang Y., and Lassar A. 1991. The myoD gene family: Nodal point during specification of the muscle cell lineage. *Science* **251:** 761–766.

Weiss M.J., Keller G., and Orkin S.H. 1994. Novel insights into erythroid development revealed through *in vitro* differentiation of GATA-1- embryonic stem cells. *Genes Dev.* **8:** 1184–1197.

Weiss M.J., Yu C., and Orkin S.H. 1997. Erythroid-cell-specific properties of transcription factor GATA-1 revealed by phenotypic rescue of a gene-targeted cell line. *Mol. Cell. Biol.* **17:** 1642–1651.

Weissman I.L. 2000. Translating stem and progenitor cell biology to the clinic: Barriers and opportunities. *Science* **287:** 1442–1446.

Yamada Y., Pannell R., Forster A., and Rabbitts T.H. 2000. The oncogenic LIM-only transcription factor Lmo2 regulates angiogenesis but not vasculogenesis in mice. *Proc. Natl. Acad. Sci.* **97:** 320–324.

Yamada Y., Warren A.J., Dobson C., Forster A., Pannell R., and Rabbitts T.H. 1998. The T cell leukemia LIM protein Lmo2 is necessary for adult mouse hematopoiesis. *Proc. Natl. Acad. Sci.* **95:** 3890–3895.

Yoder M.C. and Hiatt K. 1999. Murine yolk sac and bone marrow hematopoietic cells with high proliferative potential display different capacities for producing colony-forming cells ex vivo. *J. Hematother. Stem Cell Res.* **8:** 421–430.

Yoder M.C., Hiatt K., Dutt P., Mukherjee P., Bodine D.M., and Orlic D. 1997. Characterization of definitive lymphohematopoietic stem cells in the day 9 murine yolk sac. *Immunity* **7:** 335–344.

Zhang D.E., Hetherington C.J., Meyers S., Rhoades K.L., Larson C.J., Chen H.M., Hiebert, S.W., and Tenen D.G. 1996. CCAAT enhancer-binding protein (C/EBP) and AML1 (CBFα2) synergistically activate the macrophage colony-stimulating factor receptor promoter. *Mol. Cell. Biol.* **16:** 1231–1240.

Zhang P., Behre G., Pan J., Iwama A., Wara-Aswapati N., Radomska H.S., Auron P.E., Tenen D.G., and Sun Z. 1999. Negative cross-talk between hematopoietic regulators: GATA proteins repress PU.1. *Proc. Natl. Acad. Sci.* **96:** 8705–8710.

Zhang P., Zhang X., Iwama A., Yu C., Smith K.A., Muella B., Narravula S., Torbett B.E., Orkin S.H., and Tenen D.G. 2000. PU.1 inhibits GATA-1 function and erythroid differentiation by blockingGATA-1 DNA-binding. *Blood* (in press).

14

Hematopoietic Stem Cells: Lymphopoiesis and the Problem of Commitment Versus Plasticity

Fritz Melchers and Antonius Rolink
Basel Institute for Immunology
Basel, Switzerland

B lymphocytes, T lymphocytes, and natural killer (NK) cells (cells of the lymphoid lineages) and erythrocytes, megakaryocytes, platelets, granulocytes, monocytes, macrophages, osteoclasts, and dendritic cells (cells of the erythroid/myeloid lineages) are all descendants of a pluripotent hematopoietic stem cell (pHSC) (for recent reviews, see Fuchs and Segre 2000 and Weissman 2000). In fact, transplantation of a single pHSC can reconstitute a lethally irradiated host with all these lineages of cells. The differentiated cells of the erythroid/myeloid and lymphoid lineages, with the exception of memory B and T cells, turn over rapidly, with half-lives between days and weeks. Therefore, in order to maintain the pools of hematopoietic cells in an individual, these cells have to be continuously generated throughout life by cell division and differentiation from stem cells.

The cells of the adaptive immune system, B and T lymphocytes, rearrange V, D, and J segments during their development to form functional IgH and L-chain genes in B cells, and TCR α, β, γ, and δ genes in T cells (Tonegawa 1983). Through positive and negative selection of the original antigen-recognizing repertoires in the primary lymphoid organs, for B cells in the bone marrow, for T cells in the thymus, the repertoires are shaped by selective processes. The selected repertoires of lymphocytes become available for recognition of foreign antigens in the secondary lymphoid organs of the peripheral immune system. These processes of repertoire selection must continue to operate throughout life, as lymphocytes continue to be generated from pHSC and from progenitors through continuous V(D)J rearrangements of, respectively, the Ig and TCR gene loci, and by cellular differentiation.

Hematopoietic stem cells can be defined by at least four properties: Self-renewal, multipotency, long-term reconstitution capacity, and secondary transplantability. These properties are discussed below.

SELF-RENEWAL

Upon division of a stem cell, at least one daughter cell retains the state of this stem cell. This capacity is called self-renewal. Symmetric divisions expand the number of HSCs, whereas asymmetric divisions retain HSC potential in one daughter cell, generating further differentiated progeny in the other daughter cell. Divisions that generate two differentiated progeny daughter cells delete the HSC potential. At different times of ontogeny and in different environments, the probability of an HSC dividing either symmetrically, asymmetrically, or fully differentiating may well vary (for further discussion, see Morrison et al. 1997). It has been a matter of much debate whether the environment, recognized by the HSC through cell contacts and via cytokines and chemokines and their receptors, does influence the type of division and the potential of differentiation of the HSC (Metcalf 1991; Mayani et al. 1993; Fuchs and Segre 2000; Weissman 2000).

Clonal succession models (Kay 1965) have proposed that HSCs, once generated during embryogenesis, remain resting cells throughout life until they are called upon to enter hematopoiesis. When the progeny of the original HSC has been used up by turnover, a new HSC from the remaining pool is recruited (Lemischka et al. 1986). This model predicts that HSC potential is limited and can be used up by complete recruitment. On the other hand, models of random symmetric HSC division have been proposed that would not only provide HSCs, but also preserve them. In these models, HSCs could never be completely used up by recruitment into hematopoietic differentiation. In favor of this type of model, it has been observed that 10% of all HSCs divide symmetrically every day, so that within 1–3 months, all HSCs are called into the cell cycle at least once (Bradford et al. 1997; Cheshier et al. 1999). However, within the total population of HSCs, only the resting cells provide long-term repopulation potential (see below) (Spangrude and Johnson 1990; Fleming et al. 1993). Therefore, the cycling HSCs could be those that are about to be used up for hematopoietic differentiation. In any case, bone marrow transplantation of aged donors into young or aged recipients shows that HSC potential remains intact for most, if not all, of the life of a mouse (Rolink et al. 1993).

MULTIPOTENCY

In asymmetric or fully differentiating divisions of a single HSC, the differentiated daughter cell(s) can develop among different lineage pathways in distinct cellular steps. Their choices include erythrocytes, megakaryocytes and platelets, granulocytes, monocytes and macrophages, osteoclasts and dendritic cells, NK cells, thymocytes, T cells, and B cells. When a single HSC can give rise to all these lineages of blood cells, it is called a pluripotent HSC (pHSC). Stem cells with self-renewal capacity but with more limited potencies for hematopoietic differentiation are usually called progenitors, e.g., common lymphoid progenitor (CLP) for stem cells with B, T, and NK-lymphoid differentiation capacities; common myeloid progenitor (CMP) for stem cells with granulocyte, monocyte, macrophage, osteoclast, and dendritic cell potential; megakaryocyte and erythrocyte progenitor (MEP); and granulocyte and macrophage progenitor (GMP). Even more differentiated stages of these different lineages may have stem cell properties.

RECONSTITUTION POTENTIAL

Upon transplantation into a suitably receptive host, stem cells can home to their proper sites in the body—unless already implanted at the proper site—and establish differentiation along all or parts of the hematopoietic lineages. Reconstitution can be short term, generating differentiated cells in a wave of developmental steps in which the progenitors vanish as the more differentiated cells develop. The differentiated cells generated in such a wave will usually disappear by normal turnover from the host. Whenever the host compartments are properly filled, turnover will be of the order of days or weeks. In lymphoid development this may be different, especially when empty compartments (such as in the RAG- or SCID severe combined immunodeficient mice) are to be filled with donor cells. This may be a consequence of a different homeostasis, or because these donor lymphocytes become long-lived memory cells due to exposure to foreign antigens (Sprent et al. 1991; Neuberger 1997). The cycling pHSCs (Fig. 1A) and most of the progenitors with more limited hematopoietic potentials, i.e., the CMP, CLP, MEP, GMP, proT, and preB-I cells, all exhibit only this short-term reconstitution potential.

The exception is the progeny of preB-I cells, i.e., some of the mature B cells that develop from them in vivo. PreB-I cells from wild-type mice have short-term reconstitution potential, because they appear not to be

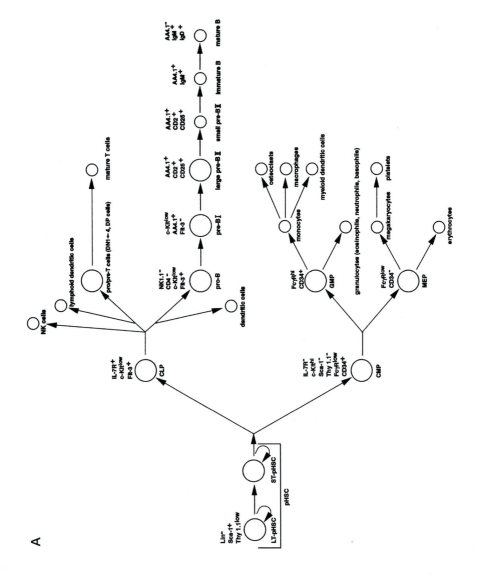

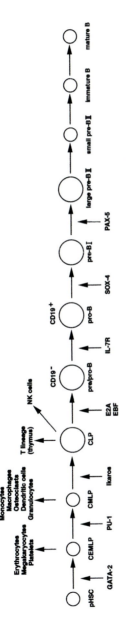

Figure 1 Hierarchies of hematopoietic cell development: (*A*) This scheme is derived from clonal progeny analyses in vitro and in vivo, after transplantation by scoring the development of differentiated progeny cells. Purification of clonable progenitors was done for long-term (LT) repopulating and short-term (ST) repopulating hematopoietic stem cells (HSC) by FACS using the markers shown with the progenitor cell. LT-pHSC are resting, ST-pHSC proliferating, cells (Morrison and Weissman 1994; Morrison et al. 1997). pHSC give rise to all lineages of hematopoiesis shown in the figure when transplanted into lethally irradiated, radioprotected hosts. Only from LT-pHSC, but not from ST-pHSC-transplantation, pHSC can be recovered from the recipient. A clonogenic progenitor for all myeloid and erythroid/megakaryocyte cells (CMP) was isolated (Akashi et al. 2000) by FACS using the markers indicated on the progenitor. The differential expression of FcγR and CD34 allowed them to subdivide to two more committed progenitors, one for megakaryocyte and erythrocyte development (MEP), the other for megakaryocyte and erythrocyte development (MEP), all assayed primarily by in vitro colony assays. Kondo et al. (1997) have defined a common lymphoid progenitor (CLP), essentially by the same techniques used for FACS and colony assays. (*B*) This scheme is derived from in vivo analyses of mutant mouse strains, defective in the genes shown in the figure. The arrows indicate the transitions from one to the next cell stage, at which a given mutant mouse strain appears to be blocked for further development, and which cell lineages remain to be made (for details see the text). Large cells (O) in the figure indicate that they are in the cell cycle, while small cells (o) show that they are resting. The expression pattern of AA4.1 in the different progenitor and precursor cells has recently been elucidated (Rolink et al. 1998). Only LT-pHSC have long-term, repopulating potential; all others, i.e., ST-pHSC, CLP, CMP, GMP, MEP, and their further differentiated progeny, only yield waves of hematopoietic development. Exceptions, as mentioned in the text, are B1-B cells and memory T and B cells.

able to home to their proper sites in the bone marrow, and because they develop in a wave of differentiation first to preB-II, then to immature, and finally to mature B cells. However, some of the mature B cells generated in this developmental wave acquire long-term reconstitution potential as individually V(D)J-rearranged clones of sIgM$^+$ B cells, particularly when these B cells are selected into the B1 lineage (Kantor et al. 1995). They not only become long-lived, but also gain long-term reconstitution potential, which is apparent when such B1 cells are transplanted into a secondary host, where they again fill the B1 compartment. These B1 cells can be considered to be V(D)J-rearranged, B-lymphocyte-committed, and B-lineage-restricted "stem" cells that, upon symmetric divisions, generate daughter cells with the same properties. It is suspected that their longevity and continuously activated cell cycle status are a consequence of chronic exposure to autoantigens and/or to cross-reactive foreign antigens from infectious agents (for review, see Potter and Melchers 2000).

Clones of IgG-producing B cells, i.e., derived by T-cell-dependent stimulation, which may be from conventional B cells, have also been seen to have long-term reconstitution potential. Again, this potential may be dependent on the presence of a stimulating antigen (Askonas and Williamson 1972; Manz et al. 1997; Slifka et al. 1998).

The only known long-term reconstituting early hematopoietic cell is the resting pHSC. The resting population of pHSCs (Fig. 1A) home to their proper sites, e.g., in the bone marrow, stably populate them in normal numbers, and continuously generate cell lineages of hematopoietic cell development. Successful migration and seeding into the proper niches of pHSCs depends on an intact environment of reticular cells, stromal cells, and vascular endothelium. It is likely that this environment develops only in interactions with the hematopoietic progenitors, as it has been seen in the development of the thymus (van Ewijk et al. 1994; Boehm et al. 1995; Holländer et al. 1995). Further development of the transplanted pHSCs to cells that fill the compartments of the different committed lineages of hematopoiesis can also be aided when these further differentiated compartments are missing as a consequence of mutation arresting that development in the transplanted host. As one example, defects in the V(D)J rearrangement machinery, such as the RAG$^{-/-}$ and SCID severe combined immunodeficiencies, arrest B- and T-lymphocyte development at the preT- and preB-cell stages (Fig. 1). Drug treatment or high-dose irradiation destroys the preT and preB cells and their progenitors, allowing the seeding of donor pHSCs and their progeny so that the T- and B-lymphoid compartments are filled with donor lymphocytes. Similarly, hosts that are defective in the gene encoding the common γ chain of the IL2/IL7-receptor lack NK cells and therefore support some in vivo cell development from donor pHSCs and their progeny (DiSanto et al. 1995). Furthermore, c-fos-deficient mice, lacking osteoclast development, are suitable recipients to develop these osteoclasts from transplanted donor cells (Wang et al. 1992; Grigoriadis et al. 1994).

pHSCs and their progenitors may also possess different properties to reconstitute different hematopoietic lineages, dependent on a genetic makeup of the donor that is currently being analyzed (Müller-Sieburg and Riblet 1996; de Haan and Van Zant 1997). This strength is measured by producing mixed chimeras from graded numbers of progenitors from two genetically different hosts, which are transplanted together. Transgenic expression of bcl-2 increases both the numbers of pHSCs and their repopulation potential (Domen et al. 2000), whereas mice homozygous for an Ikaros-transcription factor null-mutation have a 30-fold reduced number of LT-pHSC units. The generalized defect in all hematopoietic lineages appears to be, in part, compensated by unknown genetic factors in the erythroid/megakaryocytic cell lineage. A reduced expression of the tyrosine kinases c-kit and flt-3 on early progenitors (Fig. 1A) may account for some of the hematopoietic defects in this Ikaros null-mutant mouse strain (Nichogiannopoulou et al. 1999).

The capacity of pHSCs to home to the right environment is one of the essential prerequisites for successful reconstitution of the transplanted host. This migratory capacity of pHSC is first played out during embryogenesis. The earliest site of pHSC generation is the splanchnopleura of the aorta-gonad-mesonephros (AGM) region, and its anterior part in the mouse embryo between day 8 and 9 of gestation, when embryonic blood circulation is established (Cumano et al. 1995; Cumano et al. 1996; Godin et al. 1995; Medvinsky and Dzierzak 1996). pHSCs are expected to migrate from the AGM region first to sites where primitive hematopoiesis takes place, e.g., in the yolk sac. Later, they must arrive at sites of definite hematopoiesis, and of myeloid and lymphoid cell development, e.g., in the fetal liver, omentum, bone marrow, and, subsequently, in the thymus (for review, see Melchers and Rolink 1999). Molecules involved in adhesion, e.g., β1-integrin (Potocnik 2000), or chemoattraction, e.g., the chemokine SDF-1 and its receptor (for references, see Ma et al. 1999), might be involved in the direction of pHSC traffic. It might well be that pHSCs of adults still use the same molecular modes to migrate to their proper niches, e.g., in bone marrow, and it is certain that most of these molecular modes of pHSC traffic still need to be discovered.

SECONDARY AND SUBSEQUENT RECONSTITUTION POTENTIAL

When a pHSC has populated the proper sites in the transplanted host, it should, in principle, be transplantable again in a secondary host, and thereafter even in subsequent hosts. In practice, however, the efficiency of secondary pHSC transplantation has been found to drop substantially (Spangrude et al. 1995).

Two factors may contribute to such losses of reconstitution potential: loss of environmental contact and/or loss of telomeres. When removed from their normal environment of stromal cells, epithelial cells and vascular endothelium pHSC could well enter differentiation and thereby lose reconstitution potential, because they are no longer exposed to the proper cell-to-cell contacts and no longer receive stimuli from the right cytokines and chemokines to keep them in the state of a pHSC. This might easily happen while pHSC are isolated from the tissue, are transplanted, and have to migrate until they reach the proper site. In addition, a larger number of cell divisions (symmetric or asymmetric) may result in telomere shortening, whenever telomerase activity is decreased or absent (Allsopp et al. 1992, 1995; Vaziri et al. 1994; Hiyama et al. 1995; Lee et al. 1998; Hodes 1999).

In fact, pHSCs can be separated into two subpopulations, one with high (LT-pHSC), the other with low (ST-pHSC) long-term reconstitution potential (Bradford et al. 1997; Cheshier et al. 1999). LT-pHSCs have been found to have as much telomerase activity as cancer cells do, while ST-pHSCs have less, suggesting that telomeres in pHSCs are kept at a constant, unshortened length when they enter cell cycle only occasionally and are usually resting. They lose their telomeres when they continue to proliferate (Broccoli et al. 1995; Morrison et al. 1996). Human pHSCs shorten their telomere lengths with age (Vaziri et al. 1994), and telomere length in mouse pHSCs still needs to be measured. It is conceivable that parts of the signals given to pHSCs by their proper environment keep telomerase activity up-regulated.

MODELS OF HEMATOPOIESIS

Models of the hierarchies of hematopoeitic differentiation pathways have been proposed either on the basis of cellular development from progenitors to differentiated, mature cells observed in in vitro cultures and colony assays, and in in vivo transplantation experiments, or on the basis of developmental arrests in hematopoiesis introduced by targeted disruption of a series of genes mostly encoding transcription factors.

With the help of characteristic marker genes expressed in specific combinations in and on pHSCs, progenitors, and mature cells of the different lineages, the branched development pictured in Figure 1A has been developed. In principle, this hierarchy has been deduced from in vitro cultures and colony assays, and from in vivo transplantation experiments, in which a given progenitor was isolated by cell sorting with the help of fluorescent-labeled monoclonal antibodies detecting a characteristic combination of surface markers. Either the purified cell populations were then mass-cultured, or colonies were grown from single cells transplanted into appropriately receptive hosts as genetically distinct donor cells. The differentiated progeny were thereafter analyzed and detectable in the transplanted host with their genetically determined markers (for a review of experiments supporting this scheme, see Weissman 2000).

Targeted disruption of genes encoding the transcription factors GATA-2 (Tsai et al. 1994), Spi-1 encoding PU.1 (McKercher et al. 1996; Singh 1996; Tondravi et al. 1997), Ikaros (Georgopoulos et al. 1994), E2A encoding E12 and E47 (Bain et al. 1994, 1997; Zhuang et al. 1994; Choi et al. 1996; O'Riordan and Grosschedl 1999), EBF (Lin and Grosschedl 1995), SOX-4 (van de Wetering et al. 1993; Schilham et al. 1996), PAX-5 (Urbanek et al. 1994), and the IL-7 receptor α chain (IL7Rα, Peschon et al. 1994) were found to arrest hematopoiesis at the points indicated in Figure 1B, resulting in a complete arrest of all lineages of hematopoiesis (GATA-2), allowing only erythropoiesis and megakaryocyte/platelet formation (PU.1), allowing erythroid and myeloid, but not lymphoid development (Ikaros), blocking B-cell development before $D_H J_H$-rearrangements and expression of sterile transcripts of the μH-chain gene (E2A, EBF), blocking B-cell development at the CD19$^-$ partially $D_H J_H$-rearranged stage (IL-7R), arresting B-cell development before the preB-I cell stage (SOX-4), or blocking the development of $V_H D_H J_H$-rearranged large preB-II cells from preB-I cells (PAX-5) (Nutt et al. 1997; for review, see Melchers and Rolink 1999). These experiments have suggested a linear developmental model of hematopoiesis (Fig. 1B) (Singh 1996).

One major difference in the two models outlined in Figure 1A and B is the way by which B and T lymphocytes are generated from pHSCs. This becomes an issue if a hematopoietic cell of a given lineage could not only proceed along a given pathway in one direction of differentiation, but could also reverse its track and dedifferentiate from one type of committed cell, e.g., a precursor B cell, back to an earlier progenitor, and then assume redifferentiation along another lineage of hematopoiesis. If the same pathways were used in both directions, a precursor B cell would have to dedifferentiate as far back as a pHSC in model 1 (Fig. 1A) before it could redifferentiate to a myeloid cell. In contrast, in model 2 (Fig. 1B), dedifferentiation to only the common myeloid/lymphoid progenitor would suffice.

Both models of hematopoiesis are supported by limited experimental evidence. Against model 1 it can always be argued that the proper physiological conditions of in vivo hematopoietic differentiation of progenitors and precursors are not met in vitro because certain cytokines, chemokines, or cell contacts and their proper dosage and application with time of differentiation are missing or wrong for a given lineage to develop. Even in vivo differentiation after progenitor transplantation may be limited by the inability of a given progenitor to find its right environment, either because it cannot home to that site, or because the site has not developed properly.

Different mutant forms of the same transcription factor can elicit quite different phenotypes of hematopoietic defects. Examples are the two types of mutants that have been generated for the PU.1 encoding SPI-1 gene, and the Ikaros gene (Molnar and Georgopoulos 1994). In both cases either the whole gene, or only the DNA-binding domain of it, have been deleted in the germ line of mice. Deleting only the DNA-binding domain generates in both cases dominant-negative forms that block hematopoietic differentiation as severely as shown in Figure 1B. With age, some thymocytes develop in both the PU.1 and the Ikaros mutated mice. This suggests that very rare successes to overcome these developmental blocks are most strongly used for T-cell development.

In contrast, in PU.1$^{-/-}$ mice only the formation of macrophages and osteoclasts is inhibited (Tondravi et al. 1997). Ikaros$^{-/-}$ mice are defective in fetal B- and T-cell development, and in adult B cell development. They also lack a large proportion of the NK cells, some subsets of γ/δ TCR T cells, and thymic dendritic cells. However, postnatally CD4$^+$ T cells appear to expand in almost normal numbers (Wang et al. 1996).

These results suggest that it is easier to complement a given transcription factor in a complex of factors which regulates the expression of key target genes involved in the commitment to different hematopoietic lineages when that factor is absent, than in a complex that still contains the factor, capable of interactions within the complex, but not with DNA. If the target genes of the mutated transcription factor include those that control homing and/or attachment to the proper environment, then the observed mutant phenotypes are no more informative for the hierarchies of hematopoiesis than the in vitro and in vivo assays with progenitors.

DIFFERENTIATION, DEDIFFERENTIATION, AND REDIFFERENTIATION OF HEMATOPOIETIC CELLS: PLASTICITY VERSUS DIRECTIONAL COMMITMENT

In normal hematopoiesis, cells proceed most probably in unidirectional steps through sequential stages that commit these cells to a given differentiated type of lineage. At the same time, they become more and more restricted to that chosen lineage, with fewer and fewer options to enter other lineages. These pathways of increasing commitments are experimentally observed either by in vitro or in vivo assays of cell development without detectable dedifferentiation or redifferentiation into other pathways (Fig. 1). As cells become committed, even the exposure to different environmental influences, such as cell-to-cell contacts, cytokines and chemokines, at best only stops further development but usually does not lead to redifferentiation. One example of such commitment, studied in detail in our laboratory, is the commitment of early progenitors to B-lineage lymphocytes (for review, see Melchers and Rolink 1999).

The earliest cell with B-lineage potential is a $B220^+$, $CD19^-$, $AA4.1^+$, $ckit^{low}$, $flt-3^+$, surrogate light (SL) chain progenitor that develops with high clonal proliferative capacity in vitro on stromal cells in the presence of interleukin-7 (IL-7) to preB-I cells (Ogawa et al. 2000). Both the ligands for ckit and for flt-3 are involved in the stimulation of this development as they, together with IL-7, are provided by the stromal cells of this hematopoietic environment.

These progenitors develop via a SL-chain$^+$ $CD19^-$ intermediate to $B220^+$, $CD19^+$, $AA4.1^+$, $ckit^{low}$, $flt-3^-$ SL chain$^+$, $CD43^+$ preB-I cell. During this cellular development both Ig heavy (H)-chain alleles become $D_H J_H$-rearranged, so that every preB-I cell has a characteristic set of individually $D_H J_H$-rearranged H-chain alleles. As preB-I cells, they retain the capacity to proliferate extensively on stromal cells in the presence of IL-7 so that the individual $D_H J_H$-rearranged alleles become clonal markers of the progeny of this proliferative expansion (Rolink et al. 1991). As long as IL-7 is present, preB-I cells will not differentiate further along the B-lineage pathway. Removal of IL-7 induces V_H to $D_H J_H$ rearrangements on the H-chain locus, and V_L to J_L rearrangements. Whenever both IgH and IgL chain loci have been rearranged productively, $sIgM^+$ immature B cells are formed. They are then selected negatively as well as positively to generate the peripheral, mature B-cell pools reactive to foreign antigens.

The cellular stages of this stepwise repertoire development of B cells can be distinguished by the expression of characteristic surface markers.

PreB-cell-receptor-expressing, i.e., $V_H D_H J_H$-rearranged μH chain$^+$/SL chain$^+$ proliferating preB-II cells, are ckit$^-$CD25$^+$AA4.1$^+$, while immature sIgM$^+$ B cells lose CD25 expression, and AA4.1 expression is lost as immature B cells become sIgM$^+$/sIgD$^+$ mature B cells (Rolink et al. 1998, 1999; Melchers and Rolink 1999).

Progenitor B and preB-I cells from wild-type mice have a strong unidirectional tendency to develop along this pathway of differentiation to B cells. Thus, either induced in vitro, first on stromal cells and IL-7, subsequently by the removal of IL-7, or by transplantation into lymphocyte-deficient RAG$^{-/-}$ or SCID hosts in vivo, only B-lineage cells, but no T cells nor myeloid cells, can be seen to develop from these pro and preB-I cells. Culturing preB-I cells in the absence of IL-7, and in the presence of cytokines capable of inducing myeloid cell differentiation, does not induce such myeloid differentiation.

COMMITMENT TO B LYMPHOPOIESIS

Transcription factors appear to control the commitment of progenitors along different lineages. Three such factors have been identified for the commitment to the B-lymphocyte lineage (E2A, EBF, PAX-5). Targeted disruption of either the E2A or the EBF gene results in an arrest of B lymphopoiesis at the stage shown in Figure 1B. E2A$^{-/-}$ and EBF$^{-/-}$ mutant mice show an arrest before any rearrangements of either IgH or IgL chain gene segments are initiated (Zhuang et al. 1994; Lin and Grosschedl 1995). Target genes controlled by E2A and EBF are RAG1 and RAG2, Igα and Igβ, VpreB and λ5, as well as the intron enhancer of the μH chain locus (Eμ) controlling sterile transcription of the μH chain locus (for review, see Busslinger et al. 2000). Transgenic expression of E2A-encoded E47 activates some of these target genes even in fibroblasts (Choi et al. 1996). E2A and EBF also appear to control the expression of PAX-5 (O'Riordan and Grosschedl 1999).

PAX-5$^{-/-}$ mutant mice are arrested at a later stage of B-lineage development, i.e., at a preB-I-like state, in which the cells have $D_H J_H$ rearranged both IgH chain alleles, but continue to express earlier markers, such as the flt-3 receptor tyrosine kinase. Hence, it may well be that their cellular arrest is at the earlier, proB-cell stage (Fig. 1) but that D_H to J_H rearrangements continue in these PAX-5$^{-/-}$ cells. PAX-5$^{-/-}$ preB-I cells, like wild-type pro- and preB-I cells, proliferate for long periods of time on stromal cells in the presence of IL-7, and can be cloned as individually $D_H J_H$-rearranged cell clones. PAX-5$^{-/-}$ mice are blocked in B-cell development at the transition of $D_H J_H$-rearranged preB-I to $V_H D_H J_H$-

rearranged large preB-II cells (Urbanek et al 1994; Nutt et al. 1999a). Hence, whereas withdrawal of IL-7 from wild-type preB-I cell cultures results in the development of sIgM$^+$ immature and mature B cells (Rolink et al. 1991), this development is blocked for PAX-5$^{-/-}$ preB-I cells. PAX-5 is expressed monoallelically from the earliest proB cell to the stage of an immature B cell, where it changes to biallelic expression (Nutt et al. 1999b). PAX-5$^{-/-}$ preB-I cells express almost all of the proB-cell-specific genes (with the exception of CD19). Several genes expressed in other myeloid or lymphoid lineage cells are also expressed in PAX-5$^{-/-}$ preB-I cells, although some at very low levels, such as preTα (lymphoid-related), perforin (NK-cell-related), myeloperoxidase and M-GSF receptor (myeloid-related). It has been suggested that PAX-5 not only positively controls B-lineage development but, at the same time, represses myeloid and T-lymphoid lineage development (Busslinger et al. 2000). PAX-5 could, in fact, act like a traffic sign. When it is on, traffic of hematopoiesis will proceed along the B-lineage way; when it is off, traffic is routed into the myeloid and T-lymphoid directions.

PLASTICITY OF PAX-5$^{-/-}$ PREB-I CELLS

It had previously been observed that preB-I cells from the fetal liver of wild-type mice could be grown on stromal cells in the presence of IL-7 for more than 60 divisions without losing their capacity to develop to sIgM$^+$ B cells in vitro and in vivo. In contrast, wild-type preB-I cells from bone marrow tend to cease to proliferate after 4–6 weeks; i.e., after 30–50 divisions. Bone-marrow-derived preB-I cells of PAX-5$^{-/-}$ mice appear to proliferate as well as wild-type cells from fetal liver. Clones of these cells have now been expanded for at least 100 divisions; hence, one PAX-5$^{-/-}$ preB-I cell can, in principle, be expanded to 10^{30} cells.

It was a surprise to discover that PAX-5$^{-/-}$ preB-I cells, in fact, possess stem cell-like properties. Not only are they self-renewing (for up to 100 divisions), they are also pluripotent (with the exception that B-cell development is blocked, and that erythroid and megakaryocyte development has so far not been observed) (Nutt et al. 1999a,b; Rolink et al. 1999a,b), and they home back to the bone marrow, from where they can be reisolated as preB-I cells. Therefore, they have long-term reconstituting capacity (Rolink et al. 1999a,b).

The pluripotency of PAX-5$^{-/-}$ preB-I cells is documented in the following experiments. Clones of these cells develop into macrophages when IL-7 is removed and M-CSF is added to in vitro cultures. Removal of IL-7, followed by exposure to IL-3/IL-6 and SCF first and G-CSF later, develops granulocytes. Exposure of the IL-7-deprived cells to M-CSF and GM-CSF generates antigen-representing dendritic cells, exposure to IL-2 generates NK cells, and cultures on stromal cells expressing TRANCE lead to osteoclast development (Nutt et al. 1999a,b). The last two lineages of hematopoiesis can also be induced in vivo by transplanting PAX-5$^{-/-}$ preB-I cells into mice that are deficient in the common γ chain of the IL-2/IL-7-receptor (γc$^{-/-}$) and into c-fos-deficient mice, respectively. In the γc$^{-/-}$-deficient mice, endogenous NK-cell development is defective. It is replenished by NK cells derived from the PAX-5$^{-/-}$ preB-I cells, and the same PAX-5$^{-/-}$ preB-I cells become the source of osteoclast generation in the osteoclast-deficient c-fos$^{-/-}$ mice.

Equally impressive is the complete reconstitution of T-cell development in lymphocyte-deficient RAG$^{-/-}$ hosts by the transplantation of as little as 5×10^4 ex vivo isolated, or 5×10^6 in vitro grown, PAX-5$^{-/-}$ preB-I cells (Rolink et al. 1999a,b). All stages of thymocyte development in the recipient thymus, i.e., double-negative (DN) stage 1–4, double-positive and single-positive thymocytes, as well as peripheral T cells, all develop in normal numbers and retain this homeostatic potential for many months. T cells expressing α/β TCR as well as γ/δ TCR develop normally. Positive and negative selection on MHC class I and class II is normal, and the peripheral, mature T-cell repertoire reacts normally in cytolytic and helper responses to alloantigens and foreign antigens (Melchers and Rolink 1999).

These experiments show that the apparently pluripotent PAX-5$^{-/-}$ preB-I cells can fill vacant hematopoietic compartments in the transplanted, partially deficient host. They also show that a single PAX-5$^{-/-}$ preB-I cell genetically marked by a characteristic set of $D_H J_H$-rearranged IgH chain alleles generates all these different hematopoietic lineages, thereby endowing every progeny cell of these lineages with the same set of $D_H J_H$ rearrangements. Furthermore, they show that neither the expression of surrogate L chain, nor of Igβ, nor the $D_H J_H$ rearrangements irreversibly commit a hematopoietic cell to the B-lineage pathway. Finally, repeated isolation of the transplanted, clonal PAX-5$^{-/-}$ preB-I cells from the bone marrow of the recipient followed each time by in vitro and in vivo induction to the different hematopoietic lineages demonstrates, for at least 100 divisions, a surprisingly strong long-term reconstitution capacity.

At present, we do not know to what extent the earliest progenitor of the B-lineage pathway (the B220$^+$, CD19$^-$, AA4.1$^+$, ckit^{low}, flt-3$^+$, pro-/pre-B cell shown in Fig. 1) bears similarities in cellular behavior to PAX-5$^{-/-}$ preB-I-like cells. In particular, do they respond similarly to inductive signals by cytokines, and are they inducible into different directions? The rearrangement status of the IgH chain locus may not be a reliable marker for B cells of mutant mice, as they have been found in macrophages and T cells (Born et al. 1988). Thus, the plasticity of earlier stages of hematopoiesis may be greater, as previously thought, and influenced by the environment, rather than only autonomously determined by the hematopoietic cell.

It is clear that targeted deletion of the PAX-5 gene can hardly be called a normal state. However, if PAX-5 acts as a traffic signal, so that myeloid and T cells are made when PAX-5 is "off," and B cells are made when PAX-5 is "on," then one could imagine that the regulation of PAX-5 expression by end cells and/or their products could, for instance, influence which of the two routes of traffic is generated. Myeloid and T cells and/or their secreted products would feed back on the earlier progenitor to stop further production of cells of this lineage by up-regulating PAX-5 expression, whereas B cells and/or their secreted products would do the opposite; namely, turn off PAX-5 expression to stop further B-cell production (Fig. 2). Depending on whether hematopoiesis occurs as shown in Figure 1A or Figure 1B, the target cell of this homeostatic regulation of myeloid and lymphoid cell production would be pHSC or the CMLP, respectively.

PRACTICAL CONSEQUENCES

It is important to realize that all hematopoietic lineages developed from the PAX-5$^{-/-}$ preB-I cells generate cells that have been found to function normally. This could be expected, since only early progenitors and B-lineage cells, but no other hematopoietic cells, express PAX-5. Therefore, PAX-5$^{-/-}$ preB-I cell clones offer the exciting possibility to study, and genetically influence, the development of all these normal hematopoietic pathways. The PAX-5$^{-/-}$ preB-I cells can be transgenically modified, since they can be infected with high efficiencies by a retrovirus (Rolink et al. 1999a,b). Transfection of genes, or homologous recombination following such transfections, has so far not been possible. Retroviral infection allows us to mark the cells; e.g., the expression of a fluorescent protein gene, a procedure that facilitates the identification and FACS purification of progeny cells in vitro and in the transplanted host. Retroviral infection of PAX-5$^{-/-}$ preB-I cells by promoter- or polyA-tail trap vectors opens the possibilities for a genetic and functional screening of mutations; i.e., of genes that are active and functional at a given stage of development of T cells, NK cells, or myeloid cells. By analogy, retroviral infection of wild-type preB-I cells can be used for such a mutational analysis of genes active in B-cell development.

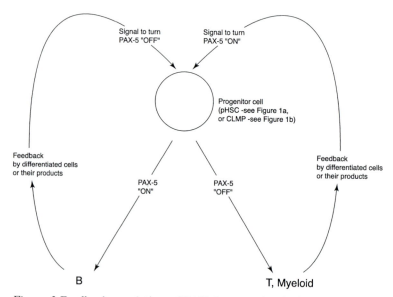

Figure 2 Feedback regulation of PAX-5 expression in hematopoietic progenitor cells, resulting in balanced homeostasis of the B-cell, T-cell, and myeloid-cell compartments (for details, see text).

By crossing the PAX-5$^{-/-}$ mutation onto other hematopoietically defective mutant mice, it should be possible to use preB-I cells of double mutant mice for the study of the detailed structure–function relationships of such a defective gene.

It is predictable that the genetic programs controlling the development and the interactions of cells of different hematopoietic lineages with their environment, self, or non-self, will involve many genes. If homologous recombination of such genes into PAX-5$^{-/-}$ preB-I cells becomes an experimental possibility, this will obviate the need to construct "knock-out" and "knock-in" strains of mice for these genes. Still more exciting are the prospects that a human preB-I cell could even proliferate in tissue culture like its counterpart from mice, and that homologous recombination with an exogenously inducible, normally repressed form of the human PAX-5 gene on both alleles could create a human PAX-5$^{-/-}$ preB-I cell.

ACKNOWLEDGMENTS

The Basel Institute for Immunology was founded and is supported by F. Hoffmann-La Roche Ltd, CH 4002-Basel.

REFERENCES

Akashi K., Traver D., Miyamoto T., and Weissman I. 2000. A clonogenic common myeloid progenitor that gives rise to all myeloid lineages. *Nature* **404:** 193–198.

Allsopp R.C., Chang E., Kashefi-Aazam M., Rogaev E.I., Piatyszek M.A., Shay J.W., and Harley C.B. 1995. Telomere shortening is associated with cell division in vitro and in vivo. *Exp. Cell. Res.* **220:** 194–200.

Allsopp R.C., Vaziri H., Patterson C., Goldstein S., Younglai E.V., Futcher A.B., Greider C.W., and Harley C.B. 1992. Telomere length predicts replicative capacity of human fibroblasts. *Proc. Natl. Acad. Sci.* **89:** 10114–10118.

Askonas B.A. and Williamson A.R. 1972. Factors affecting the propagation of a B cell clone forming antibody to the 2,4-dinitrophenyl group. *Eur. J. Immunol.* **2:** 487–493.

Bain G., Robanus Maandag E.C., te Riele H.P., Feeney A.J., Sheehy A., Schlissel M., Shinton S.A., Hardy R.R., and Murre C. 1997. Both E12 and E47 allow commitment to the B cell lineage. *Immunity* **6:** 145–154.

Bain G., Maandag E.C., Izon D.J., Amsen D., Kruisbeek A.M., Weintraub B.C., Krop I., Schlissel M.S., Feeney A.J., van-Roon M., van der Valk M., te Riele H.P.J., Berns A., and Murre C. 1994. E2A proteins are required for proper B cell development and initiation of immunoglobulin gene rearrangements. *Cell* **79:** 885–892.

Boehm T., Nehls M., and Kyewski B. 1995. Transcription factors that control development of the thymic microenvironment. *Immunol. Today* **16:** 555–556.

Born W., White J., Kappler J., and Marrack P. 1988. Rearrangement of IgH genes in normal thymocyte development. *J. Immunol.* **140:** 3228–3232.

Bradford G.B., Williams B., Rossi R., and Bertoncello I. 1997. Quiescence, cycling, and turnover in the primitive hematopoietic stem cell compartment. *Exp. Hematol.* **25:** 445–453.

Broccoli D., Young J.W., and de Lange T. 1995. Telomerase activity in normal and malignant hematopoietic cells. *Proc. Natl. Acad. Sci.* **92:** 9082–9086.

Busslinger M., Nutt S.L., and Rolink A.G. 2000. Lineage commitment in lymphopoiesis. *Curr. Opin. Immunol.* **12:** 151–158.

Cheshier S.H., Morrison S.J., Liao X., and Weissman I.L. 1999. In vivo proliferation and cell cycle kinetics of long-term self-renewing hematopoietic stem cells. *Proc. Natl. Acad. Sci.* **96:** 3120–3125.

Choi J.K., Shen C.P., Radomska H.S., Eckhardt L.A., and Kadesch T. 1996. E47 activates the Ig-heavy chain and TdT loci in non-B cells. *EMBO J.* **15:** 5014–5021.

Cumano A., Dieterlen-Lievre F., and Godin I. 1996. Lymphoid potential, probed before circulation in mouse, is restricted to caudal intraembryonic splanchnopleura. *Cell* **86:** 907–916.

Cumano A., Garcia-Porrero J., Dieterlen-Lievre F., and Godin I. 1995. [Intra-embryonic hematopoiesis in mice]. *C.R. Seances Soc. Biol. Fil.* **189:** 617–627.

de Haan G. and Van Zant G. 1997. Intrinsic and extrinsic control of hemopoietic stem cell numbers: Mapping of a stem cell gene. *J. Exp. Med.* **186:** 529–536.

DiSanto J.P., Muller W., Guy-Grand D., Fischer A., and Rajewsky K. 1995. Lymphoid development in mice with a targeted deletion of the interleukin-2 receptor γ chain. *Proc. Natl. Acad. Sci.* **92:** 377–381.

Domen J., Cheshier S.H., and Weissman I.L. 2000. The role of apoptosis in the regulation of hematopoietic stem cells: Overexpression of Bcl-2 increases both their number and repopulation potential. *J. Exp. Med.* **191:** 253–264.

Fleming W.H., Alpern E.J., Uchida N., Ikuta K., Spangrude G.J., and Weissman I.L. 1993.

Functional heterogeneity is associated with the cell cycle status of murine hematopoietic stem cells. *J. Cell. Biol.* **122:** 897–902.

Fuchs E., and Segre J.A. 2000. Stem cells: A new lease on life. *Cell* **100:** 143–155.

Georgopoulos K., Bigby M., Wang J.H., Molnár Á., Wu P., Winandy S., and Sharpe A. 1994. The Ikaros gene is required for the development of all lymphoid lineages. *Cell* **79:** 143–156.

Godin I., Dieterlen-Lievre F., and Cumano A. 1995. Emergence of multipotent hemopoietic cells in the yolk sac and paraaortic splanchnopleura in mouse embryos, beginning at 8.5 days postcoitus (erratum in *Proc. Natl. Acad. Sci.* [1995] **92:** 10815). *Proc. Natl. Acad. Sci.* **92:** 773–777.

Grigoriadis A.E., Wang Z.Q., Cecchini M.G., Hofstetter W., Felix R., Fleisch H.A., and Wagner E.F. 1994. c-Fos: A key regulator of osteoclast-macrophage lineage determination and bone remodeling. *Science* **266:** 443–448.

Hiyama K., Hirai Y., Kyoizumi S., Akiyama M., Hiyama E., Piatyszek M.A., Shay J.W., Ishioka S., and Yamakido M. 1995. Activation of telomerase in human lymphocytes and hematopoietic progenitor cells. *J. Immunol.* **155:** 3711–3715.

Hodes R.J. 1999. Telomere length, aging, and somatic cell turnover. *J. Exp. Med.* **190:** 153–156.

Holländer G.A., Wang B., Nichogiannopoulou A., Platenburg P.P., van Ewijk W., Burakoff S.J., Gutierrez-Ramos J.C., and Terhorst C. 1995. Developmental control point in induction of thymic cortex regulated by a subpopulation of prothymocytes. *Nature* **373:** 350–353.

Kantor A.B., Stall A.M., Adams S., Watanabe K., and Herzenberg L.A. 1995. *De novo* development and self-replenishment of B cells. *Int. Immunol.* **7:** 55–68.

Kay H. 1965. How many cell-generations? *Lancet II:* 418–419.

Kondo M., Weissman I.L., and Akashi K. 1997. Identification of clonogenic common lymphoid progenitors in mouse bone marrow. *Cell* **91:** 661–672.

Lee H.W., Blasco M.A., Gottlieb G.J., Horner II, J.W., Greider C.W., and DePinho R.A. 1998. Essential role of mouse telomerase in highly proliferative organs. *Nature* **392:** 569–574.

Lemischka I.R., Raulet D.H., and Mulligan R.C. 1986. Developmental potential and dynamic behavior of hematopoietic stem cells. *Cell* **45:** 917–927.

Lin H. and Grosschedl R. 1995. Failure of B-cell differentiation in mice lacking the transcription factor EBF. *Nature* **376:** 263–267.

Ma Q., Jones D., and Springer T.A. 1999. The chemokine receptor CXCR4 is required for the retention of B lineage and granulocytic precursors within the bone marrow microenvironment. *Immunity* **10:** 463–471.

Manz R.A., Thiel A., and Radbruch A. 1997. Lifetime of plasma cells in the bone marrow (letter). *Nature* **388:** 133–134.

Mayani H., Dragowska W., and Lansdorp P.M. 1993. Lineage commitment in human hemopoiesis involves asymmetric cell division of multipotent progenitors and does not appear to be influenced by cytokines. *J. Cell. Physiol.* **157:** 579–586.

McKercher S., Torbett B.E., Anderson K.L., Henkel G.W., Vestal D.J., Barbault H., Klemsz M., Feeney A.J., Wu G.E., Paige C.J., and Maki R.A. 1996. Targeted disruption of the PU.1 gene results in multiple hematopoietic abnormalities. *EMBO J.* **15:** 5647–5658.

Medvinsky A. and Dzierzak E. 1996. Definitive hematopoiesis is autonomously initiated by the AGM region. *Cell* **86:** 897–906.

Melchers F. and Rolink A. 1999. B-lymphocyte development and biology. In *Fundamental immunology,* 4th edition (ed. W.E. Paul), pp. 183–224. Lippincott-Raven, Philadelphia, Pennsylvania.

Metcalf D. 1991. Lineage commitment of hemopoietic progenitor cells in developing blast cell colonies: Influence of colony-stimulating factors. *Proc. Natl. Acad. Sci.* **88:** 11310–11314.

Molnar A. and Georgopoulos K. 1994. The Ikaros gene encodes a family of functionally diverse zinc finger DNA binding proteins. *Mol. Cell. Biol.* **14:** 8292–8303.

Morrison S.J., Shah N.M., and Anderson D.J. 1997. Regulatory mechanisms in stem cell biology. *Cell* **88:** 287–298.

Morrison S.J., Prowse K.R., Ho P., and Weissman I.L. 1996. Telomerase activity in hematopoietic cells is associated with self-renewal potential. *Immunity* **5:** 207–216.

Morrison S.J. and Weissman I.L. 1994. The long-term repopulating subset of hematopoietic stem cells is deterministic and isolatable by phenotype. *Immunity* **1:** 661–673.

Müller-Sieburg C.E. and Riblet R. 1996. Genetic control of the frequency of hematopoietic stem cells in mice: Mapping of a candidate locus to chromosome 1. *J. Exp. Med.* **183:** 1141–1150.

Neuberger M.S. 1997. Antigen receptor signaling gives lymphocytes a long life (comment). *Cell* **90:** 971–973.

Nichogiannopoulou A., Trevisan M., Neben S., Friedrich C., and Georgopoulos K. 1999. Defects in hemopoietic stem cell activity in *Ikaros* mutant mice. *J. Exp. Med.* **190:** 1201–1214.

Nutt S.L., Heavey B., Rolink A.G., and Busslinger M. 1999a. Commitment to the B-lymphoid lineage depends on the transcription factor Pax5 (see comments). *Nature* **401:** 556–562.

Nutt S.L., Urbanek P., Rolink A., and Busslinger M. 1997. Essential functions of Pax5 (BSAP) in pro-B cell development: Difference between fetal and adult B lymphopoiesis and reduced V-to-DJ recombination at the IgH locus. *Genes Dev.* **11:** 476–491.

Nutt S.L., Vambrie S., Steinlein P., Kozmik Z., Rolink A., Weith A., and Busslinger M. 1999b. Independent regulation of the two Pax5 alleles during B-cell development. *Nat. Genet.* **21:** 390–395.

Ogawa M., ten Boekel E., and Melchers F. 2000. Identification of CD19⁻ B220⁺cKit⁺Flt3/Flk-2⁺ cells as early B lymphoid precursors before pre-B-I cells in juvenile mouse bone marrow. *Int. Immunol.* **12:** 313–324.

O'Riordan M., and Grosschedl R. 1999. Coordinate regulation of B cell differentiation by the transcription factors EBF and E2A. *Immunity* **11:** 21–31.

Peschon J.J., Morrissey P.J., Grabstein K.H., Ramsdell F.J., Maraskovsky E., Gliniak B.C., Park L.S., Ziegler S.F., Williams D.E., Ware C.B., et al. 1994. Early lymphocyte expansion is severely impaired in interleukin 7 receptor-deficient mice. *J. Exp. Med.* **180:** 1955–1960.

Potocnik A. 2000. Role of β1 integrin for hemato-lymphopoiesis in mouse development. *Curr. Top. Microbiol. Immunol.* **251:** 43–50.

Potter M. and Melchers F. 2000. Opinions on the nature of B-1 cells and their relationship to B cell neoplasia. *Curr. Top. Microbiol. Immunol.* **252:** (in press).

Rolink A.G., Andersson J., and Melchers F. 1998. Characterization of immature B cells by a novel monoclonal antibody, by turnover and by mitogen reactivity. *Eur. J. Immunol.* **28:** 3738–3748.

Rolink A., Haasner D., Nishikawa S.I., and Melchers F. 1993. Changes in frequencies of clonable preB cells during life in different lymphoid organs of mice. *Blood* **81:** 2290–2300.

Rolink A., Kudo A., Karasuyama H., Kikuchi Y., and Melchers F. 1991. Long-term proliferating early pre B cell lines and clones with the potential to develop to surface Ig-positive, mitogen reactive B cells *in vitro* and *in vivo*. *EMBO J.* **10:** 327–336.

Rolink A., Ntt S., Melchers F., and Busslinger M. 1999a. Long-term in vivo reconstitution of T-cell development by Pax5-deficeint B-cell progenitors. *Nature* **401:** 603–606.

Rolink A., Nutt S., Busslinger M., ten Boekel E., Seidl T., Andersson J., and Melchers F. 1999b. Differentiation, dedifferentiation and redifferentiation of B-lineage lymphocytes: The roles of the surrogate light chain and the PAX-5 gene. *Cold Spring Harbor Symp. Quant. Biol.* **64:** 21–25.

Schilham M.W., Oosterwegel M.A., Moerer P., Ya J., de Boer P.A.J., van de Wetering M., Verbeek S., Lamers W.H., Kruisbeek A.M., Cumano A., and Clevers A. 1996. Defects in cardiac outflow tract formation and pro-B-lymphocyte expansion in mice lacking Sox-4. *Nature* **380:** 711–714.

Singh H. 1996. Gene targeting reveals a hierarchy of transcription factors regulating specification of lymphoid cell fates. *Curr. Opin. Immunol.* **8:** 160–165.

Slifka M.K., Antia R., Whitmire J.K., and Ahmed R. 1998. Humoral immunity due to long-lived plasma cells. *Immunity* **8:** 363–372.

Spangrude G.J. and Johnson G.R. 1990. Resting and activated subsets of mouse multipotent hematopoietic stem cells. *Proc. Natl. Acad. Sci.* **87:** 7433–7437.

Spangrude G.J., Brooks D.M., and Tumas D.B. 1995. Long-term repopulation of irradiated mice with limiting numbers of purified hematopoietic stem cells: In vivo expansion of stem cell phenotype but not function. *Blood* **85:** 1006–1016.

Sprent J., Schaefer M., Hurd M., Surh C.D., and Ron Y. 1991. Mature murine B and T cells transferred to SCID mice can survive indefinitely and many maintain a virgin phenotype. *J. Exp. Med.* **174:** 717–728.

Tondravi M.M., McKercher S.R., Anderson K., Erdmann J.M., Quiroz M., Maki R., and Teitelbaum S.L. 1997. Osteopetrosis in mice lacking haematopoietic transcription factor PU.1. *Nature* **386:** 81–84.

Tonegawa S. 1983. Somatic generation of antibody diversity. *Nature* **302:** 575–581.

Tsai F.Y., Keller G., Kuo F.C., Weiss M., Chen J., Rosenblatt M., Alt F.W., and Orkin S.H. 1994. An early haematopoietic defect in mice lacking the transcription factor GATA-2. *Nature* **371:** 221–226.

Urbanek P., Wang Z.Q., Fetka I., Wagner E.F., and Busslinger M. 1994. Complete block of early B cell differentiation and altered patterning of the posterior midbrain in mice lacking Pax5/BSAP (see comments). *Cell* **79:** 901–912.

van de Wetering M., Oosterwegel M., van Norren K., and Clevers H. 1993. Sox-4, an Sry-like HMG box protein, is a transcriptional activator in lymphocytes. *EMBO J.* **12:** 3847–3854.

van Ewijk W., Shores E.W., and Singer A. 1994. Crosstalk in the mouse thymus. *Immunol. Today* **15:** 214–217.

Vaziri H., Dragowska W., Allsopp R.C., Thomas T.E., Harley C.B., and Lansdorp P.M. 1994. Evidence for a mitotic clock in human hematopoietic stem cells: Loss of telomeric DNA with age. *Proc. Natl. Acad. Sci.* **91:** 9857–9860.

Wang J.H., Nichogiannopoulou A., Wu L., Sun L., Sharpe A.H., Bigby M., and Georgopoulos K. 1996. Selective defects in the development of the fetal and adult lymphoid system in mice with an Ikaros null mutation. *Immunity* **5:** 537–549.

Wang Z.Q., Ovitt C., Grigoriadis A.E., Mohle-Steinlein U., Ruther U., and Wagner E.F. 1992. Bone and haematopoietic defects in mice lacking c-fos. *Nature* **360:** 741–745.

Weissman I.L. 2000. Stem cells: Units of development, units of regeneration, and units in evolution. *Cell* **100:** 157–168.

Zhuang Y., Soriano P., and Weintraub H. 1994. The helix-loop-helix gene E2A is required for B cell formation. *Cell* **79:** 875–884.

15

The Hemangioblast

Gordon Keller
Institute for Gene Therapy and Molecular Medicine
Mount Sinai School of Medicine
New York, New York 10029-6514

HISTORICAL PERSPECTIVE

The name hemangioblast was first introduced by Murray (1932) to describe discrete cell masses that developed in chick embryo cultures and displayed both hematopoietic and endothelial potential. Although originally used to describe groups of cells, the name hemangioblast is now used exclusively in reference to a single cell, the hypothetical precursor of the hematopoietic and endothelial lineages. The concept that these two lineages share a common precursor arose from observations of early embryos which indicated that the respective precursor populations develop in close spatial and temporal proximity in the yolk sac (Sabin 1920; Haar and Ackerman 1971). Detailed histological analysis revealed that commitment to the hematopoietic and endothelial lineages begins with the proliferation of a single layer of mesodermal cells in the presumptive yolk sac that results in the formation of cell clusters, known as mesodermal cell masses (Haar and Ackerman 1971). Cells within these mesodermal masses differentiate quickly and give rise to angioblasts, precursors of the endothelial lineage, and primitive erythroblasts, the first committed hematopoietic cells. As these populations mature further, the angioblasts generate endothelial cells which rapidly establish the first vascular structure that surrounds the primitive erythroblasts. These clusters of developing endothelial and erythroid cells within the yolk sac, commonly referred to as blood islands, are found by the headfold stage of embryonic development in the mouse (day 8.0 of gestation) and represent the first site of hematopoietic and vascular differentiation (Haar and Ackerman 1971).

Since the hypothesis of the hemangioblast was first put forward, a number of studies have provided evidence in support of its existence. Despite this large body of evidence, however, a cell with the characteristics of the hemangioblast has not yet been isolated from developing embryos. The strongest evidence in support of the hemangioblast has come from studies using a model system based on the capacity of embryonic stem (ES) cells to generate differentiated progeny in culture.

The goal of this chapter is to review the evidence supporting the existence of the hemangioblast and to outline a number of issues relating to the developmental status of a precursor with this potential. These issues include the site or sites of hemangioblast development, the relationship of the hemangioblast to mesodermal cells, the relationship of the hemangioblast to the hematopoietic stem cell, and the developmental potential of the hemangioblast with respect to primitive and definitive hematopoiesis. As the hemangioblast is the putative ancestor of the hematopoietic and endothelial lineages, it should be present at sites in the embryo where both of these lineages develop. Thus, as part of the discussion of the hemangioblast, it is important to review the sites and stages of hematopoietic and endothelial development in the embryo.

DEVELOPMENT OF THE HEMATOPOIETIC AND ENDOTHELIAL LINEAGES: POTENTIAL SITES OF HEMANGIOBLAST DEVELOPMENT

The Yolk Sac, an Extraembryonic Site of Hematopoiesis

As indicated above, the blood islands in the yolk sac represent the first site of both hematopoietic and endothelial development in the embryo. Although the timing of blood island development was initially defined through histological analysis, the kinetics of hematopoietic commitment within the yolk sac has been analyzed more precisely through the use of sensitive colony-forming assays that measure precursor populations (Wong et al. 1986; Palis et al. 1999). This approach is advantageous because it defines cells by their potential to generate a colony in culture rather than by their morphology and therefore can identify a precursor before it displays any distinguishing characteristics of a maturing hematopoietic cell. On the basis of precursor analysis, it was found that hematopoietic commitment takes place in the developing yolk sac as early as day 7.0 of gestation at the mid-primitive streak stage of development, ~24 hours earlier than the appearance of the blood islands (Palis et al. 1999).

As expected, precursors of the primitive erythroid lineage, the lineage present in the blood islands, are among the first to develop in the early yolk sac. Kinetic analysis revealed that these precursors are generated for a limited period of time (48 hours) and then are no longer detected in the yolk sac nor in any other tissue at any other stage of development (Palis et al. 1999). This short yolk-sac-restricted stage of erythroid development is known as primitive hematopoiesis. All other hematopoietic activity, regardless of the site, is considered to be definitive hematopoiesis. Erythrocytes generated during the primitive hematopoietic stage of development are characterized by their large size, by the retention of their nuclei, and by the production of embryonic forms of globin (Barker 1968; Brotherton et al. 1979; Russel 1979). In contrast, definitive erythroid cells that are generated during the fetal liver and adult bone marrow stages of hematopoiesis are small, enucleated, and produce adult globins (Barker 1968; Brotherton et al. 1979; Russel 1979). With the onset of circulation, the yolk-sac-derived primitive erythrocytes enter the blood system where they persist until approximately day 16 of gestation.

Although primitive erythroid cells represent the predominant mature hematopoietic population in the yolk sac, they are not the only hematopoietic cells generated in this tissue. Precursors of the macrophage lineage can be detected in low numbers as early as those of the primitive erythroid lineage (Palis et al. 1999). Definitive erythroid precursors are found by the 1–7 somite pairs (sp) stage of development (8.25 days), and those of the mast cell lineage by the 9–16 sp stage (8.5 days) (Palis et al. 1999). Unlike the primitive erythroid precursors, the definitive precursors, for the most part, do not undergo complete maturation in the yolk sac environment. This population of definitive precursors likely migrates from the yolk sac and differentiates in other sites, possibly the fetal liver.

The development of precursors from multiple lineages in the yolk sac suggests that multipotential stem cells with repopulating capacity should be present in this tissue. However, transplantation studies have shown that the early yolk sac contains few, if any, cells able to repopulate adult animals (Müller et al. 1994). Repopulating stem cells are not readily detected in the yolk sac until day 11 of gestation, shortly following their appearance in the embryo proper (Müller et al. 1994). These findings suggest either that stem cells do not exist in the yolk sac of the early embryo or that cells with this potential are present but, due to their embryonic stage of development, are unable to function in an adult environment. Evidence to support the latter interpretation has been provided by the transplantation studies of Yoder et al. (1997). These investigators transplanted CD34$^+$/c-Kit$^+$ yolk sac cells from 9-day-old embryos into the livers of newborn pups, reasoning that this environment retains fetal properties and therefore could be better suited to support the growth and development of these embryonic cells. Using this strategy, they were able to demonstrate that the CD34$^+$/c-Kit$^+$ yolk sac population could repopulate the hematopoietic lineages of these pups and that these transplanted cells persisted into adult life. When bone marrow from these animals was transplanted into secondary adult recipients, yolk-sac-derived stem cells were able to function in this environment and provide repopulation. In contrast, when the CD34$^+$/c-Kit$^+$ yolk sac cells were transplanted directly into adult animals, they failed to show any repopulating potential. These findings strongly suggest that stem cells with repopulating potential are present in the yolk sac, but that they have to undergo specific maturation steps before they can function in an adult environment.

Morphological analysis and gene expression studies have shown that the endothelial lineage is established at the same time as the early hematopoietic populations in the developing yolk sac (Sabin 1920; Haar and Ackerman 1971; Drake and Fleming 2000). The development of endothelial cells from mesodermal precursors at this site occurs through a process known as vasculogenesis and results in the establishment of the primary vascular system (Risau and Flamme 1995).

The pattern of hematopoietic and endothelial development observed in the yolk sac provides the basis for several predictions regarding the putative hemangioblast. First, this precursor should be present prior to the development of these two lineages, sometime before or on day 7.0 of gestation. Second, it should have the potential to generate both the primitive and definitive hematopoietic lineages in addition to the endothelial lineage.

Intraembryonic Sites of Hematopoiesis

Hematopoietic activity shifts from the yolk sac to the developing fetal liver between days 10 and 12 of gestation, and with this shift, the system undergoes a change from one that generates a single mature lineage to one that displays multilineage differentiation (Metcalf and Moore 1971). Unlike yolk sac hematopoiesis where precursors develop in situ from mesoderm, fetal liver hematopoiesis is thought to be established by cohorts of stem/precursor cells that migrate into this tissue from other sites (Moore and Metcalf 1970; Metcalf and Moore 1971). Given that the yolk sac is the first site of hematopoiesis, it was assumed for many years that yolk-sac-derived precursors seed the liver (Moore and Metcalf 1970). Although it is likely that some hematopoietic activity found early in the fetal liver is of yolk sac origin, there is a considerable body of evidence which suggests that hematopoietic sites within the embryo proper, rather than the yolk sac, may be the major source of precursors that establish the fetal program (for review, see Dzierzak et al. 1998).

Studies carried out, initially in the chick (Dieterlen-Lièvre 1975) and more recently in the mouse (Godin et al. 1993; Medvinsky et al. 1993), have defined a region near the aorta that displays hematopoietic potential at specific stages of development. This region is known as the para-aortic splanchnopleura (P-Sp) between 8.5 and 10 days of gestation and as the aorta-gonad-mesonephros (AGM) from days 10.5 to 12. Analysis of the hematopoietic potential of the P-Sp/AGM has demonstrated the presence of multipotential precursors as early as day 8.5 (Godin et al. 1995; Godin et al. 1999) and stem cells capable of repopulating adult recipients by day 10.5 (Müller et al. 1994). Stem cells that are able to repopulate newborn pups have been detected in P-Sp/AGM by day 9.0 of gestation (Yoder et al. 1997). Recent mapping studies have localized the hematopoietic potential of the AGM region to the aorta (Godin et al. 1999; de Bruijn et al. 2000). Although it is clear that the P-Sp/AGM contains multipotential progenitors and repopulating stem cells, extensive analyses have failed to detect significant numbers of committed precursors in this region (Godin et al. 1999; Palis et al. 1999). This suggests that the P-Sp/AGM may represent an unusual site of hematopoietic development in that it supports the generation of multipotential precursors and stem cells, but not their maturation and terminal differentiation. An alternative interpretation is that these precursors and stem cells do not develop in the P-Sp/AGM but rather have migrated to it from elsewhere, possibly the yolk sac. As all analyses of the yolk sac and P-Sp/AGM stem cell potential have been carried out following the onset of circulation, the ultimate origin of these populations is not yet resolved and remains an area of active investigation.

The observation that the hematopoietic potential of the AGM associates with the aorta suggests that this region could be a second site of hemangioblast development. The endothelial cells that give rise to the aorta begin to develop at approximately day 8 of gestation just prior to the appearance of the hematopoietic precursors in the embryo (Coffin et al. 1991; Garcia-Porrero et al. 1995; Pardanaud et al. 1996). Studies in the chick have shown that the aorta is a mosaic tissue, composed of endothelial precursors derived from different mesodermal sites. The endothelial cells that form the roof and the sides of the aorta develop from paraxial mesoderm, whereas those found on the floor derive from the splanchnopleural mesoderm (Pardanaud et al. 1996). Histological studies in the chick (Dieterlen-Lièvre and Martin 1981), mouse (Garcia-Porrero et al. 1995), and human (Tavian et al. 1996) have demonstrated the presence of clusters of hematopoietic cells in close association with, and often adhering to, the endothelial cells on the ventral surface (floor) of the aorta. The hematopoietic nature of these clusters has been defined by surface markers and by the observation that they are absent in Cbfa2$^{-/-}$ mice that lack all definitive hematopoietic potential (Tavian et al. 1996; Wood et al. 1997; North et al. 1999). The observation that the appearance of these clusters coincides with the onset of hematopoietic activity at this site suggests that they are developing stem cells and precursors. As with the endothelial cells in this region of the aorta, the hematopoietic cells that form these clusters also appear to be derived from splanchnopleural mesoderm (Pardanaud et al. 1996). In addition to the aorta, hematopoietic clusters have also been identified in the vitelline and umbilical arteries, indicating that intraembryonic hematopoietic development may be associated with the major arterial regions of the embryo (Garcia-Porrero et al. 1995; Wood et al. 1997; de Bruijn et al. 2000). The structure of these intraembryonic clusters differs from that of the yolk sac blood islands, but the close association of the hematopoietic and endothelial lineages in these regions of the embryo has led to speculation that they could be sites of hemangioblast development. These intraembryonic hemangioblasts would likely differ from their counterparts in the yolk sac in that they should be restricted to the definitive hematopoietic system, as there is no detectable primitive erythroid potential outside of the yolk sac (Palis et al. 1999).

IN VITRO DIFFERENTIATION OF ES CELLS: A MODEL FOR EMBRYONIC HEMATOPOIESIS AND ENDOTHELIAL DEVELOPMENT

Given the fact that hematopoietic precursors are present in the yolk sac as early as day 7.0 of gestation, the search for the hemangioblast should focus on this or slightly earlier stages of development. A significant problem in isolating the yolk sac hemangioblast is the fact that the embryo is extremely small and difficult to access at this stage.

As an alternative approach to studying early embryonic events, a number of groups have focused on the in vitro differentiation potential of ES cells as a model of yolk sac hematopoietic and endothelial development (Risau et al. 1988; Lindenbaum and Grosveld 1990; Burkert et al. 1991; Schmitt et al. 1991; Wiles and Keller 1991; Wang et al. 1992; Keller et al. 1993; Nakano et al. 1994; Vittet et al. 1996). In appropriate culture conditions, ES cells will spontaneously differentiate and form colonies known as embryoid bodies (EBs) that contain many different types of precursors, including those of the hematopoietic and endothelial lineages (Doetschman et al. 1985; Keller 1995). A number of different studies have demonstrated that the hematopoietic and endothelial lineages develop in a highly reproducible pattern within the differentiating EBs (Keller et al. 1993; Vittet et al. 1996). These reproducible patterns of lineage commitment enable one to access the respective precursors at specific stages of differentiation.

Although the ES/EB system does provide the advantage of precursor accessibility, it is only a useful model if it recapitulates the developmental programs found in the normal embryo. Although it is difficult to investigate all aspects of this issue, the following observations support the interpretation that the early events in hematopoietic and endothelial commitment within the EBs are similar to those found in the developing embryo in utero. First, precursor analysis has demonstrated that the primitive erythroid and macrophage lineages appear within the EBs prior to those of the definitive erythroid and other myeloid lineages, a developmental pattern which parallels that found in early yolk sac (Keller et al. 1993). Moreover, as observed in the yolk sac, primitive erythropoiesis within the EBs is a transient developmental program. Second, expression studies on developing EBs have shown that mesoderm-specific genes are expressed earlier than those associated with hematopoietic and endothelial precursors, which in turn precede those that define specific hematopoietic lineages (Keller et al. 1993; Robertson et al. 2000). This temporal pattern of gene expression is consistent with the fact that the hematopoietic and endothelial lineages develop from mesoderm. Third, molecular analysis of endothelial development within the EBs indicates that genes essential to the early stages of lineage commitment are expressed prior to those that are involved in later stages of growth and differentiation (Vittet et al. 1996). Fourth, gene-targeting studies have provided strong evidence indicating that similar molecular programs are involved in the development of the hematopoietic and endothelial lineages in the embryo and EBs (Tsai et al. 1994; Weiss et al. 1994; Porcher et al.1996; Elefanty et al. 1997; Robertson et al. 2000). Taken together, these observations strongly suggest that the early events involved in the establishment of the hematopoietic and endothelial lineages within the EBs are comparable, if not identical, to that of the yolk sac in the early embryo. As such, the ES/EB system provides an ideal model for the identification and characterization of the hemangioblast.

DOES THE HEMANGIOBLAST EXIST?

Since the concept of the hemangioblast was first introduced, findings from numerous studies have provided evidence in support of its existence. This evidence ranges from observations that are consistent with the existence of the hemangioblast to studies that directly demonstrate the presence of cells with both hematopoietic and endothelial potential. In addition to studies that provide support for the concept of the hemangioblast, there is also experimental evidence that is difficult to incorporate into a model in which the hematopoietic and endothelial lineages share a common precursor. In the following section, I review the experimental evidence for and against the existence of the hemangioblast.

Evidence Supporting the Existence of the Hemangioblast

One piece of evidence that is often used in support of the hemangioblast is the observation that the hematopoietic and endothelial lineages express a number of different genes in common, including CD34 (Young et al. 1995), flk-1 (Millauer et al. 1993; Eichmann et al. 1997; Kabrun et al. 1997), flt-1 (Fong et al. 1996), TIE2 (Takakura et al. 1998), scl/tal-1 (Kallianpur et al. 1994), GATA-2 (Orkin 1992), and PECAM-1 (Watt et al. 1995). The fact that these lineages co-express these genes, many of which encode growth factor receptors or transcription factors, is not only consistent with the notion that they share a common precursor, but also suggests that similar molecular programs and growth regulatory mechanisms are involved in their development from it. Analyses of specific mouse and zebrafish mutants have provided evidence in support of this interpretation. In mice, gene-targeting studies have demonstrated that flk-1 (Shalaby et al. 1995, 1997), sclL/tal-1 (Robb et al. 1995; Shivdasani et al. 1995), and TGFβ1 (Dickson et al. 1995) are essential for the normal development and growth of both lineages. In zebrafish the mutation known as *cloche* disrupts the development of hematopoietic lineages as well as the endocardium in the embryo (Stainier et al. 1995).

A more direct approach to the identification of the hemangioblast utilizes surface markers as a means to isolate it. The following group of studies has begun to pursue this strategy and has provided further evidence in support of the existence of this precursor. However, none has yet identified a single cell that can give rise to both the hematopoietic and endothelial lineages. Eichmann et al. (1997) sorted VEGF receptor 2^+ (Flk-1^+) cells from the mesoderm of the early chick gastrula and found that this population could generate both hematopoietic and endothelial progeny, suggesting that it contains the hemangioblast. Analyses of single sorted cells, however, demonstrated that they could generate either hematopoietic or endothelial progeny, but not both, as different conditions were required for the development of these lineages. Consequently, it is difficult to determine from this study whether this Flk-1^+ population contains a mixture of lineage-restricted precursors or the bi-potential heman-gioblast. Nishakawa et al. (1998b) isolated mouse embryo yolk sac and P-Sp/AGM cells based on VE-cadherin expression and demonstrated multilineage hematopoietic potential in these populations. Because VE-cadherin was considered to be a marker of endothelial cells, these find-ings were interpreted as evidence that hematopoietic cells can develop from a specific subpopulation of endothelial cells with hemangioblast potential. Although these findings are consistent with the interpretation of a common cell for these lineages, this study failed to demonstrate any endothelial potential of the isolated VE-cadherin$^+$ cells. Consequently, similar results would be obtained if a subpopulation of hematopoietic-restricted precursors also expressed VE-cadherin. Using an antibody against the receptor tyrosine kinase TEK, Hamaguchi et al. (1999) isolat-ed precursors from the AGM of day-10.5 embryos that could generate hematopoietic cells as well as cells with endothelial characteristics as defined by PECAM-1 expression. Given that single cells were analyzed, these findings suggest that these AGM-derived TEK$^+$ precursors are hemangioblasts. One concern with this interpretation is that hematopoiet-ic cells also express PECAM-1 (Watt et al. 1995). Consequently, a more in-depth characterization of the adherent cells, with a number of different markers, will be required to demonstrate that they are of the endothelial lineage and thus prove that these AGM-derived cells are indeed heman-gioblasts. In a more recent study, Hara et al. (1999) demonstrated that AGM cells isolated on the basis of podocalyxin-like protein 1 (PCLP1) expression displayed both hematopoietic stem cell and endothelial poten-tial, suggesting that this molecule could be a marker of the heman-gioblast. However, as clonal analysis was not carried out in this study, it is difficult to distinguish between the presence of restricted hematopoiet-ic and endothelial precursors and hemangioblasts in the population. Finally, cells with endothelial and hematopoietic potential have recently been isolated from the mobilized peripheral blood of humans using the marker AC133 (Gehling et al. 2000). Again, the lack of clonal analysis in this study does not allow one to distinguish between a population that contains restricted precursors and one that contains the hemangioblast.

As an alternative approach to identifying the hemangioblast, Jaffredo et al. (1998) used marking studies to analyze the relationship of intraem-bryonic endothelial and hematopoietic cells. These investigators labeled endothelial cells in chick embryos with acetylated low-density lipoprotein (AcLDL) and then followed the fate of the marker over a 24-hour period. AcLDL uptake is a characteristic of endothelial cells and macrophages (Traber et al. 1981; Voyta et al. 1984). Hematopoietic cells were characterized based on expression of CD45, and the appearance of CD45$^+$ LDL$^+$ cells was taken as evidence that hematopoietic cells developed from the marked endothelial cells. Although these findings are consistent with this interpretation, it is difficult to exclude the possibility that CD45$^-$ or CD45^{lo} immature macrophages or macrophage precursors took up the AcLDL independent of the endothelial cells and contributed to the CD45$^+$ LDL$^+$ population. Direct proof of a precursor/progeny relationship between these lineages will require clonal analysis.

Taken together, these observations provide strong support for the concept that the hematopoietic and endothelial lineages develop from a common precursor. They do not, however, prove that such a cell exists, because the same observations would support the interpretation that these lineages develop from separate precursors that express similar markers.

The only direct evidence for the hemangioblast has been provided by studies which have incorporated clonal analysis and directly demonstrate that cells with hematopoietic and endothelial characteristics can develop from the same precursor. The most detailed analysis to date has come from studies using the ES cell in vitro differentiation system. We identified a cell population in EBs at day 3.0–3.5 of differentiation that could generate colonies of undifferentiated blast cells in the presence of vascular endothelial growth factor (VEGF) (Kennedy et al. 1997; Choi et al. 1998). Functional analysis showed that these blast cell colonies contained primitive and definitive hematopoietic precursors as well as endothelial precursors. Cell mixing and limiting dilution studies demonstrated that these bi-lineage colonies derived from a single cell, the blast colony-forming cell (BL-CFC), which is present in EBs immediately prior to the onset of primitive erythropoiesis (Choi et al. 1998). The developmental potential of the BL-CFC is consistent with the interpretation that it represents the in vitro equivalent of the yolk sac hemangioblast. Using a somewhat different approach, Nishakawa et al. (1998a) demonstrated that single Flk-1$^+$ precursors isolated from ES differentiation cultures were able to generate cells with both hematopoietic and endothelial characteristics. These precursors, like the BL-CFC, appear to have the capacity to generate both primitive and definitive hematopoietic progeny. The recent demonstration that BL-CFC are Flk-1$^+$ (Faloon et al. 2000) suggests that the populations in the two studies are the same.

Although these studies have provided the most direct evidence for the existence of the hemangioblast, they have both utilized a model system that may or may not accurately reflect the early events in the normal embryo with respect to the development of this precursor. Applying the information obtained from these studies to the normal embryo should provide the answer as to whether or not the hemangioblast does exist in vivo.

Evidence against the Existence of the Hemangioblast

The previous section outlined a large body of experimental evidence which supports the concept that the hematopoietic and endothelial lineages develop from a common precursor. However, the fact that precursors with hemangioblast potential have not yet been isolated from developing embryos raises the possibility that this cell does not exist. At least one recent study has provided evidence that is inconsistent with the concept of the hemangioblast. Kinder et al. (1999) mapped the fate of cells in the primitive streak isolated from the early, mid, and late stages of the mouse gastrula and found that mesoderm precursors that generate erythropoietic cells emerge earlier than those that establish the endothelial lineage. Simultaneous contribution to both the erythroid and endothelial populations in the same region of the yolk sac was rarely observed, suggesting that these lineages arise from restricted precursors that develop within the primitive streak. If these precursors are truly restricted as they emerge from the primitive streak, the existence of the hemangioblast in the yolk sac would certainly be brought into question. However, in this particular study, the erythroid and endothelial populations were defined only by morphological criteria, and the fate of the cells was followed for a relatively short period of time. Consequently, the possibility remains that immature cells of either lineage were not recognized or that other potentials would have developed beyond the time frame of the study.

REGULATION OF HEMANGIOBLAST DEVELOPMENT

Given the limited data demonstrating the existence of the hemangioblast, it may be somewhat premature to discuss the regulation of this precursor. Nevertheless, it is useful to review several aspects of the regulation of hematopoietic and endothelial lineage development, as these studies can provide insights into possible approaches for further characterization of the elusive hemangioblast. Although molecules involved in the generation and specification of mesoderm will certainly affect hematopoietic and endothelial development, the discussion in this section is limited to two specific genes, flk-1 and scl/tal-1, that appear to act at the earliest stages of commitment and differentiation of these lineages, possibly at the level of the putative hemangioblast.

Flk-1, the VEGFR2 receptor, is required for the development of the hematopoietic and endothelial lineages in the early embryo, as mice lacking the receptor are unable to generate yolk sac blood islands (Shalaby et al. 1995). The defect in these animals is thought to result from the inability of Flk-1$^{-/-}$ mesodermal cells and/or hemangioblasts to migrate to the appropriate regions of the yolk sac rather than from a specific block in the developmental pathway of these lineages. This interpretation is supported by the following observations. First, analysis of chimeric embryos demonstrated that Flk-1$^{-/-}$ ES-derived cells were unable to colonize the yolk sac, but rather accumulated on the surface of the amnion, a position where they are not normally found (Shalaby et al. 1997). Second, Flk-1$^{-/-}$ ES cells are able to generate hematopoietic cells following their differentiation to embryoid bodies in culture, a system in which cell migration and movement are less extensive than in the embryo (Schuh et al. 1999). Third, Flk-1$^{-/-}$ embryos were found to contain hematopoietic precursors when assayed at day 7.5 of gestation, indicating that the hematopoietic lineage is generated in vivo (Schuh et al. 1999). Taken together, these findings suggest that Flk-1 is expressed initially on a subpopulation of mesodermal cells and/or hemangioblasts that normally migrate to and differentiate within the developing yolk sac. The primary role of Flk-1 at this stage appears to be in the migration of these cells to the appropriate environment.

The second gene known to play a role at the early stages of hematopoietic and endothelial development is scl/tal-1, a member of the helix-loop-helix family of transcription factors (Begley and Green 1999). Its role in the development of the putative hemangioblast is derived from the following observations. First, gene targeting studies have shown that scl/tal-1 is essential for the development of both primitive and definitive hematopoiesis as well as for the proper establishment of the primary capillary plexus in the yolk sac (Robb et al. 1995; Shivdasani et al. 1995; Visvader et al. 1998; Elefanty et al. 1999). Second, overexpression of scl/tal-1 in zebrafish embryos results in the expansion of cell populations expressing hematopoietic and endothelial markers (Gering et al. 1998). Third, overexpression of scl/tal-1 is able to rescue the hematopoietic and endothelial defects in zebrafish *cloche* mutant embryos (Liao et al. 1998). Fourth, in vitro differentiation of scl/tal-1$^{-/-}$ ES cells demonstrated that they are unable to generate hemangioblast-derived blast colonies (Faloon et al. 2000; Robertson et al. 2000). The developmental block appears to be just prior to the BL-CFC, as the scl/tal-1$^{-/-}$ ES cells are able to generate colonies referred to as transitional colonies that display pre-blast colony characteristics. These observations are consistent with the notion that scl/tal-1 plays a pivotal role in the development of the hemangioblast and that it could provide one of the earliest markers for this cell.

QUESTIONS TO BE ADDRESSED IN FUTURE STUDIES

As is evident from this review, the field encompassing the identification and characterization of the hemangioblast is an active area of research that is still very much in its infancy. Consequently, there are a large number of issues and questions regarding the hemangioblast that need to be addressed in future studies.

The first relates to the sites of hemangioblast development. Where does this precursor develop in the embryo, and is it restricted to embryonic development? Clearly, the early yolk sac would be the first site of hemangioblast development. Kinetic studies defining the onset of hematopoiesis predict that the hemangioblast should be present within the developing yolk sac at approximately day 7.0 of gestation. Preliminary studies from our lab have shown that precursors able to generate blast colonies with primitive and definitive hematopoietic potential do indeed exist in the yolk sac at this stage of development (J. Palis and G. Keller, unpubl.). Further studies will be required to determine whether or not these colonies also have endothelial potential. A second embryonic site of hemangioblast development would be the AGM. The findings summarized above, demonstrating the presence of hematopoietic clusters associated with the floor of the aorta and the expression of the same markers on hematopoietic and endothelial cells isolated from this region, support this interpretation. Future studies, incorporating clonal analysis and detailed functional studies on the progeny of single AGM-derived cells, will be required to demonstrate that the hemangioblast exists at this site. Other potential sites of hemangioblast development could be the fetal liver and adult bone marrow, tissues that support multilineage hematopoiesis. Evidence that adult human hematopoietic stem cells express KDR, the human equivalent of Flk-1 (Ziegler et al. 1999), and that both endothelial and hematopoietic precursors in mobilized peripheral blood express A133 (Gehling et al. 2000) are consistent with this notion. However, as with the embryonic populations, clonal analysis demonstrating both hematopoietic and endothelial potential will be required to prove the existence of the hemangioblast in the adult bone marrow.

The second major issue relates to developmental potential of the hemangioblast. If hemangioblasts develop at different sites, do they have different potential? What is the relationship of the hemangioblast to mesodermal precursors? What is the relationship of the hemangioblast to the long-term repopulating hematopoietic stem cell?

With respect to potential, the possibility that the yolk sac and the P-Sp/AGM are both sites of hemangioblast development suggests that subpopulations of these precursors exist. The yolk sac hemangioblast would be expected to generate both primitive and definitive hematopoietic progeny, whereas the hemangioblast that develops in the P-Sp/AGM would likely be restricted to the definitive lineages (Fig. 1). Alternatively, there may be a single population of hemangioblasts whose potential is regulated by the microenvironment in which it develops. This cell would generate both primitive and definitive hematopoietic cells in the yolk sac, but only definitive cells in the intraembryonic environments. A prediction of this model would be that the "definitive" hemangioblasts might be able to generate primitive erythroid cells, if placed back into a yolk sac environment. Evidence to support this interpretation has been provided by Geiger et al. (1998), who demonstrated that adult hematopoietic stem cells, when introduced into an embryonic environment, could reactivate embryonic globin gene expression. Although this study did not address this question at the level of a putative hemangioblast, it does raise the possibility that cells with primitive erythroid potential may exist outside the yolk sac.

The rapid commitment to the hematopoietic and endothelial lineages in the developing yolk sac following the onset of gastrulation indicates that the distinction between mesoderm and the hemangioblast may be subtle and difficult to define. Expression of Flk-1 within a subpopulation of mesoderm may represent the first commitment step toward the endothelial and hematopoietic lineages. As these Flk-1$^+$ mesodermal cells migrate toward the extraembryonic region that will form the yolk sac, they may undergo differentiation to the hemangioblast and subsequently to angioblasts and primitive erythroid precursors. If this proposed sequence of events is accurate, it is possible that the hemangioblast stage is very short-lived and takes place before the cells actually colonize the region of the developing yolk sac that will give rise to the blood islands. Consequently, a detailed analysis of different Flk-1$^+$ regions of the embryo at various stages of early development might be required to iden-

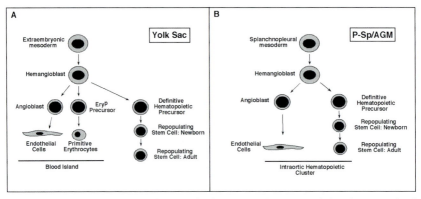

Figure 1 A model depicting hemangioblast commitment and development in the yolk sac (*A*) and the P-Sp/AGM (*B*).

tify the hemangioblast in vivo.

Given the fact that the hemangioblast is hypothesized to develop earlier than other hematopoietic lineages, it should in theory represent the precursor to all hematopoietic cells including the long-term repopulating stem cell. As such, it can be considered a pre-stem cell. The developmental progression observed in both the yolk sac and P-Sp/AGM, whereby cells able to repopulate a newborn pup appear before those that can function in an adult animal, would support the notion that pre-hematopoietic stem cells do exist and that the adult long-term repopulating stem cell is not the most immature in the system. If the hemangioblast represents the most immature precursor within the hematopoietic system, it likely would not display any repopulating potential, at least in an adult environment. The hemangioblast would first have to undergo a series of maturation events to generate the newborn repopulating stem cell, which in turn would give rise to the adult repopulating stem cell (Fig. 1). Given this predicted potential, the hemangioblast would represent an outstanding source of hematopoietic stem cells. Studies aimed at identifying the hemangioblast at different stages of development will determine whether this model is correct.

ACKNOWLEDGMENT

I thank Marion Kennedy, Jim Palis, and Liz Zahradka for critically reading the manuscript.

REFERENCES

Barker J. 1968. Development of the mouse hematopoietic system I. Types of hemoglobin produced in embryonic yolk sac and liver. *Dev. Biol.* **18:** 14–29.

Begley C.G. and Green A.R. 1999. The SCL gene: From case report to critical hematopoietic regulator. *Blood* **93:** 2760–2770.

Brotherton T., Chui D., Gauldie J., and Patterson M. 1979. Hemoglobin ontogeny during normal mouse fetal development. *Proc. Natl. Acad. Sci.* **76:** 2853–2857.

Burkert U., von Ruden T., and Wagner E.F. 1991. Early fetal hematopoietic development from in vitro differentiated embryonic stem cells. *New Biol.* **3:** 698–708.

Choi K., Kennedy M., Kazarov A., Papadimitriou J.C., and Keller G. 1998. A common precursor for hematopoietic and endothelial cells. *Development* **125:** 725–732.

Coffin J.D., Harrison J., Schwartz S., and Heimark R. 1991. Angioblast differentiation and morphogenesis of the vascular endothelium in the mouse embryo. *Dev. Biol.* **148:** 51–62.

de Bruijn M.F., Speck N.A., Peeters M.C., and Dzierzak E. 2000. Definitive hematopoietic stem cells first develop within the major arterial regions of the mouse embryo. *EMBO J.* **19:** 2465–2474.

Dickson M.C., Martin J.S., Cousins F.M., Kulkarni A.B., Karlsson S., and Akhurst R.J. 1995. Defective haematopoiesis and vasculogenesis in transforming growth factor-β 1 knock out mice. *Development* **121:** 1845–1854.

Dieterlen-Lièvre F. 1975. On the origin of haemopoietic stem cells in the avian embryo: An experimental approach. *J. Embryol. Exp. Morphol.* **33:** 607–619.

Dieterlen-Lièvre F., and Martin C. 1981. Diffuse intraembryonic hemopoiesis in normal and chimeric avian development. *Dev. Biol.* **88:** 180–191.

Doetschman T.C., Eistetter H., Katz M., Schmidt W., and Kemler R. 1985. The in vitro development of blastocyst-derived embryonic stem cell lines: Formation of visceral yolk sac, blood islands and myocardium. *J. Embryol. Exp. Morphol.* **87:** 27–45.

Drake C.J. and Fleming P.A. 2000. Vasculogenesis in the day 6.5 to 9.5 mouse embryo. *Blood* **95:** 1671–1679.

Dzierzak E., Medvinsky A., and de Bruijn M. 1998. Qualitative and quantitative aspects of haematopoietic cell development in the mammalian embryo. *Immunol. Today* **19:** 228–236.

Eichmann A., Corbel C., Nataf V., Vaigot P., Breant C., and Le Douarin N.M. 1997. Ligand-dependent development of the endothelial and hemopoietic lineages from embryonic mesodermal cells expressing vascular endothelial growth factor receptor 2. *Proc. Natl. Acad. Sci.* **94:** 5141–5146.

Elefanty A.G., Robb L., Birner R., and Begley C.G. 1997. Hematopoietic-specific genes are not induced during in vitro differentiation of *scl*-null embryonic stem cells. *Blood* **90:** 1435–1447.

Elefanty A.G., Begley C.G., Hartley L., Papaevangeliou B., and Robb L. 1999. SCL expression in the mouse embryo detected with a targeted *lacZ* reporter gene demonstrates its localization to hematopoietic, vascular, and neural tissues. *Blood* **94:** 3754–3763.

Faloon P., Arentson E., Kazarov A., Deng C.X., Porcher C., Orkin S., and Choi K. 2000. Basic fibroblast growth factor positively regulates hematopoietic development. *Development* **127:** 1931–1941.

Fong G.H., Klingensmith J., Wood C.R., Rossant J., and Breitman M.L. 1996. Regulation of flt-1 expression during mouse embryogenesis suggests a role in the establishment of vascular endothelium. *Dev. Dyn.* **207:** 1–10.

Garcia-Porrero J.A., Godin I.E., and Dieterlen-Lièvre F. 1995. Potential intraembryonic hemogenic sites at pre-liver stages in the mouse. *Anat. Embryol.* **192:** 425–435.

Gehling U.M., Ergün S., Schumacher U., Wagener C., Pantel K., Otte M., Schuch G., Schafhausen P., Mende T., Kilic N., Kluge K., Schäfer B., Hossfeld D.K., and Fiedler W. 2000. In vitro differentiation of endothelial cells from AC133-positive progenitor cells. *Blood* **95:** 3106–3112.

Geiger H., Sick S., Bonifer C., and Müller A.M. 1998. Globin gene expression is reprogrammed in chimeras generated by injecting adult hematopoietic stem cells into mouse blastocysts. *Cell* **93:** 1055–1065.

Gering, M., Rodaway A.R., Gottgens B., Patient R.K., and Green A.R. 1998. The *SCL* gene specifies haemangioblast development from early mesoderm. *EMBO J.* **17:** 4029–4045.

Godin I., Dieterlen-Lièvre F., and Cumano A. 1995. Emergence of multipotent hemopoietic cells in the yolk sac and paraaortic splanchnopleura in mouse embryos, beginning at 8.5 days postcoitus. *Proc. Natl. Acad. Sci.* **92:** 773–777.

Godin I., Garcia-Porrero J.A., Dieterlen-Lièvre F., and Cumano A. 1999. Stem cell emergence and hemopoietic activity are incompatible in mouse intraembryonic sites. *J. Exp. Med.* **190:** 43–52.

Godin I.E., Garcia-Porrero J.A., Coutinho A., Dieterlen-Lièvre F., and Marcos M.A. 1993. Para-aortic splanchnopleura from early mouse embryos contains B1a cell progenitors. *Nature* **364:** 67–70.

Haar J.L., and Ackerman G.A. 1971. A phase and electron microscopic study of vasculogenesis and erythropoiesis in the yolk sac of the mouse. *Anat. Rec.* **170:** 199–223.

Hamaguchi I., Huang X.L., Takakura N., Tada J., Yamaguchi Y., Kodama H., and Suda T. 1999. In vitro hematopoietic and endothelial cell development from cells expressing TEK receptor in murine aorta-gonad-mesonephros region. *Blood* **93:** 1549–1556.

Hara T., Nakano Y., Tanaka M., Tamura K., Sekiguchi T., Minehata K., Copeland N.G., Jenkins N.A., Okabe M., Kogo H., Mukouyama Y., and Miyajima A. 1999. Identification of podocalyxin-like protein 1 as a novel cell surface marker for hemangioblasts in the murine aorta-gonad-mesonephros region. *Immunity* **11:** 567–578.

Jaffredo T., Gautier R., Eichmann A., and Dieterlen-Lièvre F. 1998. Intraaortic hemopoietic cells are derived from endothelial cells during ontogeny. *Development* **125:** 4575–4583.

Kabrun N., Buhring H.J., Choi K., Ullrich A., Risau W., and Keller G. 1997. Flk-1 expression defines a population of early embryonic hematopoietic precursors. *Development* **124:** 2039–2048.

Kallianpur A.R., Jorda J.E., and Brandt S.J. 1994. The SCL/Tal-1 gene is expressed in progenitors of both the hematopoietic and vascular systems during embryogenesis. *Blood* **83:** 1200–1208.

Keller G. 1995. In vitro differentiation of embryonic stem cells. *Curr. Opin. Cell Biol.* **7:** 862–869.

Keller G., Kennedy M., Papayannopoulou T., and Wiles M. 1993. Hematopoietic commitment during embryonic stem cell differentiation in culture. *Mol. Cell. Biol.* **13:** 473–486.

Kennedy M., Firpo M., Choi K., Wall C., Robertson S., Kabrun N., and Keller G. 1997. A common precursor for primitive erythropoiesis and definitive haematopoiesis. *Nature* **386:** 488–493.

Kinder S.J., Tsang T.E., Quinlan G.A., Hadjantonakis A.K., Nagy A., and Tam P.P. 1999. The orderly allocation of mesodermal cells to the extraembryonic structures and the anteroposterior axis during gastrulation of the mouse embryo. *Development* **126:** 4691–4701.

Liao E.C., Paw B.H., Oates A.C., Pratt S.J., Postlethwait J.H., and Zon L.I. 1998. SCL/tal-1 transcription factor acts downstream of *cloche* to specify hematopoietic and vascular progenitors in zebrafish. *Genes Dev.* **12:** 621–626.

Lindenbaum M.H. and Grosveld F. 1990. An in vitro globin gene switching model based on differentiated embryonic stem cells. *Genes Dev.* **4:** 2075–2085.

Medvinsky A.L., Samoylina N.L., Müller A.M., and Dzierzak E.A. 1993. An early pre-liver intra-embryonic source of CFU-S in the developing mouse. *Nature* **364:** 64–67.

Metcalf D., and Moore M. 1971. Haemopoietic cells. In *Frontiers in biology* (eds. A. Neuberger and E.L. Tatum), North-Holland Publishing, London, United Kingdom.

Millauer B., Wizigmann-Voos S., Schnurch H., Martinez R., Moller N.P., Risau W., and Ullrich A. 1993. High affinity VEGF binding and developmental expression suggest Flk-1 as a major regulator of vasculogenesis and angiogenesis. *Cell* **72:** 835–846.

Moore M. and Metcalf D. 1970. Ontogeny of the hematopoietic system: Yolk sac origin of in vivo and in vitro colony forming cells in the developing mouse embryo. *Br. J. Hematol.* **18:** 279–296.

Müller A.M., Medvinsky A., Strouboulis J., Grosveld F., and Dzierzak E. 1994. Development of hematopoietic stem cell activity in the mouse embryo. *Immunity* **1:** 291–301.

Murray P.D.F. 1932. The development in vitro of the blood of the early chick embryo. *Proc. Roy. Soc.* **111:** 497–521.

Nakano T., Kodama H., and Honjo T. 1994. Generation of lymphohematopoietic cells from embryonic stem cells in culture. *Science* **265:** 1098–1101.

Nishikawa S.I., Nishikawa S., Hirashima M., Matsuyoshi N., and Kodama H. 1998a. Progressive lineage analysis by cell sorting and culture identifies FLK1$^+$VE-cadherin$^+$ cells at a diverging point of endothelial and hemopoietic lineages. *Development* **125:** 1747–1757.

Nishikawa S.I., Nishikawa S., Kawamoto H., Yoshida H., Kizumoto M., Kataoka H., and Katsura Y. 1998b. In vitro generation of lymphohematopoietic cells from endothelial cells purified from murine embryos. *Immunity* **8:** 761–769.

North T., Gu T.L., Stacy T., Wang Q., Howard L., Binder M., Marin-Padilla M., and Speck N.A. 1999. *Cbfa2* is required for the formation of intra-aortic hematopoietic clusters. *Development* **126:** 2563–2575.

Orkin S. 1992. GATA-binding transcription factors in hematopoietic cells. *Blood* **80:** 575–581.

Palis J., Robertson S., Kennedy M., Wall C., and Keller G. 1999. Development of erythroid and myeloid progenitors in the yolk sac and embryo proper of the mouse. *Development* **126:** 5073–5084.

Pardanaud L., Luton D., Prigent M., Bourcheix L.M., Catala M., and Dieterlen-Lièvre F. 1996. Two distinct endothelial lineages in ontogeny, one of them related to hemopoiesis. *Development* **122:** 1363–1371.

Porcher C., Swat W., Rockwell K., Fujiwara Y., Alt F. W., and Orkin S.H. 1996. The T cell leukemia oncoprotein SCL/tal-1 is essential for development of all hematopoietic lineages. *Cell* **86:** 47–57.

Risau W., and Flamme I. 1995. Vasculogenesis. *Annu. Rev. Cell. Dev. Biol.* **11:** 73–91.

Risau W., Sariola H., Zerwes H. G., Sasse J., Ekblom P., Kemler R., and Doetschman T. 1988. Vasculogenesis and angiogenesis in embryonic-stem-cell-derived embryoid bodies. *Development* **102:** 471–478.

Robb L., Lyons I., Li R., Hartley L., Kontgen F., Harvey R. P., Metcalf D., and Begley C.G. 1995. Absence of yolk-sac hematopoiesis from mice with a targeted disruption of the scl gene. *Proc. Natl. Acad. Sci.* **92:** 7075–7079.

Robertson S.M., Kennedy M., Shannon J.M., and Keller G. 2000. A transitional stage in the commitment of mesoderm to hematopoiesis requiring the transcription factor SCL/tal-1. *Development* **127:** 2447–2459.

Russel E. 1979. Hereditary anemias of the mouse: A review for geneticists. *Adv. Genet.* **20:** 357–459.

Sabin F.R. 1920. Studies on the origin of blood vessels and of red corpuscles as seen in the living blastoderm of the chick during the second day of incubation. *Contrib. Embryol.* **9:** 213–262.

Schmitt R., Bruyns E., and Snodgrass H. 1991. Hematopoietic development of embryonic stem cells in vitro: Cytokine and receptor gene expression. *Genes Dev.* **5:** 728–740.

Schuh A.C., Faloon P., Hu Q.L., Bhimani M., and Choi K. 1999. In vitro hematopoietic and endothelial potential of *flk-1*$^{(-/-)}$ embryonic stem cells and embryos. *Proc. Natl. Acad. Sci.* **96:** 2159–2164.

Shalaby F., Rossant J., Yamaguchi T.P., Gertsenstein M., Wu X.F., Breitman M.L., and Schuh A.C. 1995. Failure of blood-island formation and vasculogenesis in Flk-1-deficient mice. *Nature* **376:** 62–66.

Shalaby F., Ho J., Stanford W.L., Fischer K.D., Schuh A.C., Schwartz L., Bernstein A., and Rossant J. 1997. A requirement for Flk1 in primitive and definitive hematopoiesis and vasculogenesis. *Cell* **89:** 981–990.

Shivdasani R., Mayer E., and Orkin S.H. 1995. Absence of blood formation in mice lacking the T-cell leukemia oncoprotein tal-1/SCL. *Nature* **373:** 432–434.

Stainier D.Y., Weinstein B.M., Detrich III, H.W., Zon L.I., and Fishman M.C. 1995. *cloche*, an early acting zebrafish gene, is required by both the endothelial and hematopoietic lineages. *Development* **121:** 3141–3150.

Takakura N., Huang X., Naruse T., Hamaguchi I., Dumont D.J., Yancopoulos G.D., and Suda T. 1998. Critical role of the TIE2 endothelial cell receptor in the development of definitive hematopoiesis. *Immunity* **9:** 677–686.

Tavian M., Coulombel L., Luton D., Clemente H.S., Dieterlen-Lièvre F., and Peault B. 1996. Aorta-associated CD34$^+$ hematopoietic cells in the early human embryo. *Blood* **87:** 67–72.

Traber M.G., Defendi V., and Kayden H.J. 1981. Receptor activities for low-density lipoprotein and acetylated low-density lipoprotein in a mouse macrophage cell line (IC21) and in human monocyte-derived macrophages. *J. Exp. Med.* **154:** 1852–1867.

Tsai F.Y., Keller G., Kuo F.C., Weiss M., Chen J., Rosenblatt M., Alt F.W., and Orkin S.H. 1994. An early haematopoietic defect in mice lacking the transcription factor GATA-2. *Nature* **371:** 221–226.

Visvader J.E., Fujiwara Y., and Orkin S.H. 1998. Unsuspected role for the T-cell leukemia protein SCL/tal-1 in vascular development. *Genes Dev.* **12:** 473–479.

Vittet D., Prandini M.H., Berthier R., Schweitzer A., Martin-Sisteron H., Uzan G., and Dejana E. 1996. Embryonic stem cells differentiate in vitro to endothelial cells through successive maturation steps. *Blood* **88:** 3424–3431.

Voyta J.C., Via D.P., Butterfield C.E., and Zetter B.R. 1984. Identification and isolation of endothelial cells based on their increased uptake of acetylated-low density lipoprotein. *J. Cell Biol.* **99:** 2034–2040.

Wang R., Clark R., and Bautch V.L. 1992. Embryonic stem cell-derived cystic embryoid bodies form vascular channels: An in vitro model of blood vessel development. *Development* **114:** 303–316.

Watt S.M., Gschmeissner S.E., and Bates P.A. 1995. PECAM-1: Its expression and function as a cell adhesion molecule on hemopoietic and endothelial cells. *Leuk. Lymphoma* **17:** 229–244.

Weiss M., Keller G., and Orkin S. 1994. Novel insights into erythroid development revealed through in vitro differentiation of GATA-1$^-$ embryonic stem cells. *Genes Dev.* **8:** 1184–1197.

Wiles M., and Keller G. 1991. Multiple hematopoietic lineages develop from embryonic stem (ES) cells in culture. *Development* **111:** 259–267.

Wong P., Chung S., Chui D., and Eaves C. 1986. Properties of the earliest clonogenic hemopoietic precursor to appear in the developing murine yolk sac. *Proc. Natl. Acad. Sci.* **83:** 3851–3854.

Wood H.B., May G., Healy L., Enver T., and Morriss-Kay G.M. 1997. CD34 expression patterns during early mouse development are related to modes of blood vessel formation and reveal additional sites of hematopoiesis. *Blood* **90:** 2300–2311.

Yoder M.C., Hiatt K., Dutt P., Mukherjee P., Bodine D.M., and Orlic D. 1997. Characterization of definitive lymphohematopoietic stem cells in the day 9 murine yolk sac. *Immunity* **7:** 335–344.

Young P.E., Baumhueter S., and Lasky L.A. 1995. The sialomucin CD34 is expressed on hematopoietic cells and blood vessels during murine development. *Blood* **85:** 96–105.

Ziegler B.L., Valtieri M., Porada G.A., De Maria R., Muller R., Masella B., Gabbianelli M., Casella I., Pelosi E., Bock T., Zanjani E.D., and Peschle C. 1999. KDR receptor: A key marker defining hematopoietic stem cells. *Science* **285:** 1553–1558.

16

Mesenchymal Stem Cells of Human Adult Bone Marrow

Mark F. Pittenger
Osiris Therapeutics Inc.
Baltimore, Maryland 21231

Daniel R. Marshak
Cambrex Corp.
Walkersville, Maryland 21793 and
Johns Hopkins School of Medicine
Baltimore, Maryland 21205

We define stem cells broadly as those cells that give rise to progeny with more than one differentiated phenotype and that may be greatly expanded in an undifferentiated form. This differs from a "progenitor cell," which gives rise to a single cell lineage only. Human mesenchymal stem cells (hMSCs) are isolated from bone marrow and expanded ex vivo. Flow cytometry using many different surface markers has demonstrated the expanded population to be >98% homogeneous and in defined in vitro assays these cells readily differentiate to multiple connective tissue lineages, including osteoblasts, chondrocytes, and adipocytes (Fig. 1) (Pittenger et al. 1999). In vivo implantation of these cells at orthotopic sites will also yield tissues in these lineages. Additionally, cultured hMSCs either produce, or can be induced to produce, cytokines for support of hematopoietic cells (Majumdar et al. 1998; Cheng et al. 2000). Cocultures of the MSCs with hematopoietic stem cells (HSCs) demonstrated that hMSCs or adipogenic hMSCs can support the in vitro maintenance, and even expansion, of HSCs, suggesting hMSCs serve as functional stroma (Thiede et al. 2000). In addition, conditions that produce myogenic differentiation of rat MSCs have been reported (Saito et al. 1995), and hMSCs show similar behavior but perhaps less efficiently. MSCs with similar potential have been isolated from other species as well, and those isolated from rabbits differentiated to tenocytes to produce a suitable replacement for severed tendon with excellent biome-

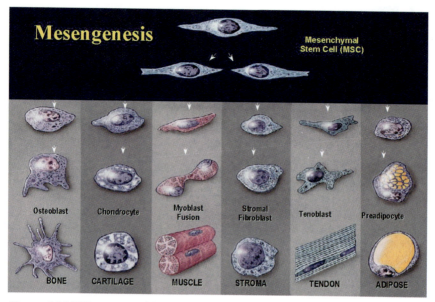

Figure 1 hMSCs are capable of differentiating into multiple mesenchymal lineages. This diagram depicts the lineages into which hMSCs have been shown to differentiate and shows that the cells move through stages of differentiation that involve several layers of commitment and alterations in gene expression before becoming a mature differentiated cell type.

chanical stability (Young et al. 1998). The rabbit MSCs were also shown to form suitable cartilaginous grafts when implanted in defects in the femoral condyle (Wakitani et al.1994). We therefore refer to the adherent, marrow-derived human cells which can be expanded ex vivo as a homogeneous population shown to give rise to multiple differentiated connective cell types, as human mesenchymal stem cells (hMSCs), a term first used by Arnold Caplan (1991). In this chapter, we present a discussion of the development of hMSC technology and offer some perspectives for the future.

HISTORICAL BACKGROUND

Medical interest in the mechanisms of wound healing is long-standing. The body's limited ability to regenerate damaged tissue has engendered interest in the nature of cells involved in wound repair. The appearance of a repair blastema in the amputated amphibian, the remodeling granulation tissue familiar to the surgeon, and the bone callus formation that follows a fracture all involve extensive expansion of unstructured disorganized cells, followed by a period of remodeling. Historically, experimental research for the purpose of defining the cellular events that occur at a wound site have been conducted for well over a century. Early experimental work was limited to histology and microscopic observation of repairing or transplanted tissues, because tissue culture methods were quite limited.

Very early, it was recognized that there were at least two classes of cells at a wound—blood cells and fibroblasts. Leukocyte diapedesis, the movement of cells out of blood vessels and into tissues, was proposed to be a source of repair cells (Cohnheim 1890), but other researchers maintained that repair cells arose from within the damaged tissue. Early this century, Marchand (1901) described in detail the histological changes that take place during wound healing, and local, tissue-dwelling, inactive fibroblasts referred to as fibrocytes were implicated to contribute to regenerating connective tissues (Maximow 1928). Other investigators have reviewed and updated what is known of the cellular events in a regenerating wound (see Arey 1936; Harvey 1949; Allgöwer 1956). In experimental work on new bone formation, Huggins (1931) described the generation of bone when fascia tissue was transplanted to the bladder epithelium. The histology revealed new bone tissue, again raising the question of which cell types were responsible for the new tissue. Cell-based experimentation prior to established cell culture methods and antibiotics was limited, and a lack of standardized reagents, such as antibodies for cell characterization, was another obstacle in early studies of tissue regeneration. Nevertheless, many of the concepts and fundamental questions about regenerative healing, dedifferentiation of functional cells, and the mobilization of quiescent resident cells had been framed by the early part of the 20th century.

Experiments on the biological effects of radiation gave clues to potential sources of regenerative cells. The experiments of Jacobson et al. (1949) showed that shielding the spleen from radiation allowed the survival of lethally irradiated animals. Subsequently, it was shown that a similar effect could be achieved by providing an injection of spleen or bone marrow cells to the irradiated animals, thus preventing hematological insufficiency (Lorenz et al. 1951). Such work continued through the 1960s and 1970s, leading to the development of therapeutic bone marrow transplantation (for review, see Thomas and Blume 1999). The identification and characterization of the transplantable cells in bone marrow responsible for survival implicated the nonadherent, hematopoietic stem cells as necessary to provide the functional myeloid and lymphoid lineage cells needed throughout the life of an individual (Chapter 13). These experiments demonstrated that bone marrow contained regenerative cells for the hematopoietic system but did not address the source of cells for connective tissue regeneration. This work also suggested that, in adult mammals, stem cells responsible for connective tissue regeneration are distinct from hematopoietic stem cells.

Early experimental evidence that a multipotential connective tissue stem cell exists and could be isolated and cultured from mammalian tissue came from mouse studies. In these experiments, testes-derived murine teratomas were transplanted into the peritoneal cavity of recipient mice (Stevens 1959). Here the transplanted tissue formed organized embryoid bodies containing a variety of tissue types. Stevens pursued the cells that could produce these teratomas and identified the primordial germ cells of the genital ridge as the source of the cells (Stevens 1970). These cells were the first cells to be named pluripotent embryonic stem cells, later referred to more commonly as embryonal carcinoma (EC) cells. These EC cells were propagated as an ascites tumor for many years. Mintz and Illmensee (1975) injected these EC cells into developing blastocysts and, remarkably, produced healthy mosaic mice. The cells could be found in most tissues and expressed gene products not previously seen in the teratomas, demonstrating that they retained potential beyond that seen in vitro. The use of teratocarcinomas to study developmental processes has become a well-developed experimental system (see Robertson 1987). The fact that cloned EC cell lines produced multiple types of mesenchymal tissues also suggested the presence of a normal mammalian cell with the potential to differentiate to multiple mesenchymal lineages.

Other experiments performed in the 1950s and 1960s, involving the transplantation of whole bone marrow to ectopic sites, demonstrated the dramatic osteogenic potential of cells from this tissue (Urist and McLean 1952; Tavassoli and Crosby 1968). Bone marrow stroma is a well-organized sinusoidal tissue composed of several cell types. It is found throughout the medullary cavities of long bones, vertebral spongiosa, hip bone, and ribs and forms one of the largest tissues in the body. At the time of this research, scientists had not cultured cells from bone marrow for the generation of differentiated cells and tissue.

Alexander Friedenstein and colleagues pursued the isolation of the bone marrow cells responsible for this osteogenic response. In a series of papers, they reported the characterization of fibroblast colony-forming cells (FCFC) from the bone marrow of guinea pig (Friedenstein et al. 1966, 1968, 1970; Friedenstein 1976). These cells could be cultured in vitro and were subsequently tested in vivo for their osteogenic potential. The cultured population of fibroblastic cells was placed into diffusion chambers, to rule out the host tissue as a source of progenitor cells, and implanted intraperitoneally. Following several weeks of in vivo culture, the researchers were able to demonstrate histologically that the cultured fibroblastic marrow cells gave rise to bone. They were able to attribute the ectopic osteogenesis to the bone marrow cells and termed them osteogenic precursor cells (OPCs). Thus, fibroblastic, adherent bone marrow cells were recognized to form bone.

Prominent work by Maureen Owen and colleagues further developed this concept. These researchers isolated rabbit bone marrow stromal cells and consistently showed the generation of bone and cartilage in diffusion chambers implanted intraperitoneally in host animals (Ashton et al. 1980). The osteocytes and chondrocytes derived from the cultured bone marrow fibroblasts were indistinguishable in appearance from those found in the skeleton in vivo. Many believed that the presence of cartilage with bone was indicative of osteogenic activity, rather than separate activities.

At about this time, Castro-Malaspina et al. (1980) isolated FCFC from human bone marrow and characterized their in vitro characteristics. The human fibroblastic marrow cells had strong adherence properties, similar to bone marrow monocytes, but were not phagocytic, and were therefore distinguished from macrophages. Culturing with tritiated thymidine of high specific activity immediately after attachment failed to reduce the number of cell colonies, showing that, at isolation, the cells were not actively cycling. The marrow fibroblasts did not produce factor VIII, basement membrane collagen, Weibel-Palade bodies, or growth factors supporting granulocytes and macrophages, thus distinguishing them from endothelial cells. Their cellular characterization substantiated for human bone marrow fibroblasts, also called colony forming units-fibroblastic (CFU-F), many of the findings of cells from guinea pig and rabbit bone marrow. However, they did not investigate the differentiation of the isolated CFU-F.

The stem cells of the bone marrow stroma are generally thought to be in a resting state and have a low turnover. As well as stem cells, it is thought that bone marrow contains committed progenitor cells for specific cell types that take part in tissue renewal. There may be situations where trauma stimulates tissue regeneration. As Friedenstein points out, there is a special problem in identifying stem cells in resting marrow, as well as in regenerating tissues where stem cells and progenitor cells in the microenvironment both take part in the renewal process (Friedenstein 1976). The histology tools remain largely inadequate to distinguish stem cell parent and immediate offspring in most tissues. Exceptions to this are epithelial tissue, such as skin, and the intestinal brush border, where the organized position of cells explains their history (see Chapters 19 and 22).

MARROW STROMAL CELLS OR MESENCHYMAL STEM CELLS

Bone marrow stroma is a complex tissue with the function of supporting hematopoiesis. It encompasses a number of cell types and maintains the undifferentiated HSC and supports differentiation of erythroid, myeloid, and lymphoid lineages. There are adherent macrophages and other mononuclear cells of hematopoietic lineage, including some phagocytic cells and other antigen-presenting (dendritic) cells. There are mesenchymal cells, such as osteoblasts, adipoblasts, and more differentiated forms of these. There are endothelial cells, which may arise from a hemangioblast or other endothelial cell precursor. Bone marrow stroma promotes cellular differentiation to these specific lineages while also maintaining stem and progenitor cells. For example, erythrocytes and megakaryocytes are actively produced in bone marrow stroma, whereas many mesenchymal tissues, such as muscle, tendon, ligament, and articular cartilage, are not produced here. Therefore, bone marrow may actively maintain the undifferentiated state of HSCs and MSCs. "Marrow stromal cells" infers a complex mixture of uncharacterized cells. Therefore, the name human mesenchymal stem cell or hMSC more accurately reflects the potential of the isolated, culture-expanded cells we study.

Over the years, a number of investigators have isolated and cultured fibroblastic cells from bone marrow, and the name marrow stromal cell has been used frequently. Although the source may be the bone marrow, it is important to characterize the isolated cells, and it is unlikely that all fibroblastic cells grown from bone marrow are either marrow stromal cells or mesenchymal stem cells. These names imply functional roles that need to be demonstrated, in order to properly define their cellular phenotype or potential. The identity or interrelated nature of cells isolated in different labs should be tested with the same methods and reagents, to the extent possible.

SURFACE MARKERS ON hMSCs

The expression of cell-surface proteins is often used in the characterization of different cell types. These surface molecules are variously responsible for hetero- and homotypic interactions among cell types and also serve as receptors for growth factors, cytokines, or extracellular matrices. We have extensively analyzed the expression of cell-surface receptors on hMSCs by reverse transcriptase-polymerase chain reaction (RT-PCR) analysis of mRNA and confirmed the results by flow cytometry. Many classes of cell surface molecules were present, and a partial list of hMSC surface molecules is shown in Figure 2. The absence of certain surface molecules also helps to characterize the hMSCs. Notable is the lack of expression on the culture-expanded hMSCs of the hematopoietic markers CD14, CD34, and CD45, or the endothelial markers von Willebrand factor and P-selectin. Although no specific surface molecule has been found

Cytokine Receptors
 IL-1R, IL-3R, IL-4R, IL-6R, IL-7R

Extracellular Matrix Receptors
 ICAM-1, ICAM-2, VCAM-1, ALCAM, Endoglin, Hyaluonate Receptor
 Integrins α1, α2, α3, αA, αV, β1, β2, β3, β4

Growth Factor Receptors
 BFGFR, PDGFR

Other Receptors
 Thy-1, IFNγR, TGFβR, TNFR

Figure 2 hMSC surface markers. The expression of surface molecules on hMSCs was first tested by RT-PCR and then confirmed by using fluorescent antibodies and flow cytometry. This is a partial list of positive results.

that unequivocally identifies the hMSC, the list of surface molecules gives clues to the signals and interactions that may stimulate responses and cellular differentiation.

CLONAL GROWTH OF MSCs

The intrinsic growth potential of MSCs has been investigated by analyzing the clonal growth of the isolated marrow cells. CFU-F is probably the most commonly used name associated with clonal studies of marrow-derived cells, but other names have been used, including FCFC, OPC, and marrow stromal cell. It has been recognized that explanted marrow stromal cells attached to a culture surface establish colonies only slowly (several days). This may happen for several reasons: the cells being quiescent initially upon explantation, or needing to overcome the explant stress or adjust to in vitro culture conditions. Perhaps there is a negative cell cycle regulator present in the dormant MSC in situ that must undergo turnover before rounds of mitosis can begin in the explanted cells. Explant cultures of bone marrow stroma may contain small groups of cells that are initially dormant, but which then begin rapid proliferation (Friedenstein 1976). Data presented recently also demonstrated that at low cell densities, single hMSCs in culture may undergo apoptotic cell death prior to colony formation (Van den Bos et al.1998). Therefore, there may be autocrine and paracrine factors produced by hMSCs, or elements of the stromal environment in situ, that provide survival signals to the cells. Apoptosis is an important and normal process in mesenchymal cells during embryonic development and is known to occur during digit development and endochondral ossification (Zou and Niswander 1996; Amling et al. 1997).

Despite the possibility of apoptotic events, many researchers have isolated clones of marrow stromal cells in order to study their intrinsic properties. Colony formation by marrow stromal cells has been extensively studied in guinea pig and rabbit (Friedenstein et al. 1970; Friedenstein 1976; Ashton et al. 1980; Owen et al. 1987; Owen and Friedenstein 1988). Clonal analysis of rabbit marrow stromal cells indicated epidermal growth factor would increase colony size and reduce the spontaneous expression of the osteogenic marker alkaline phosphatase (Owen et al. 1987). A number of investigators have found difficulty in isolating homogeneous populations of mouse MSCs while Phinney and coworkers have reported on their success with certain strains of mice (Phinney et al. 1999). Using serum-deprived conditions, dexamethasone and L-ascorbate were found to be required for colony formation of human bone marrow-derived stromal cells, and their growth was most responsive to platelet-derived growth factor and epidermal growth factor (Gronthos and Simmons 1995). Quarto and colleagues demonstrated that their primary cultures of human osteogenic precursors (referred to as bone marrow stromal cells) grown in the presence of FGF-2 expanded faster and retained a strong osteogenic phenotype (Martin et al. 1997). Robey and colleagues isolated 34 individual clones from marrow-derived cells and utilized in vivo differentiation to evaluate their osteogenic potential (Kuznetsov et al. 1997). These investigators found that 20 clones, or 58%, produced bone after 8 weeks when seeded onto porous ceramic carriers and implanted, suggesting that perhaps not all human CFU-F from bone marrow will become osteocytes.

We demonstrated that cells isolated from bone marrow were homogeneous for multiple surface receptors and that they would differentiate with high fidelity to either the osteogenic, adipogenic, or chondrogenic lineages. Other experiments demonstrated that these cells could serve a stroma role for the support of HSCs. However, there was still the formal possibility that unrecognized subpopulations of cells were giving rise to the differentiated phenotypes. Therefore, we utilized clonally derived hMSCs and the osteogenic, adipogenic, and chondrogenic differentiation assays to demonstrate that clonally derived hMSCs undergo differentiation to these three lineages. Of 6 clonally derived populations that were tested, 3, or 50%, of these differentiated to all three lineages, whereas 2 went to the adipo and osteo lineages, and 1 became osteogenic. That at least half of the highly expanded cell populations went to all three lineages established that they were derived from true multipotential stem cells for at least these mesenchymal lineages (Pittenger et al. 1999) and warrant the name human mesenchymal stem cells. The fact that not all clonally derived populations differentiated to the three lineages may be due to many factors related to clonal expansion and the very late passage number of these highly expanded cells, and further improvements may be possible. In other experiments utilizing clonally derived hMSCs, Seuven and colleagues noted that all 24 clonally derived populations analyzed were osteogenic, 16 of them also showed adipogenic differentiation, and 12 of these were chondrogenic as well (C. Halleux et al., pers. comm.).

Colony-forming ability of hMSCs has been used to assess propagation and predict their differentiation ability (DiGirolamo et al. 1999). Interestingly, the initial growth rate of some marrow-derived progenitor cells was seen to be affected by the plating density, and very low cell density gave a rapid expansion of at least some cells (Colter et al. 2000).

As stem cells, hMSCs can be expanded many fold and retain their ability to differentiate. Expanding a single hMSC to one million cells represents 21 population doublings, and the progeny of at least some of the cells initiating colonies retain their multipotentiality. We have analyzed the karyotype of passage12 hMSCs that have undergone ~30 population doublings and found no chromosomal aberrations. Can hMSCs be expanded indefinitely? Currently, there are limitations on the expansion of hMSCs, as noticed in the slowing of their overall growth rate and changes in the population of these highly expanded cells, the emergence of large flattened cells that do not appear to divide. Whether conditions can be found that allow unlimited expansion of hMSCs remains to be determined. However, for research or clinical purposes, it is not necessary, as large numbers of multipotential hMSCs can be isolated with current procedures. We have used a 25-ml bone marrow aspirate to produce as many as one billion hMSCs by passage 3, and further expansion is certainly possible (Pittenger et al. 1999).

One hypothesis of the aging process and the failure to regenerate damaged tissue in aged individuals is that stem cells are lost as part of aging. Clonal growth also has been used to assess the abundance of progenitor cells in aging populations (Quarto et al. 1995; Oreffo et al. 1998), and formation of CFU-F colonies from bone marrow in these persons appears to be consistent with this decrease in progenitor cells in the later decades of life.

OSTEOGENESIS IN POROUS CERAMIC IMPLANTS

Early experiments using diffusion chambers that excluded the host cells demonstrated that the implanted cultured marrow cells produced the mesenchymal tissues found therein, but the chambers often showed fibrous tissue rather than bone or cartilage. An alternative approach was offered by Caplan and colleagues, who utilized porous ceramic materials composed of hydroxyapatite/tricalcium phosphate similar to normal bone as a vehicle for the cultured cells (Goshima et al. 1989). Ceramic material, on which rat bone marrow-derived cells were seeded, was implanted subcutaneously and consistently produced bone when harvested at 4 weeks or later, and cartilage was sometimes noted as well. Implants with cultured skin or muscle fibroblasts produced only fibrous tissue with no discernible bone or cartilage. A similar assay was utilized to isolate adherent human marrow cells with the potential to form bone and cartilage, enabling further characterization of the human MSC (Haynesworth et al. 1992). Triffitt and colleagues showed that marrow-derived cells implanted on ceramic carriers were reproducibly osteogenic, whereas the cells in their implanted diffusion chambers rarely produced bone unless they were cultured in the presence of dexamethasone (Gundle et al. 1995). Thus, the use of the osteoconductive ceramic implants provided a more reproducible method to characterize properties of the isolated hMSCs and served as an assay for the selection of fetal calf serum that supports the selective growth of hMSCs (Haynesworth et al. 1992; Lennon et al. 1996). We have used the appearance of cartilage and bone in these in vivo implants, as well as results of in vitro chondrogenic, adipogenic, and osteogenic assays, to score fetal bovine serum lots from several vendors. Until a composition of growth factors and cytokines is defined for the in vitro selection and expansion of multipotential hMSCs, this rather tedious method of screening lots of serum will continue.

OSTEOGENIC DIFFERENTIATION OF hMSCs

The culture of bone marrow-derived fibroblastic cells has allowed assessment of their osteogenic potential by using diffusion chambers and implantation. In vitro approaches to osteogenic assessment have been developed as well and allow greater experimental manipulation of the cells under study. Avioli and coworkers isolated human bone marrow stromal cells and tested the effects of dexamethasone on their osteogenic differentiation as measured by the increase in alkaline phosphatase activity, calcium mineralization of the extracellular matrix, and responses to parathyroid hormone (Cheng et al. 1994). Kim et al. (1999) also investigated the dexamethasone response on the secretion of cytokines by marrow-derived osteogenic cells. The responsiveness of the cells to dexamethasone demonstrated the effects that glucocorticoids may have on maturation of osteogenic cells and glucocorticoid-induced bone loss. Bruder and colleagues have investigated the in vitro conditions producing osteogenic differentiation of hMSCs (Jaiswal et al. 1997). They also studied osteogenic differentiation following extensive in vitro cultivation and cyropreservation (Bruder et al. 1997). These studies demonstrated that the hMSCs could be cultivated for more than 35 population doublings before slowing their growth rates or becoming enlarged and flattened, telltale signs of cellular aging. The osteogenic potential of the cells was retained into late culture, suggesting that hMSCs may provide a source of osteoblastic cells over one's lifetime. Furthermore, cyropreservation in liquid nitrogen maintained the differentiation potential of the hMSCs, opening up the potential for an expanded, preserved hMSC preparation for therapeutic purposes.

To test the feasibility of healing a substantial bone defect in vivo, Bruder et al. (1998b) removed a section in the femur of athymic rats and implanted a ceramic carrier seeded with human MSCs. A substantial repair blastema was seen by x-ray, and the healing progressed over 8–12 weeks to create new bone histologically. The hMSC-repaired femurs were subjected to biomechanical torsion testing and found to have excellent mechanical properties.

CHONDROGENIC DIFFERENTIATION OF hMSCs

Formation of cartilage by bone marrow stromal cells was initially demonstrated by placing in-vitro-cultured guinea pig marrow-derived cells in diffusion chambers and implanting them in the peritoneal cavity (Friedenstein et al. 1968). A few of the chambers showed the presence of cartilage histologically. Similarly, the use of ceramic carriers with cultured marrow stromal cells also produced mostly bone with some cartilage. It was suggested that cells in the closed-end pores of the carrier would tend to form cartilage while cells in the interconnected pores favored bone formation. Osteogenic differentiation may be aided by invasion of the carrier by host blood vessels and hematopoietic elements, which does not seem to occur in the dead end pores.

Primary chondrocytes can be isolated from explants of articular cartilage. In culture, chondrocytes lose their characteristic phenotype, lose collagen type II expression, adopt a fibroblastic appearance, and proliferate. Dedifferentiated chondrocytes in culture can be induced to resume a chondrogenic phenotype in vitro by a variety of methods. When applied to the hMSCs, these methods worked poorly. However, Ballock and Reddi (1994) described an effective system for investigating hypertrophic dif-

ferentiation of rat chondrocytes that proved effective for inducing chondrogenic differentiation of rabbit MSCs (Johnstone et al. 1998) or hMSCs
(Barry et al. 1997; Mackay et al. 1998; Yoo et al. 1998). In this method,
the cultured hMSCs are placed in suspension in a polypropylene culture
tube and gently spun in a centrifuge. The hMSCs do not attach to the
polypropylene, but adhere to one another to form a single cell mass after
24 hours that can be resuspended and free-floating. When cultured in a
serum-free medium containing TGFβ3 for 2–3 weeks, the cells express an
extensive extracellular matrix rich in cartilaginous proteoglycans and type
II collagen. Our work initially utilized low-glucose medium for growth as
well as hMSC differentiation to the osteo- or adipogenic lineages.
However, we found that switching from low-glucose (1 g/l) to high-glu-
cose (4.5 g/l) medium in this high-density pellet culture system resulted
in greater cell survival and yielded a consistent and robust chondrogenic
response for hMSCs (Mackay et al. 1998). Moreover, the hMSCs could
be further induced to undergo hypertrophic differentiation, reminiscent of
in vivo events in maturing cartilage. Therefore, whereas osteogenic or
adipogenic differentiation of hMSCs occurs in monolayer culture in the
presence of fetal bovine serum, chondrogenic differentiation conditions

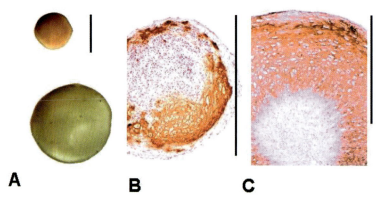

A   **B**   **C**

Figure 3 The hMSCs undergo chondrogenic differentiation in a consolidated
micromass culture. The hMSCs are subjected to gentle centrifugation in a
polypropylene culture tube in a serum-free medium containing 10 nM TGFβ3.
The cells consolidate in about 24 hr to form a cell pellet about 1 mm in diame-
ter, as shown in the upper part of *A*. Over 2–3 weeks, the pellet becomes enlarged
due to the expression and accumulation of chondrocytic extracellular matrix molecules (lower part of *A*). When the pellet is sectioned at about 2 weeks and
stained for the expression of type II collagen (*B*), differentiation begins at several sites. Later, the expression of type II collagen can be seen throughout the cartilaginous cell pellet with the center region the last to differentiate (*C*). Bars in
each panel, 1 mm.

utilize three-dimensional cultures at high cell density, TGFβ3, dexamethasone, and the absence of serum.

It is interesting to note the progression of chondrogenic differentiation of hMSCs in the pelleted cell mass over a 3-week period. As seen in Figure 3, histological sections show there is an outer flattened layer of cells perhaps 5–10 cell layers thick, and inside this layer the cells appear amorphous. The first MSCs to stain positive for type II collagen are the cells that lie at the interface between the outer flattened cells and the amorphous inner cells, and differentiation begins at multiple sites simultaneously. During the first week, there is little change in the size of the cell pellets, but during the second and third weeks of culture, the pellets usually enlarge 2- to 3-fold. Chondrogenesis appears to expand from the sites of initiation. The outer flattened cells, reminiscent of a perichondrium, become positive for type II collagen and the cells at the center appear to be the last to differentiate.

Chondrogenic differentiation in pellet culture is limited to between 50,000 and 300,000 hMSCs, the higher number producing an initial cell mass about 1 mm across. Larger masses tended to fragment. An alternative is to culture the MSCs in an alginate or hyaluronan matrix in the medium described above (K. Kavalkovich and F. Barry, pers. comm.). This method is capable of producing a layer of chondrogenic hMSCs that is amenable to biomechanical testing, as well as biochemical analysis. The robust chondrogenic differentiation of hMSCs in vitro suggests that they will prove useful for the development of therapeutic treatments for cartilage damaged by trauma or disease.

OSTEOGENESIS–ADIPOGENESIS RELATIONSHIP

Adipocytes are mesenchymal in origin. We have investigated the potential of isolated hMSCs to differentiate to this lineage (Pittenger 1998; Pittenger et al. 1999). There is a fascinating relationship between the osteogenic and adipogenic lineages, which has been recognized at the organismal and cellular levels. Virtually all loss of bone is accompanied by an increase in adipose in the bone compartment. For example, long-term medical use of glucocorticoids leads to loss of bone density through the stimulation of bone resorption by osteoclasts and the suppression of bone formation by osteoblasts (Canalis 1996). Stromal culture systems for hematopoietic stem cells contain adipocytes (Dexter 1982), and adipocytes are capable of supporting HSC or myeloid cultures (Gimble 1990; Gimble et al. 1992; Thiede et al. 2000). During aging, there is an increase in fatty marrow, although this is reversible, if there is a physiological need, such as seen upon moving to a higher altitude. Committed progenitor cells such as pre-osteoblasts or pre-adipocytes coexist in bone marrow alongside uncommitted MSCs. This raises the question of the committed nature of progenitor cells and to what level interconversion is possible. Beresford et al. (1992) investigated the plasticity of rodent adipocytes that can dedifferentiate to a proliferative cell that can become osteocytes and produce bone when placed in a diffusion chamber and implanted subcutaneously.

It was recognized by Bianco and colleagues (1988) that human bone marrow cells that were alkaline phosphatase positive, a trait associated with osteogenic cells, were also precursor cells for adipocytes. Individual colonies of rabbit bone marrow cells, presumably clonal in origin, that expressed a lipid-laden adipocytic phenotype were shown to revert to a rapidly growing fibroblastic cell type in the presence of fetal calf serum. These cells were then placed in diffusion chambers and implanted, and when they were harvested at 60 days, subsequent histology in some of the chambers showed the formation of bone (Bennett et al. 1991). Beresford et al. (1992) described the in vitro differentiation of rat marrow stromal cells to both the osteogenic and adipogenic lineages and demonstrated the ability of dexamethasone treatment to alter this ratio. Continuous treatment with the steroid resulted in increased osteogenesis, whereas if steroid was withheld initially, more adipocytes were present. Their results suggested an inverse relationship between the osteogenic and adipogenic pathways for the marrow stromal cells. A role for the bone morphogenetic protein (BMP) receptor subtype has been shown to be involved in the cell fate decision of a murine cell line to become osteoblasts or adipocytes (Chen et al. 1998) and serves as an example of BMP involvement in non-osteogenic morphogenetic pathways (Hogan 1996).

An alternative to the isolation of primary bone marrow stromal cells for study is to immortalize the cells in vitro, such as by transduction with a temperature-sensitive SV40 T antigen (Gimble 1990; Houghton et al. 1998) or isolation from a mutant p53 $^{-/-}$ mouse (Thompson et al. 1998). Then clonal populations of transformed cells can be characterized. Houghton et al. (1998) generated such cell lines from human rib marrow stromal cells and characterized one such cell line, human osteoprogenitor clone 7 (hOP7), which could be propagated indefinitely at the permissive temperature. At the nonpermissive temperature, the hOP7 cells exhibited an osteoblastic phenotype with increased alkaline phosphatase activity and produced a mineralized extracellular matrix. However, when the hOP7 cells were cultured with increasing levels of normal rabbit serum, which contains fatty acids that can stimulate an adipogenic response, the cells exhibited lipid vacuole inclusions and elevated lipoprotein lipase and glycerol 3-phosphate dehydrogenase.

Cells from adult trabecular bone explants were shown to be osteogenic and also adipogenic (Nuttall et al. 1998). The cells expressed alkaline phosphatase and osteocalcin in the presence of vitamin D_3, whereas when treated with dexamethasone and isobutylmethylxanthine (IBMX), the cultures accumulated lipid vacuoles as well as the lipogenic enzymes glycerol-3-phosphate dehydrogenase, lipoprotein lipase, and aP2. To determine whether the results were due to a mixture of osteo- and adipogenic progenitor cells present in the cultures or a population of stem cells with the potential for each lineage, the cells were grown as single-cell clones and tested. The wells containing clonal cells tested positive for elevated osteocalcin in response to vitamin D. When subsequently switched to medium containing dexamethasone and IBMX, the cells accumulated lipid-rich vacuoles, with a near absence of osteocalcin in the medium.

We used clonally isolated hMSCs and demonstrated their differentiation exclusively to the chondrogenic, osteogenic, or adipogenic pathways, depending on the in vitro culture conditions (Pittenger et al. 1999), and we then investigated the signal transduction pathways activated during osteogenic differentiation. We analyzed the role of mitogen-activated protein kinases (MAP kinases) ERK1/ERK 2, p38, and jun N-terminal kinase (JNK) during osteogenic differentiation of hMSCs. These experiments showed a strong correlation between the long-term activation of ERK2 and the osteogenic differentiation of the stem cells (Jaiswal et al. 2000). JNK and p38 likely play roles at later stages of osteogenesis of hMSCs. Interestingly, the inhibition of ERK activation by the MAP kinase kinase (MEK1 or *MAP/ERK k*inases) eliminated osteogenic differentiation and led to a concomitant and dose-dependent increase in adipogenic differentiation (see Fig. 4). This was true using either the specific MEK1 inhibitor PD98059 or transfection with a plasmid containing a dominant negative transgene of MEK1 (Yan and Templeton 1994), ruling out simple nonspecific effects of the PD compound. These signaling pathway studies further our understanding of the interrelationship between the osteoblastic and adipocytic lineages, and they suggest a role that hMSCs may play during imbalances that lead to clinical manifestations, such as osteoporosis.

EVIDENCE FOR A STROMAL FUNCTION FOR hMSCs

The hMSCs present in bone marrow are in intimate contact with HSCs and their presumed progeny. The hMSCs have also been shown to produce many factors important for the support of HSCs and their diverse

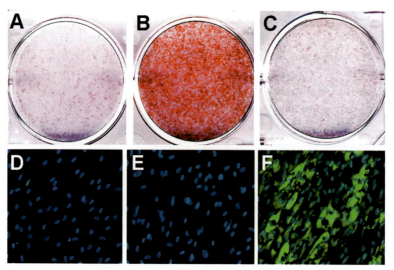

Figure 4 Inhibition of osteogenic differentiation of hMSCs leads to a pathway for adipogenic differentiation. The hMSCs in control wells (*A* and *D*), or hMSCs treated to undergo osteogenic differentiation (*B* and *E*) were compared to wells in which the hMSCs were treated with osteogenic medium containing 50 nM of the MEK1 inhibitor PD98059 (*C* and *F*). Osteogenic differentiation is accompanied by the abundant expression of alkaline phosphatase (*B*), which is not seen in the presence of the inhibitor (*C*). When the hMSCs are stained with the lipophilic dye Nile Red (*D–F*), it can be seen that the inhibitor-treated hMSCs have become adipocytes (*F*).

progeny, including interleukins (IL) IL-6, IL-7, IL-8, IL-11, IL-12, leukemia inhibitory factor, stem cell factor, Flt3 ligand, and macrophage colony-stimulating factor (Haynesworth et al. 1996; Majumdar et al. 1998; Mbalaviele et al. 1999). The hMSCs will produce additional factors in response to IL-1 and most likely other factors as well. Cultured monolayers of hMSCs, without additional cytokines, have been shown to support the maintenance of HSCs, and evidence suggests the expansion of HSCs also occurs in the cocultures (Cheng et al. 2000; Thiede et al. 2000). The therapeutic potential of hMSCs for support of HSC engraftment in patients undergoing bone marrow transplantation is under study in several settings. In early safety trials, patients in remission following treatment for breast cancer were infused with as many as 50 million autologous culture-expanded hMSCs without any adverse effects (Lazarus et al. 1995). Recent phase I–II clinical results have demonstrated the feasibility and safety of isolation of hMSCs and their autologous reinfusion, along with autologous peripheral blood progenitor cells, into advanced breast cancer patients (Koc et al. 2000).

TISSUE REGENERATION BY MSCs

Many years of work on the origins of blood cells led to the concept of the hematopoietic stem cell that could serve as a progenitor for all blood cell types. Lineage diagrams have been developed that present the interrelationship among the HSC progeny. The concept of a similar multipotential bone marrow stem cell for connective tissues was first presented by Owen (1985) and suggested that differentiated cell types found in bone marrow stroma might derive from a common progenitor, or stem cell. This concept was further developed by Caplan to include all of the mesoderm-derived lineages, including myocytes, chondrocytes, tenocytes, osteocytes, and stromal and dermal fibroblasts (Caplan 1991). More recent evidence suggests that the stroma consists of differentiated and undifferentiated cells of several lineages and that hMSCs coexist in bone marrow with progenitor cells with more limited differentiation potential.

The presence of multipotential MSCs in bone marrow is consistent with accumulated data from many labs using multiple species (Aubin et al. 1992; Pereira et al. 1995; Poliard et al. 1995; Young et al. 1995; Dennis et al. 1999; Muraglia et al. 2000). The developmental process of bone formation wherein the cartilaginous anlage is remodeled to bone following the invasion of blood vessels has been extensively studied. The common appearance of bone and/or cartilage in diffusion chambers and implanted ceramic carriers and their association in vivo suggest closely associated pathways of differentiation, although this requires the intervention of vasculature and HSCs as well (for review, see Caplan and Boyan 1994).

The marrow-derived MSCs have been used to demonstrate in vivo repair of mesenchymal tissues in critical size wounds at orthotopic sites. This includes the articular cartilage, in which Wakitani et al. demonstrated cartilage repair in the medial femoral condyle of rabbits. Bruder and Kadiyala have demonstrated MSC-driven regeneration of large segmental gaps of bone in the femurs of rats and dogs (Kadiyala et al. 1997; Bruder et al. 1998a,b). Young and colleagues showed repair of a 1-cm gap in the Achilles tendon of rabbits using MSCs, and they further showed biomechanical stability of those implants (Young et al. 1998). Caplan and coworkers showed integration of MSCs into skeletal muscles of dystrophin-deficient rats, suggesting implants of MSCs might have applications to muscular dystrophy (Saito et al. 1995).

Recently, we have turned our attention to the ability of hMSCs to engraft and differentiate in the adult heart. There are few in vitro models for cardiomyocyte development or differentiation, and therefore it is necessary to utilize in vivo models. We have introduced gene-tagged hMSCs into the hearts of immunodeficient mice through the coronary circulation and found that a percentage of the hMSCs would engraft as single cells surrounded by healthy host cardiomyocytes. The hMSCs persisted for at least 2 months. Over time, the morphology of the implanted hMSCs became indistinguishable from the surrounding cardiomyocytes, and they began to express the proteins specific for striated muscle, including desmin, α-myosin heavy chain, α-actinin, and phospholamban, at levels that were the same as the host cardiomyocytes. The expression of myoD was not detected, suggesting the cells were not differentiating to a skeletal myocyte but rather to a cardiac myocyte (C. Toma et al., in prep.). Findings were recently published for rat bone marrow stromal cells implanted into isogenic rat hearts showing expression of myosin heavy chain as well as connexin 43, the later suggesting the formation of gap junctions (Wang et al. 2000). To address the question of whether hMSCs will engraft into infarcted tissue, we have implanted cells by direct needle injection into an experimental infarct model in an athymic rat. In this system we find the hMSCs engraft in the infarct region for at least 2 months and show expression of striated muscle proteins. Additional work has begun on the porcine infarct model to develop the methods and techniques needed for human intervention (B.J. Martin et al., in prep.). Although much work remains to be done, results suggest that the hMSCs may differentiate to the cardiomyocyte phenotype and may prove useful for cellular cardiomyoplasty in ischemic or damaged heart tissue.

These demonstrations from several species further indicate that MSCs are indeed stem cells for various mesenchymal tissues. The cells are therefore not simply stromal precursors, but precursors of peripheral tissues, including those that are not vascularized, such as articular cartilage. As noted above, several of the lineages found in bone marrow are not readily evident as progeny of hMSCs, but hMSCs may have broader applications than simply stromal regeneration, and the bone marrow stroma is a complex tissue derived from several types of stem or progenitor cells.

FURTHER CLINICAL IMPLICATIONS FOR THE USE OF hMSCs

Osteogenesis imperfecta (OI) represents a debilitating genetic disease where the chromosomal defect lies in the collagen type I gene that is prominently expressed in osteocytes. Expression of the faulty gene causes systemic osteopenia resulting in bony deformities, skeletal fragility, and short stature. Recently, three infant OI patients were transfused with whole bone marrow from HLA-identical siblings, and the subsequent course of their disease was assessed during a 6-month follow-up (Horwitz et al. 1999). Osteoblasts were isolated from a bone biopsy and showed engraftment of donor mesenchymal cells. These patients had 20–37 fractures in the 6 months prior to infusion, but in the 6 months following transplantation their fractures were reduced to 2 and 3, respectively. All patients had increased total body mineral content. These patients also showed near-normal growth over this period. Although these are early results, they easily convey the promise that stem cell therapy may provide in the future.

Marrow-derived hMSCs represent a useful, easily obtained, characterized cell population to explore mesenchymal tissue regeneration, and there is good evidence to suggest the cells can be used allogeneically. The hMSCs do express small amounts of the major histocompatiblity complex (MHC) class I molecule but express little or no MHC class II or B7 costimulatory molecules. In vitro experiments with lymphocytes from unrelated donors suggest that hMSCs do not elicit proliferation of T cells and may actually suppress a mixed lymphocyte reaction, suggesting the potential for allogeneic use of hMSCs (K. McIntosh, pers. comm.). The lack of a pronounced immunological response to implanted allogeneic hMSCs and the ability to produce large numbers of cells from a small marrow aspirate open the potential to use donor-derived cells for multiple recipients. To this goal, Osiris Therapeutics has undertaken clinical trials for the use of allogeneic hMSCs to aid engraftment of matched bone marrow or mobilized peripheral blood progenitor cells. Phase I results suggest the matched hMSCs are well tolerated, and ongoing Phase II studies will provide appropriate dosage data. The pivotal Phase III multicenter trial will occur in the near future.

Vescovi and colleagues reported the reconstitution of multiple blood lineages by the engraftment of brain-derived murine neural stem cells, although the time to engraftment may have been slightly longer than seen with the use of whole bone marrrow (Bjornson et al. 1999). The recent report of purified mouse muscle satellite cells reconstituting the hematopoietic lineages of a lethally irradiated mouse (Jackson et al. 1999), or the incorporation of donor hematopoietic stem cells into muscle of affected *mdx* mice (Gussoni et al. 1999), draws further attention to the possibility that the cellular plasticity and potential of adult stem cells may be greater than previously thought. These studies, along with the landmark report of the reactivation of somatic nuclei by reinsertion into a blastocyst to produce a cloned organism (Wilmut et al. 1997), suggest the potential of stem cells to broadly contribute to tissue regeneration. Perhaps bone marrow-derived hMSCs will be used to heal not only mesodermal tissues but also ectoderm- and endoderm-derived tissues one day.

ACKNOWLEDGMENTS

We thank our Osiris colleagues and collaborators, past and present, for their interest in developing adult bone marrow-derived stem cell technology as a viable therapeutic approach to connective tissue disorders.

REFERENCES

Allgöwer M. 1956. *The cellular basis of wound repair.* Charles C. Thomas, Springfield, Illinois.
Amling M., Neff L., Tanaka S., Inoue D., Kuida K., Weir E., Philbrick W.M. Broadus A.E., and Baron R. 1997. Bcl-2 lies downstream of parathyroid related peptide in the signaling pathway that regulates chondrocyte maturation during skeletal development. *J. Cell Biol.* **136:** 205–213.
Arey L.B. 1936. Wound healing. *Physiol. Rev.* **16:** 327–405.
Ashton B.A., Allen T.D., Howlett C.R., Eaglesom C.C., Hattori A., and Owen M. 1980. Formation of bone and cartilage by marrow stromal cells in diffusion chambers *in vivo. Clin. Orthop. Relat. Res.* **151:** 294–307.
Aubin J.E., Bellows C.G., Turksen K., Liu F., and Heersche J.N.M. 1992. Analysis of the osteoblast lineage and regulation of differentiation. In *Chemistry and biology of mineralized tissues* (eds. H. Slavkin and P. Price), pp. 267–275. Elsevier, Amsterdam, The Netherlands.
Ballock R.T and Reddi A.H. 1994. Thyroxine is the serum factor that regulates morphogenesis of columnar cartilage from isolated chondrocytes in chemically defined medium. *J. Cell Biol.* **126:** 1311–1320.
Barry F.P., Johnstone B., Pittenger M.F., Mackay A.M., and Murphy J.M. 1997. Modulation of the chondrogenic potential of human bone marrow-derived mesenchymal stem cells by TGFβ$_1$ and TGFβ$_3$. *Trans. Orthop. Res. Soc.* **22:** 228.
Bennett J.H., Joyner C.J., Triffitt J.T., and Owen M.E. 1991. Adipocytic cells cultured from marrow have osteogenic potential. *J. Cell Sci.* **99:** 131–139.
Beresford J.N., Bennett J.H., Devlin C., Leboy P.S., and Owen M.E. 1992 Evidence for an inverse relationship between the differentiation of adipocytes and osteogenic cells in rat marrow stromal cell cultures. *J. Cell Sci.* **102:** 341–351.
Bianco P., Constantini M., Dearden L.C., and Bonucci E. 1988. Alkaline phosphatase positive precursors of adipocytes in the human bone marrow. *Br. J. Haematol.* **68:** 401–403.
Bjornson C.R.R., Rietze R.L., Reynolds B.A., Magli M.C., and Vescovi A.L. 1999. Turning brain into blood: A hematopoietic fate adopted by adult neural stem cells in vivo. *Science* **283:** 534–537.
Bruder S.P, Jaiswal N., and Haynesworth S.E. 1997. Growth kinetics, self-renewal, and osteogenetic potential of purified human mesenchymal stem cells during extensive subcultivation and following cryopreservation. *J. Cell. Biochem.* **64:** 278–294.
Bruder S.P., Kraus K.H., Goldberg V.M., Kadiyala S. 1998a. The effects of implants loaded with autologous mesenchymal stem cells on the healing of canine segmental bone defects. *J. Bone J. Surg. Am. Vol.* **80:** 985–996.
Bruder S.P., Kurth A.A., Shea M., Hayes W.C., Jaiswal N., and Kadiyala S. 1998b. Bone regeneration by implantation of purified, culture-expanded human mesenchymal stem

cells. *J. Orthop. Res.* **16:** 155–162.

Canalis E. 1996. Mechanisms of glucocorticoid action on bone: Implications to glucocorticoid-induced osteoporosis. *J. Clin. Endocrinol. Metab. E.* **81:** 3441–3447.

Caplan A.I. 1991. Mesenchymal stem cells. *J. Orthop. Res.* **9:** 641–650.

Caplan A.I. and Boyan B.D. 1994. Endochonadral bone formation: The lineage cascade. In *Bone: Mechanisms of bone development and growth* (ed. B. Hall), vol. 8, pp. 1–46. CRC Press, Boca Raton, Florida.

Castro-Malaspina H., Gay R.E., Resnick G., Kapoor N., Meyers P., Chiarieri D., Mckenzie S., Broxmeyer H.E., and Moore M.A.S. 1980. Characterization of human bone marrow fibroblast colony-forming cells (CFU-F) and their progeny. *Blood* **56:** 289–301.

Chen D., Ji X., Harris M.A., Feng J.Q., Karsenty G., Celeste A.J., Rosen V., Mundy G.R., and Harris S.E. 1998. Differential roles for bone morphogenetic protein (BMP) receptor type 1B and 1A in differentiation and specification of mesenchymal precursor cells to osteoblast and adipocyte lineages. *J. Cell Biol.* **141:** 295–305.

Cheng L., Qasba P., Vanguri P., and Thiede M.A. 2000. Human mesenchymal stem cells support megakaryocyte and pro-platelet formation from CD34$^+$ hematopoietic progenitor cells. *J. Cell. Physiol.* **184:** 58–69.

Cheng S.-L., Yang J.W., Rifas L., Zhang S.-F., and Avioli L.V. 1994. Differentiation of human bone marrow osteogenic stromal cells in vitro: Induction of the osteoblast phenotpye by dexamethasone. *Endocrinology* **134:** 277–286.

Colter D., Class R., DiGirolamo C.M., and Prockop D.J. 2000. Rapid expansion of recycling stem cells in cultures of plastic-adherent cells from human bone marrow. *Proc. Natl. Acad. Sci.* **97:** 3213–3218.

Cohnheim J. 1890. Lectures on general pathology (English translation). Adlard and Sons, London, United Kingdom.

Dennis J.E., Merriam A., Awadallah A., Yoo J.U., Johnstone B., and Caplan A.I. 1999. A quadripotent mesenchymal progenitor cell isolated from the marrow of mice. *J. Bone Miner. Res.* **14:** 700–709.

Dexter T.M. 1982. Stromal cell associated hematopoiesis. *J. Cell Physiol. (Suppl.)* **1:** 87–94.

DiGirolamo C.M., Stokes D., Colter D., Phinney D.G., Class R., and Prockop D.J. 1999. Propagation and senescence of human marrow stromal cells in culture: A simple colony-forming assay identifies samples with the greatest potential to propagate and differentiate. *Br. J. Haematol.* **107:** 275–281.

Friedenstein A.J. 1976. Precursor cells of mechanocytes. *Int. Rev. Cytol.* **47:** 327–355.

Friedenstein A.J., Chailakhjan R.K., and Lalykina K.S. 1970. The development of fibroblast colonies in monolayer cultures of guinea pig bone marrow and spleen cells. *Cell Tissue Kinet.* **3:** 393–403.

Friedenstein A.J., Piatetzky-Shapiro I.I., and Petrakova K.V. 1966. Osteogenesis in transplants of bone marrow cells. *J. Embryol. Exp. Morphol.* **16:** 381–390.

Friedenstein A.J., Petrakova K.V., Kurolesova A.I., and Frolova G.P. 1968. Heterotopic transplants of bone marrow: Analysis of precursor cells for osteogenic and haematopoietic tissues. *Transplantation* **6:** 230–247.

Gimble J.M. 1990. The function of adipocytes in the marrow stroma. *New Biol.* **2:** 304–312.

Gimble J.M., Youkhana K., Hua X., Bass H., Medina K., Sullivan M., Greenberger J.S., and Wang C.S. 1992. Adipogenesis in a myeloid suppporting bone marrow stroma cell line. *J. Cell. Biochem.* **50:** 73–82.

Goshima J., Goldberg V.M., and Caplan A.I. 1989. The osteogenic potential of culture expanded rat marrow mesenchymal cells as assayed in vivo in calcium phosphate ceramic blocks. *Clin. Orthop. Relat. Res.* **262:** 298–311.

Gronthos S. and Simmons P.J. 1995. The growth factor requirements of STRO-1-positive human bone marrow stromal precursors under serum-deprived conditions in vitro. *Blood* **85:** 929–940.

Gundle R., Joyner C.J., and Triffit J.T. 1995. Human bone tissue formation in diffusion chamber culture in vivo by bone-derived cells and marrow stromal fibroblastic cells. *Bone* **16:** 597–601.

Gussoni E., Soneoka Y., Strickland C.D., Buzney E.A., Khan M.K., Flint A.F., Kunkel L.M., and Mulligan R.C. 1999. Dystrophin expression in the mdx mouse restored by stem cell transplantation. *Nature* **401:** 390–394.

Harvey S.C. 1949. The healing of the wound as a biological phenomenon. *Surgery* **25:** 655–670.

Haynesworth S.E., Baber M.A., and Caplan A.I. 1996. Cytokine expression by human marrow-derived mesenchymal progenitor cells in vitro: Effects of dexamethasone and IL-1α. *J. Cell Physiol.* **166:** 585–592.

Haynesworth S.E., Goshima J., Goldberg V.M., and Caplan A.I. 1992. Characterization of cells with osteogenic potential from human bone marrow. *Bone* **13:** 81–88.

Hogan B.L.M. 1996. Bone morphogenetic proteins: Multifunctional regulators of verte-brate development. *Genes Dev.* **10:** 1580–1594.

Horwitz E.M., Prockop D.J., Fitzpatrick L.A., Koo W.W.K., Gordon P.L., Neel M., Sussman M., Orchard P., Marx J.C., Pyeritz R.E., and Brenner M.K. 1999. Transplantability and therapeutic effects of bone marrow-derived mesenchymal cells in children with osteogenesis imperfecta. *Nat. Med.* **5:** 309–313.

Houghton A., Oyajobi B.O., Foster G.A., Russell R.G., and Stronger B.M.J. 1998. Immortalization of human marrow stromal cells by retroviral transduction with a tem-perature sensitive oncogene: Identification of bipotential precursor cells capable of directed differentiation to either an osteoblast or adipocyte phenotype. *Bone* **22:** 7–16.

Huggins C.B. 1931. The formation of bone under the influence of the epithelium of the urinary tract. *Arch. Surg.* **22:** 377–408.

Jackson K.A., Tiejuan M. and Goddell M.A. 1999. Hematopoietic potential of stem cells isolated from murine skeletal muscle. *Proc. Natl. Acad. Sci.* **96:** 14482–14486.

Jacobson L.O., Marks E.K., Robson M.F., Gaston E.O., and Zirkle R.E. 1949. Effect of spleen protection on mortality following X irradiation. *J. Lab. Clin. Med.* **34:** 1538–1547.

Jaiswal N., Haynesworth S.E., Caplan A.I., and Bruder S.P. 1997. Osteogenic differentia-tion of purified, culture expanded human mesenchymal stem cells in vitro. *J. Cell. Biochem.* **64:** 295–312.

Jaiswal R.K., Jaiswal N., Bruder S.P., Mbalaviele G., Marshak D.R., and Pittenger M.F. 2000. Adult human mesenchymal stem cell differentiation to the osteogenic or adi-pogenic lineage is regulated by mitogen activated protein kinase. *J. Biol. Chem.* **275:** 9645–9652.

Johnstone B., Hering T.M., Caplan A.I. Goldberg V.M., and Yoo J. 1998. In vitro chon-drogenesis of bone marrow-derived mesenchymal progenitor cells. *Exp. Cell Res.* **238:** 265–272.

Kadiyala S., Jaiswal N., and Bruder S.P. 1997. Culture-expanded bone marrow-derived mesenchymal stem cells can regenerate a critical-sized segmental bone defect. *Tissue Eng.* **3:** 173–185.

Kim C.-H., Cheng S.-L., and Kim G.S. 1999. Effects of dexamethasone on proliferation, activity and cytokine secretion of normal human bone marrow stromal cells: Possible mechanisms of glucocorticoid-induced bone loss. *J. Endocrinol.* **162:** 371–379.

Koc O.N., Gerson S.L., Cooper B.W., Dyhouse S.M., Haynesworth S.E., Caplan A.I., and Lazarus H.M. 2000. Rapid hematopoietic recovery after coinfusion of autologous blood stem cells and culture expanded marrow mesenchymal stem cells in advanced breast cancer patients receiving high dose chemotherapy. *J. Clin. Oncol.* **18:** 307–316.

Kuznetsov S.A., Krebsbach P.H., Satomura K., Kerr J., Riminucci M., Benayahu D., and Robey P.G. 1997. Single-colony derived strains of human marrow stromal fibroblasts form bone after transplantation in vivo. *J. Bone Min. Res.* **12:** 1335–1347.

Lazarus H.M., Haynesworth S.E., Gerson S.L., Rosenthal N.S., and Caplan A.I. 1995. Ex vivo expansion and subsequent infusion of human bone marrow derived cells (mesenchymal progenitor cells): Implications for the therapeutic use. *Bone Marrow Transplant* **15:** 935–942.

Lennon D.P., Haynesworth S.E., Bruder S.P., Jaiswal N., and Caplan A.I. 1996. Human and animal mesenchymal progenitor cells from bone marrow: Identification of serum for optimal selection and proliferation. *In Vitro Cell. Dev. Biol.* **32:** 602–611.

Lorenz E., Uphoff D., Reid T.R., and Shelton T. 1951. Modification of irradiation injury in mice and guinea pigs by bone marrow injections. *J. Natl. Cancer Inst.* **12:** 197–201.

Mackay, A.M., Beck S.C., Murphy J.M., Barry F.P., Chichester C.O., and Pittenger M.F. 1998. Chondrogenic differentiation of cultured human mesenchymal stem cells from marrow. *Tissue Eng.* **4:** 415–428.

Majumdar M.K., Thiede M.A., Mosca J.D., Moorman M., and Gerson S.L. 1998. Phenotypic and functional comparison of cultures of marrow-derived mesenchymal stem cells and stromal cells. *J. Cell. Physiol.* **176:** 57–66.

Marchand F. 1901. Der prozess der Wundheilung mit Einschluss der Transplantationen. Enke, Stuttgart.

Martin I., Muraglia A., Campanile G., Cancedda R., and Quarto R. 1997. Fibroblast growth factor-2 supports ex vivo expansion and maintenance of osteogenic precursors from human bone marrow. *Endocrinology* **138:** 4456–4462.

Maximow A. 1928. Cultures of blood leucocytes: From lymphocytes and monocytes to connective tissue. *Arch. Exp. Zellforsch.* **5:** 169–181.

Mbalaviele, G., Jaiswal N., Meng A., Cheng L., van den Bos C., and Theide M. 1999. Human mesenchymal stem cells promote human osteoclast differentiation from $CD34^+$ bone marrow hematopoietic progenitors. *Endocrinology* **140:** 3736–3743.

McCulloch E.A. and Till J.E. 1964. Proliferation of hematopoietic colony-forming cells transplanted into irradiated mice. *Rad. Res.* **22:** 383–387.

Mintz B. and Illmensee K. 1975. Normal genetically mosaic mice produced from malignant teratocarcinoma cells. *Proc. Natl. Acad. Sci.* **72:** 3585–3589.

Muraglia A., Cancedda R., and Quarto R. 2000. Clonal mesenchymal progenitors from human bone marrow differentiate in an hierarchical model. *J. Cell Sci.* **13:** 1161–1166.

Nuttall M.E., Patton, A.J., Oliviera D.L., Nadeau D.P., and Gowen M. 1998. Human trabecular bone cells are able to express both osteoblastic and adipocytic phenotype: Implications for osteopenic disorders. *J. Bone Min. Res.* **13:** 371–382.

Oreffo R.O.C., Bord S., and Triffitt J.T. 1998. Skeletal progenitor cells and ageing human populations. *Clin. Sci.* **94:** 549–555.

Owen M. 1985. Lineage of osteogenic cells and their relationship to the stromal system. In *Bone and mineral research 3* (ed. W.A. Peck) pp. 1–25. Elsevier, Amsterdam, The Netherlands.

Owen M.E. and Friedenstein A.J. 1988. Stromal stem cells: Marrow-derived osteogenic precursors. *Ciba Found. Symp.* **136:** 42–60.

Owen M.E., Cave J., and Joyner C.J. 1987. Clonal analysis in vitro of osteogenic differentiation of marrow CFU-F. *J. Cell Science* **87:** 731–738.

Pereira R.F., Halford K.W., O'Hara M.D., Leeper D.B., Sokolov B.P., Pollard M.D., Bagasra O., and Prockop D.J. 1995. Cultured adherent cells from marrow can serve as long lasting precursor cells for bone, cartilage, and lung in irradiated mice. *Proc. Natl. Acad. Sci.* **92:** 4857–4861.

Phinney D.G., Kopen G., Isaacson R.L., and Prockop D.J. 1999. Plastic adherent stromal cells from the bone marrow of commonly used strains of inbred mice: Variations in yield, growth and differentiation. *J. Cell. Biochem.* **72:** 570–585.

Pittenger M.F. 1998. Adipogenic differentiation of human mesenchymal stem cells. U.S. Patent #5,827,740.

Pittenger M.F., Mackay A.M., Beck S.C., Jaiswal R.K., Douglas R., Mosca J.D., Moorman M.A., Simonetti D.W., Craig S., and Marshak D.R. 1999. Multilineage potential of adult human mesenchymal stem cells. *Science* **284:** 143–147.

Poliard A., Nifuji A., Lamblin D., Plee E., Forest C., and Kellerman O. 1995. Controlled conversion of an immortalized mesodermal progenitor cell towards the osteogenic, chondrogenic, or adipogenic pathways. *J. Cell Biol.* **130:** 1461–1472.

Quarto R.C., Thomas D., and Liang T. 1995. Bone progenitor cell deficits and the age-associated decline in bone repair capacity. *Calcif. Tissue Int.* **56:** 123–129.

Robertson E. 1987. *Teratocarcinomas and embryonic stem cells.* IRL Press, Oxford, United Kingdom.

Saito T., Dennis J.E., Lennon D.P., Young R.G., and Caplan A.I. 1995. Myogenic expression of mesenchymal stem cells within myotubes of *mdx* mice in vitro and in vivo. *Tissue Eng.* **4:** 327–342.

Stevens L.C. 1959. Embryology of testicular teratomas in strain 129 mice. *J. Natl. Cancer Inst.* **23:** 1249–1295.

———. 1970. The development of transplantable teratocarcinomas from intratesticular grafts of pre- and postimplantation mouse embryos. *Dev. Biol.* **21:** 364–382.

Tavassoli M. and Crosby W.H. 1968. Transplantation of marrow to extramedullary sites. *Science* **161:** 548–556.

Thiede M.A., Pittenger M.F., and Mbalaviele G. 2000. In vitro maintenance of hematopoietic stem cells. U.S. Patent #6,030,836.

Thomas E.D. and Blume K.G. 1999. Historical markers in the development of allogeneic hematopoietic cell transplantation. *Biol. Blood Marrow Transplant.* **5:** 341–346.

Thompson D.L., Lum K.D., Nygaard S.C., Kuestner R.E., Kelly K.A., Gimble J.M., and Moore E.E. 1998. Derivation and characterization of stromal cell lines from the bone marrow of p53–/– mice: New insights into osteoblast and adipocyte differentiation. *J. Bone Min. Res.* **13:** 195–204.

Urist M.R. and McLean F.C. 1952. Osteogenic potence and new bone formation by induction in transplants to the anterior chamber of the eye. *J. Bone Joint Surg. Am. Vol.* **34:** 443–470.

van den Bos C., Silverstetter S., Murphy M., and Connolly T. 1998. P21 rescues human mesenchymal stem cells from apoptosis induced by low density culture. *Cell Tissue Res.* **293:** 463–470.

Wakatani S., Goto T., Pineda S.J., Young R.G., Mansour J.M., Caplan A.I., and Goldberg V.M. 1994. Mesenchymal cell-based repair of large, full-thickness defects of articular cartilage. *J. Bone Joint Surg. Am. Vol.* **76:** 579–592.

Wang J.-S., Shum-Tim D., Galipeau J., Chedrawy E., Eliopoulos N., and Chiu R.J.-C. 2000. Marrow stromal cells for cellular cardiomyoplasty: Feasibility and potential clinical advantages. *J. Thorac. Surg.* **120:** 999–1006.

Wilmut I., Schnieke A.E., McWhir J., Kind A.J., and Campbell K.H. 1997. Viable offspring derived from fetal and adult mammalian cells. *Nature* **385:** 810–813.

Yan M. and Templeton D.J. 1994. Identification of the 2 serine residues of MEK-1 that are differentially phosphorylated during activation by raf and MEK kinase. *J. Biol. Chem.* **269:**19067–19073.

Yoo J.U., Barthel T.S., Nishimura K., Solchaga L., Caplan A.I., Goldberg V.M., and Johnstone B. 1998. The chondrogenic potential of human bone marrow derived mesenchymal progenitor cells. *J. Bone Joint Surg. Am. Vol.* **80:** 1745–1757.

Young H.E., Mancini M.L., Wright R.P., Smith J.C., Black A.C., Reagan C.R., and Lucas P.A. 1995. Mesenchymal stem cells reside within connective tissues of many organs. *Dev. Dyn.* **202:** 137–144.

Young R.G., Butler D.L., Weber W., Caplan A.I., Gordon S.L., and Fink D.J. 1998. Use of mesenchymal stem cells in a collagen matrix for achilles tendon repair. *J. Ortho. Res.* **16:** 406–413.

Zou H. and Niswander L. 1996. Requirement for BMP signaling in interdigital apoptosis and scale formation. *Science* **272:** 738–741.

17

Fate Mapping of Stem Cells

Alan W. Flake
Department of Surgery
The Children's Institute of Surgical Science
Children's Hospital of Philadelphia
Philadelphia, Pennsylvania 19104-4318

STEM CELL FATE MAPPING: GENERAL CONSIDERATIONS

To discuss stem cell "fate," a working definition of a stem cell must be utilized. For the purposes of this discussion, a practical definition is *a cell with the capacity for prolonged or unlimited self-renewal, combined with the capacity to produce at least one type of highly differentiated progeny.* In the context of that definition, the term "stem cell fate mapping" implies that a stem cell has a specific fate that can be discovered in experimental systems directed toward fate mapping, and once discovered, the same fate can be extrapolated to other stem cells of that type. Short of the ultimate common fate of cell death, however, stem cells may have widely variable fates depending on the parameters and conditions imposed by the mapping system. This is one of the current challenges to our understanding of stem cell biology, and a primary source of controversy regarding the identity and potential of specific stem cells. There is increasing evidence for remarkable plasticity in some stem cells even when derived from adult tissues. To cite one of many recent examples, it appears that hematopoietic stem cells give rise to muscle under circumstances of muscle injury or disease (Ferrari et al. 1998; Gussoni et al. 1999). A few years ago, this would have been heretical based on data from previously utilized fate mapping systems. It is clear that as new fate mapping systems are utilized, the currently accepted map for many stem cell candidate populations may need to be changed.

Nevertheless, it seems intuitive that in biological systems, specific stem cells do have defined and predictable fates. This may range from true pluripotentiality for embryonic stem cells to a relatively limited fate, under normal biologic circumstances, for multipotential stem cells in tissues of nonembryonic origin. Perhaps for the purpose of this discussion, the definition of fate mapping should be restricted to determining a "normal" fate for a defined stem cell, i.e., *determination of the fate that a stem cell would be expected to have in its normal environment under the regulatory influences of homeostasis.* These fates would include the participation of the cell in normal development and the response of the cell to biologic perturbations such as tissue injury, senescence of the organism, and disease. It follows that a complete mapping system of the normal fate of a stem cell would require recapitulation of all of the variables to which that cell might be exposed, during the lifetime of the organism, a daunting task for all but the simplest biological systems.

From this discussion, it is apparent that the reductionism inherent in in vitro systems is fundamentally flawed for fate mapping applications and could misrepresent the normal fate of a stem cell. For example, if long-term bone marrow cultures were used for fate mapping of hematopoietic stem cells (HSC), a skewed, predominantly myelopoietic perspective of HSC fate would be assumed. Rather than reductionism, the conceptual framework of network theory (Capra 1996; Kelly 1994) is much more relevant to fate mapping applications. A stem cell is a single unit in a complex biologic network of other stem cells. The maintenance of the stem cell compartment and provision of differentiated progeny depend on a myriad of cell-autonomous regulators modulated by external regulatory signals. Stem cell quiescence or induction of symmetric or asymmetric cell division is the result of the summation of these regulatory inputs. It is obvious that the complexity of a biologic network can only be reproduced by an in vivo system. The problem is that, at the present time, such systems are beyond our analytical capacity. In the future, analytical methods applicable to networks will evolve and allow prediction of stem cell behavior in the context of normal or abnormal perturbations in the network, i.e., true fate mapping. Until network theory is applicable to analysis of biological systems, fate mapping will be intrinsically analogous to assessment of a few frames of a feature-length film. Interpretation of the map will depend on which frames are selected, i.e., the mapping system utilized.

Within the confines of our current capabilities, how can one determine the fate, or multitude of fates, of an individual stem cell? One of two general strategies has been most frequently applied: (1) in situ labeling and subsequent fate mapping of a resident population of cells or (2) transplantation of a labeled cell population with subsequent mapping of its fate. In both strategies, labeling may be based on specific cell markers, or extrinsically applied labels such as retroviral transduction with a marker gene or labeling with thymidine or bromodeoxyuridine (BrdU). Each approach has its relative strengths and weaknesses, and the results must be taken in appropriate context. A major limitation of both strategies is that the readout is dependent on the ability to label a single or homogeneous population of stem cells. The in situ approach has been useful in the rare circumstances where stem cells can be identified precisely by their morphology or location, for instance in the *Drosophila* gonad or peripheral nervous system where stem cells and their non-stem progeny have a well-defined orientation relative to surrounding cells (Jan and Jan 1998; Lu et al. 1998; Xie and Spradling 1998). Although stem cell markers may be useful in some instances to label stem cells in situ (Jones and Watt 1993; Jones et al. 1995; Jensen et al. 1999), a hallmark of most stem cells is the lack of expression of a specific stem cell marker. The use of marker genes or BrdU is limited by the low efficiency of labeling quiescent stem cell populations and nonspecificity of cell type labeled, and by down-regulation with terminal differentiation (marker genes) or dilution by multiple cell divisions (BrdU). Similarly, strategies to map the fate of a stem cell after transplantation ideally would transplant either a single definitively isolated stem cell or a homogeneous population of stem cells. Since, in general, current methodology lacks the sensitivity for extreme low-frequency analysis, cell populations rather than single cells must generally be used as the stem cell input. The ability to extrapolate fate mapping results to a single cell within a population is dependent on the homogeneity of the starting cell population. In reality, cell populations isolated using current approaches are rarely, if ever, homogeneous. It therefore becomes critically important to recognize the limitations of current mapping systems in the context of the input population and to interpret the results as a population readout, rather than a single cell readout.

A second limitation is the receptive environment. Even if a single cell or completely homogeneous cell population is transplanted, one must ask whether the receptive environment perturbs the normal stem cell fate. The concept of external control of stem cell fate mediated by microenvironmental signals present in a stem cell "niche" is well established (Hall and Watt 1989; Quesenberry and Becker 1998). Therefore, normal control of stem cell fate would require engraftment in the appropriate niche. The primary advantage of an in situ strategy is that the cell is labeled in a normal environment without the need for cell processing or transplantation, either of which might affect cell fate. However, the in situ approach is not applicable to analysis of human stem cells, for obvious reasons. Therefore, surrogate biological systems need to be developed for assessment of normal human cell potential. In the remainder of the chapter, I discuss one such system as applied to fate mapping of the human hematopoietic and mesenchymal stem cell.

THE HUMAN–SHEEP SYSTEM FOR FATE MAPPING OF HUMAN STEM CELLS

The use of surrogate animal systems for the study of human cell biology has had variable success. The primary problems with this approach are the immune response against xenogeneic antigen, and issues of species specificity of microenvironmental factors that affect donor cell function. The immune response can be avoided by the use of sufficiently immunodeficient animal models, most notably the nude mouse, SCID mouse, or NOD/SCID mouse (Dick 1994; Larochelle et al. 1996; Dorrell et al. 2000). Unfortunately, the mouse is relatively short-lived, making long-term assessment, even under the ideal circumstances of long-term human cell engraftment, impossible. In addition, the mouse models as an assay of human hematopoiesis remain problematic with respect to the long-term maintenance of multilineage, balanced hematopoiesis. Even when human microenvironments have been co-transplanted as in the SCID-hu systems (McCune et al. 1988; Carballido et al. 2000), the models have not proven to be a reliable reflection of normal human hematopoiesis.

An alternative immunodeficient environment is that of the early gestational fetus. Since the classic observations by Billingham and Medawar (Billingham et al. 1953) of "acquired" immunologic tolerance, the phenomenon of fetal tolerance has been recognized. Evidence is now overwhelming that the fetal thymic microenvironment plays a primary role in determination of self-recognition and repertoire of response to foreign antigen. Pre-T-cells undergo positive and negative selection during a series of maturational steps in the fetal thymus that are controlled by thymic stromal cells (Sprent 1995; Goodnow 1996). The end result is deletion of T-cell clones with high affinity for self-antigen in association with self-MHC, and preservation of a T-cell repertoire against foreign antigen. Therefore, theoretically at least, introduction of foreign antigen prior to thymic processing should result in presentation of donor antigen in the thymus with clonal deletion of alloreactive T-cells. Although less well defined than the mouse system, the immunology of the fetal sheep has been investigated. The fetal sheep is immunologically tolerant of allogeneic skin grafts (Silverstein et al. 1964) or of allogeneic (Flake et al. 1986) or xenogeneic (Zanjani et al. 1994) hematopoietic cells, prior to 75 days gestation, avoiding the immunologic barriers present in postnatal models. In addition to immunologic tolerance, there may be other advantages for the fetal sheep model as a fate mapping system. No irradiation or other conditioning regimen is used, so there is no perturbation of the normal receptive environment. The transplantation of cells during development may offer a maximal opportunity for distribution of stem cells into normal niches, as it recapitulates the developmental process of hematogenous distribution and migration of hematopoiesis into developing hematopoietic environments. The sheep lives for many years, allowing true long-term assessment of transplanted cell populations. Finally, because human and sheep DNA and proteins are widely disparate with respect to sequence homology, human-specific markers can be utilized for the unequivocal detection and characterization of human cells by a variety of methodologies.

FATE MAPPING OF HUMAN HEMATOPOIETIC STEM CELLS IN THE FETAL SHEEP MODEL

The HSC has been rigorously defined as a multipotential cell capable of both self-replication and differentiation into all of the hematopoietic lineages. Implicit in this definition is the capacity for long-term, multilineage repopulation of primary and secondary recipients following transplantation. The isolation of HSCs by physical, functional, and phenotypic characteristics has made tremendous progress over the past few decades with characterization of human HSC paralleling, but lagging somewhat behind, that in the mouse for practical reasons (Goodell et al. 1997; Morrison et al. 1997). A primary obstacle to validation of human HSC candidate populations has been the absence of biologically relevant in vivo assay systems to rigorously assess HSC content. In part to address this need, we have investigated the fetal sheep as an engraftment model for human HSCs.

We initially assessed the ability of human fetal liver-derived HSC to engraft early gestational fetal sheep and demonstrated long-term multipotential human chimerism in the bone marrow and peripheral blood (Zanjani et al. 1992). We subsequently separated human HSC from long-term chimeric animal bone marrow and demonstrated multilineage engraftment of second-generation recipients for over 1 year, proving unequivocally that human HSC engraft in the sheep bone marrow (Zanjani et al. 1994). In subsequent studies, for the sake of efficiency, the assay has been abbreviated so that human cells are harvested just before term (~2 months after transplantation) and retransplanted into second-generation fetal sheep (Fig. 1). In this abbreviated assay, multilineage

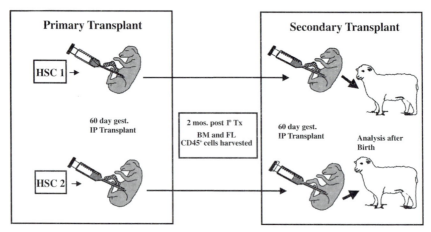

Figure 1 Schematic for the typical experimental design of the abbreviated assay for human HSC in the human–sheep model. HSC1 and HSC2 represent stem cell candidate populations for comparison, or dose comparisons of the same population (for limiting dilution). Populations containing HSC will demonstrate multi-lineage engraftment at 2 months after birth in second-generation recipients. The assay can therefore be completed in around 6 months. Human HSC are harvested by positive selection for CD45 by immunomagnetic beads. Analysis after birth can be performed by flow cytometry for human-specific markers or by fluorescence in situ hybridization and PCR using human-specific probes. In addition, colony assay for human progenitors can be performed by culture in conditions favoring human colony growth.

engraftment of the second-generation animal that persists for 2 months or more after transplantation confirms the presence of human HSC in the donor population (Civin et al. 1996). The assay has now been utilized to assess a number of human cell sources and adult bone-marrow-derived HSC candidate populations and has demonstrated excellent sensitivity as an HSC assay (Civin et al. 1996; Kawashima et al. 1996; Shimizu et al. 1998; Srour et al. 1993; Sutherland et al. 1996; Uchida et al. 1996; Yin et al. 1997; Zanjani et al. 1998, 1999). Human HSC demonstrate balanced multilineage engraftment with lymphoid, myeloid, and erythroid expression at the bone marrow progenitor level. Peripheral blood analysis using lineage markers confirms circulating multilineage human cells in the first few years after birth. In contrast to mouse models, the human–sheep model of xenogeneic hematopoietic chimerism after in utero transplantation has allowed assessment of the durability of chimerism with analysis of some animals ongoing at nearly 10 years after transplantation. The results from experiments directed toward assaying the presence of HSC have obvious implications for the model as a fate mapping system for other stem cells.

An interesting aspect of the model relevant to all xenogeneic surrogate systems is the species specificity of the receptive microenvironment. On in vitro assessment, human cells are minimally responsive to sheep cytokines (with the exception of erythropoietin) and vice versa. The administration of human recombinant cytokines IL-3/GM-CSF (Zanjani et al. 1992) or SCF (Flake et al. 1995) to long-term chimeric sheep results in dramatic increases in human hematopoiesis. These findings suggest that the sheep microenvironmental milieu is capable of long-term support of human HSC viability, but incapable of normal support of definitive hematopoiesis, at least at a level that is competitive with host hematopoiesis (Flake and Zanjani 1999). It also raises the interesting possibility that the microenvironment can be manipulated, for instance by co-transplantation of normal or genetically manipulated human stromal elements (Almeida-Porada et al. 1999), to create normal or perturbed "human" receptive environments. Such strategies may further improve the utility of the model for human HSC fate mapping and allow unique insight into microenvironmental control of fate decisions.

MESENCHYMAL STEM CELLS

The existence of a population of multipotent mesenchymal stem cells (MSCs) that reside in adult tissues and are capable of participation in repair of tissue injury related to disease, aging, or trauma was championed by Caplan as the concept of "mesangenesis" (Caplan 1991, 1994). Supporting evidence that such a cell exists has been drawn primarily from studies on cells isolated from bone marrow by plastic adherence. Freidenstein et al. (1987, 1992; Friedenstein 1995) originally described such a population isolated by placing whole bone marrow in plastic culture dishes and pouring off the nonadherent (hematopoietic) cells after 4 hours. This left a heterogeneous population of cells, the most tightly adherent of which were spindle-shaped and formed foci of 2–4 cells. These cells remained dormant for 2–4 days and then began to multiply rapidly, ultimately, after several passages, giving rise to confluent layers that were more uniformly spindle cell in appearance. Most importantly, these cells had the ability to differentiate into colonies that resembled small deposits of bone or cartilage. Subsequent studies by other investigators with cells isolated by protocols similar to Freidenstein's confirmed that this population of cells could be induced to differentiate in vitro into a variety of mesenchymal tissues, including fat, bone, cartilage, bone marrow stroma, and myotubules (Grigoriadis et al. 1988; Leboy et al. 1991; Cassiede et al. 1996; Dennis and Caplan 1996a,b; Haynesworth et al. 1996; Kadiyala et al. 1997). The conditions required for induction of differentiation varied somewhat between species. Nevertheless, mesenchymal progenitors could be isolated from mouse, rat, rabbit, and human bone marrow that readily gave rise to adipocytes, chondrocytes, and osteoblasts under specific conditions. Most studies that have been performed with mesenchymal progenitors have been performed with these relatively heterogeneous cell populations. Athough efforts have been made to isolate a more homogeneous MSC population (Simmons and Torok-Storb 1991; Gronthos et al. 1994; Gronthos and Simmons 1995; Zohar et al. 1997), in most cases it remains to be proven whether these more highly purified populations maintain the full multipotentiality of those isolated by simple plastic adherence.

It has been assumed that these heterogeneous mesenchymal progenitor populations contain a subpopulation of true mesenchymal stem cells, and the term stem cell has been loosely applied in many of these studies. In reality, the mesenchymal stem cell has not yet been isolated or definitively characterized. For practical purposes, however, a definition for MSC that is presently applied is *adult bone-marrow-derived populations enriched for progenitors that can be induced by specific in vitro conditions to commit to differentiated mesenchymal cell phenotypes and/or tissues.* Obviously, this definition does not have the rigor required for the definition of many other populations of stem cells discussed in this text. On the other hand, it took years to define the hematopoietic stem cell with the rigor currently applied, and the previous definitions were steps toward our current understanding. Nevertheless, from the perspective of fate mapping of the mesenchymal stem cell, this definition leaves much to be desired. From the perspective of the input cell, the populations are crudely heterogeneous. From the perspective of the mapping system, the in vitro potential may or may not represent a "normal" in vivo fate for MSCs.

There is some information available regarding the behavior of MSC populations in vivo. Much of the information lies in the realm of tissue engineering and is more applicable to the question of what MSCs will do when placed directly into an in vivo site, with or without a biosynthetic construct, than to what the normal fate of an MSC might be. Experiments utilizing porous diffusion chambers or ceramic cubes have documented the capacity of MSCs to form fibrous tissue, cartilage, or bone in vivo (Goshima et al. 1991; Cassiede et al. 1996; Kadiyala et al. 1997). For instance, autologous canine MSCs isolated from bone marrow, grown in culture, and loaded onto porous ceramic cylinders resulted in healing of induced bone defects that would otherwise result in non-union (Kadiyala et al. 1997; Bruder et al. 1998). Another interesting study documents astroglial differentiation of murine MSC after direct injection into the lateral ventricles of neonatal mice (Kopen et al. 1999). Although such evidence implies that MSCs may participate in such processes in vivo, it in no way proves that they, in fact, normally do so. In a separate system, the osteochondrogenic behavior of MSCs in vivo on subcutaneous ceramic implants was found to be independent of their in vitro osteochondrogenic behavior (Cassiede et al. 1996), once again demonstrating that the environment in which the MSCs are assayed modulates their ultimate fate.

There are a number of reports documenting donor-derived stromal elements after bone marrow transplantation (Keating et al. 1982; Piersma et al. 1983; Anklesaria et al. 1987; Perkins and Fleischman 1988), indirectly supporting the presence of a non-hematopoietic stem cell in whole bone marrow that gives rise to stromal supporting elements. Similarly, a report documenting donor-derived skeletal muscle in a muscle injury model after bone marrow transplantation (Ferrari et al. 1998) supports a bone marrow resident stem cell with mesenchymal differentiative capacity. Further indirect evidence supporting the presence of osteoprogenitors in bone marrow was recently reported by Horwitz et al. (1999) demonstrating clinical evidence of improvement in three patients with osteogenesis imperfecta after standard bone marrow transplantation with documentation of 1.5–2% donor-derived osteoblasts in two of the patients. All of these studies utilized whole bone marrow as a donor source rather than a defined stem cell population and thus can only be used as indirect support for the existence of a multipotent MSC that has the normal fate of stromal cell, myocyte, or osteocyte differentiation. More recently, Gussoni et al. have reported muscle reconstitution in irradiated *mdx* mice after transplantation of highly enriched hematopoietic stem cells (Gussoni et al. 1999). Their findings suggest that the MSC may be an intermediate population and that the hematopoietic stem cell is more pluripotent than previously appreciated. Once again, however, the use of irradiation in a mouse model of ongoing muscle damage may induce transdifferentiation that is not a normal fate of an HSC.

Of greater relevance to this discussion are studies that have followed the fate of MSC-containing populations after systemic transplantation. There have been two studies in mice in which cultured mouse-adherent cell populations have been transplanted systemically and documented to persist following transplantation. In the first, cells from transgenic mice expressing a human minigene for collagen I were used as mesenchymal progenitor donors, and the fate of the cells was followed after transplantation into irradiated mice (Pereira et al. 1995). Donor cells were detected in bone marrow, spleen, bone, cartilage, and lung up to 5 months later by PCR for the human minigene, and a PCR in situ assay on lung indicated that the donor cells diffusely populated the parenchyma. Reverse transcription-PCR assays indicated that the marker collagen I gene was expressed in a tissue-specific manner. A second study transplanted either cultured adherent cells or whole bone marrow into irradiated mice with a phenotype of fragile bones resembling osteogenesis imperfecta caused by expression of the human minigene for type I collagen (Pereira et al. 1998). With either source of cells, a similar distribution of engraftment was documented as observed in the previous study and, in addition, fluorescense in situ hybridization assays for the Y chromosome indicated that, after 2.5 months, donor male cells accounted for 4–19% of the fibroblasts or fibroblast-like cells obtained in primary cultures of the lung, calvaria, cartilage, long bone, tail, and skin. Although these studies suggest the presence of a mesenchymal stem cell, no immunohistochemical assessment was performed to assess what the engrafted donor cells actually were. The use of a mouse population of MSC is inherently problematic, since it is exceedingly difficult to eradicate hematopoietic elements from the culture. In the absence of immunohistochemical characterization, the presence of contaminating hematopoietic elements and fibroblasts in the donor cell preparation could account for the observed distribution of donor cells. In addition, the requirement for radiation in the model could potentially alter the receptive microenvironment, influencing the observed cell fate.

FATE MAPPING OF HUMAN MSC

From the preceding discussion, it is clear that there are significant gaps in our understanding of MSCs and MSC fate. Basic questions of what constitutes an MSC and how it can be defined, where it resides, and what biologic developmental and homeostatic mechanisms it participates in remain to be defined. Similarly, the clinically important questions of the transplantability of MSCs, their ability to home and engraft to appropriate sites, their ultimate capacity to differentiate and function after transplantation, their immunogenicity, and the regulatory factors that control MSC proliferation and differentiation are relatively unknown. To approach these questions one needs, at a minimum, to have a defined input population and an appropriate assay system for fate analysis.

In the studies discussed above, a major problem has been the lack of homogeneity and degree of characterization with respect to multipotentiality of the input populations used. Although a true MSC remains to be defined, much less isolated, it is clear that a greater degree of characterization and homogeneity can be currently achieved in some species than in others. Murine MSCs, for instance, have been exceptionally difficult to isolate and expand in culture, without contaminating hematopoietic elements, whereas human MSC are relatively easy to isolate and expand. As described in the preceding chapter, human MSCs have been relatively well characterized by their ability to proliferate in culture with homogeneous morphology, by the uniform presence of a consistent set of surface marker proteins, and by their consistent differentiation into multiple mesenchymal lineages under controlled in vitro conditions (Pittenger et al. 1999). Analysis of colonies derived from individual cells from cultured human MSCs confirms the presence of a subpopulation of cells with at least tripotential differentiative capacity (bone, cartilage, and fat) (Pittenger et al. 1999). Thus, from a fate mapping perspective, the use of a relatively defined, although undoubtedly heterogeneous, input population can be achieved with available human MSC.

However, the use of human MSCs involves obvious practical limitations with respect to the fate mapping system. Ideally, one would want to place MSCs into an unperturbed system that is immunologically inert and in which MSC would engraft in their normal locations and subsequently respond to normal growth and regulatory signals. One would also need to have donor discriminatory markers to identify the MSC and their differentiated progeny. We have developed a system that satisfies some of these requirements.

We reasoned that the fetal sheep model might also offer advantages for the engraftment of human MSC. We have therefore modified the model for the analysis of engraftment and ultimate cell fate of human MSCs. Figure 2 is a schematic depiction of the experimental design. Human MSCs were transplanted into fetal sheep at either 65 days gestation (term = 145 days) or 85 days gestation. These time points were chosen to assess the effect of two developmental events on MSC distribution and engraftment. First, hematopoiesis is derived entirely from the liver in the fetal sheep at 65 days with only minimal development of the bone marrow. By 85 days, the bone marrow is densely populated with hematopoietic cells. Following in utero hematopoietic cell transplantation, it has been observed that donor cells preferentially home to the fetal liver up until the time of bone marrow formation, after which they home almost exclusively to the bone marrow (Zanjani et al. 1993). Therefore, in the case of hematopoietic engraftment, the receptive environments strongly influence the distribution of engraftment. The second event is the development of immunologic competence for

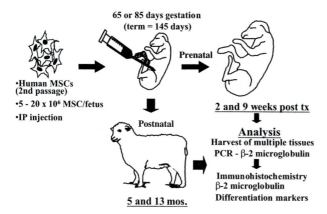

Figure 2 Schematic of the human–sheep model modified for analysis of human mesenchymal stem cells. Second-passage human MSCs obtained from Osiris Therapeutics, Inc. (Baltimore, Maryland) were transplanted into 65 or 85 day gestation sheep fetuses at a dose of 1×10^8 to 2×10^8 cells/kg/fetal weight. Recipient tissues were harvested at various intervals and analyzed for human cell engraftment using human-specific methodologies.

rejection of skin grafts or hematopoietic grafts. Fetal sheep develop the capacity to reject allogeneic skin grafts (Silverstein et al. 1964) and demonstrate allogeneic or xenogeneic hematopoietic engraftment failure (Zanjani et al. 1997), which appears to be immunologically mediated, after 75 days gestation. In view of evidence that MSCs have the capacity to ablate allogeneic and xenogeneic response in vitro (McIntosh et al. 1999), we wondered whether they might be immunomodulatory in vivo.

Distribution of Engrafted Human MSCs in the Sheep Model

To assess distribution of engraftment, and to screen for human cell engraftment in tissues prior to immunohistochemical assessment, we utilized PCR for human-specific β_2-microglobulin DNA sequences. Multiple tissues were harvested at intervals of 2 weeks, 2 months, 5 months, or 13 months after in utero transplantation. Human cells were widely distributed in most tissues assessed by PCR at 2 weeks after transplantation, including liver, spleen, bone marrow, thymus, lung, brain, muscle, heart, and blood. After 2 months, human DNA was still detected in all tissues examined from fetuses transplanted at 65 days gestation, including cartilage, with the exception of brain. In fetuses transplanted at 85 days gestation, human DNA was detected after 2 months in the spleen, bone marrow, thymus, heart, and blood. Five months after in utero transplantation (3 months after birth), human DNA was detected in the bone marrow, thymus, spleen, lung, cartilage, and blood of fetuses transplanted at 65 days and in the heart, brain, skeletal muscle, and blood of fetuses transplanted at 85 days. In two animals transplanted at 85 days gestation 13 months earlier, human cells could still be detected by PCR in liver, bone marrow, heart, cartilage, and blood. The pattern of engraftment differed between animals, but in total, 28 of 29 injected animals demonstrated engraftment of human cells in one or more tissues.

From these results, it can be surmised that MSCs, despite their very large size, can be transplanted and are capable of engraftment in multiple tissues, even when transplanted into the fetal peritoneal cavity. This requires migration across endothelial barriers, integration into host tissue microenvironments, and survival with available growth and regulatory signals. Our findings of a variable pattern of long-term MSC engraftment, following detection of MSCs at 2 weeks in nearly all tissues studied, supports a model of nonselective hematogenous distribution, with subsequent selective long-term survival in specific tissues. This may be a function of the ability of specific microenvironments to support the engraftment and differentiation of MSC, or alternatively, the loss of engraftment from some tissues may be due to heterogeneity of the transplanted population with respect to differentiation potential or replicative capacity and longevity. A third possibility is that the xenogeneic microenvironment can support the viability and differentiation of human MSCs, but not their self-replication.

Does the distribution of MSCs observed in this model replicate the distribution of MSCs under normal circumstances? The answer will be unknown until the distribution of MSCs in human tissues is understood. If, in fact, MSCs are distributed to multiple tissues early in gestation (see below) to engraft and remain resident for repair of tissue injury, then in utero transplantation may recapitulate that ontogenic event. The fact that MSCs were found in most organs, including the bone marrow, is supportive of such a model.

The results of our DNA PCR were confirmed by immunohistochemistry using antihuman β_2-microglobulin (Figs. 3 and 4). Negative controls consisted of tissues of transplanted sheep that were PCR negative, or the same tissues from non-transplanted, age-matched controls. In all but a few tissues, immunohistochemistry confirmed the presence of human cells, and all of the negative control tissues were negative by immunohistochemistry. Many human MSCs were seen in pre- and postnatal hematopoietic and lymphopoietic tissues, including the fetal liver, bone marrow, spleen, and thymus (Fig. 3). Multiple human MSCs could often be appreciated in a single high-power field in these tissues. Human cells were also identified in non-lymphohematopoietic sites, including the heart, skeletal muscle, cartilage, and lung. Five and thirteen months after transplantation, human cells continued to be present in multiple tissues, including the bone marrow, thymus, cartilage, heart, skeletal muscle, and brain.

Site-specific Differentiation of MSCs in the Sheep Model

The obvious next question was, What had the human MSCs become? Differentiation of human MSCs in various tissues was assessed by one of three techniques: (1) characteristic morphology with antihuman β_2-microglobulin staining; (2) immunohistochemical double staining for

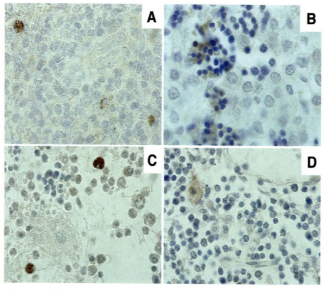

Figure 3 Engraftment in hematopoietic tissues detected by immunohistochemical staining with antihuman β_2-microglobulin and biotinylated secondary antibody developed by chromagen 3,3′-diaminobenzidine (*brown stain*) and light counterstaining with hematoxylin. (*A*) Frozen section of fetal spleen 2 weeks after transplantation showing engraftment of large human cells. (*B*) Fetal liver at 2 months after transplantation (transplanted at 65 days gestation) demonstrating large human cells in clusters of hematopoiesis. Magnification, 100x. (*C*) Bone marrow 5 months after transplantation showing large human cells with stromal morphology. (*D*) Thymus at 5 months after transplantation showing large human cell with thymic stromal morphology. Magnification, *A,C,D*, 40x.

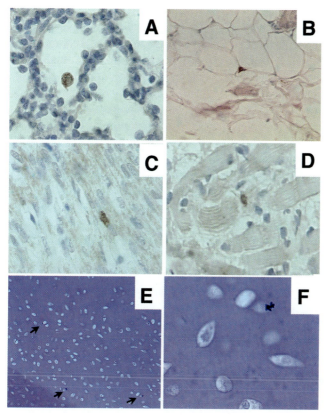

Figure 4 Engraftment of human cells in nonhematopoietic tissues by antihuman β₂-microglobulin staining. (*A*) Human cell in the alveolar space of the lung at 2 months after transplantation (prenatal). (*B*) Human adipocyte in pericardial fat at 13 months after transplantation. (*C*) Human cell in myocardium with cardiomyocyte morphology at 5 months after transplantation. (*D*) Human cell in skeletal muscle 5 months after transplantation. (*E,F*) Low- and high- magnification views of human-specific anti-β₂-microglobulin staining of PCR positive articular cartilage demonstrating human cells in three separate lacunae of the cartilage (*arrows, E*). Higher magnification confirms one of the cells to be in a lacuna in an otherwise acellular background (*F*). The particulate appearance of the staining is a result of the nickel chloride developing technique.

anti-human β₂-microglobulin and a second nonhuman-specific differentiation marker; or (3) when available, positive staining with human-specific differentiation markers proven not to cross-react with sheep cells. Using these techniques, site-specific differentiation was confirmed for human cardiomyocytes, chondrocytes, adipocytes, bone marrow stromal

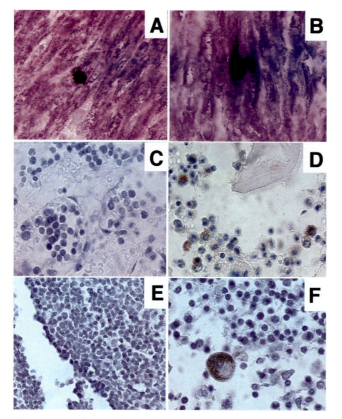

Figure 5 Further evidence of site-specific differentiation using double staining or human specific differentiation markers. (*A,B*) 100× and oil immersion views of human cells in the heart identified by anti-β_2-microglobulin (*dark brown*) and counter-stained (*pink*) with anti-Smooth Endoplasmic Reticulum Calcium ATPase-2 (SERCA-2), a cytoplasmic marker for muscle. The human cell cytoplasm stains with SERCA-2 and is uniformly incorporated into the sheep cardiac muscle, supporting cardiomyocyte differentiation. (*C,D*) Bone marrow of normal age-matched sheep (*C*, negative control) and chimeric sheep stained with antihuman CD23, a marker of stromal differentiation. Note the large size of the human cells. Antihuman CD45 staining of the bone marrow was negative, confirming that these cells are not of hematopoietic origin (not shown). (*E,F*) Negative control thymus (*E*) and thymus positive for a human cell that stains with antihuman CD74, a thymic stromal marker. The cell has epithelial morphology suggestive of a thymic epithelial cell.

cells, thymic stromal cells, and skeletal myocytes (Figs. 4 and 5). Although PCR results suggested that human cells were engrafted in the CNS, double-staining immunohistochemistry using antihuman β_2-microglobulin and anti-GFAP (glial fibrillary acid protein) showed that the human cells were not differentiated glial cells, but rather were perivascular cells surrounding blood vessels in the gyral sulci.

The results show that MSCs are capable of site-specific, multipotential differentiation and tissue integration following transplantation. Human MSCs have been shown in vitro to differentiate into adipocytic, chondrocytic, or osteocytic lineages (Pittenger et al. 1999). Less well characterized MSC populations from other species have been induced in vitro toward myocytic differentiation. Our study confirms in vivo chondrocytic differentiation and for the first time clearly demonstrates cardiomyocytic and myocytic differentiation of a defined human MSC population. MSCs derived from bone marrow from multiple species have been demonstrated to support hematopoiesis with equal or greater efficacy than stromal layers formed in long-term Dexter cultures. Our study upholds the role of MSCs in stromal support of hematopoiesis, both in the fetal liver and postnatal bone marrow. We found multiple large human cells intimately associated with clusters of hematopoiesis in the fetal liver at 2 and 9 weeks after transplantation. In addition, large cells that stained positively for human-specific CD23 were identified in the bone marrow at 9 and 22 weeks after transplantation. CD23 has been identified as a low-affinity IgE receptor as well as a functional CD21 ligand (Aubry et al. 1994; Huang et al. 1995) present on a variety of hematopoietic cells and bone marrow stromal cells (Fourcade et al. 1992). Our interpretation of CD23-positive cells in this study as "stromal" is based on the large size of the cells and the absence of human hematopoietic cells in either the donor cell population or the recipient bone marrow.

A relatively surprising finding was the presence of large thymic cells that stained positive for human-specific β_2-microglobulin and CD74. CD74 is a cell-surface MHC class II-associated invariant chain molecule that is expressed on B cells, Langerhans cells, dendritic cells, activated T cells, and thymic epithelium (Schlossman et al. 1995). The morphology of CD74[+] cells in this study appears similar to the ovine thymic epithelial cells in the surrounding thymus. The precursor of thymic dendritic cells is thought to be the HSC, whereas the origin of the thymic epithelial cell is controversial. Our data support a mesenchymal origin for the thymic epithelial cell as a "stromal" supporting cell in the thymus.

The persistence of human cells observed in this xenogeneic model, even when transplanted after the development of immunocompetence in the sheep fetus, is intriguing. Potential mechanisms for tolerance include failure of immune recognition, local immune suppression, or thymic deletional tolerance. Human MSCs are known to express class I HLA antigen but do not express class II, which may limit immune recognition. Although thymic stromal cells are known to participate in thymocyte positive and negative selection (Sha et al. 1988; Schwartz 1989), and host thymic antigen-presenting cells are capable of facilitating clonal deletion of donor-reactive lymphocytes after in utero HSC transplantation (Kim et al. 1999), neither mechanism would account for tolerance after the appearance of mature lymphocytes in the peripheral circulation. In vitro, MSCs added to mixed lymphocyte cultures, however, have been shown to nonspecifically ablate alloreactivity by an as-yet-unknown mechanism. We speculate that the persistence of MSCs in this model results from a combination of minimal immunogenicity and local immune suppression.

These results support the in vivo multipotentiality of human MSCs when transplanted into a developing receptive environment. The engraftment observed in multiple tissues with site-specific differentiation supports the concept that the fate of MSCs is determined by the environment in which they engraft rather than by an intrinsically programmed fate. Is this the full repertoire of MSC fate? Probably not. We observed a number of cells in a variety of tissues that we are currently unable to characterize. The most interesting of these are perivascular cells that persist as long as 13 months after transplantation in multiple tissues. These maintain fibroblast-like morphology and may represent the undifferentiated tissue resident MSC that has been postulated. We also have not observed CNS engraftment or glial differentiation of the MSCs used in this study. This could be a function of restriction of engraftment by the blood–brain barrier, or the cell population we are utilizing may not have neural potential.

Our results also support, but do not prove, the hypothesis that MSCs are distributed hematogenously during ontogeny to receptive tissues where they reside and ultimately differentiate. An intriguing observation relevant to this hypothesis is that circulating "stromal" elements can be isolated from human fetal blood up to but not beyond 15 weeks gestation (Campagnoli et al. 1999). These cells on early characterization have many properties analogous to MSCs and may prove to be the early cells that "seed" tissues, including hematopoietic stromal environments with stromal and mesenchymal progenitors.

The current results provide little insight into the normal regulation of MSC fate in vivo. What regulatory signals cause MSCs to proliferate and differentiate? Do they participate in normal tissue repair? Can they "rejuvenate" to any degree organs or tissues as they age? Do they respond to tissue injury in a beneficial manner? Our hope in the future is to utilize the sheep system to explore stimuli that may induce MSC response and to investigate other populations of MSC, such as those derived from the early gestational human fetus, in our model to determine whether developmental age of MSCs affects their fate. An improved understanding of the regulation of MSCs in vivo will help determine strategies to manipulate MSCs for therapeutic benefit. It is clear that in order to utilize MSCs for tissue engineering, cellular, and gene therapy applications, we will need to understand how to deliver a large number of MSCs to specific sites and induce appropriate differentiation. This will require further insight into the normal and disease-induced regulation of MSC proliferation and differentiation, the transplant immunology of MSCs, as well as the development of strategies for diffuse or site-specific delivery for specific applications.

The fate mapping of MSCs as well as other stem cell types is currently rudimentary and is inherently limited by our current methodologic and analytical capabilities. Future advances in stem cell understanding will require better characterization of stem cell populations, further definition of the signaling pathways that regulate stem cell behavior and the interaction between intrinsic and extrinsic regulatory influences, and advances in our ability to analyze complex biologic systems. The development of in vivo surrogate systems that can accurately recapitulate the normal biologic events in the life of a stem cell will be essential for unraveling the intricacies of stem cell fate. The human–sheep model may be particularly useful for such studies, as it represents a relatively unperturbed developmental model that has thus far demonstrated long-term engraftment and multipotential differentiation of two human stem cell types.

REFERENCES

Almeida-Porada G., Flake A.W., Glimp H.A., and Zanjani E.D. 1999. Cotransplantation of stroma results in enhancement of engraftment and early expression of donor hematopoietic stem cells in utero. *Exp. Hematol.* **27:** 1569–1575.

Anklesaria P., Kase K., Glowacki J., Holland C.A., Sakakeeny M.A., Wright J.A., FitzGerald T.J., Lee C.Y., and Greenberger J.S. 1987. Engraftment of a clonal bone marrow stromal cell line in vivo stimulates hematopoietic recovery from total body irradiation. *Proc. Natl. Acad. Sci.* **84:** 7681–7685.

Aubry J.P., Pochon S., Gauchat J.F., Nueda-Marin A., Holers V.M., Graber P., Siegfried C., and Bonnefoy J.Y. 1994. CD23 interacts with a new functional extracytoplasmic domain involving N-linked oligosaccharides on CD21. *J. Immunol.* **152:** 5806–5813.

Billingham R., Brent L., and Medawar P.B. 1953. Actively acquired tolerance of foreign cells. *Nature* **172:** 603–607.

Bruder S.P., Kraus K.H., Goldberg V.M., and Kadiyala S. 1998. The effect of implants loaded with autologous mesenchymal stem cells on the healing of canine segmental bone defects. *J. Bone Joint Surg. Am. Vol.* **80:** 985–996.

Campagnoli C., Fisk N., Tocci A., Bennet P., and Roberts I.A.G. 1999. Circulating stromal cells in first trimester fetal blood. *Blood* (Suppl. 1) **94**: 38a (Abstr. 157).

Caplan A.I. 1991. Mesenchymal stem cells. *J. Orthop. Res.* **9**: 641–650.

———. 1994. The mesengenic process. *Clin. Plastic Surg.* **21**: 429–435.

Capra F. 1996. *The web of life. A new scientific understanding of living systems,* p. 347. Anchor Books, New York.

Carballido J.M., Namikawa R., Carballido-Perrig N., Antonenko S., Roncarolo M.G., and de Vries J.E. 2000. Generation of primary antigen-specific human T- and B-cell responses in immunocompetent SCID-hu mice. *Nat. Med.* **6**: 103–106.

Cassiede P., Dennis J.E., Ma F., and Caplan A.I. 1996. Osteochondrogenic potential of marrow mesenchymal progenitor cells exposed to TGF-beta 1 or PDGF-BB as assayed in vivo and in vitro. *J. Bone Miner. Res.* **11**: 1264–1273.

Civin C.I., Almeida-Porada G., Lee M.J., Olweus J., Terstappen L.W., and Zanjani E.D. 1996. Sustained, retransplantable, multilineage engraftment of highly purified adult human bone marrow stem cells in vivo. *Blood* **88**: 4102–4109.

Dennis J.E. and Caplan A.I. 1996a. Analysis of the developmental potential of conditionally immortal marrow-derived mesenchymal progenitor cells isolated from the H-2Kb-tsA58 transgenic mouse. *Connect Tissue Res.* **35**: 93–99.

———. 1996b. Differentiation potential of conditionally immortalized mesenchymal progenitor cells from adult marrow of a H-2Kb-tsA58 transgenic mouse. *J. Cell Physiol.* **167**: 523–538.

Dick J.E. 1994. Future prospects for animal models created by transplanting human haematopoietic cells into immune-deficient mice. *Res. Immunol.* **145**: 380–384.

Dorrell C., Gan O.I., Pereira D.S., Hawley R.G., and Dick J.E. 2000. Expansion of human cord blood CD34($^+$)CD38($^-$) cells in ex vivo culture during retroviral transduction without a corresponding increase in SCID repopulating cell (SRC) frequency: Dissociation of SRC phenotype and function. *Blood* **95**: 102–110.

Ferrari G., Cusella-De Angelis G., Coletta M., Paolucci E., Stornaiuolo A., Cossu G., and Mavilio F. 1998. Muscle regeneration by bone marrow-derived myogenic progenitors. *Science* **279**: 1528–1530.

Flake A.W. and Zanjani E.D. 1999. In utero hematopoietic stem cell transplantation: Ontogenic opportunities and biologic barriers. *Blood* **94**: 2179–2191.

Flake A.W., Harrison M.R., Adzick N.S., and Zanjani E.D. 1986. Transplantation of fetal hematopoietic stem cells in utero: The creation of hematopoietic chimeras. *Science* **233**: 776–778.

Flake A.W., Hendrick M.H., Rice H.E., Tavassoli M., and Zanjani E.D. 1995. Enhancement of human hematopoiesis by mast cell growth factor in human-sheep chimeras created by the in utero transplantation of human fetal hematopoietic cells. *Exp. Hematol.* **23**: 252–257.

Fourcade C., Arock M., Ktorza S., Ouaaz F., Merle-Beral H., Mentz F., Kilchherr E., Debre P., and Mossalayi M.D. 1992. Expression of CD23 by human bone marrow stromal cells. *Eur. Cytokine Netw.* **3**: 539–543.

Friedenstein A.J. 1995. Marrow stromal fibroblasts. *Calcif. Tissue Int.* **56**: S17.

Friedenstein A.J., Chailakhyan R.K., and Gerasimov U.V. 1987. Bone marrow osteogenic stem cells: In vitro cultivation and transplantation in diffusion chambers. *Cell Tissue Kinet.* **20**: 263–272.

Friedenstein A.J., Latzinik N.V., Gorskaya Yu F., Luria E.A., and Moskvina I.L. 1992. Bone marrow stromal colony formation requires stimulation by haemopoietic cells. *Bone Miner.* **18**: 199–213.

Goodell M.A., Rosenzweig M., Kim H., Marks D.F., DeMaria M., Paradis G., Grupp S.A., Sieff C.A., Mulligan R.C., and Johnson R.P. 1997. Dye efflux studies suggest that hematopoietic stem cells expressing low or undetectable levels of CD34 antigen exist in multiple species. *Nat. Med.* **3:** 1337–1345.

Goodnow C. 1996. Balancing immunity and tolerance: Deleting and tuning lymphocyte repertoires. *Proc. Natl. Acad. Sci.* **93:** 2264–2271.

Goshima J., Goldberg V.M., and Caplan A.I. 1991. The osteogenic potential of culture-expanded rat marrow mesenchymal cells assayed in vivo in calcium phosphate ceramic blocks. *Clin. Orthop. Relat. Res.* **262:** 298–311.

Grigoriadis A.E., Heersche J.N., and Aubin J.E. 1988. Differentiation of muscle, fat, cartilage, and bone from progenitor cells present in a bone-derived clonal cell population: Effect of dexamethasone. *J. Cell Biol.* **106:** 2139–2151.

Gronthos S. and Simmons P.J. 1995. The growth factor requirements of STRO-1-positive human bone marrow stromal precursors under serum-deprived conditions in vitro. *Blood* **85:** 929–940.

Gronthos S., Graves S.E., Ohta S., and Simmons P.J. 1994. The STRO-1+ fraction of adult human bone marrow contains the osteogenic precursors. *Blood* **84:** 4164–4173.

Gussoni E., Soneoka Y., Strickland C.D., Buzney E.A., Khan M.K., Flint A.F., Kunkel L.M., and Mulligan R.C. 1999. Dystrophin expression in the mdx mouse restored by stem cell transplantation. *Nature* **401:** 390–394.

Hall P.A. and Watt F.M. 1989. Stem cells: The generation and maintenance of cellular diversity. *Development* **106:** 619–633.

Haynesworth S.E., Baber M.A., and Caplan A.I. 1996. Cytokine expression by human marrow-derived mesenchymal progenitor cells in vitro: Effects of dexamethasone and IL-1 alpha. *J. Cell Physiol.* **166:** 585–592.

Horwitz E.M., Prockop D.J., Fitzpatrick L.A., Koo W.W., Gordon P.L., Neel M., Sussman M., Orchard P., Marx J.C., Pyeritz R.E., and Brenner M.K. 1999. Transplantability and therapeutic effects of bone marrow-derived mesenchymal cells in children with osteogenesis imperfecta. *Nat. Med.* **5:** 309–313.

Huang N., Kawano M.M., Mahmoud M.S., Mihara K., Tsujimoto T., Niwa O., and Kuramoto A. 1995. Expression of CD21 antigen on myeloma cells and its involvement in their adhesion to bone marrow stromal cells. *Blood* **85:** 3704–3712.

Jan Y.N. and Jan L.Y. 1998. Asymmetric cell division. *Nature* **392:** 775–778.

Jensen U.B., Lowell S., and Watt F.M. 1999. The spatial relationship between stem cells and their progeny in the basal layer of human epidermis: A new view based on whole-mount labelling and lineage analysis. *Development* **126:** 2409–2418.

Jones P.H. and Watt F.M. 1993. Separation of human epidermal stem cells from transit amplifying cells on the basis of differences in integrin function and expression. *Cell* **73:** 713–724.

Jones P.H., Harper S., and Watt F.M. 1995. Stem cell patterning and fate in human epidermis. *Cell* **80:** 83–93.

Kadiyala S., Young R.G., Thiede M.A., and Bruder S.P. 1997. Culture expanded canine mesenchymal stem cells possess osteochondrogenic potential in vivo and in vitro. *Cell Transplant.* **6:** 125–134.

Kawashima I., Zanjani E.D., Almaida-Porada G., Flake A.W., Zeng H., and Ogawa M. 1996. CD34+ human marrow cells that express low levels of Kit protein are enriched for long-term marrow-engrafting cells. *Blood* **87:** 4136–4142.

Keating A., Singer J.W., Killen P.D., Striker G.E., Salo A.C., Sanders J., Thomas E.D.,

Thorning D., and Fialkow P.J. 1982. Donor origin of the in vitro haematopoietic microenvironment after marrow transplantation in man. *Nature* **298:** 280–283.

Kelly K. 1994. Hive mind. In *Out of control. The new biology of machines, social systems, and the economic world,* pp. 5–28. Addison-Wesley, Reading, Massachusetts.

Kim H.B., Shaaban A.F., Milner R., Fichter C., and Flake A.W. 1999. In utero bone marrow transplantation induces tolerance by a combination of clonal deletion and anergy. *J. Pediatr. Surg.* **34:** 726–730.

Kopen G.C., Prockop D.J., and Phinney D.G. 1999. Marrow stromal cells migrate throughout forebrain and cerebellum, and they differentiate into astrocytes after injection into neonatal mouse brains. *Proc. Natl. Acad. Sci.* **96:** 10711–10716.

Larochelle A., Vormoor J., Hanenberg H., Wang J.C., Bhatia M., Lapidot T., Moritz T., Murdoch B., Xiao X.L., Kato I., Williams D.A., and Dick J.E. 1996. Identification of primitive human hematopoietic cells capable of repopulating NOD/SCID mouse bone marrow: Implications for gene therapy. *Nat. Med.* **2:** 1329–1337.

Leboy P.S., Beresford J.N., Devlin C., and Owen M.E. 1991. Dexamethasone induction of osteoblast mRNAs in rat marrow stromal cell cultures. *J. Cell Physiol.* **146:** 370–378.

Lu B., Jan L.Y., and Jan Y.N. 1998. Asymmetric cell division: Lessons from flies and worms. *Curr. Opin. Genet. Dev.* **8:** 392–399.

McCune J.M., Namikawa R., Kaneshima H., Shultz L.D., Lieberman M., and Weissman I.L. 1988. The SCID-hu mouse: Murine model for the analysis of human hematolymphoid differentiation and function. *Science* **241:** 1632–1639.

McIntosh K., Klyushnenkova E., Shustova V., Moseley A., and Deans R. 1999. Suppression of alloreactive T cell responses by human mesenchymal stem cells involves CD8$^+$ cells. *Blood* (Suppl. 1) **94:** 133a. (Abstr. 587).

Morrison S.J., Wright D.E., Cheshier S.H., and Weissman I.L. 1997. Hematopoietic stem cells: Challenges to expectations. *Curr. Opin. Immunol.* **9:** 216–221.

Pereira R.F., Halford K.W., O'Hara M.D., Leeper D.B., Sokolov B.P., Pollard M.D., Bagasra O., and Prockop D.J. 1995. Cultured adherent cells from marrow can serve as long-lasting precursor cells for bone, cartilage, and lung in irradiated mice. *Proc. Natl. Acad. Sci.* **92:** 4857–4861.

Pereira R.F., O'Hara M.D., Laptev A.V., Halford K.W., Pollard M.D., Class R., Simon D., Livezey K., and Prockop D.J. 1998. Marrow stromal cells as a source of progenitor cells for nonhematopoietic tissues in transgenic mice with a phenotype of osteogenesis imperfecta. *Proc. Natl. Acad. Sci.* **95:** 1142–1147.

Perkins S., and Fleischman R. 1988. Hematopoietic microenvironment. Origin, lineage, and transplantability of the stromal cells in long-term bone marrow cultures from chimeric mice. *J. Clin. Invest.* **81:** 1072–1080.

Piersma A.H., Ploemacher R.E., and Brockbank K.G. 1983. Transplantation of bone marrow fibroblastoid stromal cells in mice via the intravenous route. *Br. J. Haematol.* **54:** 285–290.

Pittenger M.F., Mackay A.M., Beck S.C., Jaiswal R.K., Douglas R., Mosca J.D., Moorman M.A., Simonetti D.W., Craig S., and Marshak D.R. 1999. Multilineage potential of adult human mesenchymal stem cells. *Science* **284:** 143–147.

Quesenberry P.J. and Becker P.S. 1998. Stem cell homing: Rolling, crawling, and nesting. *Proc. Natl. Acad. Sci.* **95:** 15155–15157.

Schlossman S., Bloumsell L., and Gilks W. 1995. *Leukocyte typing. V. White cell differentiation antigens.* Oxford University Press, New York.

Schwartz R. 1989. Acquisition of immunologic self tolerance. *Cell* **57:** 1073–1081.

Sha W.C., Nelson C.A., Newberry R.D., Kranz D.M., Russell J.H., and Loh D.Y. 1988. Positive and negative selection of an antigen receptor on T cells in transgenic mice. *Nature* **336:** 73–76.

Shimizu Y., Ogawa M., Kobayashi M., Almeida-Porada G., and Zanjani E.D. 1998. Engraftment of cultured human hematopoietic cells in sheep. *Blood* **91:** 3688–3692.

Silverstein A.M., Prendergast R.A., and Kraner K.L. 1964. Fetal response to antigenic stimulus. IV. Rejection of skin homografts by the fetal lamb. *J. Exp. Med.* **119:** 955–964.

Simmons P.J. and Torok-Storb B. 1991. Identification of stromal cell precursors in human bone marrow by a novel monoclonal antibody, STRO-1. *Blood* **78:** 55–62.

Sprent J. 1995. Central tolerance of T cells. *Int. Rev. Immunol.* **13:** 95–105.

Srour E.F., Zanjani E.D., Cornetta K., Traycoff C.M., Flake A.W., Hedrick M., Brandt J.E., Leemhuis T., and Hoffman R. 1993. Persistence of human multilineage, self-renewing lymphohematopoietic stem cells in chimeric sheep. *Blood* **82:** 3333–3342.

Sutherland D.R., Yeo E.L., Stewart A.K., Nayar R., DiGiusto R., Zanjani E., Hoffman R., and Murray L.J. 1996. Identification of CD34$^+$ subsets after glycoprotease selection: Engraftment of CD34$^+$Thy-1$^+$Lin$^-$ stem cells in fetal sheep. *Exp. Hematol.* **24:** 795–806.

Uchida N., Combs J., Chen S., Zanjani E., Hoffman R., and Tsukamoto A. 1996. Primitive human hematopoietic cells displaying differential efflux of the rhodamine 123 dye have distinct biological activities. *Blood* **88:** 1297–1305.

Xie T. and Spradling A.C. 1998. Decapentaplegic is essential for the maintenance and division of germline stem cells in the *Drosophila* ovary. *Cell* **94:** 251–260.

Yin A.H., Miraglia S., Zanjani E.D., Almeida-Porada G., Ogawa M., Leary A.G., Olweus J., Kearney J., and Buck D.W. 1997. AC133, a novel marker for human hematopoietic stem and progenitor cells. *Blood* **90:** 5002–5012.

Zanjani E.D., Ascensao J.L., and Tavassoli M. 1993. Liver-derived fetal hematopoietic stem cells selectively and preferentially home to the fetal bone marrow. *Blood* **81:** 399–404.

Zanjani E., Almeida-Porada G., Ascensao J., MacKintosh F., and Flake A. 1997. Transplantation of hematopoietic stem cells in utero. *Stem Cells* **15:** 79–93.

Zanjani E.D., Almeida-Porada G., Livingston A.G., Flake A.W., and Ogawa M. 1998. Human bone marrow CD34$^-$ cells engraft in vivo and undergo multilineage expression that includes giving rise to CD34$^+$ cells. *Exp. Hematol.* **26:** 353–360.

Zanjani E.D., Almeida-Porada G., Livingston A.G., Porada C.D., and Ogawa M. 1999. Engraftment and multilineage expression of human bone marrow CD34$^-$ cells in vivo. *Ann. N.Y. Acad. Sci.* **872:** 220–231.

Zanjani E.D., Flake A.W., Rice H., Hedrick M., and Tavassoli M. 1994. Long-term repopulating ability of xenogeneic transplanted human fetal liver hematopoietic stem cells in sheep. *J. Clin. Invest.* **93:** 1051–1055.

Zanjani E.D., Pallavicini M.G., Flake A.W., Ascensao J.L., Langlois R.G., Reitsma M., MacKintosh F.R., Stutes D., Harrison M.R., and Tavassoli M. 1992. Engraftment and long-term expression of human fetal hemopoietic stem cells in sheep following transplantation in utero. *J. Clin. Invest.* **89:** 1178–1188.

Zohar R., Sodek J., and McCulloch C.A. 1997. Characterization of stromal progenitor cells enriched by flow cytometry. *Blood* **90:** 3471–3481.

18

Stem Cells and Neurogenesis

Mitradas M. Panicker[1] and Mahendra Rao[2]

[1,2]Department of Neurobiology and Anatomy
University of Utah Medical School
Salt Lake City, Utah 84132
[1]National Centre for Biological Sciences
UAS, GKVK Campus
GKVK PO, Bellary Road
Bangalore 560 065, India

NEURAL DEVELOPMENT DURING EMBRYOGENESIS

Neural differentiation is an early embryonic event that occurs soon after germ layer specification. The newly formed ectoderm undergoes further patterning to separate into two identifiable components, the presumptive neural ectoderm and the presumptive epidermis. Neural tissue segregates as a clearly demarcated epithelium termed the neuroepithelium (or neuroectoderm). The neuroepithelium generates the central nervous system (CNS) whereas cells at the margins of the neuroepithelium will generate the peripheral nervous system (PNS). Two groups of cells contribute to the PNS. Neural crest stem cells differentiate at the neuroectodermal/epithelial junction, and placodal precursors differentiate from cranial ectoderm that lies more laterally than the zone that generates neural crest (Fig. 1). Precursors that generate the PNS also contribute to nonneural structures, including pigment cells of the skin and craniofacial mesenchyme (for review, see Le Douarin and Kalchem 1999).

Undifferentiated neural precursor cells, whether in the CNS, neural crest, or the placodes, proliferate, differentiate, and migrate to appropriate locations. Cells undergo further maturation and become postmitotic. Neuronal cells go on to project to appropriate targets, make synapses, and acquire the correct rostrocaudal and dorsoventral identity. Seminal work by a number of laboratories has led to rapid advances in our understanding of phenotypic specification (for review, see Rao 1999). An accumulating body of evidence suggests that neurogenesis follows a pattern of development similar to developmental patterns described in the liver, skin, and the hematopoietic system (Edlund and Jessell 1999; Rao 1999;

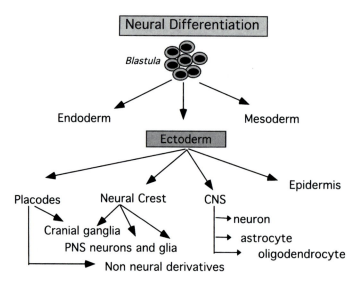

Figure 1 Neural differentiation during development. ES cells undergo differentiation in vitro and in vivo to generate ectodermal, endodermal, and mesodermal
derivatives. The ectoderm subsequently undergoes differentiation to generate the
CNS and PNS. Precursor cells arise from three different domains and generate
distinct but overlapping derivatives.

Weissman 2000). In each of these systems, tissue-specific stem cells are
generated and undergo a series of developmental restrictions to generate
more restricted progeny that ultimately give rise to fully differentiated
cells.

In this chapter, we discuss recent advances in our understanding of
stem cells in the developing nervous system, their isolation, characterization, and role in normal development. We also discuss how some of the
cell fate transitions may be achieved in vitro and the potential fates of
these cells in vivo. More recently, increased interest and study of embryonic stem cells has allowed the generation of specific cell types including
neurally restricted precursors and differentiated neural precursor cells.
These cells have great potential both in understanding basic developmental programs and in therapeutic applications.

MULTIPOTENT STEM CELLS IN NORMAL DEVELOPMENT

The early neuroepithelium that will generate the CNS undergoes further
growth to form a closed neural tube with a central canal either by folding
or by aggregation and subsequent cavitation (see Jacobson 1991).

Initially, the neural tube consists of proliferating, morphologically homogeneous cells termed neuroepithelial (NEP) stem cells (Kalyani et al. 1997). NEP cells or neural stem cells (NSCs) are initially present in a single layer of pseudostratified epithelium spanning the entire distance from the central canal to the external limiting membrane (Sauer and Chittenden 1959; Sauer and Walker 1959). NEP cells continue to proliferate, and are patterned over several days in vivo to generate mature neurons, oligodendrocytes, and astrocytes (see Fig. 2) in a characteristic spatial and temporal pattern (Hamburger 1948; Nornes and Das 1974; Hirano and Goldman 1988; Phelps et al. 1988). Mitotic activity in the proliferating ventricular zone is accompanied by nuclear translocation within the cytoplasm. While the cells remain attached to the basal lamina, the nuclei move away from the lumen during the S phase of the mitotic cycle, and return near to the lumen when undergoing division, a process termed interkinetic nuclear migration (Seymour and Berry 1975). Detailed analysis has suggested that the abventricular translocation occurs in the G_1/S transition (Takahashi et al. 1994), whereas adventricular transitions occur predominantly in the M/G_1 transition (Fig. 3). Cell cycle time for the ventricular zone has been studied. It changes during development and cells appear synchronized with few differences in cell cycle times. Small changes in

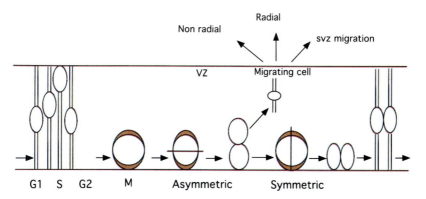

Figure 2 Nuclear translocation and symmetric and asymmetric differentiation. Stem cells present in the ventricular zone undergo characteristic interkinetic nuclear translocation and can divide both symmetrically and asymmetrically to generate either another stem cell and a differentiated daughter cell or two stem cells or two differentiated daughter cells (not shown) with a consequent diminution of the proliferating cell pool. The ratio of symmetric and asymmetric divisions changes during development with a consequent reduction in the number of multipotent stem cells present in the adult.

MULTIPOTENT NEURAL PRECURSOR

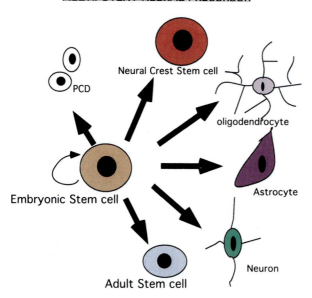

Figure 3 Neural stem cells during development. Early fetal stem cells express characteristic markers, can undergo self-renewal, die by a process of programmed cell death, differentiate into neuronal and nonneuronal derivatives, or mature to form adult stem cells that differ from early multipotent stem cells in growth factor dependence, cell cycle kinetics, migration, and differentiation potential (see text for details).

cell cycle kinetics can change the total number of cells generated significantly (Cai et al. 1997; Mione et al. 1997). Cell cycle kinetics are regulated by extrinsic growth factors, and differential growth of stem cells may serve to sculpt the developing brain. Programmed cell death (PCD) may be important in regulating stem cell number (for review, see Gilmore et al. 2000; Raoul et al. 2000), although details of its exact role are not known. Stem cells generate differentiated progeny that lose their attachment to the basal lamina and rapidly migrate to the overlying layers of the cortex. Progenitor cells begin to express differentiation markers while migrating and can be distinguished from stem cells by such expression. Multipotent cells in the ventricular zone undergo both symmetrical and asymmetrical divisions. Cai et al. (1997) used retroviral labeling to show that approximately 48% of labeled cells formed clusters located entirely within the ventricular zone, suggesting self-renewal via symmetrical divisions. Approximately 20% of cells, however, appeared to generate cells in both the ventricular zone and the mantle, suggesting at least some asymmetrical divisions. Whether a cell will undergo symmetric or asymmetric divisions depends on whether molecules asymmetrically distributed within the cytoplasm are differentially partitioned into the two daughter cells (for review, see Temple 2000). It has been suggested that notch, numb, and possibly other molecules are distributed apically or basally (for review, see Morrison et al. 1997). Divisions in the horizontal plane will result in asymmetrical localization of notch and numb to the two daughter cells with consequent differences in cell fate. Divisions in an oblique or perpendicular plane will result in a more equal partitioning with a greater likelihood of symmetric divisions (see Fig. 3). How the axis of cell division is determined is a subject of study, and possible mechanisms are discussed by Jan and Jan (1998). The relationship between nuclear migration and symmetric and asymmetric cell division has been studied primarily in the telencephalic neuroepithelium (Chenn and McConnell 1995; Zhong et al. 1997; Chenn et al. 1998; for review, see Jan and Jan 1998), but it is likely that similar relationships are also important in the spinal cord.

As development proceeds, the ventricle becomes significantly diminished in size and the characteristics of the cells present in the ventricular zone change. It is thought that the ependymal cells represent the remnants of the ventricular zone stem cells, although some cells persist as undifferentiated cells in or near the subependymal layer (Smart 1961; Morshead and van der Kooy 1992). Proliferating cells are seen in an additional zone of precursor cells termed the subventricular zone (svz), which is derived from the ventricular zone during embryonic development (Reznikov et al. 1997) and persists throughout life. The svz contains a mixed population of precursor cells that can generate neurons and glia (Reynolds and Weiss 1992; Lois and Alvarez-Buylla 1993; Craig et al. 1996; Doetsch and Alvarez-Buylla 1996). This zone may contribute to ongoing neurogenesis that continues throughout life. A svz is not present in the spinal cord, hindbrain, or cerebellum, and little postnatal neurogenesis is seen in these brain regions (Gilbert 1988; Jacobson 1991; Horner et al. 2000). Within the cerebellum there exists a separate zone of proliferating precursors termed the external granule cell layer (egl). The egl is a transient layer of proliferating precursors derived from the ventricular zone of the midbrain and hindbrain that disappears in the early postnatal period (for review, see Hatten and Heintz 1995) and generates the granule cells of the cerebellum.

Characteristics of cells present in each of these developmental zones have been described (for review, see Mayer-Proschel and Rao 2000). Much of the focus has been on the cortical ventricular zone, although pluripotent stem cells that self-renew and generate neurons, astrocytes, and oligodendrocytes (see Fig. 3) have been identified from the entire neural axis. Evidence of pluripotentiality includes retroviral labeling (see, e.g., Price et al. 1991; Levison and Goldman 1997), transplantation of clonal cell populations (McKay 1992), and characterizing stem cells in clonal and mass culture (Johe et al. 1996; Reynolds and Weiss 1996; Kalyani et al. 1997; Qian et al. 1997). Fetal precursor cells appear to express certain characteristic features. They require fibroblast growth factor (FGF) for their proliferation in vivo and in vitro and express nestin and additional markers (summarized in Table 1). An emerging consensus is that although cells present in all of these different regions are multipotent and display common features, they are nevertheless distinguishable from each other in growth factor dependence, cell cycle time, markers, and ability to differentiate (for review, see Rao 1999). Stem cells isolated from the spinal cord and early stages of embryogenesis appear to require FGF for their survival, whereas stem cells isolated from more rostral regions at later developmental stages seem equally responsive to FGF and/or epidermal growth factor (EGF) (for review, see Rao 1999). The cell cycle time progressively lengthens as the embryo matures and, in the adult, stem cells can be detected in multiple regions, including the cortex. Cortical stem cells express polysialated N-CAM whereas cells that remain in the adult svz express glial fibrillary acid protein (GFAP) immunoreactivity (Marmur et al. 1998; Doetsch et al. 1999). Stem cells in vivo also express rostrocaudal positional markers (for review, see

Table 1 Multiple types of multipotent cells are present in the nervous system

Classification	Characteristics
Embryonic stem cells	FGF-dependent, nestin-immunoreactive cells present in the ventricular zone along the entire rostrocaudal axis including the cerebellum, midbrain, and hindbrain
Adult stem cells	EGF-dependent, nestin-immunoreactive cells present in the subventricular zone, spinal cord, and cortex
Retinal stem cells	nestin-immunoreactive, Chx10-expressing, dividing cells that are biased toward retinal differentiation
Hypothalamic-pituitary stem cells	nestin-immunoreactive, dividing cells that require NOS for activity
Neural crest stem cells, stem cells	nestin, p75, HNK-1-immunoreactive
Placodal stem cells	nestin-immunoreactive

Some examples of stem cells present in the nervous system are listed, and their salient characteristics are summarized. Refer to text for details and their potential lineage relationship.

Rubenstein and Rakic 1999), and these markers are maintained in culture. Response to neurotransmitters is also different. Ventricular zone stem cells proliferate in response to glutamate whereas subventricular zone stem cells respond to glutamate with a reduction in proliferation (P. Rakic, pers. comm.). Transplant studies have also suggested a bias in differentiation potential. For example, cells present in the lateral ganglionic eminence (LGE) differ in their migration and differentiation properties from cells present in the medial ganglionic eminence (MGE) (Wichterle et al. 1999).

The available data do not allow us to draw any strong conclusions about how these differences arise. Either a common multipotent stem cell undergoes specification as development proceeds or multiple classes of multipotent cells arise at an early developmental age. Distinguishing between these possibilities, except in select instances, has been difficult. In the case of embryonic FGF-dependent neuroepithelial stem cells and later arising EGF-dependent neurospheres, a direct lineage relationship has been established. Early rat multipotent stem cells present from E10 onward are FGF-dependent (Kalyani et al. 1997). FGF-dependent cells undergo maturation and begin to respond to EGF by proliferation (Ciccolini and Svendsen 1998; Tropepe et al. 1999). The EGF-responsive cells can be maintained solely in EGF and appear to be present from E14 onward. At early developmental ages, both EGF- and FGF-dependent stem cells are present and likely continue to coexist in the adult. Proof that FGF-dependent stem cells generate EGF-dependent cells came from culture experiments and the use of chimeric mice (Tropepe et al. 1999). In these experiments, initially only an FGF-dependent population of stem cells was present, but later in development FGF-dependent and EGF-dependent cells (which arise from FGF-dependent cells) are both present.

Stem cells have now been isolated from proliferating ventricular and subventricular zones of the developing forebrain as well as from the spinal cord, cortex, midbrain, and hindbrain. In addition, stem cells have also been identified in another area of the mammalian CNS, the neuro-hypophyseal system of the endocrine hypothalamus. Stem cells emerge from the subependymal regions of the third cerebral ventricle, migrate, generate neurons, and repopulate the region after hypophysectomy. Up-regulation of nitric oxide synthase (NOS) seems to be essential for this process (Scott and Hansen 1997). Another specialized region of the brain from which stem cells have been identified is the neural retina. Two laboratories have independently isolated and characterized retinal stem cells (Ahmad et al. 2000; Tropepe et al. 2000). Both groups showed that embryonic and adult retinas contain a multipotent, self-renewing stem cell. This cell is preferentially localized to the ciliary margin and requires FGF, and perhaps EGF, for survival. Individual retinal stem cells are multipotent and can generate retinal derivatives in mass and clonal culture. The retinal stem cell differed from CNS stem cells in the expression of retinal-specific genes such as Chx-10 and appears to preferentially differentiate into retinal cells.

Overall, the available evidence shows that stem cells exist in multiple regions of the developing and adult brain, and specialized stem cells exist in specific regions. These multipotent cells are present at the appropriate time and place to play a role in normal development and can be distinguished on the basis of growth factor dependence, time of isolation, cell surface receptors, transcription factors expressed, and their ability to differentiate into specific subtypes of cells.

RESTRICTED PRECURSORS

Multipotent stem cells do not appear to migrate extensively and are largely localized to the ventricular zones (however, see cortical stem cells above), but their derivatives do migrate. During development, differentiating cells lose their attachment to the basal lamina and migrate from the ventricular zone to appropriate target sites. Migrating neuronal precursor cells express markers of differentiation and follow radial glial and nonradial glial pathways of migration to terminal sites. Glial precursors do not appear to require radial glia for migration, and their exact mode of migration remains to be determined. In the spinal cord the first postmitotic cells to differentiate are ventral motoneurons, followed by more dorsal neuronal phenotypes. In the cortex, differentiation is layer-specific, with early-born neurons being present in the lowest layers. Neuronal precursors migrate past formed layers to form successively more superficial layers (see, e.g., McConnell 1988). Neurogenesis, except in certain specific regions, persists from E11 to E17 in rats (Nornes and Das 1974; Altman and Bayer 1984; Phelps et al. 1988) and precedes (but overlaps) differentiation of oligodendrocytes and astrocytes (Abney et al. 1981; Miller et al. 1985; Frederiksen and McKay 1988; Hirano and Goldman 1988). A variety of evidence suggests that multipotent stem cells generate differentiated mature neurons via the generation of more restricted precursors.

Bromodeoxyuridine (BrdU) labeling studies have shown that some cell division occurs in migrating cells as well as in white matter, suggesting that cells may continue to divide after leaving the ventricular zone. These migrating precursors have been isolated and shown to possess at least limited self-renewal potential and retain the ability to generate multiple derivatives. We have termed these cells restricted precursors and classified them on the basis of their differentiation ability. Thus, neuronal restricted precursors can generate multiple classes of neurons, but not astrocytes or oligodendrocytes, under conditions in which multipotent stem cells generate such derivatives. Multiple classes of such precursors have been identified and are discussed below (also see Fig. 5).

By analogy to the hematopoietic system, these cells would be termed blast cells or restricted progenitor cells. Compared to multipotent stem cells, they have a more limited self-renewing ability and are more restricted in their ability to differentiate. In the hematopoietic system, where prolonged self-renewal is a necessary requisite for therapy, blast cells are of limited therapeutic value. In the nervous system, however, cellular replacement is not an ongoing requirement, and thus replacement by cells that have a more limited self-renewal ability may be preferred. Transplanting cells with a restricted differentiation potential would reduce the chance of tumor formation or heterotopias. Furthermore, it is more likely that cues for normal differentiation would be present, and more differentiated cells would be far more likely to respond to cues present in the adult. Finally, the availability of more restricted precursor cells may provide the ability to replace selected populations of cells. In the following section, we describe some of the lineage-restricted precursors that have been characterized and discuss their therapeutic potential.

Neuron-restricted Precursors

A number of in vivo and in vitro experiments over the years have provided evidence that NRPs are present and play an important role in normal development. Strong evidence for the existence of NRPs in vivo came from retroviral-labeling experiments (Luskin et al. 1988; Parnavelas et al. 1991; Price et al. 1991; Grove et al. 1992; Lavdas et al. 1996; Levison and Goldman 1997). Labeled single cells and their progeny gave rise to clones that comprised solely neurons. Clones that contained a single class of neurons as well as clones that contained multiple kinds of neurons were identified, suggesting precursors exist that could undergo at least limited self-renewal and generate solely neurons. Progeny arising from these clones were present in clusters or were widely dispersed, suggesting that they could undertake radial and nonradial migration (Luskin 1994; Price and Thurlow 1988). Since in the same experiments other clones could be identified that generated solely glial cells, it appeared likely that the restriction seen was intrinsic to the cells and that the environment at this stage could support both neuronal and glial differentiation (Grove et al.

1993). The generation of restricted precursors appears to be a late developmental event as analysis in vivo and in vitro at early embryonic ages generated largely multipotent clones, whereas at later stages, primarily unipotent clones were seen (Temple 1989; Williams and Price 1995; Lavdas et al. 1996; Levison and Goldman 1997). If cells were followed at later stages of development, most precursor cells gave rise to either neurons or oligodendrocytes or astrocytes (Luskin et al. 1988). Few mixed clones were detected, suggesting that initially multipotent stem cells generate differentiated cells via the generation of more restricted precursors.

The existence of NRPs (Fig. 4) has also been corroborated by in vitro culture assays. Early work by Gensburger et al. (1987) had shown the presence of neurofilament-positive cells from 13-day-old rat embryos that proliferate in culture in response to bFGF. Other investigators have maintained dividing neuronal precursors from a number of regions of the mammalian brain (Temple 1989; Cattaneo and McKay 1990; Deloulme et al. 1991; Gao et al. 1991; Ray and Gage 1994; Palmer et al. 1995; Shihabuddin et al. 1997; Brewer 1999; Mujtaba et al. 1999) although, except in selected cases, the cultures were not pure NRP populations. Other experiments (Blass-Kampmann et al. 1994) suggested that embryonal N-CAM was expressed by neuronal and astrocytic precursors and could be used to isolate these cells. Mayer-Proschel and colleagues (Mayer-Proschel et al. 1997; Kalyani et al. 1998; Mujtaba et al. 1999; Yang et al. 2000) used antibody panning to isolate a pure population of NRP cells that could differentiate into multiple classes of neurons. They did not differentiate into astrocytes and oligodendrocytes, even in conditions where multipotent stem cells or glial precursors did. The authors have termed these cells NRP cells and have shown that, when transplanted in vivo, they remain restricted to differentiate into neurons. Although restricted to neuronal differentiation, these early NRPs could differentiate into excitatory, inhibitory, and cholinergic neurons (Yang et al. 2000). Direct isolation of neuronal precursors, which do not generate glial cells, has been achieved by fluorescence sorting after transfection with GFP constructs under the control of the Tα1 tubulin early promoter (Wang et al. 1998).

Equally important are recent results that clearly establish a lineage relationship between multipotent stem cells and more restricted precursor cells. Neuroepithelial precursors (NEP) from the spinal cord have been shown to give rise to NRPs (Kalyani et al. 1997; Mayer-Proschel et al. 1997). NEP cells generate E-NCAM-immunoreactive cells that can further differentiate into neurons of multiple phenotypes in culture, including some that are not normally observed in the spinal cord. They do not give rise to oligodendrocytes or astrocytes (Kalyani et al. 1998). NRP cells iso-

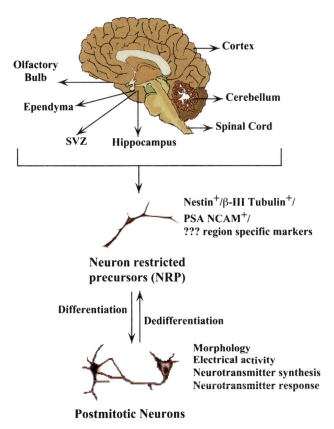

Figure 4 Neuron-restricted precursors. Cells that generate primarily neurons have been isolated from multiple regions of the brain. These cells share many characteristics but are likely to differ in the expression of region-specific markers and their ability to differentiate into specific subclasses of neurons. Differentiated neurons have been classified based on their morphology, neurotransmitter profile, response to neurotransmitters, and electrophysiological response to excitatory or inhibitory input.

lated from NEP cells seem identical to those generated directly from the developing spinal cord (Ray and Gage 1994; Mayer-Proschel et al. 1997; Kalyani et al. 1998; Mujtaba et al. 1999). Vescovi et al. (1993) have also showed that transient exposure to bFGF can cause the differentiation of EGF-responsive precursors into secondary progenitors, some of which give rise to neurons alone (Vescovi et al. 1993). It is important to emphasize here that work with cultured precursor cells from the embryonic CNS has been consistent with much of the in vivo observations. In particular, the retroviral labeling of cells in vivo or following single cells in culture has allowed the unambiguous delineation of lineage and potential of proliferating precursors (Temple 1989; Kilpatrick and Bartlett 1993).

Neuronal precursors have also been isolated from the developing human brain by fluorescence sorting after transfection with GFP constructs under the control of the Tα1 tubulin promoter. Goldman and colleagues have recently reported the successful use of neuronal promoter-targeted screening techniques to obtain neuronal precursors from adult human hippocampus. These precursors divide in vitro and mature to form physiologically active neurons (Roy et al. 2000b). Using the same technique, neuronal precursors have been isolated from the adult ventricular zone (Roy et al. 2000a). Not surprisingly, a human immortalized and neuron-restricted spinal precursor cell line (HSP-1) has been identified. This cell line may represent the equivalent of NRPs in humans, an idea strongly supported by the fact that it does not differentiate into astrocytes or oligodendrocytes under conditions where they are usually generated (Li et al. 2000).

Are There Subclasses of NRPs?

When marked SVZa cells from postnatal mice are transplanted in utero into the ventricles of E15 mice, they integrate at multiple levels throughout the neuraxis and form neurons. Interestingly, the migration is not uniform into all areas of the brain. Transplanted cells were not seen in the cortex or the hippocampus of the recipient (Lim et al. 1997). Stem cells from the adult forebrain of rats also could be directed to increased generation of neurons in the presence of insulin-like growth factor 1 (IGF-1) and heparin (Brooker et al. 2000). External cues as well as intrinsic potential, therefore, seem to play a role. Similarly, Luskin and coworkers have shown that the origin of the precursor cells seems to be important in determining the efficiency with which NRPs integrate in a homotypic or heterotypic site (Zigova et al. 1996). Embryonic neurons from the medial ganglionic eminence seem to be more widely dispersed and differentiate in multiple areas of the adult brain in comparison to cells from the lateral ganglionic eminence (Wichterle et al. 1999).

Progenitor cells, isolated from postnatal mouse hippocampus, cultured in the presence of EGF, divide, and on addition of brain-derived neurotrophic factor, give rise to pyramidal-like neurons (Shetty and Turner 1998). When transplanted into the cerebellum, however, these progenitors do not give rise to neurons, and when introduced into the rostral olfactory tract, only a few cells migrated into the olfactory bulb to give tyrosine hydroxylase (TH)-positive neurons (Suhonen et al. 1996). Thus, multipotent precursors isolated from different regions of the developing brain are likely to differ depending on the developmental stage and region from which they were isolated.

Glial-restricted Precursors

Radial glia are the first identified glial population to develop, followed by glial precursors, followed by astrocytes and oligodendrocytes (Rakic 1972). Unlike most neurons, which cease to divide postnatally, astrocytes continue to be generated in adults (Altman 1966; Sturrock 1982). Oligodendrocytes do not divide, dedifferentiate, or reenter the cell cycle (for review, see Blakemore and Keirstead 1999; for an alternate viewpoint, see Grinspan et al. 1994). However, precursors to oligodendrocytes exist and their division persists, albeit at a slow rate, throughout life (Bensted et al. 1957; Fujita 1965). Extrinsic signals can modulate cell division, and the rate of oligodendrocyte differentiation is increased after demyelinating lesions (McMorris et al. 1986; Gensert and Goldman 1996). Current evidence suggests that glial cells differentiate from multipotential stem cells by sequential stages of restriction in developmental potential, and several types of glial precursors (Fig. 5) have been identified (for review, see Rao 1999; Lee et al. 2000).

Glial precursors are first seen at E13 in mice and E14.5 in rats in multiple restricted foci (Spassky et al. 1998). In the developing caudal neural tube, glial precursors arise in ventral regions and migrate both dorsally and ventrally, and differentiate into oligodendrocytes (Timsit et al. 1995; Miller 1996; Hardy 1997; Spassky et al. 1998). Astrocyte differentiation is first observed in the dorsal region although the location of astrocyte precursors within the neural tube remains to be determined (Fok-Seang and Miller 1994; Pringle et al. 1998).

Rao and colleagues have suggested that the early precursor identified on the basis of A2B5 immunoreactivity, the expression of PLP-DM20 and Nkx2.2, and the absence of platelet-derived growth factor receptor-α (PDGFR-α) immunoreactivity, is the precursor for both astrocytes and oligodendrocytes. These investigators used immunopanning to isolate A2B5 immunoreactive cells and showed that these cells differed from multipotent stem cells and NRPs and that these glial precursors could generate astrocytes and oligodendrocytes both in vitro and in vivo. The investigators termed these cells glial restricted precursors (GRPs) and showed that they differentiated from multipotent stem cells, thereby establishing a direct relationship between these two precursor populations (Rao and Mayer-Proschel 1997; Rao et al. 1998).

Mayer-Proschel and colleagues have further characterized the process of differentiation. They have shown that GRP cells acquire PDGFR-α

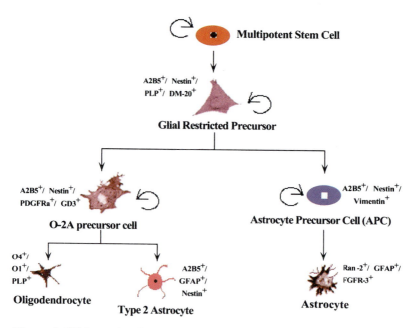

Figure 5 Glial-restricted precursors. A potential lineage relationship between multipotent stem cells, glial precursors, and even more restricted unipotent precursors is shown. It is important to emphasize that only some of these relationships have been directly demonstrated. The relationship between GRPs and aldynoglia remains to be established.

immunoreactivity and PDGF dependence upon prolonged culture. GRP cells can generate more differentiated precursors that do not generate astrocytes in vivo but can generate oligodendrocytes and thus resemble the well-characterized O2A progenitor cell (M. Mayer-Proschel, pers. comm.). This transition is also likely to occur in vivo. Mengsheng Qiu and colleagues have used Nkx2.2 expression to follow glial precursors and were able to show that glial precursors do not initally express PDGFR-α immunoreactivity but acquire it within 2 days of developmental time (Qiu et al. 1998). Spassky and colleagues have likewise shown that when the expression of LacZ is driven by the PLP promoter, they see multiple foci of expression that match regions of A2B5 immunoreactivity and do not overlap regions of PDGFR-α immunoreactivity (Spassky et al. 1998). Cells isolated at this early stage appear capable of differentiating into both astrocytes and oligodendrocytes, providing independent confirmation of the existence of an oligodendrocyte–astrocyte precursor.

Another class of glial precursors found in a structure termed the oligosphere has been described by Avellana-Adalid et al. (1996).

Oligospheres are floating aggregates, generated from neonatal rat brains, containing presumably homogeneous populations of A2B5 immunoreactive cells. These aggregates can be propagated as undifferentiated cells for long periods of time and can differentiate into oligodendrocytes and astrocytes in culture or after transplantation (Zhang et al. 1998; Brüstle et al. 1999). Similar cultures of oligospheres have been obtained from the subependymal striata of adult rats and canines (Zhang et al. 1998; Brüstle 1999).

Apart from precursors that can generate both astrocytes and oligodendrocytes, more restricted precursors have been isolated. The best characterized of all such precursors is the O2A or oligodendrocyte type-2 astrocyte precursor cell. This cell was initially isolated from the optic nerve (Raff et al. 1983) and has been subsequently shown to exist in multiple brain regions (Raine et al. 1981; Prabhakar et al. 1995; Scolding et al. 1995). Unlike the GRP cell, it does not differentiate into astrocytes when transplanted in vivo and thus appears more restricted in its differentiation potential. It is likely that at least some O2A cells arise from GRP cells, but it is not clear whether additional pathways of glial differentiation exist. A variety of astrocyte precursors have also been identified. One such population is the astrocyte precursor cell (APC) that gives rise to astrocytes alone (Mi and Barres 1999). These have been isolated from embryonic and P1 rat optic nerves by immunopanning with an astrocyte-lineage-specific anti-neuroepithelial antibody (C5) (Miller et al. 1984). In culture, APCs differentiate into type-1 astrocytes alone. APCs have an antigenic phenotype that is GFAP$^-$, A2B5$^+$, and Pax2$^+$, whereas type-1 astrocytes are GFAP$^+$, A2B5$^-$, and Pax2$^+$. APCs are different from O2A cells, since no oligodendrocytes are obtained. Levels of the A2B5 antigen are found to be lower in APCs than in other precursors. Astrocytes have been generated from the dorsal spinal cord, which suggests the existence of an astrocyte precursor (Hall et al. 1996; Pringle et al. 1998). A2B5$^+$ cells have also been identified in the dorsal spinal cord. This raises the possibility that cells similar to APCs exist in the spinal cord. Seidman et al. (1997) have also described an immortalized astrocyte-restricted precursor cell line. This cell line, isolated from E16 mouse cerebellum, proliferates in response to EGF and, upon EGF withdrawal and the addition of bFGF, develops the morphology and expression pattern of a fibrous astrocyte.

Specialized glia such as Bergmann glia or Muller glia provide a different view of glial cell production and differentiation. Recently, Gudino-Cabrera and Nieto-Sampedro have suggested that Muller glia and olfactory ensheathing cells belong to a third glial population, distinguished on the basis of antigenic and functional criteria. This population of glial cells, termed aldynoglia (Gudino-Cabrera and Nieto-Sampedro 1999), includes olfactory ensheathing cells, tanycytes, pituocytes, pineal glial, Muller glial, and Bergman glial cells. These cells are distinguished from astrocytes and oligodendrocytes in that they concomitantly express O4, GFAP, P75, and estrogen receptor α. Differentiating these cells from other glial populations is primarily their potential functional importance. They appear to have dramatic growth- and regeneration-promoting properties. In particular, transplanted olfactory ensheathing cells have shown remarkable ability to promote axonal regeneration and functional recovery (Ramon-Cueto et al. 2000). How these cells are lineally related to the more prevalent glial populations present in the brain is not known. Muller glia, a specialized retinal glial cell, is one of the last cell types to mature in the retina. It does not seem to arise from a glial-restricted precursor, but rather from a multipotential precursor that also gives rise to neurons (Turner et al. 1990). It has been suggested that Muller glia can dedifferentiate to give rise to retinal stem cells in amphibian and avian retina (Reh and Levine 1998). More recently, stem cells have been identified in the mammalian retina that give rise to Muller glia in culture (Tropepe et al. 2000). Another specialized glial cell type is the intrafascicular ensheathing cells in the olfactory bulb, which ensheathe olfactory axons. They are unique in that they seem to have a mixture of astrocytic and oligodendrocytic properties (Doucette 1993). These cells may arise from the olfactory placode and express the homeoprotein Otx-2 (Mallamaci et al. 1996; Ramon-Cueto and Avila 1998). Thus, these specialized glia, although functionally similar, may have distinct embryological origins. Of interest, however, is a recent observation by Blakemore and colleagues on the differentiation of CNS glial precursors. They isolated CNS glial precursors and showed that they generated Schwann-like cells in addition to astrocytes and oligodendrocytes (Keirstead et al. 1999). This result raises the possibility that some aldynoglia share a common lineage with other glial precursors. In conclusion, the recent identification of GRPs and the relationship between different glial cell types has led to a clearer understanding of gliogenesis. The molecular mechanisms involved await further studies.

Neural Crest Stem Cells

The neural crest is a late development in the evolution of vertebrates and is of importance because of the variety of derivatives that arise from this specialized population of cells (Northcutt and Gans 1983). Crest cells segregate from the developing neural tube at or around the time of neural tube closure. The exact process of delamination is species dependent. In mice, cells begin to delaminate before the tube has completely closed (Nieto et al. 1992), whereas in the chick, a premigratory form of crest exists and can be reconstituted from surrounding tissue (Scherson et al. 1993).

Crest stem cells differ from CNS stem cells discussed earlier because of their extensive migration ability, their epithelial to mesenchymal transition, and the phenotypes that they can differentiate into (for review, see Ayer-Le Lievre and Le Douarin 1982; Douarin 1983; Anderson et al. 1997; Baker and Bronner-Fraser 1997; LaBonne and Bronner-Fraser 1998). The neural crest stem cell (NCSC) has been isolated and characterized in multiple species and, although it is a transient population, it nevertheless fulfills all the criteria of a stem cell (Morrison et al. 1999). The NCSC cell is multipotent, undergoes self-renewal, and can generate multiple phenotypes that include craniofacial mesoderm, melanocytes, and the neurons and glia of the PNS (for review, see Ayer-Le Lievre and Le Douarin 1982; Douarin 1983; Bronner-Fraser 1995a,b). It is important to note that NCSC, like mesodermal stem cells (Bianco and Cossu 1999; Seale and Rudnicki 2000), can generate mesodermal derivatives including bone, cartilage, smooth muscle, etc. The potential of neural crest to generate craniofacial mesenchyme was initially thought to be limited to the cranial crest, but several groups have shown that crest from more caudal regions is equally capable of differentiating into nonneural derivatives. What restricts this developmental potential in more caudal regions of the embryo remains undefined.

Evidence from chick embryo experiments at early developmental stages suggests that NCSC and differentiated CNS cells share a common progenitor (Bronner-Fraser and Fraser 1988, 1989; Sanes 1989; Leber et al. 1990; Scherson et al. 1993; Artinger et al. 1995; Mujtaba et al. 1998). Additional evidence that the CNS and the PNS share a common precursor comes from chick neural fold ablation experiments which demonstrate that cells of the remaining neural tube have the regulative capacity to compensate for the ablated neural crest cells (Scherson et al. 1993). These results suggest that neuroepithelial cells normally destined to form the CNS have the ability to regulate their prospective fates to generate PNS derivatives. Recent work from two different laboratories has shown that FGF-dependent multipotent CNS stem cells likely represent the common CNS-PNS precursor in rats. Mujtaba and colleagues (1998) have shown that NEP cells can generate p75/nestin immunoreactive cells that are morphologically and antigenically similar to previously characterized NCSCs (Stemple and Anderson 1992; Ito et al. 1993; Rao and Anderson 1997). NEP-derived p75 immunoreactive cells differentiate into peripheral neurons, smooth muscle, and Schwann cells in both mass and clonal culture. More importantly, clonal analysis indicates that individual NEP cells could generate both CNS and PNS derivatives, providing evidence for the first time of a direct lineage relationship between these two distinct cell types. In addition, McKay and colleagues have shown that cortical stem cells which were isolated at a stage well after neural crest migration has taken place still retain their ability to differentiate into PNS derivatives (Hazel et al. 1997). No data regarding the ability of EGF-dependent neurosphere cells to generate crest or PNS derivatives exist. Although the NEP cell can generate NCSCs, it is unclear whether NCSCs can differentiate into CNS derivatives. Transplants of neural crest into the spinal cord result in Schwann cell differentiation but not into CNS derivatives, suggesting that the NCSC is a restricted precursor cell.

NCSCs isolated during crest migration have a characteristic phenotype but may not represent the sole kind of multipotent crest precursor (see Fig. 6). Multiple classes of stem cells are likely to be present, and in this respect, PNS differentiation may be similar to CNS differentiation. Initial results have suggested that there is some rostrocaudal patterning that distinguishes crest cells from each other and thus biases their differentiation potential. For example, the ability to contribute to heart development is normally restricted to a specific rostrocaudal level (for review, see Kirby 1990; Creazzo et al. 1998).Clonal assays have suggested, however, that even caudal crest can differentiate into smooth muscle and when transplanted will migrate to the heart (M.S. Rao and M. Bronner-Fraser, unpubl.). Sommer and colleagues have identified a subpopulation of crest precursors that, unlike most NCSCs, express PMP-22 (Hagedorn et al. 1999). These cells, nevertheless, are multipotent by the same criteria that have been used to establish the stem cell potential of neural crest.

Like the CNS stem cell, it is likely that the NCSC also generates differentiated progeny via the generation of more restricted precursors. Although a detailed description of the multiple classes of more restricted precursors identified is beyond the scope of this chapter, several restricted precursors have been identified. Of interest are Schwann cell precursors that appear to be the equivalent of PNS glial restricted precursors (Mirsky and Jessen 1996). Schwann cells perform the functions of both astrocytes and oligodendrocytes and are known to be important in promoting axonal regeneration and recovery in peripheral nerves. A melanocyte precursor may also exist, and Weston and colleagues have suggested the existence of such restricted precursors (Weston 1991). Anderson and colleagues have immortalized a sympathoadrenal precursor that makes sympathetic neurons and adrenal chromaffin cells (Vandenbergh et al. 1991). The enteric nervous system may also be pop-

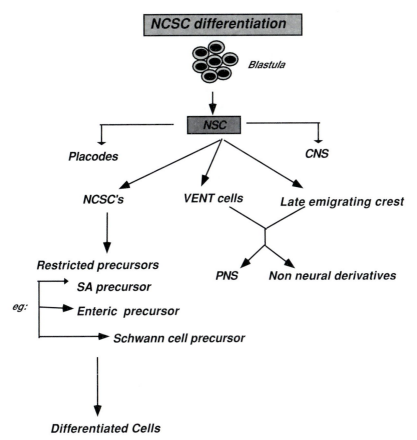

Figure 6 Neural crest stem cells. A potential lineage of crest cells is illustrated. ES cells and CNS stem cells have both been shown to generate melanocytes and other crest derivatives. A variety of evidence suggests that a common CNS-PNS precursor exists at early stages of embryonic development and that at later stages PNS derivatives are derived from VENT cells and late emigrating neural crest populations.

ulated by more restricted precursors (for review, see Gershon 1997). Thus, NCSCs represent a lineage-restricted precursor cell that can generate PNS but not CNS derivatives. As in the CNS, differentiation appears to progress through sequential stages of more differentiated cells. Although such classes of cells have been identified, these cells have not been characterized in as much detail due to the limited numbers of cells available for analysis and the small number of stage-specific markers available.

Two other populations of cells that contribute to the developing PNS have been described. Both appear to differentiate later than NCSCs and migrate along characteristic pathways. One population, termed the late emigrating crest cell population (Korade and Frank 1996; Sharma et al. 1995), emigrates along dorsal nerve roots along the rostrocaudal axis and can contribute neurons and glia to the sensory ganglia. Frank and colleagues have shown that this population may also contribute to pigment cell development and perhaps to sensory neuron derivatives (Sharma et al. 1995). Sohal and colleagues have described yet another population of cells that arise from the neural tube and migrate through the ventral roots of cranial nerves (Sohal et al. 1996, 1998; Poelmann and Gittenberger-de Groot 1999) and contribute to a variety of tissues. These cells have been termed ventrally emigrating neural cells or VENT cells. VENT cells differ from neural crest in that they arise later from ventral neural tube and do not express HNK-1 immunoreactivity (a marker for emigrating neural crest), and the repertoire of their phenotypes is distinct. Sohal and colleagues used replication-deficient retrovirus to label VENT cells and follow their differentiation. VENT cells followed nerve roots of the cranial ganglia and could be localized to a variety of tissue that included the trigeminal ganglion, heart, cartilage, vascular smooth muscle, and liver (for review, see Erickson and Weston 1999). These results suggest that neural precursor cells are more pluripotent than previously supposed and may be capable of generating ectodermal and mesodermal cells. The developmental significance of these populations of late emigrating cells is unclear. No specific ablation experiments have been performed, and the importance of discrete multipotent populations that contribute to the same developing structure remains to be determined. The existence of these populations, however, needs to be taken into account as a potential atypical source of cells for cellular replacement strategies.

Adult Precursor Cells

Recent data have suggested that both neurogenesis and gliogenesis persist in the adult and can be modulated by external environmental influences. It is not clear from the available data whether this represents activation of a quiescent population of multipotent stem cells, activation of more restricted neuronal or glial precursors (see below), or dedifferentiation of postmitotic cells (Brewer 1999). Evidence demonstrating the presence of multipotent cells in the adult suggests that multipotent stem cells may contribute to some of the ongoing neuro-gliogenesis. Controversy exists as to the location of adult stem cells, and multipotent cells may be present in the ependymal, subventricular, and cortical regions. The structure of the subependymal region has been characterized and at least five different classes of cells (see Table 2) have been described (Doetsch et al. 1997). Which of these cells represents the putative stem cell remains unclear. Johansson et al. (1999) have argued that the ependymal cells represent the adult stem cell population. These authors showed that ependymal cells are a quiescent population that generates a more rapidly dividing cell (termed transit amplifying cell), which then generates neurons and astrocytes. Conversely, van der Kooy and colleagues have argued that in their in vitro culture system only subependymal cells (and not ependymal cells) can self-renew and generate multipotent cells (Chiasson et al. 1999). Which subependymal population represents the true stem cell is still under investigation. Doetsch and others have suggested that type C cells represent a stem cell (Morshead et al. 1994; Doetsch et al. 1999), as they express nestin but no other differentiation markers and are rapidly proliferating. More recently, Alvarez Buylla and colleagues (Garcia-Verdugo et al. 1998) have postulated that type B1 cells may represent the adult stem cell population. Using a retroviral label, they have shown that a GFAP immunoreactive cell is present in the subventricular zone and that this cell fulfills the criteria of a stem cell (Doetsch et al. 1999). Marmur and colleagues have suggested that in the adult, stem cells may be present not only in the remnants of ventricular or subventricular zones, but also as a quiescent population throughout the cortex. These investigators have shown that polysialated NCAM immunoreactivity can be used to isolate multipotent cortical stem cell populations (Marmur et al. 1998). Similarly, Gage and coworkers have isolated multipotent neural progenitors from adult hippocampus (Palmer et al. 1997).

Localizing stem cells in the adult is important for detailed analysis in vivo as well as for future therapeutic uses. There has been a tremendous

Table 2 Localization of multipotent stem cells in the adult svz

Classification	Characteristics
Type A	neuronal markers, rapidly dividing, limited self-renewal
Type B1	GFAP-immunoreactive, rapidly dividing cells
Type B2	GFAP-immunoreactive, slow dividing cells
Type C	nestin-immunoreactive, dividing cells
Type D	tanycytes, possess microvilli and are GFAP-immunoreactive
Type E	ependymal cell, villi, nestin, and vimentin-immunoreactive

Cells present in the adult subventricular zone are listed and their salient properties described. Each of these cell populations may represent a stem cell population. It is important to note that this classification may not be complete and further subpopulations may be identified based on additional antigenic criteria. (Modified from Doestch et al. 1997.)

excitement in the field because the presence of significant numbers of stem cells in the adult was not expected. The ability to maintain these cells in culture for prolonged periods using genetic or epigenetic means has provided the potential for virtually unlimited numbers of cells for therapy. The development of techniques to obtain stem cells from small pieces of human tissue has further heightened expectations that stem cells will be clinically useful (for review, see Vescovi and Snyder 1999). Although the excitement is warranted, caution should be maintained, as several questions need to be resolved before therapeutic transplants can be attempted. An important issue that still remains is whether the environment contains the requisite signals to direct differentiation of pluripotent cells to the desired cell type. In most reported transplant experiments, a majority of the transplanted multipotent stem cells fail to differentiate, suggesting the absence of instructive cues (see, e.g., Svendsen et al. 1996, 1997; Winkler et al. 1998; Quinn et al. 1999). Indeed, the best examples of differentiation and migration are usually in regions of ongoing neurogenesis such as the hippocampus and olfactory bulb. Little differentiation is seen in the spinal cord (Quinn et al. 1999) where there is no ongoing neurogenesis (Horner et al. 2000). Likewise, the ability to migrate in response to endogenous signals appears limited. Neuronal precursors (see below) readily migrate but multipotent stem cells when transplanted to the same region fail to do so (Zigova et al. 1996). Indeed, several investigators have suggested that transplanting predifferentiating stem cells may be a better option (for review, see Mayer-Proschel and Rao 2000).

Adult NRPs

It had been widely believed that neurogenesis in the mammalian brain ceases after early postnatal life (Raedler and Raedler 1978; Rakic and Nowakowski 1981). In fact, postnatal neurogenesis was believed to be an anomaly occurring in exceptional areas of the avian and rodent brain (Altman and Das 1965; Kaplan and Hinds 1977; Kaplan 1983). Considerable evidence has now accumulated that neurogenesis in the adult primate (including human) brain is possible (Eriksson et al. 1998; Gould et al. 1999a,b; Kornack and Rakic 1999). Therefore, there must be stem cells that divide and generate neurons in the adult mammalian brain. What is not clear is whether these are multipotent stem cells biased toward neuronal differentiation or NRPs. Even dedifferentiation of mature neurons may occur, as has been dramatically demonstrated in the hippocampus (Brewer 1999). It is likely that NRPs exist in at least two regions where there is ongoing adult neurogenesis: the ependymal/subependymal zone and the dentate gyrus of the hippocampus (Kaplan and Hinds 1977; Bayer et al. 1982; Lois and Alvarez-Buylla 1993; Kuhn et al. 1996). Neuronal progenitors from this region, in particular the anterior part often termed SVZ(a), give rise to neurons exclusively (Brock et al. 1998). They migrate along the rostral olfactory tract and terminally differentiate to form interneurons of the olfactory bulb (Okano et al. 1993; Lois and Alvarez-Buylla 1994). Labeling of the dentate gyrus cells by BrdU in adult humans and in rats in vivo has been observed with dramatic increases seen post-seizure (Kuhn et al. 1996; Parent et al. 1997; Eriksson et al. 1998).

Using the early neuronal Tα1 tubulin promoter to drive the expression of GFP, Goldman and coworkers have isolated cells from 3-month-old rat forebrain that were morphologically neuronal and expressed MAP-2 and b-III tubulin after a week in culture (Wang et al. 2000). This promoter is active in early neuronal precursors and, as expected, these precursors differentiate into neurons in vitro but do not generate any glial cells (Wang et al. 1998). Fewer than 5% of the cells sorted exhibited astrocytic markers. The cells also incorporated BrdU in culture, indicating that they were capable of replication. All the recent data, therefore, suggest that in the hippocampus, neuronal precursors either already exist or can be induced, and these precursor cells can repopulate some regions of the adult or fetal nervous system.

It is increasingly evident that neurogenesis can take place in the adult brain and that new neurons are generated and can integrate into the existing network and establish synapses. This has raised the possibility that, rather than transplanting cells for therapy, it may be possible to enhance endogenous stem cell proliferation or bias their differentiation by providing extrinsic cues. Several investigators have reported on the ability to alter neuronal generation. These include providing an enriched environment in juvenile or adult mice (Kempermann et al. 1997,1998) or infusion of growth factors (Zigova et al. 1998). Increased neurogenesis may not be beneficial and has been noted in seizures both in vivo (Parent et al. 1999) and in vitro (Pincus et al. 1997). In response to ischemia, there is a 12-fold increase in neurogenesis in the dentate gyrus of gerbils (Liu et al. 1998). The endogenous proliferation may lead to heterotopias and increased chances of seizures. Not all regions exhibit ongoing or regulated neurogenesis; the spinal cord is a notable example. Dividing glial cells have been observed (Horner et al. 2000). Transplants of embryonic neurons, on the other hand, survive in the adult spinal cord (Foster et al. 1989), and new neurons are generated from newborn and adult rat spinal cords in culture (Kehl et al. 1997), as determined by BrdU incorporation. This de novo generation of neurons suggests that a quiescent population of multipotent stem cells may exist in the spinal cord.

ES Cells and Neural Precursors

The neural precursor cells that have been described above are derived from tissues of the advanced embryo and adult. In normal development, these neural precursor cells must arise from earlier, more undifferentiated cells, and it should be possible to isolate neural precursors from such undifferentiated cells in vitro. Indeed, neural precursors have been isolated from ES cells and primordial germ cells.

The idea that ES cells can be used as a reservoir of cells from which differentiated cells can be harvested has been validated in rodent models. Several groups have shown that cell surface markers (Mujtaba et al. 1999), manipulation of culture conditions (Okabe et al. 1996), or utilizing tissue-specific promoters (Li et al. 1998) can be used to isolate neural stem cells or more restricted precursors (Fig. 7). Recently transplanted oligodendrocyte precursor cells isolated from ES cells have been shown to generate new myelin in a rat model of demyelination (Brüstle et al. 1999). McKay and colleagues (Okabe et al. 1996) have manipulated culture conditions to isolate multipotent stem cells from ES cell cultures, and Li et al. (1998) have used an elegant selection strategy to isolate neural precursor cells. Using cell-type-specific markers, we have isolated neuronal and glial restricted precursors from mouse ES cells and have shown that these cells are antigenically and phenotypically identical to restricted precursors isolated from fetal tissue (Mujtaba et al. 1999). Data on isolation of specific neural precursor types from human ES cell cultures are not available. However, preliminary results (Dr. M.K. Carpenter, pers. comm.) suggest that markers utilized to isolate neuron and glial precursor populations from rodent ES cells are also expressed by differentiating human ES cell cultures (Fig. 8). Thus, it is likely that human ES cells could also serve a reservoir function.

One potential therapeutic advantage of neurons, glia, or precursor cells derived from ES cells is that they may not be regionally specified and thus may be more capable of site-specific integration. Furthermore, since it is possible to obtain regionally specific phenotypes by manipulating ES cell culture conditions, it may be possible to obtain appropriately specified phenotypes. Thus, ES-cell-derived precursors may be preferable to fetal or adult precursor cells. McDonald and colleagues have presented suggestive evidence that ES-cell-derived cells may be useful in spinal cord injury. When ES-cell-derived neural cells were transplanted in a spinal cord injury model, significant functional improvement was seen (McDonald et al. 1999). Suggestive evidence that neural cells derived from human ES cells will prove useful in spinal cord injury is provided by experiments using a NRP cell derived from a human embryonic carci-

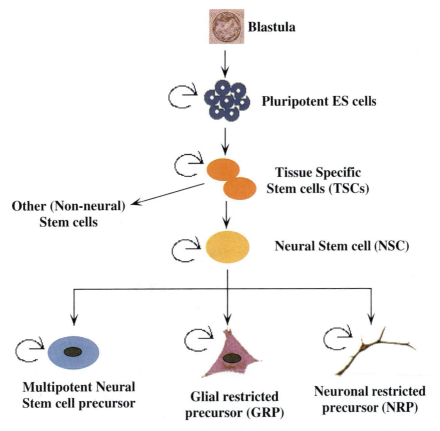

Figure 7 Neural precursors isolated from ES cell culture. Mouse ES cells have been differentiated in culture and several classes of neural stem cells have been isolated (Okabe et al. 1996; Li et al. 1998; McDonald et al. 1999; Brustle et al. 1999; Mujtaba et al. 1999). These include multipotent stem cells, neuron-restricted and glial-restricted precursors. In general, the method of differentiation for neuronal and glial precursors is similar and is based on the protocols devised by Bain et al. (1995).

noma cell line. Trojanowski and colleagues isolated a subclone (HNT-2) from a human embryonic carcinoma that showed exclusive differentiation into neurons. Neurons derived from this subclone were used in rat models of spinal cord injury. Transplanted cells differentiate into neurons that send long axonal projections, which even project into the nerve roots. No tumors have been seen in any of the transplants done so far (Trojanowski et al. 1997). These results suggest that it will be possible to obtain NRPs from human ES cell lines and that these are likely to be functionally useful. Several other classes of precursors have been isolated (for review, see Rao 1999). The recent demonstration that melanocytes and potential neural crest precursors can be directly isolated from ES cells (Yamane et al. 1999) is of great interest. Melanocytes were generated from ES cells by co-culturing them with a bone marrow-derived stromal cell line, dexamethasone, and the steel factor. All the above results taken together sug-

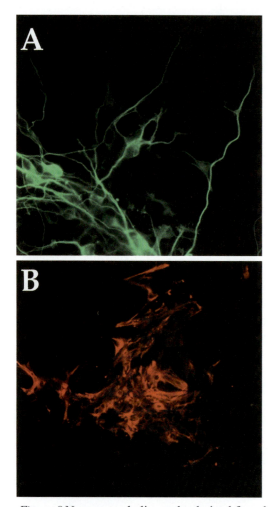

Figure 8 Neurons and glia can be derived from human ES cell lines. An example of neurons derived from human ES cell lines is shown. These ES cell lines have been maintained in culture for over a year, are karyotypically normal, and can differentiate into derivatives of all three germ layers. Photo and data are courtesy of Geron, Inc.

gest that it should be possible to obtain both CNS and PNS derivatives from differentiating ES cells.

Are Tissue-specific Stem Cells Irreversibly Determined?

Although we have discussed the ability of neural stem cells to generate CNS derivatives, data from several groups have suggested that these cells are more plastic than previously proposed and perhaps it is premature to classify stem cells based on the tissue from which they were isolated. Recent studies have shown that neural stem cells, when transplanted in the bone marrow of irradiated mice, will generate hematopoietic derivatives (Bjornson et al. 1999). Similarly, in an impressive demonstration of pluripotentiality, Frisen and colleagues (Clarke et al. 2000) injected adult neural stem cells into chick embryos and mouse blastocysts and showed that neural stem cells contributed to ectodermal, endodermal, and mesodermal tissue. Contributions to tissue were large and occasionally comprised as much as 30% of the entire organ. These data suggest that neural stem cells are capable of contributing to multiple tissues, and under appropriate conditions this contribution may be very large. Thus, the term neural may be too restrictive. It should be noted, however, that this ability to contribute to other tissues appears restricted to multipotent neural stem cells. Available data suggest that more restricted neural precursor cells do not transdifferentiate in a similar fashion.

Likewise, mesenchymal stem cells and bone marrow cells will generate astrocytes and possibly neurons when infused into the brain (Eglitis and Mezey 1997; Kopen et al. 1999). Since these precursor cells usually generate mesodermal derivatives, their ability to generate neuroectodermal derivatives is somewhat surprising. These and other trans-tissue differentiation results (Jackson et al. 1999; Petersen et al. 1999) suggest that tissue-specific stem cells may be more pluripotent than previously thought or still may retain the ability to dedifferentiate. Whether this ability is simply a by-product of the plasticity of these early cells or whether this ability has some developmental significance remains to be determined.

Ectoderm to mesoderm transformation is normally seen in neural crest differentiation. Indeed, neural crest cells have been shown to generate muscle, bone, cartilage melanocytes, fibroblasts, and smooth muscle as well as neural components of the PNS (for review, see Douarin 1983; Rao 1999). Thus, a potential pathway for dedifferentiation from mesoderm to ectoderm or vice versa may exist (Fig. 9). Quiescent neural stem cells present in ectopic neural tissue transplants may generate neural crest that subsequently can generate bone, cartilage, and smooth and striated

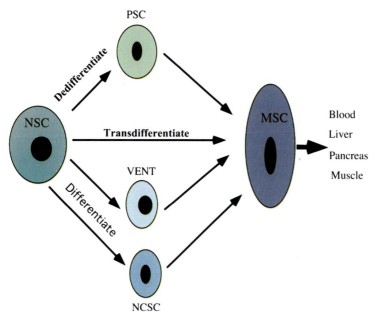

Figure 9 Generation of nonneural derivatives from stem cells. Hypothetical pathways by which neural stem cells could generate hematopoietic stem cells, skeletal muscle, liver, or other derivatives. Cells could dedifferentiate or transdifferentiate to generate other classes of tissue-specific stem cells. Alternatively, neural stem cells could generate neural crest or VENT cells that can differentiate into many of the same derivatives as a normal pathway of differentiation (see text). Yet another alternative is that rare totipotent cells are present in all tissues and it is these cells rather than neural stem cells that generate other tissue derivatives (see Weissman 2000).

muscle. Alternatively, an additional neural derivative, VENT cells (ventrally emigrating neural cells), which have also been shown to contribute to cartilage, bone, heart muscle, and hepatocytes (Ali et al. 1999; Sohal et al. 1999a,b,c) during normal development, may be present in neural tissue. These cells are distinct from crest cells and appear to have a truly broad spectrum of differentiation. Thus, the ability of neuroectoderm to differentiate into mesodermal derivatives may reflect an activation of this VENT cell differentiation pathway or a neural crest differentiation pathway. Finally, it is possible that rare totipotent cells are present in all tissues, and it is these cells rather than tissue-specific stem cells that generate nonneural derivatives. The possibilities are summarized in Figure 9.

It is interesting to note that mesodermal to ectodermal transformation is a normal aspect of some organ development. In kidney, for example, mesodermal cells undergo an epithelial transformation to generate kidney tubules. Mesodermal stem cells or mesenchymal stem cells (MSC) have also been identified. It is possible that these MSCs can generate all mesodermal derivatives (including hematopoietic lineages) as well as undergo an ectodermal transformation to generate ectodermal derivatives. Alternatively, quiescent neural crest stem cells (or VENT cells) may persist in peripheral tissue and be activated when transplanted into the CNS. Most transplants have not utilized a homogeneous population of cells. Irrespective of the source of cells, it should be noted that the effectiveness of neuronal differentiation has been relatively modest (Eglitis and Mezey 1997; Kopen et al. 1999), and it is unclear whether these results merely illustrate the plasticity of stem cells or whether they provide a novel therapeutic source of cells. Additional experiments are clearly required to refine our understanding of the extent and limitation of the differentiation potential of stem cells isolated from different tissues. It is unlikely, in our opinion, that cells derived from the adult or late fetal stages can contribute to all germ layers and also contribute to germ-line cells (ES cell equivalents). However, in the absence of direct evidence to the contrary, this remains a formal possibility that should be tested.

REFERENCES

Abney E.R., Bartlett P.P., and Raff M.C. 1981. Astrocytes, ependymal cells, and oligodendrocytes develop on schedule in dissociated cell cultures of embryonic rat brain. *Dev. Biol.* **83:** 301–310.

Ahmad I., Tang L., and Pham H. 2000. Identification of neural progenitors in the adult mammalian eye. *Biochem. Biophys. Res. Commun.* **270:** 517–521.

Ali A.A., Ali M.M., Dai D., and Sohal G.S. 1999. Ventrally emigrating neural tube cells differentiate into vascular smooth muscle cells. *Gen. Pharmacol.* **33:** 401–405.

Altman J. 1966. Proliferation and migration of undifferentiated precursor cells in the rat during postnatal gliogenesis. *Exp. Neurol.* **16:** 263–278.

Altman J. and Bayer S.A. 1984. The development of the rat spinal cord. *Adv. Anat. Embryol. Cell. Biol.* **85:** 1–164.

Altman J. and Das G.D. 1965. Autoradiographic and histological evidence of postnatal hippocampal neurogenesis in rats. *J. Comp. Neurol.* **124:** 319–335.

Anderson D.J., Groves A., Lo L., Ma Q., Rao M., Shah N.M., and Sommer L. 1997. Cell lineage determination and the control of neuronal identity in the neural crest. *Cold Spring Harbor Symp. Quant. Biol.* **62:** 493–504.

Artinger K.B., Fraser S., and Bronner-Fraser M. 1995. Dorsal and ventral cell types can arise from common neural tube progenitors. *Dev. Biol.* **172:** 591–601.

Avellana-Adalid V., Nait-Oumesmar B., Lachapelle F., and Baron-Van Evercooren A. 1996. Expansion of rat oligodendrocyte progenitors into proliferative "oligospheres" that retain differentiation potential. *J. Neurosci. Res.* **45:** 558–570.

Ayer-Le Lievre C.S. and Le Douarin N.M. 1982. The early development of cranial sensory ganglia and the potentialities of their component cells studied in quail-chick chimeras. *Dev. Biol.* **94:** 291–310.

Bain G., Kitchens D., Yao M., Huettner J.E., and Gottlieb D.I. 1995. Embryonic stem cells express neuronal properties in vitro. *Dev. Biol.* **168:** 342–357.

Baker C.V. and Bronner-Fraser M. 1997. The origins of the neural crest. Part I: Embryonic induction. *Mech. Dev.* **69:** 3–11.

Bayer S.A., Yackel J.W., and Puri P.S. 1982. Neurons in the rat dentate gyrus granular layer substantially increase during juvenile and adult life. *Science* **216:** 890–892.

Bensted J., Dobbing J., Morgan R., Reid R., and Wright G. 1957. Neuroglial development and myelination in the spinal cord of the chick embryo. *J. Embryol. Exp. Morphol.* **5:** 428–437.

Bianco P. and Cossu G. 1999. Uno, nessuno e centomila: Searching for the identity of mesodermal progenitors. *Exp. Cell. Res.* **251:** 257–263.

Bjornson C.R., Rietze R.L., Reynolds B.A., Magli M.C., and Vescovi A.L. 1999. Turning brain into blood: A hematopoietic fate adopted by adult neural stem cells in vivo (see comments). *Science* **283:** 534–537.

Blakemore W.F. and Keirstead H.S. 1999. The origin of remyelinating cells in the central nervous system. *J. Neuroimmunol.* **98:** 69–76.

Blass-Kampmann S., Reinhardt-Maelicke S., Kindler-Rohrborn A., Cleeves V., and Rajewsky M.F. 1994. In vitro differentiation of E-NCAM expressing rat neural precursor cells isolated by FACS during prenatal development. *J. Neurosci. Res.* **37:** 359–373.

Brewer G.J. 1999. Regeneration and proliferation of embryonic and adult rat hippocampal neurons in culture (see comments). *Exp. Neurol.* **159:** 237–247.

Brock S.C., Bonsall J., and Luskin M.B. 1998. The neuronal progenitor cells of the forebrain subventricular zone: Intrinsic properties in vitro and following transplantation. *Methods* **16:** 268–281.

Bronner-Fraser M. 1995a. Origin of the avian neural crest. *Stem Cells* **13:** 640–646.

———. 1995b. Origins and developmental potential of the neural crest. *Exp. Cell. Res.* **218:** 405–417.

Bronner-Fraser M. and Fraser S.E. 1988. Cell lineage analysis reveals multipotency of some avian neural crest cells. *Nature* **335:** 161–164.

———. 1989. Developmental potential of avian trunk neural crest cells in situ. *Neuron* **3:** 755–766.

Brooker G.J., Kalloniatis M., Russo V.C., Murphy M., Werther G.A., and Bartlett P.F. 2000. Endogenous IGF-1 regulates the neuronal differentiation of adult stem cells. *J. Neurosci. Res.* **59:** 332–341.

Brüstle O. 1999. Building brains: Neural chimeras in the study of nervous system development and repair. *Brain Pathol.* **9:** 527–545.

Brüstle O., Jones K.N., Learish R.D., Karram K., Choudhary K., Wiestler O.D., Duncan I.D., and McKay R.D. 1999. Embryonic stem cell-derived glial precursors: A source of myelinating transplants (see comments). *Science* **285:** 754–756.

Cai L., Hayes N.L., and Nowakowski R.S. 1997. Synchrony of clonal cell proliferation and contiguity of clonally related cells: Production of mosaicism in the ventricular zone of developing mouse neocortex. *J. Neurosci.* **176:** 2088–2100.

Cattaneo E. and McKay R. 1990. Proliferation and differentiation of neuronal stem cells regulated by nerve growth factor. *Nature* **347:** 762–765.

Chenn A. and McConnell S.K. 1995. Cleavage orientation and the asymmetric inheritance of Notch1 immunoreactivity in mammalian neurogenesis. *Cell* **82:** 631–641.

Chenn A., Zhang Y.A., Chang B.T., and McConnell S.K. 1998. Intrinsic polarity of mammalian neuroepithelial cells. *Mol. Cell. Neurosci.* **11**: 183–193.

Chiasson B.J., Tropepe V., Morshead C.M., and van der Kooy D. 1999. Adult mammalian forebrain ependymal and subependymal cells demonstrate proliferative potential, but only subependymal cells have neural stem cell characteristics. *J. Neurosci.* **19**: 4462–4471.

Ciccolini F. and Svendsen C.N. 1998. Fibroblast growth factor 2 (FGF-2) promotes acquisition of epidermal growth factor (EGF) responsiveness in mouse striatal precursor cells: Identification of neural precursors responding to both EGF and FGF-2. *J. Neurosci.* **18**: 7869–7880.

Clarke D.L., Johansson C.B., Wilbertz J., Veress B., Nilsson E., Karlstrom H., Lendahl U., and Frisen J. 2000. Generalized potential of adult neural stem cells. *Science* **288**:1660–1663.

Craig C.G., Tropepe V., Morshead C.M., Reynolds B.A., Weiss S., and van der Kooy D. 1996. In vivo growth factor expansion of endogenous subependymal neural precursor cell populations in the adult mouse brain. *J. Neurosci.* **16**: 2649–2658.

Creazzo T.L., Godt R.E., Leatherbury L., Conway S.J., and Kirby M.L. 1998. Role of cardiac neural crest cells in cardiovascular development. *Annu. Rev. Physiol.* **60**: 267–286.

Deloulme J.C., Baudier J., and Sensenbrenner M. 1991. Establishment of pure neuronal cultures from fetal rat spinal cord and proliferation of the neuronal precursor cells in the presence of fibroblast growth factor. *J. Neurosci. Res.* **29**: 499–509.

Doetsch F. and Alvarez-Buylla A. 1996. Network of tangential pathways for neuronal migration in adult mammalian brain. *Proc. Natl. Acad. Sci.* **93**: 14895–14900.

Doetsch F., García-Verdugo J.M., and Alvarez-Buylla A. 1997. Cellular composition and three-dimensional organization of the subventricular germinal zone in the adult mammalian brain. *J. Neurosci.* **17**: 5046–5061.

Doetsch F., Caillé I., Lim D.A., García-Verdugo J.M., and Alvarez-Buylla A. 1999. Subventricular zone astrocytes are neural stem cells in the adult mammalian brain. *Cell* **97**: 703–716.

Douarin L. 1983.*The neural crest*. Cambridge: Cambridge University Press, Cambridge, United Kingdom.

Doucette R. 1993. Glial cells in the nerve fiber layer of the main olfactory bulb of embryonic and adult mammals. *Microsc. Res. Tech.* **24**: 113–130.

Edlund T. and Jessell T.M. 1999. Progression from extrinsic to intrinsic signaling in cell fate specification: A view from the nervous system. *Cell* **96**: 211–224.

Eglitis M.A. and Mezey E. 1997. Hematopoietic cells differentiate into both microglia and macroglia in the brains of adult mice. *Proc. Natl. Acad. Sci.* **94**: 4080–4085.

Erickson C.A. and Weston J.A. 1999. VENT cells: A fresh breeze in a stuffy field? *Trends Neurosci.* **22**: 486–488.

Eriksson P.S., Perfilieva E., Bjork-Eriksson T., Alborn A.M., Nordborg C., Peterson D.A., and Gage F.H. 1998. Neurogenesis in the adult human hippocampus (comments). *Nat. Med.* **4**: 1313–1317.

Fok-Seang J. and Miller R.H. 1994. Distribution and differentiation of A2B5+ glial presursors in the developing rat spinal cord. *J. Neurosci. Res.* **37**: 219–235.

Foster G.A., Roberts M.H., Wilkinson L.S., Bjorklund A., Gage F.H., Hokfelt T., Schultzberg M., and Sharp T. 1989. Structural and functional analysis of raphe neurone implants into denervated rat spinal cord. *Brain Res. Bull.* **22**: 131–137.

Frederiksen K. and McKay R.D. 1988. Proliferation and differentiation of rat neuro-epithelial precursor cells in vivo. *J. Neurosci.* **8:** 1144–1151.

Fujita S. 1965. An autoradiographic study on the origin and fate of subpial glioblasts in the embryonic chick spinal cord. *J. Comp. Neurol.* **124:** 51–60.

Gao W.O., Heintz N., and Hatten M.E. 1991. Cerebellar granule cell neurogenesis is regulated by cell-cell interactions in vitro. *Neuron* **6:** 705–715.

Garcia-Verdugo J.M., Doetsch F., Wichterle H., Lim D.A., and Alvarez-Buylla A. 1998. Architecture and cell types of the adult subventricular zone: In search of the stem cells. *J. Neurobiol.* **36:** 234–248.

Gensburger C., Labourdette G., and Sensenbrenner M. 1987. Brain basic fibroblast growth factor stimulates the proliferation of rat neuronal precursor cells in vitro. *FEBS Lett.* **217:** 1–5.

Gensert J.M. and Goldman J.E. 1996. In vivo characterization of endogenous proliferating cells in adult rat subcortical white matter. *Glia* **17:** 39–51.

Gershon M.D. 1997. Genes and lineages in the formation of the enteric nervous system. *Curr. Opin. Neurobiol.* **7:** 101–109.

Gilbert S.F. 1988. *Developmental biology.* Sinauer, Sunderland, Massachusetts.

Gilmore E.C., Nowakowski R.S., Caviness V.S., Jr., and Herrup K. 2000. Cell birth, cell death, cell diversity and DNA breaks: How do they all fit together? *Trends Neurosci.* **23:** 100–105.

Gould E., Reeves A.J., Graziano M.S., and Gross C.G. 1999a. Neurogenesis in the neocortex of adult primates. *Science* **286:** 548–552.

Gould E., Reeves A.J., Fallah M., Tanapat P., Gross C.G., and Fuchs E. 1999b. Hippocampal neurogenesis in adult Old World primates. *Proc. Natl. Acad. Sci.* **96:** 5263–5267.

Grinspan J.B., Stern J.L., Franceschini B., and Pleasure D. 1994. Trophic effects of basic fibroblast growth factor (bFGF) on differentiated oligodendroglia: A mechanism for regeneration of the oligodendroglial lineage. *J. Neurosci. Res.* **36:** 672–680.

Grove E.A., Kirkwood T.B., and Price J. 1992. Neuronal precursor cells in the rat hippocampal formation contribute to more than one cytoarchitectonic area. *Neuron* **8:** 217–229.

Grove E.A., Williams B.P., Li D.Q., Hajihosseini M., Friedrich A., and Price J. 1993. Multiple restricted lineages in the embryonic rat cerebral cortex. *Development* **117:** 553–561.

Gudino-Cabrera G. and Nieto-Sampedro M. 1999. Estrogen receptor immunoreactivity in Schwann-like brain macroglia. *J. Neurobiol.* **40:** 458–470.

Hagedorn L., Suter U., and Sommer L. 1999. P0 and PMP22 mark a multipotent neural crest-derived cell type that displays community effects in response to TGF-β family factors. *Development* **126:** 3781–3794.

Hall A., Giese N.A., and Richardson W.D. 1996. Spinal cord oligodendrocytes develop from ventrally derived progenitor cells that express PDGF alpha-receptors. *Development* **122:** 4085–4094.

Hamburger V. 1948. The mitotic patterns in the spinal cord of chick embryo and their relationship to the histogenetic process. *J. Comp. Neurol.* **88:** 221–284.

Hardy R.J. 1997. Dorsoventral patterning and oligodendroglial specification in the developing central nervous system. *J. Neurosci. Res.* **50:** 139–145.

Hatten M.E. and Heintz N. 1995. Mechanisms of neural patterning and specification in the developing cerebellum. *Annu. Rev. Neurosci.* **18:** 385–408.

Hazel T.G., Panchision D.M., Warriner D.G., and McKay R.D.G. 1997. Regional plasticity of multipotent precursors from the developing CNS. *Soc. Neurosci. Abstr.,* p. 319.

Hirano M. and Goldman J.E. 1988. Gliogenesis in rat spinal cord: Evidence for origin of astrocytes and oligodendrocytes from radial precursors. *J. Neurosci. Res.* **21:** 155–167.

Horner P.J., Power A.E., Kempermann G., Kuhn H.G., Palmer T.D., Winkler J., Thal L.J., and Gage F.H. 2000. Proliferation and differentiation of progenitor cells throughout the intact adult rat spinal cord. *J. Neurosci.* **20:** 2218–2228.

Ito K., Morita T., and Sieber-Blum M. 1993. In vitro clonal analysis of mouse neural crest development. *Dev. Biol.* **157:** 517–525.

Jackson K.A., Mi T., and Goodell M.A. 1999. Hematopoietic potential of stem cells isolated from murine skeletal muscle (comments). *Proc. Natl. Acad. Sci.* **96:** 14482–14486.

Jacobson M. 1991. *Developmental neurobiology.* Plenum Press, New York.

Jan Y.N. and Jan L.Y. 1998. Asymmetric cell division. *Nature* **392:** 775–778.

Johansson C.B., Momma S., Clarke D.L., Risling M., Lendahl U., and Frisen J. 1999. Identification of a neural stem cell in the adult mammalian central nervous system. *Cell* **96:** 25–34.

Johe K.K., Hazel T.G., Muller T., Dugich-Djordjevic M.M., and McKay R.D. 1996. Single factors direct the differentiation of stem cells from the fetal and adult central nervous system. *Genes Dev.* **10:** 3129–3140.

Kalyani A., Hobson K., and Rao M.S. 1997. Neuroepithelial stem cells from the embryoinc spinal cord: Isolation, characterization and clonal analysis. *Dev. Biol.* **187:** 203–226.

Kalyani A.J., Piper D., Mujtaba T., Lucero M.T., and Rao M.S. 1998. Spinal cord neuronal precursors generate multiple neuronal phenotypes in culture. *J. Neurosci.* **18:** 7856–7868.

Kaplan M.S. 1983. Proliferation of subependymal cells in the adult primate CNS: Differential uptake of DNA labelled precursors. *J. Hirnforschung* **24:** 23–33.

Kaplan M.S. and Hinds J.W. 1977. Neurogenesis in the adult rat: Electron microscopic analysis of light radioautographs. *Science* **197:** 1092–1094.

Kehl L.J., Fairbanks C.A., Laughlin T.M., and Wilcox G.L. 1997. Neurogenesis in postnatal rat spinal cord: A study in primary culture. *Science* **276:** 586–589.

Keirstead H.S., Ben-Hur T., Rogister B., O'Leary M.T., Dubois-Dalcq M., and Blakemore W.F. 1999. Polysialylated neural cell adhesion molecule-positive CNS precursors generate both oligodendrocytes and Schwann cells to remyelinate the CNS after transplantation. *J. Neurosci.* **19:** 7529–7536.

Kempermann G., Kuhn H.G., and Gage F.H. 1997. More hippocampal neurons in adult mice living in an enriched environment. *Nature* **386:** 493–495.

———. 1998. Experience-induced neurogenesis in the senescent dentate gyrus. *J. Neurosci.* **18:** 3206–3212.

Kilpatrick T.J. and Bartlett P.F. 1993. Cloning and growth of multipotent neural precursors: Requirements for proliferation and differentiation. *Neuron* **10:** 255–265.

Kirby M.L. 1990. Alteration of cardiogenesis after neural crest ablation. *Ann. N.Y. Acad. Sci.* **588:** 289–295.

Kopen G.C., Prockop D.J., and Phinney D.G. 1999. Marrow stromal cells migrate throughout forebrain and cerebellum, and they differentiate into astrocytes after injection into neonatal mouse brains. *Proc. Natl. Acad. Sci.* **96:** 10711–10716.

Korade Z. and Frank E. 1996. Restriction in cell fates of developing spinal cord cells transplanted to neural crest pathways. *J. Neurosci.* **16:** 7638–7648.

Kornack D.R. and Rakic P. 1999. Continuation of neurogenesis in the hippocampus of the adult macaque monkey. *Proc. Natl. Acad. Sci.* **96:** 5768–5773.

Kuhn H.G., Dickinson-Anson H., and Gage F.H. 1996. Neurogenesis in the dentate gyrus of the adult rat: Age-related decrease of neuronal progenitor proliferation. *J. Neurosci.* **16:** 2027–2033.

LaBonne C. and Bronner-Fraser M. 1998. Induction and patterning of the neural crest, a stem cell-like precursor population. *J. Neurobiol.* **36:** 175–189.

Lavdas A.A., Mione M.C., and Parnavelas J.G. 1996. Neuronal clones in the cerebral cortex show morphological and neurotransmitter heterogeneity during development. *Cereb. Cortex* **6:** 490–497.

Leber S.M., Breedlove S.M., and Sanes J.R. 1990. Lineage, arrangement, and death of clonally related motoneurons in chick spinal cord. *J. Neurosci.* **10:** 2451–2462.

Le Dourain N.M. and Kalcheim C. 1999. *The neural crest,* 2nd edition. Cambridge University Press, Cambridge, United Kingdom.

Lee J., M. Mayer-Proschel and Rao M. 2000. Gliogenesis in the central nervous system. *Glia* **30:** 105–121.

Levison S.W. and Goldman J.E. 1997. Multipotential and lineage restricted precursors coexist in the mammalian perinatal subventricular zone. *J. Neurosci. Res.* **48:** 83–94.

Li M., L. Pevny, R. Lovell-Badge, and A. Smith. 1998. Generation of purified neural precursors from embryonic stem cells by lineage selection. *Curr. Biol.* **8:** 971–974.

Li R., Thode S., Zhou J.Y., Richards N., Pardinas J., Rao M.S., and Sah D.W.Y. 2000. Motoneuron differentiation of immortalized human spinal cord cell lines. *J. Neurosci. Res.* **59:** 342–352.

Lim D.A., Fishell G.J., and Alvarez-Buylla A. 1997. Postnatal mouse subventricular zone neuronal precursors can migrate and differentiate within multiple levels of the developing neuraxis. *Proc. Natl. Acad. Sci.* **94:** 14832–14836.

Liu J., Solway K., Messing R.O., and Sharp F.R. 1998. Increased neurogenesis in the dentate gyrus after transient global ischemia in gerbils. *J. Neurosci.* **18:** 7768–7778.

Lois C. and Alvarez-Buylla A. 1993. Proliferating subventricular zone cells in the adult mammalian forebrain can differentiate into neurons and glia. *Proc. Natl. Acad. Sci.* **90:** 2074–2077.

———. 1994. Long-distance neuronal migration in the adult mammalian brain. *Science* **264:** 1145–1148.

Luskin M.B. 1994. Neuronal cell lineage in the vertebrate central nervous system. *FASEB J.* **8:** 722–730.

Luskin M.B., Pearlman A.L., and Sanes J.R. 1988. Cell lineage in the cerebral cortex of the mouse studies in vivo and in vitro with a recombinant retrovirus. *Neuron* **1:** 635–647.

Mallamaci A., Di Blas E., Briata P., Boncinelli E., and Corte G. 1996. OTX2 homeoprotein in the developing central nervous system and migratory cells of the olfactory area. *Mech. Dev.* **58:** 165–178.

Marmur R., Mabie P.C., Gokhan S., Song Q., Kessler J.A., and Mehler M.F. 1998. Isolation and developmental characterization of cerebral cortical multipotent progenitors. *Dev. Biol.* **204:** 577–591.

Mayer-Proschel M. and Rao M.S. 2000. Lineage restricted precursors for transplantation. *Prog. Brain Res.* **128:** 273–292.

Mayer-Proschel M., Kalyani A.J., Mujtaba T., and Rao M.S. 1997. Isolation of lineage-restricted neuronal precursors from multipotent neuroepithelial stem cells. *Neuron* **19:** 773–785.

McConnell S.K. 1988. Development and decision-making in the mammalian cerebral cortex. *Brain Res.* **472:** 1–23.

McDonald J.W., Liu X.Z., Qu Y., Liu S., Mickey S.K., Turetsky D., Gottlieb D.I., and Choi D.W. 1999. Transplanted embryonic stem cells survive, differentiate and promote recovery in injured rat spinal cord. *Nat. Med.* **5:** 1410–1412.

McKay R. 1992. Reconstituting animals from immortal precursors. *Curr. Opin. Neurobiol.* **2:** 582–585.

McMorris F.A., Smith T.M., DeSalvo S., and Furlanetto R.W. 1986. Insulin-like growth factor I/somatomedin C: A potent inducer of oligodendrocyte development. *Proc. Natl. Acad. Sci.* **83:** 822–826.

Mi H. and Barres B. 1999. Purification and characterization of astrocyte precursor cells in the developing rat optic nerve. *J. Neurosci.* **19:** 1049–1061.

Miller R.H. 1996. Oligodendrocyte origins. *Trends Neurosci.* **19:** 92–96.

Miller R.H., Williams B., Cohen J., and Raff M.C. 1984. A4: An antigenic marker for neural-tube derived cells. *J. Neurocytol.* **13:** 329–338.

Miller R.H., David S., Patel R., Abney E.R., and Raff M.C. 1985. A quantitative immunohistochemical study of macroglial cell development in the rat optic nerve: In vivo evidence for two distinct astrocyte lineages. *Dev. Biol.* **111:** 35–41.

Mione M.C., Cavanagh J.F.R., Harris B., and Parnavelas J.G. 1997. Cell fate specification and symmetrical/asymmetrical divisions in the developing cerebral cortex. *J. Neurosci.* **17:** 2018–2029.

Mirsky R. and Jessen K.R. 1996. Schwann cell development, differentiation and myelination. *Curr. Opin. Neurobiol.* **6:** 89–96.

Morrison S.J., Shah N.M., and Anderson D.J. 1997. Regulatory mechanism in stem cell biology. *Cell* **88:** 287–298.

Morrison S.J., White P.M., Zock C., and Anderson D.J. 1999. Prospective identification, isolation by flow cytometry, and in vivo self-renewal of multipotent mammalian neural crest stem cells. *Cell* **96:** 737–749.

Morshead C.M. and van der Kooy D. 1992. Postmitotic death is the fate of constitutively proliferating cells in the subependymal layer of the adult mouse brain. *J. Neurosci.* **12:** 249–256.

Morshead C.M., Reynolds B.A., Craig C.G., McBurney M.W., Staines W.A., Morassutti D., Weiss S., and van der Kooy D. 1994. Neural stem cells in the adult mammalian forebrain: A relatively quiescent subpopulation of the subependymal cells. *Neuron* **13:** 1071–1082.

Mujtaba T., Mayer-Proschel M., and Rao M.S. 1998. A common neural progenitor for the CNS and PNS. *Dev. Biol.* **200:** 1–15.

Mujtaba T., Piper D.R., Kalyani A., Groves A.K., Lucero M.T., and Rao M.S. 1999. Lineage-restricted neural precursors can be isolated from both the mouse neural tube and cultured ES cells. *Dev. Biol.* **214:** 113–127.

Nieto M.A., Bradley L.C., Hunt P., Das Gupta R., Krumlauf R., and Wilkinson D.G. 1992. Molecular mechanisms of pattern formation in the vertebrate hindbrain. *Ciba Found. Symp.* **165:** 92–102.

Nornes H.O. and Das G.D. 1974. Temporal pattern of neurogenesis in the spinal cord of rat. I. An autoradiographic study—Time and sites of origin and migration and settling patterns of neuroblasts. *Brain Res.* **73:** 121–138.

Northcutt R.G. and Gans C. 1983. The genesis of neural crest and epidermal placodes: A reinterpretation of vertebrate origins. *Q. Rev. Biol.* **58:** 1–28.

Okabe S., Forsberg-Nilsson K., Spiro A.C., Segal M., and McKay R.D. 1996. Development of neuronal precursor cells and functional postmitotic neurons from embryonic stem cells in vitro. *Mech. Dev.* **59:** 89–102.

Okano H.J., Pfaff D.W., and Gibbs R.B. 1993. RB and Cdc2 expression in brain: Correlations with 3H-thymidine incorporation and neurogenesis. *J. Neurosci.* **13:** 2930–2938.

Palmer T.D., Ray J., and Gage F.H. 1995. FGF-2-responsive neuronal progenitors reside in proliferative and quiescent regions of the adult rodent brain. *Mol. Cell. Neurosci.* **6:** 474–486.

Palmer T.D., Takahashi J., and Gage F.H. 1997. The adult rat hippocampus contains primordial neural stem cells. *Mol. Cell. Neurosci.* **8:** 389–404.

Parent J.M., Tada E., Fike J.R., and Lowenstein D.H. 1999. Inhibition of dentate granule cell neurogenesis with brain irradiation does not prevent seizure-induced mossy fiber synaptic reorganization in the rat. *J. Neurosci.* **19:** 4508–4519.

Parent J.M., Yu T.W., Leibowitz R.T., Geschwind D.H., Sloviter R.S., and Lowenstein D.H. 1997. Dentate granule cell neurogenesis is increased by seizures and contributes to aberrant network reorganization in the adult rat hippocampus. *J. Neurosci.* **17:** 3727–3738.

Parnavelas J.G., Barfield J.A., Franke E., and Luskin M.B. 1991. Separate progenitor cells give rise to pyramidal and nonpyramidal neurons in the rat telencephalon. *Cereb. Cortex* **1:** 463–468.

Petersen B.E., Bowen W.C., Patrene K.D., Mars W.M., Sullivan A.K., Murase N., Boggs S.S., Greenberger J.S., and Goff J.P. 1999. Bone marrow as a potential source of hepatic oval cells. *Science* **284:** 1168–1170.

Phelps P.E., Barber R.P., and Vaughn J.E. 1988. Generation patterns of four groups of cholinergic neurons in rat cervical spinal cord: A combined tritiated thymidine autoradiographic and choline acetyltransferase immunocytochmeical study. *J. Comp. Neurol.* **273:** 459–472.

Pincus D.W., Harrison-Restelli C., Barry J., Goodman R.R., Fraser R.A., Nedergaard M., and Goldman S.A. 1997. In vitro neurogenesis by adult human epileptic temporal neocortex. *Clin. Neurosurg* **44:** 17–25.

Poelmann R.E. and Gittenberger-de Groot A.C. 1999. A subpopulation of apoptosis-prone cardiac neural crest cells targets to the venous pole: Multiple functions in heart development? *Dev. Biol.* **207:** 271–286.

Prabhakar S., D'Souza S., Antel J.P., McLaurin J., Schipper H.M., and Wang E. 1995. Phenotypic and cell cycle properties of human oligodendrocytes in vitro. *Brain Res.* **672:** 159–169.

Price J. and Thurlow L. 1988. Cell lineage in the rat cerebral cortex: A study using retroviral-mediated gene transfer. *Development* **104:** 473–482.

Price J., Williams B., and Grove E. 1991. Cell lineage in the cerebral cortex. *Development* (Suppl.) **2:** 23–28.

Pringle N.P., Guthrie S., Lumsden A., and Richardson W.D. 1998. Dorsal spinal cord neuroepithelium generates astrocytes but not oligodendrocytes. *Neuron* **20:** 883–893.

Qian X., Davis A.A., Goderie S.K., and Temple S. 1997. FGF2 concentration regulates the generation of neurons and glia from multipotent cortical stem cells. *Neuron* **18:** 81–93.

Qiu M., Shimamura K., Sussel L., Chen S., and Rubenstein J.L. 1998. Control of anteroposterior and dorsoventral domains of Nkx-6.1 gene expression relative to other Nkx genes during vertebrate CNS development. *Mech. Dev.* **72:** 77–88.

Quinn S.M., Walters W.M., Vescovi A.L., and Whittemore S.R. 1999. Lineage restriction of neuroepithelial precursor cells from fetal human spinal cord. *J. Neurosci. Res.* **57:** 590–602.

Raedler E. and Raedler A. 1978. Autoradiographic study of early neurogenesis in rat neocortex. *Anat. Embryol.* **154:** 267–284.

Raff M.C., Miller R.H., and Noble M. 1983. A glial progenitor cell that develops in vitro into an astrocyte or an oligodendrocyte depending on the culture medium. *Nature* **303:** 390–396.

Raine C.S., Scheinberg L., and Waltz J.M. 1981. Multiple sclerosis. Oligodendrocyte survival and proliferation in an active established lesion. *Lab. Invest.* **45:** 534–546.

Rakic P. 1972. Mode of cell migration to the superficial layers of fetal monkey neocortex. *J. Comp. Neurol.* **145:** 61–83.

Rakic P. and Nowakowski R.S. 1981. The time of origin of neurons in the hippocampal region of the rhesus monkey. *J. Comp. Neurol.* **196:** 99–128.

Ramon-Cueto A. and Avila J. 1998. Olfactory ensheathing glia: Properties and function. *Brain Res. Bull.* **46:** 175–187.

Ramon-Cueto A., Cordero M.I., Santos-Benito F.F., and Avila J. 2000. Functional recovery of paraplegic rats and motor axon regeneration in their spinal cords by olfactory ensheathing glia. *Neuron* **25:** 425–435.

Rao M.S. 1999. Multipotent and restricted precursors in the central nervous system. *Anat. Rec.* **257:** 137–148.

Rao M.S. and Anderson D.J. 1997. Immortalization and controlled in vitro differentiation of murine multipotent neural crest stem cells. *J. Neurobiol.* **32:** 722–746.

Rao M.S. and Mayer-Proschel M. 1997. Glial restricted precursors are derived from multipotent neuroepithelial stem cells. *Dev. Biol.* **188:** 48–63.

Rao M.S., Noble M., and Mayer-Proschel M. 1998. A tripotential glial precursor cell is present in the developing spinal cord. *Proc. Natl. Acad. Sci.* **95:** 3996–4001.

Raoul C., Pettmann B., and Henderson C.E. 2000. Active killing of neurons during development and following stress: A role for p75(NTR) and Fas? *Curr. Opin. Neurobiol.* **10:** 111–117.

Ray J. and Gage F.H. 1994. Spinal cord neuroblasts proliferate in response to basic fibroblast growth factor. *J. Neurosci.* **14:** 3548–3564.

Reh T.A. and Levine E.M. 1998. Multipotential stem cells and progenitors in the vertebrate retina. *J. Neurobiol.* **36:** 206–220.

Reynolds B.A. and Weiss S. 1992. Generation of neurons and astrocytes from isolated cells of the adult mammalian central nervous system. *Science* **225:** 1707–1710.

———. 1996. Clonal and population analyses demonstrate that an EGF-responsive mammalian embryonic CNS precursor is a stem cell. *Dev. Biol.* **175:** 1–13.

Reznikov K., Acklin S.E., and van der Kooy D. 1997. Clonal heterogeneity in the early embryonic rodent cortical germinal zone and the separation of subventricular from ventricular zone lineages. *Dev. Dyn.* **210:** 328–343.

Roy N.S., Benraiss A., Wang S., Fraser R.A., Goodman R., Couldwell W.T., Nedergaard M., Kawaguchi A., Okano H., and Goldman S.A. 2000a. Promoter-targeted selection and isolation of neural progenitor cells from the adult human ventricular zone. *J. Neurosci. Res.* **59:** 321–331.

Roy N.S., Wang S., Jiang L., Kang J., Benraiss A., Harrison-Restelli C., Fraser R.A., Couldwell W.T., Kawaguchi A., Okano H., Nedergaard M., and Goldman S.A. 2000b. In vitro neurogenesis by progenitor cells isolated from the adult human hippocampus. *Nat. Med.* **6:** 271–277.

Rubenstein J.L. and Rakic P. 1999. Genetic control of cortical development. *Cereb. Cortex* **9:** 521–523.

Sanes J.R. 1989. Analysing cell lineages with a recombinant retrovirus. *Trends Neurosci.* **12:** 21–28.

Sauer M.E. and Chittenden A.C. 1959. Deoxyribonucleic acid content of cell nuclei in the neural tube of the chick embryo: Evidence for intermitotic migration of nuclei. *Exp. Cell Res.* **16:** 1–6.

Sauer M.E. and Walker B.E. 1959. Radioautographic study of interkinetic nuclear migration in the neural tube. *Proc. Soc. Exp. Biol. Med.* **101:** 557–560.

Scherson T., Serbedzija G., Fraser S., and Bronner-Fraser M. 1993. Regulative capacity of the cranial neural tube to form neural crest. *Development* **118:** 1049–1062.

Scolding N.J., Rayner P.J., Sussman J., Shaw C., and Compston D.A. 1995. A proliferative adult human oligodendrocyte progenitor. *NeuroReport* **6:** 441–445.

Scott D.E. and Hansen S.L. 1997. Post-traumatic regeneration, neurogenesis and neuronal migration in the adult mammalian brain. *Va. Med. Q.* **124:** 249–261.

Seale P. and Rudnicki M.A. 2000. A new look at the origin, function, and "stem-cell" status of muscle satellite cells. *Dev. Biol.* **218:** 115–124.

Seidman K.J., Teng A.L., Rosenkopf R., Spilotro P., and Weyhenmeyer J.A. 1997. Isolation, cloning and characterization of a putative type-1 astrocyte cell line. *Brain Res.* **753:** 18–26.

Seymour R.M. and Berry M. 1975. Scanning and transmission electron microscope studies of interkinetic nuclear migration in the cerebral vesicles of the rat. *J. Comp. Neurol.* **160:** 105–125.

Sharma K., Korade Z., and Frank E. 1995. Late-migrating neuroepithelial cells from the spinal cord differentiate into sensory ganglion cells and melanocytes. *Neuron* **14:** 143–152.

Shetty A.K. and Turner D.A. 1998. In vitro survival and differentiation of neurons derived from epidermal growth factor-responsive postnatal hippocampal stem cells: Inducing effects of brain-derived neurotrophic factor. *J. Neurobiol.* **35:** 395–425.

Shihabuddin L.S., Ray J., and Gage F.H. 1997. FGF-2 is sufficient to isolate progenitors found in the adult mammalian spinal cord. *Exp. Neurol.* **148:** 577–586.

Smart I. 1961. The subependymal layer of the mouse brain and its cell production as shown by radioautography after thymidine-H3 injection. *J. Comp. Neurol.* **116:** 325–347.

Sohal G.S., Ali A.A., and Ali M.M. 1998. Ventral neural tube cells differentiate into craniofacial skeletal muscles (erratum *Biochem. Biophys. Res. Commun.* [1999] **254:** 515). *Biochem. Biophys. Res. Commun.* **252:** 675–678.

Sohal G.S., Ali M.M., Ali A.A., and Bockman D.E. 1999a. Ventral neural tube cells differentiate into hepatocytes in the chick embryo. CMLS *Cell. Mol. Life Sci.* **55:** 128–130.

Sohal G.S., Ali M.M., Ali A.A., and Dai D. 1999b. Ventrally emigrating neural tube cells contribute to the formation of Meckel's and quadrate cartilage. *Dev. Dyn.* **216:** 37–44.

———. 1999c. Ventrally emigrating neural tube cells differentiate into heart muscle. *Biochem. Biophys. Res. Commun.* **254:** 601–604.

Sohal G.S., Bockman D.E., Ali M.M., and Tsai N.T. 1996. DiI labeling and homeobox gene islet-1 expression reveal the contribution of ventral neural tube cells to the formation of the avian trigeminal ganglion. *Int. J. Dev. Neurosci.* **14:** 419–427.

Spassky N., Goujet-Zalc C., Parmantier E., Olivier C., Martinez S., Ivanova A., Ikenaka

K., Macklin W., Cerruti I., Zalc B., and Thomas J.L. 1998. Multiple restricted origin of oligodendrocytes. *J. Neurosci.* **18:** 8331–8343.

Stemple D.L. and Anderson D.J. 1992. Isolation of a stem cell for neurons and glia from the mammalian neural crest. *Cell* **71:** 973–985.

Sturrock R.R. 1982. Gliogenesis in the prenatal rabbit spinal cord. *J. Anat.* **134:** 771–793.

Suhonen J.O., Peterson D.A., Ray J., and Gage F.H. 1996. Differentiation of adult hippocampus-derived progenitors into olfactory neurons in vivo. *Nature* **383:** 624–627.

Svendsen C.N., Clarke D.J., Rosser A.E., and Dunnett S.B. 1996. Survival and differentiation of rat and human epidermal growth factor-responsive precursor cells following grafting into the lesioned adult central nervous system. *Exp. Neurol.* **137:** 376–388.

Svendsen C.N., Caldwell M.A., Shen J., ter Borg M.G., Rosser A.E., Tyers P., Karmiol S., and Dunnett S.B. 1997. Long-term survival of human central nervous system progenitor cells transplanted into a rat model of Parkinson's disease. *Exp. Neurol.* **148:** 135–146.

Takahashi T., Nowakowski R.S., and Caviness V.S., Jr. 1994. Mode of cell proliferation in the developing mouse neocortex. *Proc. Natl. Acad. Sci.* **91:** 375–379.

Temple S. 1989. Division and differentiation of isolated CNS blast cells in microculture. *Nature* **340:** 471–473.

Temple S. 2000. Defining neural stem cells and their role in normal development of the nervous system. In *Stem cells and the nervous system* (ed. M.S. Rao), pp. 1–29. Humana Press, Totowa, New Jersey.

Timsit S., Martinez S., Allinquant B., Peyron F., Puelles L., and Zalc B. 1995. Oligodendrocytes originate in a restricted zone of the embryonic ventral neural tube defined by DM-20 mRNA expression. *J. Neurosci.* **15:** 1012–1024.

Trojanowski J.Q., Kleppner S.R., Hartley R.S., Miyazono M., Fraser N.W., Kesari S., and Lee V.M. 1997. Transfectable and transplantable postmitotic human neurons: A potential platform for gene therapy of nervous system diseases. *Exp. Neurol.* **144:** 92–97.

Tropepe V., Sibilia M., Ciruna B.G., Rossant J., Wagner E.F., and van der Kooy D. 1999. Distinct neural stem cells proliferate in response to EGF and FGF in the developing mouse telencephalon. *Dev. Biol.* **208:** 166–188.

Tropepe V., Coles B.L., Chiasson B.J., Horsford D.J., Elia A.J., McInnes R.R., and van der Kooy D. 2000. Retinal stem cells in the adult mammalian eye. *Science* **287:** 2032–2036.

Turner D.L., Snyder E.Y., and Cepko C.L. 1990. Lineage-independent determination of cell type in the embryonic mouse retina. *Neuron* **4:** 833–845.

Vandenbergh D.J., Mori N., and Anderson D.J. 1991. Co-expression of multiple neurotransmitter enzyme genes in normal and immortalized sympathoadrenal progenitor cells. *Dev. Biol.* **148:** 10–22.

Vescovi A.L. and Snyder E.Y. 1999. Establishment and properties of neural stem cell clones: Plasticity in vitro and in vivo. *Brain Pathol.* **9:** 569–598.

Vescovi A.L., Reynolds B.A., Fraser D.D. and Weiss S. 1993. bFGF regulates the proliferative fate of unipotent (neuronal) and bipotent (neuron/astroglial) EGF-generated CNS progenitor cells. *Neuron* **11:** 951–966.

Wang S., Roy N.S., Benraiss A., and Goldman S.A. 2000. Promoter-based isolation and fluorescence-activated sorting of mitotic neuronal progenitor cells from the adult mammalian ependymal/subependymal zone. *Dev. Neurosci.* **22:** 167–176.

Wang S., Wu H., Jiang J., Delohery T.M., Isdell F., and Goldman S.A. 1998. Isolation of neuronal precursors by sorting embryonic forebrain transfected with GFP regulated by the Tα1 tubulin promoter (erratum *Nat. Biotechnol.* [1998] **16:** 478). *Nat. Biotechnol.* **16:** 196–201.

Weissman I.L. 2000. Stem cells: Units of development, units of regeneration, and units in evolution. *Cell* **100:** 157–168.

Weston J.A. 1991. Sequential segregation and fate of developmentally restricted intermediate cell populations in the neural crest lineage. *Curr. Top. Dev. Biol.* **25:** 133–153.

Wichterle H., Garcia-Verdugo J.M., Herrera D.G., and Alvarez-Buylla A. 1999. Young neurons from medial ganglionic eminence disperse in adult and embryonic brain. *Nat. Neurosci.* **2:** 461–466.

Williams B.P. and Price J. 1995. Evidence for multiple precursor cell types in the embryonic rat cerebral cortex. *Neuron* **14:** 1181–1188.

Winkler C., Fricker R.A., Gates M.A., Olsson M., Hammang J.P., Carpenter M.K., and Bjorklund A. 1998. Incorporation and glial differentiation of mouse EGF-responsive neural progenitor cells after transplantation into the embryonic rat brain. *Mol. Cell. Neurosci.* **11:** 99–116.

Yamane T., Hayashi S., Mizoguchi M., Yamazaki H., and Kunisada T. 1999. Derivation of melanocytes from embryonic stem cells in culture. *Dev. Dyn.* **216:** 450–458.

Yang T., Mujtaba T., Venkatraman G., Yuan W., Rao M.S., and Luskin M. 2000. Region-specific-differentiation of rodent neuron restricted precursor cells after heterotopic transplantation. *Proc. Natl. Acad. Sci.* **21:** 97(24): 13366–13371.

Zhang S.C., Lipsitz D., and Duncan I.D. 1998. Self-renewing canine oligodendroglial progenitor expanded as oligospheres. *J. Neurosci. Res.* **54:** 181–190.

Zhong W., Jiang M.M., Weinmaster G., Jan L.Y., and Jan Y.N. 1997. Differential expression of mammalian Numb, Numblike and Notch1 suggests distinct roles during mouse cortical neurogenesis. *Development* **124:** 1887–1897.

Zigova T., Pencea V., Wiegand S.J., and Luskin M.B. 1998. Intraventricular administration of BDNF increases the number of newly generated neurons in the adult olfactory bulb. *Mol. Cell. Neurosci.* **11:** 234–245.

Zigova T., Betarbet R., Soteres B.J., Brock S., Bakay R.A., and Luskin M.B. 1996. A comparison of the patterns of migration and the destinations of homotopically transplanted neonatal subventricular zone cells and heterotopically transplanted telencephalic ventricular zone cells. *Dev. Biol.* **173:** 459–474.

19

Epidermal Stem Cells

Fiona M. Watt
Keratinocyte Laboratory
Imperial Cancer Research Fund
London WC2A 3PX, United Kingdom

The epidermis of mammals forms the outer covering of the skin and comprises both the interfollicular epidermis and the adnexal structures, such as the hairs and sebaceous glands (Odland 1991). The major cell type in the epidermis is an epithelial cell called a keratinocyte. Interfollicular epidermis is made up of multiple layers of keratinocytes. The basal layer of cells, attached to the underlying basement membrane, contains keratinocytes that are capable of dividing, and cells that leave the basal layer undergo a process of terminal differentiation as they move toward the surface of the skin. The end point of this pathway is an anucleate cell, called a squame, which is filled with insoluble, transglutaminase-crosslinked protein and provides an effective barrier between the environment and the underlying living layers of the skin. The basal layer of interfollicular keratinocytes is continuous with the basal layer of keratinocytes that form the hair follicles and sebaceous glands; once again, the end point of terminal differentiation is a dead, highly specialized cell, forming the hair shaft or the lipid-filled sebocytes.

If stem cells are defined as cells with the capacity for unlimited self-renewal and also the ability to generate daughter cells that undergo terminal differentiation (Hall and Watt 1989; Watt 1998; Watt and Hogan 2000), then the epidermis is one of the tissues in which a stem cell compartment must be present. Throughout adult life there is a requirement for the production of new interfollicular keratinocytes to replace the squames that are continually being shed from the surface of the skin, and there is also a need to produce new hairs to replace those lost at the end of each hair growth cycle.

It seems likely that there is a single, pluripotential, stem cell compartment in the epidermis and that the differentiation pathway selected by stem cell progeny is determined by the microenvironment in which they find themselves (Watt and Hogan 2000). The earliest evidence for this came from wound-healing studies in which it was found that hair follicle keratinocytes could migrate out of the follicle and repopulate interfollicular epidermis (Al-Bawari and Potten 1976). Conversely, when interfollicular keratinocytes are grafted into an empty hair follicle, they can differentiate to produce a normal hair (Reynolds and Jahoda 1992). There is also a report that sweat gland cells can produce interfollicular epidermis; whether this reflects the pluripotential nature of the epidermal stem cell compartment or a process of transdifferentiation remains to be investigated (Miller et al. 1998).

Keratinocytes have not featured in the numerous recent accounts of the plasticity of stem cells in a variety of tissues (Watt and Hogan 2000). Two observations suggest, however, that some plasticity exists. First of all, the process of keratinocyte terminal differentiation can be reversed by introduction of a viral oncogene (Barrandon et al. 1989). Second, metaplasia of epithelial cells, including keratinocytes, is not uncommon: This is the formation of one differentiated cell type from another in postnatal life, such as the formation of ectopic intestinal epithelium in the stomach or endocervical epithelium in the vagina (Slack 2000).

PROLIFERATIVE HETEROGENEITY

Under normal conditions, each epidermal stem cell division results in one daughter to replenish the stem cell compartment and one daughter to undergo terminal differentiation. There is no evidence at present that this is achieved through invariant asymmetric divisions (Watt and Hogan 2000). Rather, there appears to be populational asymmetry, so that although on average each stem cell produces one stem and one non-stem cell daughter, individual divisions can potentially result in production of two stem cells, two terminally differentiating cells, or one stem and one non-stem daughter. This populational asymmetry allows the epidermis to respond to varying physiological need, as when the tissue is damaged through wounding.

Studies of interfollicular epidermis have demonstrated that not all dividing cells are stem cells (Potten 1981; Potten and Morris 1988). Instead, the daughter of a stem cell that is destined to undergo terminal differentiation can divide a small number of times before moving out of the basal cell layer. This dividing population, with low self-renewal capacity and high probability of undergoing terminal differentiation, is known as the transit amplifying compartment. In interfollicular epidermis, the prime function of this population is to increase the number of terminally differentiated cells generated by each stem cell division, so that although stem cells have a high capacity for proliferation, they divide infrequently.

A second potential attribute of transit amplifying cells, by analogy with the committed progenitor compartment of hematopoietic lineages, is that they have more restricted differentiation potential than the stem cells: In other words, transit amplifying cells may be committed to differentiate exclusively into squames or hair or sebocytes. The increasing use of transgenic mice to study epidermal proliferation and function should soon shed light on this issue (see, e.g., Gat et al. 1998). In the meantime, with only proliferative potential as a marker of the transit compartment, it remains possible that instead of discrete populations of stem and transit cells, there are gradients of keratinocyte proliferative and differentiative potential, with transit amplifying cells reflecting an intermediate position between stem cells (maximum self-renewal potential, minimum terminal differentiation probability) and terminally differentiated cells (minimum self-renewal capacity, maximum probability of differentiation) (Jones and Watt 1993).

ASSAYS FOR EPIDERMAL STEM CELLS

To identify epidermal stem cells, it is necessary to have assays to measure the proportion of stem cells in a given population. There are well-established techniques for growing human keratinocytes in culture (Rheinwald 1989), and confluent sheets of cultured keratinocytes have been used as autografts, primarily for the treatment of burn victims, since the late 1970s. Long-term follow-up of patients has shown that the progeny of keratinocytes expanded in culture persist and make a normal epidermis for years following grafting (Gallico et al. 1984; Compton et al. 1998). Thus, there is now doubt that stem cells can survive in culture.

In hematopoiesis, stem cells can be assayed by their ability to reconstitute all the blood cell lineages in a lethally irradiated mouse (see, e.g., Bhatia et al. 1998; Uchida et al. 1998; for review, see Hall and Watt 1989). Although human keratinocytes can reconstitute epidermis when grafted onto immunocompromised mice (see, e.g., Jones et al. 1995), it is not feasible to graft individual candidate epidermal stem cells and look for their ability to reconstitute the entire epidermis of the animal. As a result, there has been more reliance on clonal analysis in vitro, making use of the fact that human keratinocytes can be grown at clonal density on a feeder layer of mitotically inactivated mouse 3T3 embryonic fibroblasts (Rheinwald 1989).

Although the growth rate of a mixed population of human keratinocytes in culture will undoubtedly be influenced by the proportion of stem cells present (see, e.g., Gandarillas and Watt 1997; Li et al. 1998; Zhu and Watt 1999), it cannot be used as a quantitative measure of stem cells. This is because the growth rate will depend on the proportion of cells that are dividing and the length of the cell cycle. It will also depend on the proportion of terminally differentiating cells, and, to a lesser extent, on cell loss through apoptosis or in vitro senescence (see, e.g., Gandarillas et al. 1999; Gandarillas 2000). To evaluate the number of stem cells in a population of keratinocytes in vitro, it is therefore essential to carry out clonal analysis, examining the self-renewal and terminal differentiation potential of individual cells. This has been used both for interfollicular keratinocytes (see, e.g., Barrandon and Green 1987; Jones and Watt 1993) and for keratinocytes of hair follicles (Yang et al. 1993; Rochat et al. 1994).

One of the earliest, and undoubtedly the most thorough, analyses of clonal growth of human keratinocytes in culture was carried out by Barrandon and Green (1987). The importance of the study is that it depended not on the behavior of the clones founded on initial plating of keratinocytes (primary clones), but on the secondary clones that grew following disaggregation and replating of individual primary clones, thereby providing a more rigorous measure of self-renewal capacity. Three types of proliferating keratinocytes were defined on the basis of the type of clone they founded in vitro. When no secondary clones formed or all consisted of terminally differentiated cells (terminal clones) the founder clone was classified as a paraclone. When 0–5% of the clones were terminal, the clone was described as a holoclone. Meroclones were intermediate in their behavior, >5% and <100% of the secondary clones being terminal. Holoclones thus have the greatest self-renewal potential and are those most likely to be founded by stem cells. The total life span of a paraclone is no more than 15 generations prior to terminal differentiation and so could be attributable to a transit amplifying cell. Meroclones could be indicative of stem cells that generate transit amplifying cells at higher frequency than holoclones; they should still be attributed to stem cell founders, however, because epidermis from elderly people yields meroclones but few or no holoclones (Barrandon and Green 1987).

Unfortunately, the holo/mero/paraclone assay has not been used extensively, because it is time-consuming and labor-intensive when large numbers of keratinocytes are to be screened. Instead, there has been reliance on analysis of primary clones, in particular scoring terminal or abortive clones (typically, 32 cells or fewer per clone by 14 days after plating, all the cells expressing terminal differentiation markers) and attributing them to transit amplifying cells (Jones and Watt 1993; Jones et al. 1995; Gandarillas and Watt 1997; Zhu and Watt 1999; Zhu et al. 1999; Lowell et al. 2000), the remaining, actively growing, colonies being attributed to stem cell founders. Although the assignment of the abortive clones to transit amplifying cell founders is reasonably uncontroversial, it is worth noting that their proliferative potential is lower than that of the majority of paraclones (Barrandon and Green 1987) and, more importantly, that attributing all of the nonabortive clones to stem cell founders is likely to overestimate stem cell numbers.

Clonal analysis, with all its imperfections, remains the only practical way to screen for molecular markers of stem cells and for in vitro studies of factors that regulate exit from the stem cell compartment. As different subpopulations of proliferating keratinocytes become more clearly defined at the molecular level, much of the current uncertainty about the in vitro clonal behavior of the stem cell compartment should disappear.

EPIDERMAL STEM CELL MARKERS

As in other tissues, there is a clear need for molecular markers characteristic of the stem cell population, preferably cell-surface molecules that allow fluorescence-activated cell sorter (FACS) selection. There is a wealth of markers that distinguish basal from differentiating keratinocytes, with changes in keratin expression and the onset of expression of precursors of the cornified envelope that is assembled in squames being most frequently used (for review, see Watt 1989; Fuchs 1990). However, heterogeneity within the basal compartment has been harder to tackle.

The first surface marker of human epidermal stem cells to be described was $\beta 1$ integrins, receptors that bind extracellular matrix proteins. $\beta 1$ integrins are expressed by all cells in the basal layer of the epidermis, but interfollicular keratinocytes with properties of stem cells have two- to threefold higher levels than cells with properties of transit amplifying cells. Elevated expression of $\beta 1$ integrins is also a marker for stem cells in human hair follicles (Jones et al. 1995; Moll 1995; Lyle et al. 1998).

$\beta 1$ integrins can be used to enrich for stem cells, either in culture or directly from the epidermis, by FACS or differential adhesiveness to extracellular matrix-coated dishes, and to visualize the stem cells using confocal microscopy (Jones and Watt 1993; Jones et al. 1995; Jensen et al. 1999). Approximately 10% of cells in the basal epidermal layer are thought to be stem cells (Potten and Morris 1988), and the proportion of basal cells with high $\beta 1$ integrin levels varies from 25% in palm epidermis to >40% in neonatal foreskin (Jones et al. 1995). In vitro, human epidermal stem cells (defined by their ability to found actively growing clones) can be isolated to 90% purity on the basis of their adhesive properties (Jones and Watt 1993).

Human keratinocytes with the highest expression of the $\alpha2\beta1$ integrin (collagen receptor) also express the highest levels of $\alpha3\beta1$ and $\alpha5\beta1$ integrins (receptors for laminin and fibronectin, respectively), and therefore it is not possible to enrich further for stem cells by using combinations of antibodies specific for these individual integrins (Jones and Watt 1993). The relationship between log $\beta1$ integrin fluorescence and clone forming ability is linear, and this would be consistent with a continuum of keratinocyte behavior rather than discrete subpopulations of proliferative keratinocytes (Jones and Watt 1993). In mouse epidermis it is also possible to enrich for stem cells on the basis of rapid adhesion to extracellular matrix, although the integrins involved have not been defined (Bickenbach and Chism 1998).

The $\alpha6\beta4$ integrin is a component of hemidesmosomes and is essential for anchoring the epidermis to the underlying basement membrane (Dowling et al. 1996; Georges-Labouesse et al. 1996; van der Neut et al. 1996). Stem cells, like all basal keratinocytes, express $\alpha6\beta4$; however, there is no strong correlation between level of expression and proliferative potential, whether assessed in clonogenicity assays (Jones and Watt 1993; Jones et al. 1995) or by comparison with the distribution of actively cycling cells in human epidermis (Jensen et al. 1999). The "$\alpha6$ bright" population described by Li et al. (1998) as enriched for stem cells appears to correspond to total basal keratinocytes when the FACS profiles are compared with those of Jones and Watt (1993) (see also Kaur and Li 2000).

Other proposed surface markers include the antigen recognized by mAb 10G7 (Li et al. 1998), low surface expression of E-cadherin (Molès and Watt 1997), and high expression of Delta1 (Lowell et al. 2000). Disappointingly, the combination of E-cadherin or Delta1 with $\beta1$ integrins is unlikely to give greater enrichment for stem cells than $\beta1$ integrins alone, because the size and location of basal keratinocytes that are defined with each marker are similar (Molès and Watt 1997; Lowell et al. 2000).

A number of other proteins have been reported to be markers for the epidermal stem cell compartment. These include keratins 19 (Stasiak et al 1989) and 15 (Lyle et al. 1998; but see also Waseem et al. 1999), a high level of non-cadherin-associated β-catenin (Zhu and Watt 1999; but see also Molès and Watt 1997), and p63, a member of the p53 gene family (Parsa et al. 1999). Because these are intracellular proteins, they are not useful for isolating stem cells; however, they can still provide important information about stem cell properties. p63 is of particular interest, since mice which are homozygous null for the p63 gene lack all stratified squamous epithelia, including the epidermis (Mills et al. 1999; Yang et al. 1999).

Finally, it is worth pointing out that expression of some of the potential markers of epidermal stem cells may be interdependent. There is good evidence for cross-talk between integrins and cadherins in cells (see, e.g., Hodivala and Watt 1994; Monier-Ganelle and Duband 1997) and between the Notch (Delta receptor) and Wnt (upstream of β-catenin) signaling pathways (see, e.g., de Celis and Bray 1997).

EPIDERMAL STEM CELL PATTERNING

The distribution of stem cells within the epidermis is not random. In hair follicles, the keratinocytes with high proliferative potential are reported to lie in the outer root sheath at the point of insertion of the muscle ("bulge region") or lower down (Cotsarelis et al. 1990; Yang et al. 1993; Rochat et al. 1994). In mouse interfollicular epidermis, it is proposed that a single stem cell lies at the base of a column of suprabasal cells and is surrounded by transit amplifying cells and cells that are committed to terminal differentiation (Potten 1981; Potten and Morris 1988); support for this model comes from more recent lineage marking studies (see, e.g., Mackenzie 1997).

β1 integrin staining has revealed a high level of patterning of the stem cell compartment in interfollicular human epidermis (Fig. 1). The cells with high β1 levels are found in clusters that lie at the tips of the dermal papillae (where the basal epidermal layer comes closest to the skin surface) in most body sites, but at the tips of the deep rete ridges (where the basal layer projects deepest into the dermis) in palm and sole epidermis (Jones et al. 1995; Jensen et al. 1999). Consistent with this view of the epidermis, the actively cycling cells are concentrated in the areas of low β1 integrin expression, as are the cells that have initiated expression of keratin 10 and are in the process of moving out of the basal layer (Jones et al. 1995; Jensen et al. 1999). Clustering of stem cells implies some lateral migration of cells along the basement membrane, and the high β1 integrin-expressing keratinocytes are indeed less motile than the keratinocytes with lower β1 levels, whether motility is measured in isolated cells or in confluent cell sheets (Jensen et al. 1999).

The simple architecture of the epidermis lends itself to mathematical modeling. It is interesting that from biophysical considerations, adhesiveness of keratinocytes to the basement membrane is predicted to be an important determinant of movement out of the basal layer (Dubertret and Rivier 1997). The predicted topology of stem and transit cells in some

Skin surface

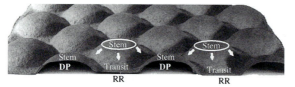

Dermis

Dermis

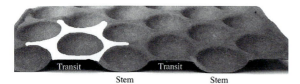

Skin surface

Figure 1 Model of the basal layer of the epidermis in body sites in which the stem cell patches (Stem) lie at the tips of the dermal papillae (DP) and the transit amplifying cells (Transit) are at the tips of the rete ridges (RR). Arrows in top panel represent movement of transit amplifying cells away from the stem cell patches. Bottom panel shows basal layer in opposite orientation to top panel and illustrates how the transit amplifying compartment forms a continuous network (highlighted in white) surrounding the stem cell patches. (Reprinted from Jensen et al. 1999.)

models of normal and hyperproliferative epidermis is consistent with the distribution of clusters of keratinocytes expressing high and low $\beta 1$ integrin levels (Iizuka et al. 1996).

REGULATION OF STEM CELL FATE

One of the most potent terminal differentiation stimuli is to place cultured keratinocytes in suspension: Both stem and transit amplifying cells initiate terminal differentiation without any further rounds of division, and by 24 hours the majority of cells are expressing markers of the differentiation pathway (Jones and Watt 1993). Suspension-induced differentiation can be partially inhibited by ligating $\beta 1$ integrins with extracellular matrix proteins or anti-integrin antibodies (Adams and Watt 1989; Watt et al. 1993). Recent experiments suggest that the integrin signal is "do not differentiate," transduced by occupied receptors, rather than a positive "differentiate" signal transduced by unoccupied receptors (Levy et al. 2000). Ligand binding is required both for integrin-mediated adhesion and integrin-regulated differentiation, but mutagenesis of the β1 cytoplasmic domain has established that the sequences which are required for differentiation control are distinct from those which are required to support extracellular matrix adhesion (Levy et al. 2000).

Integrins regulate not only the onset of overt differentiation, but also morphogenesis, down-regulation of integrin function and expression ensuring selective migration of committed cells from the basal epidermal layer (Adams and Watt 1990; Hotchin et al. 1995). In addition, high levels of β1 integrins are required for keratinocytes to remain in the stem cell compartment in vitro (Zhu et al. 1999). Introduction of a dominant negative β1 integrin into human keratinocytes in culture increases the proportion of clones attributable to transit amplifying cells. The dominant negative mutant interferes with β1 signaling to MAPK, although MAPK activation in response to growth factors or α6β4 ligation is not impaired (Zhu et al. 1999). Constitutive activation of MAPK rescues keratinocytes expressing the dominant negative integrin, decreasing the proportion of abortive clones to control levels; conversely, a dominant negative MAPKK1 construct reduces MAPK activation and increases the proportion of abortive clones (Fig. 2) (Zhu et al. 1999).

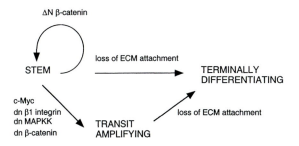

Stem cell characteristics: high β1 integrin expression;
high 'free' β-catenin pool; relatively non-motile

Figure 2 Summary of some characteristics of human epidermal stem cells and factors that regulate exit from the stem cell compartment. (ECM) Extracellular matrix; (dn) dominant negative. Data are collated from Jones and Watt (1993) (loss of ECM adhesion); Gandarillas and Watt (1997) (c-Myc); Zhu et al. (1999) (β1 integrins and MAPKK); and Zhu and Watt (1999) (β-catenin). (Reprinted, with permission, from Watt 2000).

As described above, stem cells have higher levels of non-cadherin-associated β-catenin than transit amplifying cells in vitro (Zhu and Watt 1999). Expression of a dominant negative β-catenin mutant in human keratinocytes promotes the formation of abortive, transit amplifying colonies, whereas expression of stabilized, amino-terminally truncated β-catenin increases the proportion of putative stem cells to almost 90% of the proliferative population (Zhu and Watt 1999). Interestingly, expression of stabilized amino-terminally truncated β-catenin in the basal layer of transgenic mouse epidermis causes keratinocytes to revert to a pluripotent state in which they can differentiate into hair follicles or interfollicular epidermis (Gat et al. 1998). Overexpression of stabilized β-catenin leads to ectopic formation of feather buds in developing chick skin (Normaly et al. 1999).

One of the genes that is regulated by β-catenin signaling is c-Myc (He et al. 1998). Since c-Myc promotes entry of keratinocytes into the transit amplifying compartment in vitro (Gandarillas and Watt 1997), it is possible that there is a feedback loop involving the two proteins that controls the ratio of stem to transit amplifying cells in the epidermis. Further targets of β-catenin and c-Myc in keratinocytes remain to be identified. It is, for example, possible that c-Myc down-regulates integrin expression (Hotchin et al. 1990; Gandarillas and Watt 1997; Judware and Culp 1997). Just as there may be cross-regulation of epidermal stem cell markers, the same is likely to be true for the molecules that regulate stem cell fate.

In addition to factors that act cell-autonomously to regulate epidermal stem cells, there is good evidence for a role of cell-cell interactions (see, e.g., Jones et al. 1995). One of the signaling pathways that is implicated is the pathway downstream from the transmembrane receptor Notch, which binds to transmembrane ligands such as Delta on neighboring cells (for review, see Artavanis-Tsakonas et al. 1999). Notch is expressed in all the layers of postnatal human epidermis; the Notch ligand Delta1 is confined to the basal layer and is most abundant in the clusters of cells known to express high levels of β1 integrins (Lowell et al. 2000). High Delta1 expression blocks the responsiveness of epidermal stem cells to Notch signals and may enhance cohesiveness of stem cell clusters, thereby discouraging intermingling with neighboring transit amplifying cells. Furthermore, Notch activation in cells at the edges of the stem clusters stimulates them to become transit amplifying cells (Lowell et al. 2000).

In surveying the molecules that are important for regulating epidermal stem cell fate, it is striking that the key signaling molecules, integrins, β-catenin, and Notch, play similar roles in diverse tissues and organisms (Watt and Hogan 2000).

LOOKING INTO THE FUTURE

It is possible to anticipate several advances that will both increase our understanding of epidermal stem cells and result in further therapeutic applications of keratinocytes. The use of proteomics and gene arrays should yield additional markers of the stem and transit amplifying compartments, enabling us to isolate the different cell populations to greater purity than is possible at present and providing new information about how stem cell fate is regulated. There will be increased use of lineage marking, both in vitro and in vivo, to monitor the behavior of keratinocytes in response to signals from their neighbors (see, e.g., Jensen et al. 1999; Lowell et al. 2000). There will be increased exploitation of transgenic mice to study stem cell renewal and differentiation, particularly making use of inducible transgene expression and inducible gene deletions (Pelengaris et al. 1999; Topley et al. 1999; Vasioukhin et al. 1999), and this will address the issue of whether transit amplifying cells have more restricted differentiation options than stem cells. Finally, the combination of improved retroviral vectors (Deng et al. 1997) and optimized transduction protocols (Mathor et al. 1996; Kolodka et al. 1998; Levy et al. 1998) will allow the exploitation of epidermal stem cells for gene therapy; for example, to treat inherited skin blistering diseases that result from mutation of genes encoding proteins that anchor the epidermis to the underlying dermis (Vailly et al. 1998; Seitz et al. 1999).

ACKNOWLEDGMENTS

I gratefully acknowledge the insights into epidermal stem cells provided by members of my laboratory past and present.

REFERENCES

Adams J.C. and Watt F.M. 1989. Fibronectin inhibits the terminal differentiation of human keratinocytes. *Nature* **340:** 307–309.

——.1990. Changes in keratinocyte adhesion during terminal differentiation: Reduction in fibronectin binding precedes $\alpha5\beta1$ integrin loss from the cell surface. *Cell* **63:** 425–435.

Al-Bawari S.E. and Potten C.S. 1976. Regeneration and dose-response characteristics of irradiated mouse dorsal epidermal cells. *Int. J. Radiat. Biol.* **30:** 201–216.

Artavanis-Tsakonas S., Rand M.D., and Lake R.J. 1999. Notch signaling: Cell fate control and signal integration in development. *Science* **284:** 770–776.

Barrandon Y. and Green H. 1987. Three clonal types of keratinocyte with different capacities for multiplication. *Proc. Natl. Acad. Sci.* **84:** 2302–2306.

Barrandon Y., Morgan J.R., Mulligan R.C., and Green H. 1989. Restoration of growth potential in paraclones of human keratinocytes by a viral oncogene. *Proc. Natl. Acad. Sci.* **86:** 4102–4106.

Bhatia M., Bonnet D., Murdoch B., Gan O.I., and Dick J.E. 1998. A newly discovered class of human hematopoietic cells with SCID-repopulating activity. *Nat. Med.* **4:** 1038–1045.

Bickenbach J.R. and Chism E. 1998. Selection and extended growth of murine epidermal stem cells in culture. *Exp. Cell Res.* **244:** 184–195.

Compton C.C., Nadire K.B., Regauer S., Simon M., Warland G., O'Connor N.E., Gallico G.G., and Laudry D.B. 1998. Cultured human sole-derived keratinocyte grafts re-express site-specific differentiation after transplantation. *Differentiation* **64:** 45–53.

Cotsarelis G., Sun T.-T., and Lavker R.M. 1990. Label-retaining cells reside in the bulge area of pilosebaceous unit: Implications for follicular stem cells, hair cycle, and skin carcinogenesis. *Cell* **61:** 1329–1337.

de Celis J.F. and Bray S. 1997. Feedback mechanisms affecting Notch activation at the dorsoventral boundary in the *Drosophila* wing. *Development* **124:** 3241–3251.

Deng H., Lin Q., and Khavari P.A. 1997. Sustainable cutaneous gene delivery. *Nat. Biotechnol.* **15:** 1388–1391.

Dowling J., Yu Q.C., and Fuchs E. 1996. β4 integrin is required for hemidesmosome formation, cell adhesion and cell survival. *J. Cell Biol.* **134:** 559–572.

Dubertret B. and Rivier N. 1997. The renewal of the epidermis: A topological mechanism. *Biophys. J.* **73:** 38–44.

Fuchs E. 1990. Epidermal differentiation: The bare essentials. *J. Cell Biol.* **111:** 2807–2814.

Gallico III., G.G., O'Connor N.E., Compton C.C., Kehinde O., and Green H. 1984. Permanent coverage of large skin wounds with autologous cultured epithelium. *N. Engl. J. Med.* **311:** 448–451.

Gandarillas A. 2000. Epidermal differentiation, apoptosis, and senescence: Common pathways? *Exp. Gerontol.* **35:** 53–62.

Gandarillas A. and Watt F.M. 1997. c-*Myc* promotes differentiation of epidermal stem cells. *Genes Dev.* **11:** 2869–2882.

Gandarillas A., Goldsmith L.A., Gschmeissner S., Leigh I.M., and Watt F.M. 1999. Evidence that apoptosis and terminal differentiation of epidermal keratinocytes are distinct processes. *Exp. Dermatol.* **8:** 71–79.

Gat U., Dasgupta R., Degenstein L. and Fuchs E. 1998. De novo hair follicle morphogenesis and hair tumors in mice expressing a truncated β-catenin in skin. *Cell* **95:** 605–614.

Georges-Labouesse E., Messaddeq N., Yehhia G., Cadalbert L., Dierich A., and Le Meur M. 1996. Absence of integrin α6 leads to epidermolysis bullosa and neonatal death in mice. *Nat. Genet.* **13:** 370–373.

Hall P.A. and Watt F.M. 1989. Stem cells: The generation and maintenance of cellular diversity. *Development* **106:** 619–633.

He T.-C., Sparks A.B., Rago C., Hermeking H., Zawel L., Da Costa L.T., Morin P.J., Vogelstein B., and Kinzler K.W. 1998. Identification of c-*MYC* as a target of the APC pathway. *Science* **281:** 1509–1512.

Hodivala K.J. and Watt F.M. 1994. Evidence that cadherins play a role in the downregulation of integrin expression that occurs during keratinocyte terminal differentiation. *J. Cell Biol.* **124:** 589–600.

Hotchin N.A., Gandarillas A., and Watt F.M. 1995. Regulation of cell surface β1 integrin levels during keratinocyte terminal differentiation. *J. Cell Biol.* **128:**1209–1219.

Hotchin N.A., Allday M.J., and Crawford D.H. 1990. Deregulated c-*myc* expression in Epstein-Barr-virus-immortalized B-cells induces altered growth properties and surface phenotype but not tumorigenicity. *Int. J. Cancer* **45:** 566–571.

Iizuka H., Ishida-Yamamoto A., and Honda H. 1996. Epidermal remodelling in psoriasis. *Br. J. Dermatol.* **135:** 433–438.

Jensen U.B., Lowell S., and Watt F.M. 1999. The spatial relationship between stem cells and their progeny in the basal layer of human epidermis: A new view based on whole mount labelling and lineage analysis. *Development* **126:** 2409–2418.

Jones P.H. and Watt F.M. 1993. Separation of human epidermal stem cells from transit amplifying cells on the basis of differences in integrin function and expression. *Cell* **73:** 713–724.

Jones P.H., Harper S., and Watt F.M. 1995. Stem cell patterning and fate in human epidermis. *Cell* **80:** 83–93.

Judware R. and Culp L.A. 1997. Concomitant down-regulation of expression of integrin subunits by N-*myc* in human neuroblastoma cells: Differential regulation of $\alpha 2$, $\alpha 3$, and $\beta 1$. *Oncogene* **14:** 1341–1350.

Kaur P. and Li A. 2000. Adhesive properties of human basal epidermal cells: An analysis of keratinocyte stem cells, transit amplifying cells, and postmitotic differentiating cells. *J. Invest. Dermatol.* **114:** 413–420.

Kolodka T.M., Garlick J.A., and Taichman L.B. 1998. Evidence for keratinocyte stem cells in vitro: Long term engraftment and persistence of transgene expression from retrovirus-transduced keratinocytes. *Proc. Natl. Acad. Sci.* **95:** 4356-4361.

Levy L., Broad S., Diekmann D., Evans R.D., and Watt F.M. 2000. $\beta 1$ integrins regulate keratinocyte adhesion and differentiation by distinct mechanisms. *Mol. Biol. Cell* **11:** 453–466.

Levy L., Broad S., Zhu A.J., Carroll J.M., Khazaal I., Péault B., and Watt F.M. 1998. Optimised retroviral infection of human epidermal keratinocytes: Long-term expression of transduced integrin gene following grafting onto SCID mice. *Gene Ther.* **5:** 913–922.

Li A., Simmons P.J., and Kaur P. 1998. Identification and isolation of candidate human keratinocyte stem cells based on cell surface phenotype. *Proc. Natl. Acad. Sci.* **95:** 3902–3907.

Lowell S., Jones P., Le Roux I., Dunne J., and Watt F.M. 2000. Stimulation of human epidermal differentiation by Notch/Delta signalling at the boundaries of stem cell clusters. *Curr. Biol.* **10:** 491–500.

Lyle S., Christofidou-Solomidou M., Liu Y., Elder D.E., Albelda S., and Cotsarelis G. 1998. The C8/144B monoclonal antibody recognizes cytokeratin 15 and defines the location of human hair follicle stem cells. *J. Cell Sci.* **111:** 3179–3188.

Mathor M.B., Ferrari G., Dellambra E., Cilli M., Mavilio F., Cancedda R., and De Luca M. 1996. Clonal analysis of stably transduced human epidermal stem cells in culture. *Proc. Natl. Acad. Sci.* **93:** 10371–10376.

Mackenzie I.C. 1997. Retroviral transduction of murine epidermal stem cells demonstrates clonal units of epidermal structure. *J. Invest. Dermatol.* **109:** 377–383.

Miller S.J., Burke E.M., Rader M.D., Coulombe P.A., and Lavker R.M. 1998. Re-epithelialization of porcine skin by the sweat apparatus. *J. Invest. Dermatol.* **110:** 13–19.

Mills A.A., Zheng B., Wang X.J., Vogel H., Roop D.R., and Bradley A. 1999. p63 is a p53 homologue required for limb and epidermal morphogenesis. *Nature* **398:** 708–713.

Molès J.-P. and Watt F.M. 1997. The epidermal stem cell compartment: Variation in expression levels of E-cadherin and catenins within the basal layer of human epidermis. *J. Histochem. Cytochem.* **45:** 867–874.

Moll I. 1995. Proliferative potential of different keratinocytes of plucked human hair follicles. *J. Invest. Dermatol.* **105:** 14–21.

Monier-Gavelle F. and Duband J.L. 1997. Cross talk between adhesion molecules: Control of N-cadherin activity by intracellular signals elicted by β1 and β3 integrins in migrating neural crest cells. *J. Cell Biol.* **137:** 1663–1681.

Normaly S., Freeman A., and Morgan B.A. 1999. β-catenin signalling can initiate feather bud development. *Development* **126:** 3509–3521.

Odland G.F. 1991. Structure of the skin. In *Physiology, biochemistry, and molecular biology of the skin*, 2nd edition (ed. L.A. Goldsmith), pp. 3–62. Oxford University Press, Oxford, United Kingdom.

Parsa R., Yang A., McKeon F., and Green H. 1999. Association of p63 with proliferative potential in normal and neoplastic human keratinocytes. *J. Invest. Dermatol.* **113:** 1099–1105.

Pelengaris S., Littlewood T., Khan M., Elia G., and Evan G. 1999. Reversible activation of c-Myc in skin: Induction of a complex neoplastic phenotype by a single oncogenic lesion. *Mol. Cell* **3:** 565–577.

Potten C.S. 1981. Cell replacement in epidermis (keratopoiesis) via discrete units of proliferation. *Int. Rev. Cytol.* **69:** 271–318.

Potten C.S. and Morris R.J. 1988. Epithelial stem cells *in vivo. J. Cell Sci.* **10:** 45–62.

Reynolds A.J., and Jahoda C. 1992. Cultured dermal papilla cells induce follicle formation and hair growth by transdifferentiation of an adult epidermis. *Development* **115:** 587–593.

Rheinwald J.G. 1989. Methods for clonal growth and serial cultivation of normal human epidermal keratinocytes and mesothelial cells. In *Cell growth and differentiation. A practical approach* (ed. R. Baserga), pp. 81–94. IRL Press, Oxford, United Kingdom.

Rochat A., Kobayashi K., and Barrandon Y. 1994. Location of stem cells of human hair follicles by clonal analysis. *Cell* **76:** 1063–1073.

Seitz C.S., Giudice G.J., Balding S.D., Marinkovich M.P., and Khavari P.A. 1999. BP180 gene therapy in junctional epidermolysis bullosa. *Gene Ther.* **6:** 42–47.

Slack J.M.W. 2000. Stem cells in epithelial tissues. *Science* **287:** 1431–1433.

Stasiak P.C., Purkis P.E., Leigh I.M., and Lane E.B. 1989. Keratin 19: Predicted amino acid sequence and broad tissue distribution suggest it evolved from keratinocyte keratins. *J. Invest. Dermatol.* **92:** 707–716.

Topley G.I., Okuyama R., Gonzales J.G., Conti C., and Dotto G.P. 1999. p21[WAF1/Cip1] functions as a suppressor of malignant skin tumor formation and a determinant of keratinocyte stem-cell potential. *Proc. Natl. Acad. Sci.* **96:** 9089–9094.

Uchida N., Tsukamoto A., He D., Friera A.M., Scollay R., and Weissman I.L. 1998. High doses of purified stem cells cause early hematopoietic recovery in syngeneic and allogeneic hosts. *J. Clin. Invest.* **101:** 961–966.

Vailly J., Ganoux-Palacios L., Dell'Ambra E., Romero C., Pinola M., Zambruno G., De Luca M., Ortonne J.P, and Meneguzzi G. 1998. Corrective gene transfer of keratinocytes from patients with junctional epidermolysis bullosa restores assembly of hemidesmosomes in reconstructed epithelia. *Gene Ther.* **5:** 1322–1332.

van der Neut R., Krimpenfort P., Calafat J., Niessen C.M., and Sonnenberg A. 1996. Epithelial detachment due to absence of hemidesmosomes in integrin β4 null mice.

Nat. Genet. **13:** 366–369.

Vasioukhin V., Degenstein L., Wise B., and Fuchs E. 1999. The magical touch: Genome targeting in epidermal stem cells induced by tamoxifen application to mouse skin. *Proc. Natl. Acad. Sci.* **96:** 8551–8556.

Waseem A., Dogan B., Tidman N., Alam Y., Purkis P., Jackson S., Lalli A., Machesne Y.M., and Leigh I.M. 1999. Keratin 15 expression in stratified epithelia: Downregulation in activated keratinocytes. *J. Invest. Dermatol.* **112:** 362–369.

Watt F.M. 1989. Terminal differentiation of epidermal keratinocytes. *Curr. Opin. Cell Biol.* **1:** 1107–1115.

———. 1998. Epidermal stem cells: Markers, patterning and the control of stem cell fate. *Philos. Trans. R. Soc. Lond. Biol. Sci.* **353:** 831–837.

———. 2000. Epidermal stem cells as targets for gene transfer. *Hum. Gene Ther.* **11:** 2261–2266.

Watt F.M. and Hogan B.L.M. 2000. Out of Eden: Stem cells and their niches. *Science* **287:** 1427–1430.

Watt F.M., Kubler M.-D., Hotchin N.A., Nicholson L.J., and Adams J.C. 1993. Regulation of keratinocyte terminal differentiation by integrin-extracellular matrix interactions. *J. Cell Sci.* **106:** 175–182.

Yang J.S., Lavker R.M., and Sun T.-T. 1993. Upper human hair follicle contains a sub-population of keratinocytes with superior in vitro proliferative potential. *J. Invest. Dermatol.* **101:** 652–659.

Yang A, Schweitzer R., Sun D., Kaghad M., Walker N., Bronson R.T., Tabin C., Sharpe A., Caput D., Crum C., and McKeon F. 1999. p63 is essential for regenerative prolif-eration in limb, craniofacial and epithelial development. *Nature* **398:** 714–718.

Zhu A.J. and Watt F.M. 1999. β-catenin signalling modulates proliferative potential of human epidermal keratinocytes independently of intercellular adhesion. *Development* **126:** 2285–2298.

Zhu A.J., Haase I., and Watt F.M. 1999. Signalling via β1 integrins and mitogen-activated protein kinase determines human epidermal stem cell fate in vitro. *Proc. Natl. Acad. Sci.* **96:** 6728–6733.

20
Liver Stem Cells

Markus Grompe
Department of Molecular and Medical Genetics
Oregon Health Sciences University
Portland, Oregon 97201

Milton J. Finegold
Department of Pathology
Texas Children's Hospital
Baylor College of Medicine
Houston, Texas 77030-2399

HEPATIC STEM CELLS

The adult mammalian liver contains many different cell types of various embryological origins. Nevertheless, the term liver or hepatic stem cells is used for precursors of the two epithelial liver cell types, the hepatocytes and the bile duct epithelial cells. This terminology also applies to this chapter where only hepatocyte and the bile duct stem cells are discussed.

ORGANIZATION AND FUNCTION OF ADULT MAMMALIAN LIVER

Anatomy

The liver is a large parenchymal organ consisting of several separate lobes and representing about 2% of the body weight in the human and 5% in the mouse (Desmet 1994). It is the only organ with two separate afferent blood supplies. The hepatic artery provides oxygenated blood, and the portal vein brings in venous blood rich in nutrients and hormones from the splanchnic bed (intestines and pancreas). Venous drainage is into the vena cava. The bile secreted by hepatocytes is collected in an arborized collecting system, the biliary tree, which drains into the duodenum. The gall bladder is part of the distal biliary tree and acts to store bile. The hepatic artery, portal vein, and common bile duct enter the liver in the same location, the porta hepatis.

The main cell types resident in the liver are hepatocytes, bile duct epithelium, stellate cells (formerly called Ito cells), Kupffer cells, vascular endothelium, fibroblasts, and leukocytes (Desmet 1994). Although hepatocytes are responsible for most organismal liver function and represent about 90% of the weight of the liver, they are large cells and only ~60% of total liver DNA is hepatocyte-derived. An adult mouse liver contains about 5×10^7, and an adult human liver about 80×10^9, hepatocytes. Knowledge of the microscopic structure of the liver is essential for understanding hepatic stem cell biology, and two main models for its organization have been proposed. According to one model, the hepatic lobule (illustrated in Fig. 1) is the functional unit of the liver (Mall 1906). The portal triad consisting of a small portal vein, hepatic artery branch, and bile duct is located on the perimeter. Arterial and portal venous blood enter here, mix, and flow past the hepatocytes toward the central vein in the middle of the lobule. The second model considers liver acini the basic units, with each acinus having the portal triad at the center and the "central" veins at the periphery (Rappaport et al. 1954).

We base our discussions on the lobule model. In both models, liver sinusoids are the vasculature connecting the portal triad vessels and the central vein. Unlike other capillary beds, sinusoidal vessels have a fenestrated endothelium, thus permitting direct contact between blood and the

Figure 1 (*A*) Diagram of vascular supply and sinusoidal structure of the liver lobule. Blood from the hepatic artery branch (HAb) and portal vein branch (PVb) enters the hepatic sinusoids one or two cells from the edge of the lobule, mixes in the sinusoids (S), delivers oxygen and nutrients to the liver cells, picks up carbon dioxide and metabolic products from the liver cells, and drains into the central vein branch (CV). Limiting plate (LmP) is the first row of hepatocytes that separates liver parenchyma from the portal space. Liver plate (LP) is a single layer of hepatocytes that extends from portal space to the central venule. Endothelial (En) cells form walls of the sinusoids and make openings (fenestrae) between sinusoids and hepatocytes. Kupffer cells (K) and pit cells (not shown) are located in the sinusoids, and Ito cells (fat-storing cells, FCS) are located in spaces between endothelial cells and hepatocytes (Disse's space, DS). On the opposite side from the sinusoids, hepatocytes form bile canaliculi (BC), channels that drain bile into interlobular bile ducts (BDI) in a direction opposite from the blood flow. Bile canaliculi and interlobular bile ducts are connected by bile ductules (cholangioles). Canaliculo-ductular junction (CDJ) is the region that connects bile canaliculi (last hepatocyte) and bile ductule (first biliary epithelial cell, ductular cell), and is also known as the opening or canal of Hering. (Reprinted, with permission, from Motta et al. 1978.) (*B*) Metabolic zonation of the lobule. A histological section of mouse liver was stained with an antibody to glutamine synthetase. Only zone-3 hepatocytes adjacent to the central vein (CV) express GS. (PV) Portal vein.

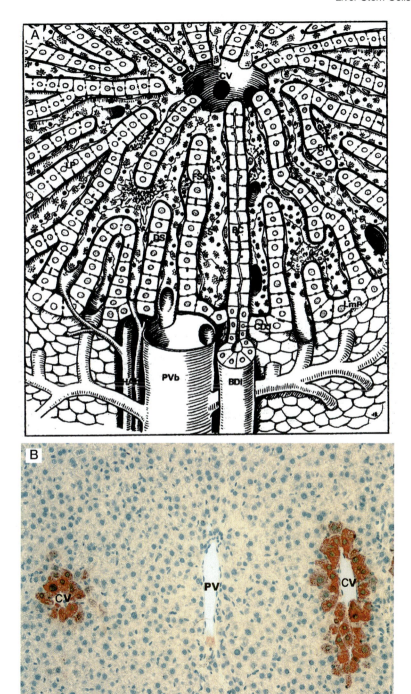

Figure 1 (See facing page for legend.)

hepatocyte cell surface (Wisse 1970). In two-dimensional images, rows of hepatocytes oriented from portal to central form a hepatic plate. A channel formed by adjacent hepatocytes forms a bile canaliculus that serves to drain secreted bile toward the bile duct in the portal triad. Hepatocytes are large, cuboidal epithelial cells with a basal and apical surface, and the apical surface is also called the canalicular surface. Hepatocytes exchange metabolites with the blood on the basal surface and secrete bile at the canalicular surface. Zone-1, -2, and -3 hepatocytes are distinguished on the basis of their relative position within the lobule. Zone-1 hepatocytes are close to the portal triad, zone-2 cells are in the middle, and zone 3 consists of cells directly adjacent to the central vein. Although somewhat variable according to species, a large proportion of adult hepatocytes are binucleated, with some nuclei being tetraploid. Thus, hepatocytes can have 2n, 4n, or 8n total DNA content (Digernes and Bolund 1979; Medvedev 1988). Bile secreted by the hepatocytes is collected in bile ducts, which are lined by duct epithelial cells. The smallest bile ducts are located in the portal zone of each hepatic lobule. The canal of Hering represents the connection between the bile canaliculi (the inter-hepatocyte space into which bile is secreted) and the bile ducts, at the interface between the lobule and the portal triad.

Stellate cells represent about 5–10% of the total number of hepatic cells. In addition to storing vitamin A, they are essential for the synthesis of extracellular matrix proteins and produce many hepatic growth factors that play an essential role in the biology of liver regeneration (Friedman 1996). They are thought to be mesodermal in origin, but very little is known about their turnover and renewal. Kupffer cells also represent about 5% of all liver cells and are resident macrophages. These cells are of hematopoietic origin (bone marrow-derived), but are capable of replicating within the liver itself. Oval cells (Sell 1994) are the apparent progenitors of liver hepatocytes and epithelial cells, and are found in regenerating liver following partial hepatectomy or chemical damage. The origin of oval cells from liver and/or other sources is discussed later in this chapter (see also Thiese et al. 1999; Alison et al. 1996).

Functions

The liver is responsible for a variety of biochemical functions. These include the intermediary metabolism of amino acids, lipids, and carbohydrates; the detoxification of xenobiotics; and the synthesis of serum proteins. In addition, the liver produces bile, which is important for intestinal absorption of nutrients, as well as the elimination of cholesterol and copper. All of these functions are primarily executed by hepatocytes. The biochemical properties and pattern of gene expression are not uniform among all hepatocytes. The term "metabolic zonation" has been coined to indicate the different properties of zone-1, zone-2, and zone-3 hepatocytes (Jungermann and Katz 1989; Jungermann and Kietzmann 1996). For example, only zone-3 hepatocytes express glutamine synthetase (Fig. 1B) and utilize ammonia to generate glutamine (Gebhardt and Mecke 1983; Wagenaar et al. 1994). In contrast, zone-1 and zone-2 hepatocytes express urea cycle enzymes and convert ammonia to urea (Moorman et al. 1989; Haussinger et al. 1992). Similarly, glycogen synthesis and glycolysis are segregated within the hepatic lobule (Wals et al. 1988).

Embryology

In the mouse, the liver develops from ventral foregut endoderm beginning at day 8 of gestation (Zaret 2000). Figure 2 schematically depicts the sequence of events. The first evidence of hepatic differentiation is the induction of albumin and α-fetoprotein mRNA in endodermal cells, even prior to their morphological differentiation (Gualdi et al. 1996). Between days 8.5 and 9.5, the hepatocyte precursors proliferate, and beginning at day 9.5, migrate toward cardiac mesoderm in the septum transversum (Cascio and Zaret 1993). Signals from the cardiac mesoderm induce the cells to increase their levels of albumin and α-fetoprotein mRNAs and to form the liver bud. Very recently some of the specific signals produced by the mesenchyme have been identified. Fibroblast growth factors (FGFs) 1, 2, and 8 were sufficient to induce the liver gene expression program in isolated murine foregut endoderm (Jung et al. 1999). FGF receptors 1 and 4 are expressed on foregut endoderm cells and are essential for this induction.

At day 10.5, the vascularization of the liver bud begins, followed by a large increase in liver mass (Zaret 1996, 2000). The early cells in the liver bud are positive for both albumin and α-fetoprotein. The more differentiated phenotypes of hepatocytes and bile duct epithelium emerge in midgestation. Definitive lineage studies have not yet been reported, but it is generally thought that bile ducts and hepatocytes emerge from common precursors, termed hepatoblasts (Shiojiri et al. 1991; Zaret 1996, 2000). It is not known whether there is only one type of hepatoblast or whether there is a hierarchy of lineage progression consisting of primitive hepatoblasts and more committed bipotential progenitors. Fetal hepatoblasts can be considered as the equivalent to a fetal liver stem cell.

Several genes that are important for the development of the liver have been identified. Many of the relevant studies have involved mouse knock-

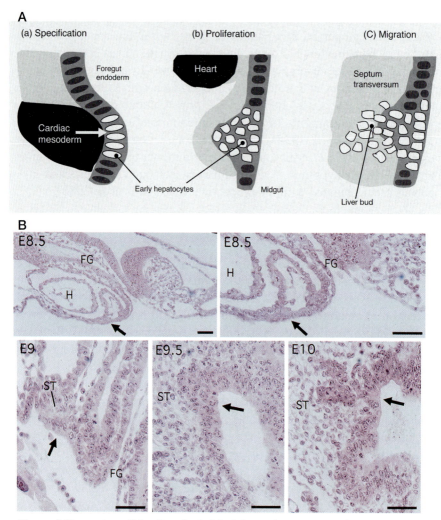

Figure 2 Formation of the liver bud. (*A*) Schematic representation. (*a*) In the ~6 somite embryo, cardiac mesoderm induces (*arrow*) the foregut endoderm to activate liver-specific genes (denoted by white blocks). (*b*) As the endoderm is pulled to the midgut during gut closure, the early hepatocytes begin to proliferate within the endoderm layer. (*c*) The early hepatocytes migrate into a region of loose mesenchyme called the septum transversum. The early hepatocytes then coalesce around sinusoids in the mesenchyme, forming the liver organ. (Reprinted, with permission, from Zaret 1998 [©Elsevier Science].) (*B*) Histology of liver bud formation in the mouse. Sagittal sections; ventral on the left; dorsal on the right. The embryonic day is given in the left upper corner. (H) heart; (FG) foregut; (ST) septum transversum; the arrow indicates the liver primordium. (Images courtesy of Nobuyoshi Shiojiri, Department of Biology, Faculty of Science, Shizuoka University, Japan.)

out models (see Table 1). Figure 3 illustrates the currently known important players. The first genes of importance are the transcription factors HNF3β and GATA-4 . These genes are essential for the specification of endoderm and also play a role in the development of other epithelial tissues such as the lung and the pancreas (Ang and Rossant 1994; Kaestner et al. 1994; Weinstein et al. 1994; Kuo et al. 1997; Molkentin et al. 1997). Presently, the factor(s) which is responsible for the onset of liver gene expression before formation of the liver bud is not known. This factor would be of obvious interest in the utilization of liver stem cells. In contrast, several factors involved in the formation of the liver bud are already known (Hentsch et al. 1996). c-jun (Hilberg et al. 1997), HGF (Schmidt et al. 1995), and c-met (Bladt et al. 1995) have all been shown to be essential for liver bud formation. Other factors such as β1-integrin act later in the development of the liver (see Fig. 3). The phenotypes of mouse embryos homozygous for targeted disruptions in genes known to play a role in liver development are listed in Table 1.

Overall, our understanding of liver development at the molecular level is still in its early stages. It is likely that many of the yet-to-be discovered mechanisms involved in liver specification during embryogenesis will also apply to progenitor-dependent liver regeneration and liver stem cell biology.

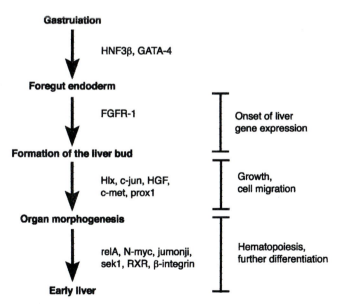

Figure 3 Genes involved in early liver development. Phases of liver development are shown with regulatory proteins required for each of the designated transitions, based on gene knockout experiments in mice. (Adapted, with permission, from Zaret 1998 [©Elsevier Science].)

Table 1 Targeted disruption of genes involved in liver development

Gene	Phenotype	Reference
HNF3β	embryonic-lethal, day 10; absent node and notochord; endodermal cells present, but gut tube doesn't form	Ang and Rossant (1994); Weinstein et al. (1994)
GATA4	embryonic-lethal, day 8–10; absent heart tube and foregut	Kuo et al. (1997); Molkentin et al. (1997); Morrisey et al. (1998)
FGF receptor-1	early-embryonic-lethal; failure of mesodermal and endodermal lineages	Ciruna et al. (1997)
prox1	embryonic-lethal, mid gestation; hepatocyte migration into the liver bud is impaired	Sosa-Pineda et al. (2000)
c-jun	embryonic-lethal, day 12–14; impaired hepatogenesis	Hilberg et al. (1997)
Hlx	embryonic-lethal, day 15; hypoplasia of liver and gut; liver begins ontogeny normally but fails to expand	Hentsch et al. (1996)
HGF	embryonic-lethal; small liver size and loss of parenchymal cells	Schmidt et al. (1995)
c-met	embryonic lethal; small liver; myogenic precursors fail to migrate to limb buds	Bladt et al. (1995)
rel-A	embryonic-lethal, day 15; hepatocyte apoptosis in utero	Beg et al. (1998)
sek1/mkk4	embryonic-lethal, day 10–12; small liver, hepatocyte apoptosis	Nishina et al. (1999)
N-myc	embryonic-lethal, day 12; hepatocyte apoptosis in utero	Giroux and Charron (1998)
jumonji	embryonic lethal; liver hypoplasia	Motoyama et al. (1997)
RXR	embryonic-lethal, day 13–16; delay in hepatocyte differentiation; hypoplastic heart	Sucov et al. (1994)

Markers of Hepatic Lineages

Most of the studies pertaining to liver stem cell biology make extensive use of specific markers for different cellular phenotypes, including differentiated hepatocytes, biliary duct epithelium, hepatoblasts, and oval cells. Some markers are based on enzyme histochemical methods, but most rely on the expression of cell-specific antigens, detectable with antibodies. Some markers are expressed only in hepatocytes, some only in bile duct epithelium, some only in oval cells, and some in combinations of these. The best antibodies have been developed against rat marker proteins, and these have been used to map the sequence of antigen expression in liver development and carcinogenesis (Hixson et al. 1990, 1996, 1997).

Not all markers are expressed similarly in all species, and some monoclonal antibodies do not cross-react. For example, α-fetoprotein is not expressed at high levels in mouse oval cells. Table 2 depicts the most important of these markers, their expression patterns, and the species in which they can be used.

Unfortunately, most of the monoclonal antibodies that have been developed are not against antigens expressed on the cell surface. Hence, fluorescence-activated cell sorting (FACS) has not been possible for phenotypic analysis of liver subpopulations.

Hepatocyte-enriched Transcription Factors

Four families of evolutionarily conserved transcription factors are involved in hepatocyte-specific gene expression (Cereghini 1996). These factors are enriched in liver but are not completely restricted to this organ. Because these factors are involved in setting up a hepatocyte program, they are also of interest in liver stem cell biology. Each family is composed of several members displaying similar DNA recognition properties. Current studies suggest a model for liver differentiation based on a regulatory network rather than a genetic hierarchy (Cereghini 1996). The four transcription factor families are (1) the variant homeodomain-containing family of hepatocyte nuclear factor 1 (HNF1) proteins, (2) the HNF3 winged helix proteins, (3) the nuclear receptor superfamily, and (4) the leucine zipper C/EBP family. These factors have been reviewed recently (Cereghini 1996).

Two different members belong to the HNF1 homeodomain family: HNF1 and variant HNF1 (vHNF1). Target genes include albumin, α-fetoprotein, and phenylalanine hydroxylase (Cereghini et al. 1988). In adult animals, HNF1 and vHNF1 are present in liver and kidney and intestinal organs (Rey-Campos et al. 1991). However, vHNF1 is primarily expressed in kidney, whereas HNF1 is abundant in the liver. Both genes are also expressed in a variety of epithelial tissues during embryogenesis (Coffinier et al. 1999). During mammalian development, vHNF1 expression occurs earlier than that of HNF1. vHNF1 can already be found at day 5 of gestation in the mouse in visceral endoderm (Cereghini et al. 1992). It is also expressed at the onset of liver development when ventral foregut

Table 2 Markers for hepatic cell types

Marker	Hepatocytes	Biliary duct epithelium	Oval cells	Reference
Albumin	+	–	+	Houssaint (1980); Shiojiri et al. (1991)
α1-Antitrypsin	+	–	+	Gauldie et al. (1980)
α-Fetoprotein	fetal only	–	+ (rat, human) – (mouse)	Shiojiri et al. (1991)
Glucose-6-phos-phatase	+	–	+	Plenat et al. (1988)
Dipeptidyl peptidase IV	canalicular	+	+	Petell et al. (1990)
Fumarylaceto-acetate hydrolase	+	–	– (mouse) ? (rat, human)	Grompe et al. (1995)
Glutamine synthetase	+ (zone 3 only)	–	–	Smith and Campbell (1988)
A6	– (mouse)	+ (mouse)	+ (mouse)	Engelhardt et al. (1990)
Cytokeratin 7	–	+	–	Shiojiri et al. (1991)
Cytokeratin 8	+	+	+	Van Eyken et al. (1988)
Cytokeratin 14	–	–	+ (human)	Haruna et al. (1996)
Cytokeratin 18	+	+	+	Van Eyken et al. (1988)
Cytokeratin 19	–	+	– (mouse) + (rat, human)	Gebhardt et al. (1988); Bouwens et al. (1994)
OV1	–	+ (rat)	+ (rat)	Dunsford and Sell (1989)
OV6	–	+	+ (rat, human)	Dunsford and Sell (1989)
OC.1	–	+ (rat)	– (rat)	Hixson and Allison (1985)
OC.2	–	+ (rat)	+ (rat)	Hixson and Allison (1985)
OC.3	–	+ (rat)	+ (rat)	Hixson and Allison (1985)
BD.1	–	+ (rat)	+ (rat)	Yang et al. (1993)
Vimentin	–	fetal only	+	Golding et al. (1995)

endoderm cells proliferate to form the liver primordium. HNF1 is first found in the yolk sac at 8 days but is expressed strongly only at later stages in more differentiated cells of the developing liver. These observations suggest that the vHNF1 may be involved in morphogenesis of organs such as the liver and kidney, whereas HNF1 may be involved in maintaining the differentiated state. Consistent with this hypothesis, HNF1 knockout mice have intact hepatic organogenesis but defects in expression of some liver-specific genes (Pontoglio et al. 1996).

The HNF3 winged helix family contains three members, HNF3α, HNF3β, and HNF3γ. The DNA-binding motif of these putative transcription factors has a high degree of similarity to a region of the *Drosophila* gene fork head, which is involved in organogenesis in the fly. The HNF3 family members are expressed during the development of the endoderm as well as in cells of the notochord and ventral neural epithelium. During embryogenesis, HNF3β comes on first, followed by HNF3α and finally HNF3γ. The three genes show different anterior boundaries but an identical posterior boundary (the hindgut) in the developing endoderm. This suggests that they are involved in the regionalization of the definitive endoderm (Ang et al. 1993). All three family members are expressed in a variety of epithelial adult organs, including the liver and the intestine. Targeted gene knockouts of some have shed some light on their specific functions. HNF3β knockout mice die at day 10 of embryogenesis because of notochord defects. Recently, a novel transcription factor HNF6 has been found to regulate expression of HNF3β. HNF6 belongs to the cut homeodomain family of transcription factors. HNF6 knockout mice lack a gall bladder and have developmental abnormalities of the intrahepatic bile ducts (Jacquemin et al. 2000).

Several orphan nuclear receptors have been identified as hepatocyte transcription factors. These include HNF4, CoupF1, and Arp-1. HNF4 was first identified by its interaction with liver-specific promoters, and its ligand is unknown (Costa et al. 1989). HNF4 is involved with diverse metabolic functions, including gluconeogenesis, cholesterol metabolism, and amino acid metabolism. In the adult, HNF4 is expressed at high levels in liver, kidney, and intestine (Sladek et al. 1991). During mouse development, it is expressed in primitive endoderm at 4.5 days and then becomes restricted to visceral endoderm at day 5.5 (Duncan et al. 1994). GATA6 is upstream of HNF4 and regulates its expression (Morrisey et al. 1998). In embryonic development, HNF4 is essential, as shown by the fact that HNF4 knockout mice die at day 6 of gestation with an endodermal defect (Chen et al. 1996). However, the embryos can be rescued later in gestation and thus show that HNF4 is essential for hepatocyte differentiation (Duncan et al. 1997; Li et al. 2000). CoupTF1 and Arp-1 are negative regulators of hepatocyte gene expression (Kimura et al. 1993; Legraverend et al. 1994; Hall et al. 1995; Lazennec et al. 1997).

The CCAAT enhancer-binding protein family (C/EBP) has four known members; C/EBPα, C/EBPβ, C/EBPδ, and C/EBPγ. These share a highly conserved terminal bipartite domain defined as a basic leucine zipper (bZIP). C/EBPα is expressed predominantly in hepatocytes, intestinal epithelial cells, and fat cells. C/EBPα knockout mice have an interesting phenotype that includes some hyperproliferation of hepatocytes and an absence of brown fat (Lee et al. 1997). Like C/EBPα, both C/EBPβ and C/EBPδ are also required for adipocyte differentiation (Tanaka et al. 1997), but all of these factors are also found at high levels in the liver (Descombes and Schibler 1991). C/EBPβ has been implicated in regulating genes of the acute-phase response and inflammation (Poli et al. 1990).

The PAR subfamily of leucine zipper transcription factors is related to the C/EBP proteins. Three members are currently known, including DBP (Mueller et al. 1990), hepatic leukemia factor (HLF) (Inaba et al. 1994), and TEF (Drolet et al. 1991). Whereas the C/EBP factors have a more relaxed specificity and bind to PAR recognition sites, PAR proteins are more selective in their recognition and bind only to a subset of C/EBP sites (Drolet et al. 1991). The PAR subfamily member DBP has the interesting property of being expressed in circadian rhythm-dependent fashion (Lavery and Schibler 1993).

Table 3 shows the phenotypes of targeted disruptions of hepatocyte-specific transcription factors.

Table 3 Gene knockouts of hepatocyte transcription factors

HNF1	viable; defective insulin secretion; impaired expression of some liver genes	Lee et al. (1998); Pontoglio et al. (1998)
HNF3α	neonatal lethal; hypoglycemia; decreased glucagon expression	Kaestner et al. (1999)
HNF3β	embryonic-lethal, day 10; absent node and notochord; endodermal cells present, but gut tube doesn't form	Ang and Rossant (1994); Weinstein et al. (1994)
HNF-3γ	viable; altered rates of transcription of hepatocyte genes	Kaestner et al. (1998)
HNF6	viable, reduced number of pancreatic endocrine cells; absent gallbladder; bile duct abnormalities	Jacquemin et al. (2000)
HNF4	embryonic-lethal, day 6; impaired gastrulation	Chen et al. (1996)
Coup-TF1	perinatal death; abnormal cranial nerves	Qiu et al. (1997)
Coup-TFII (Arp-1)	embryonic lethal; defective heart development	Pereira et al. (1999)
C/EBPα	neonatal lethal; hypoglycemia; decreased brown fat	Wang et al. (1995); Lee et al. (1997)
C/EBPβ	neonatal lethal; decreased brown fat	Tanaka et al. (1997)
C/EBPδ	neonatal lethal; decreased brown fat	Tanaka et al. (1997)

Liver Stem Cells

The ancient Greek legend of Prometheus illustrates that the phenomenon of liver regeneration has been known since antiquity. Animals (including humans) can survive surgical removal of up to 75% of the total liver mass. The original number of cells is restored within 1 week and the original tissue mass within 2–3 weeks (Bucher and Swaffield 1964; Stocker and Pfeifer 1965). This process can occur repeatedly, indicating a very high organ regenerative capacity, which is in contrast to most other parenchymal organs, such as kidney or pancreas (Stocker et al. 1973). Importantly, liver size is also controlled by prevention of organ overgrowth. Hepatic overgrowth can be induced by a variety of compounds such as HGF or peroxisome proliferators, but the liver size returns to normal very rapidly after removal of the growth-inducing signal. The role of liver stem cells in regeneration has been controversial (Fausto 1994; Sell 1994; Thorgeirsson 1996; Alison et al. 1997; Sell and Ilic 1997), but many of the disagreements can be reconciled by considering the different experimental conditions that have been used to study the process. Liver stem cells can be defined in several different ways which are: (1) cells responsible for normal tissue turnover; (2) cells that give rise to regeneration after partial hepatectomy; (3) cells responsible for progenitor-dependent regeneration; (4) transplantable liver repopulating cells; and (5) cells that result in hepatocyte and BDE phenotypes in vitro. Current evidence strongly suggests that different cell types and mechanisms are responsible for organ reconstitution, depending on the type of liver injury. In addition, tissue replacement by endogenous cells (i.e., regeneration) must be distinguished from reconstitution by transplanted donor cells (i.e., repopulation). In the following, we discuss the role of stem or progenitor cells for each of these operant definitions.

LIVER REGENERATION

Three separate mechanisms for liver regeneration are considered: (1) normal tissue turnover, (2) hepatocyte-driven regeneration after liver injury, and (3) progenitor-dependent regeneration after liver injury.

Liver Regeneration during Normal Tissue Turnover

The average life span of adult mammalian hepatocytes has been estimated to be ~200–300 days (Bucher and Malt 1971). The mechanism by which these cells are replaced has been of interest for some time. One of the main models regarding normal liver turnover was termed the "stream-ing liver" (Zajicek et al. 1985; Arber et al. 1988). According to this model, normal liver turnover is similar to regeneration in the intestine, with young hepatocytes being born in the portal zone and then migrating toward the central vein. The different patterns of gene expression in zone-1, -2, and -3 hepatocytes were explained by the aging process during this migration and thus represented a typical lineage progression. It has also been noted that the ploidy and size of hepatocytes depend on their location within the lobule. Central (zone-3) hepatocytes tend to be larger and more polyploid than their periportal counterparts. However, recent work has provided strong evidence against the streaming liver hypothesis. First, it was shown in elegant studies that the gene expression pattern in hepatocytes was dependent on the direction of blood flow (Thurman and Kauffman 1985). If blood flow was reversed such that portal blood entered the lobule through the central vein and exited via the portal vein, the pattern inverted. Therefore, the lobular zonation is best explained by metabolite-induced gene regulation, not lineage progression. Second, retroviral marking stud-ies provide clear evidence against any hepatocyte migration during normal turnover (Bralet et al. 1994; Kennedy et al. 1995). Retrovirally marked hepatocytes formed small clones that remained largely coherent and were equally distributed in zones 1, 2, and 3.

These results have been confirmed in elegant studies utilizing the mosaic pattern of X-inactivation in female mice to analyze patterns of hepatocyte growth (Shiojiri et al. 1997, 2000). Thus, current evidence strongly suggests that normal liver turnover in adult animals is mediated primarily by in situ cell division of hepatocytes themselves and not stem cells (Ponder 1996).

Regeneration after Partial Hepatectomy (Hepatocyte-driven Injury Response)

Liver regeneration after a 66% partial hepatectomy is relatively well understood in terms of molecular regulation and has been the subject of several excellent reviews (Thorgeirsson 1996; Michalopoulos and DeFrances 1997). During partial hepatectomy, specific lobes are removed intact without damage to the lobes left behind. The residual lobes grow to compensate for the mass of the resected lobes, although the removed lobes never grow back. The process is completed within one week. Again, as in normal liver turnover, there is no evidence for involvement of, or requirement for, stem cells in this process. Classic thymidine labeling studies show that virtually all hepatocytes in the remaining liver divide

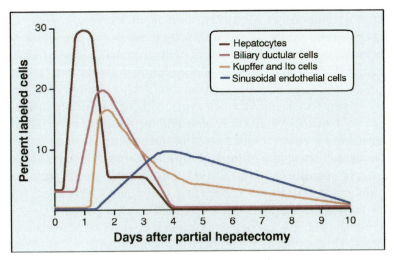

Figure 4 Time course of liver regeneration. The [³H]thymidine labeling index of different hepatic cell types after partial hepatectomy is shown. (Reprinted, with permission, from Michalopoulos and DeFrances 1997 [© American Association for the Advancement of Science].)

once or twice to restore the original cell number within 3–4 days (Bucher and Swaffield 1964; Stocker and Pfeifer 1965). The earliest labeled hepatocytes are seen 24 hours after partial hepatectomy, with the peak of thymidine incorporation occurring at 24–48 hours, depending on the species. Interestingly, there is zonal variation depending on how much tissue is removed. When only 15% of the liver is surgically removed, periportal (zone 1) hepatocytes divide preferentially, whereas cell division is seen equally in all three zones after 75% partial hepatectomy (Bucher and Swaffield 1964). Following the hepatocytes, the other hepatic cell types also undergo a wave of mitosis, thereby restoring the original number of all liver cells within 7 days (see Fig. 4).

Factors Involved in Liver Regeneration after Partial Hepatectomy

The factors that initiate and control the regenerative response after partial hepatectomy have been the subject of intense study (Michalopoulos 1994; Michalopoulos and DeFrances 1997; Fausto 2000). Obviously, some of these are likely also to be involved in the differentiation of liver stem cells and are therefore of interest in this chapter. Several critical factors for the induction of hepatocyte cell division in this system have been identified. The earliest event, occurring within one minute after the surgical removal, is a large increase in the blood level of hepatocyte growth factor (HGF) (Lindroos et al. 1991). This rapid increase cannot be explained by de novo synthesis, and it is thought that partial hepatectomy causes remodeling of extracellular matrix in the liver and release of HGF stored therein (Kim et al. 1997). HGF then binds to its receptor c-met (Bottaro et al. 1991) and activates a signal transduction pathway leading to re-entry of hepatocytes into the cell cycle. Although HGF is a primary mitogen for hepatocytes and is responsible for the early events after partial hepatectomy, other cytokine-receptor interactions are also important in the cascade leading to mitosis. Known factors include interleukin 6 (IL-6), tumor necrosis factor-α (TNFα), transforming growth factor-α (TGFα), and epidermal growth factor (EGF). IL-6 and TNFα knockout mice both show significantly delayed regeneration after partial hepatectomy (Cressman et al. 1996; Taub 1996; Yamada et al. 1997; Yamada and Fausto 1998). Although EGF is a primary mitogen for hepatocytes in tissue culture (Michalopoulos et al. 1984; Lindroos et al. 1991), its role in liver regeneration in vivo is less clear because EGF levels increase only modestly after partial hepatectomy (Noguchi et al. 1991). In contrast, TGFα mRNA and protein levels increase markedly within hours after partial hepatectomy (Mead and Fausto 1989), and TGFα overexpression can drive hepatocyte replication in vivo. Non-peptide hormones also have a significant role in the regenerative response after liver injury. Triiodothyronine (Short et al. 1980) and norepinephrine (Cruise et al. 1988; Cruise 1991) can stimulate hepatocyte replication in vivo. It is not known whether any of these factors are also important for progenitor-dependent liver regeneration or engraftment and expansion of liver stem cells (see below).

Less knowledge exists about the mechanisms by which hepatocyte cell division and liver regeneration are stopped after the appropriate liver mass has been restored. In particular, the exogenous signals (endocrine, paracrine, or autocrine) involved in sensing the overall liver cell mass and negatively regulating its size are not known. Some evidence suggests that transforming growth factor-β 1 (TGFβ1) may be important in terminating liver regeneration (Jirtle et al. 1991). Some endogenous signals are known to participate in the negative regulation of hepatocyte growth. Not surprisingly, they include general tumor suppressor genes. For example, mice lacking p53 or the p53-inducible cell cycle regulatory protein p21 have been shown to have continuous hepatocyte turnover (Wu et al. 1996; Yin et al. 1998). In addition, some more hepatocyte-specific transcription factors are also known to play a role. A hyperproliferative state was found in C/EBPα knockout mice (Wang et al. 1995; Timchenko et al. 1996).

Progenitor Cell-dependent Liver Regeneration

Oval Cells

Although neither cell replacement during normal tissue turnover nor after injury by partial hepatectomy requires stem cells for organ regeneration, this is not true for all types of liver injury. In some types of damage to the liver, small cells with a high nuclear/cytoplasmic ratio emerge in the portal zone, proliferate extensively, and migrate into the lobule. These small cells, which eventually become differentiated hepatocytes, are termed oval cells because of their initial observed morphology (Shinozuka et al. 1978). Importantly, oval cells are not derived from hepatocytes, but instead are the offspring of cells associated with the canal of Hering (Fig. 5). Oval cell proliferation therefore represents an example of progenitor-dependent liver regeneration. The cell that probably resides in the canal of Hering gives rise to oval cells and can be considered a "facultative liver stem cell" (Alison et al. 1996; Theise et al. 1999). In the rat, chronic liver injuries caused by chemicals such as DL-ethionine, galactosamine, and azo dyes represent examples of this type of liver damage (see Table 3). The toxic drugs are often combined with surgical partial hepatectomy.

A common feature of progenitor-dependent liver regeneration is that the hepatocytes themselves cannot divide normally. Thus, progenitor-dependent regeneration may be utilized when parenchymal hepatocytes are severely damaged on a chronic basis and/or unable to regenerate efficiently. Oval cells express markers of both bile duct epithelium (CK19) and hepatocytes (albumin). In the rat they also express high levels of α-fetoprotein and are thus similar to fetal hepatoblasts in their gene expression profile (Shinozuka et al. 1978). Furthermore, oval cells are bipotential and retain the ability to differentiate into both the bile duct epithelial and hepatocyte lineages in vitro (Sirica et al. 1990; Sirica 1995). Because of their similarity to hepatoblasts and their bipotentiality, oval cells have been considered early progenitors by analogy with committed hematopoietic progenitors. Thus, oval cell precursors located in the canal of Hering represent likely candidates for liver-repopulating stem cells (Fausto et al. 1993).

Several monoclonal antibodies have been raised against rat oval cells and used to study lineage progression. The cell surface marker OV6 has found wide application in a variety of studies (Hixson et al. 1997). In general, studies with these reagents have confirmed the similarity between oval cells and fetal hepatoblasts. Oval cells have been shown to express both the c-kit tyrosine kinase receptor and its ligand, stem cell factor (SCF, steele factor, MCGF) (Fujio et al. 1994). The SCF/c-kit system

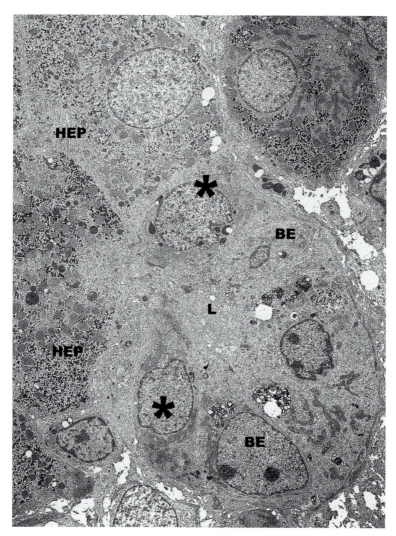

Figure 5 Electron microcopy of putative liver stem cells. A canal of Hering is shown by electron microscopy. Hepatocytes (HEP) and biliary epithelial cells (BE) join to form this transitional conduit between bile canaliculi and portal bile ducts. The interface cells (*) are thought to be oval cell precursors. (L) Lumen of the bile duct.

plays an important role in stem cell-driven hematopoiesis, melanogenesis, and gametogenesis. This has raised the issue of whether oval cells may respond to similar signals to these other stem cells.

Oval cell proliferation has also been described in a variety of human liver diseases, indicating that progenitor-dependent regeneration can be found in multiple organisms. Oval cells are found in disorders associated with chronic liver injury and are located at the edges of nodules in liver cirrhosis. As in the rat, OV6 is a useful marker for these cells in humans (Crosby et al. 1998). Interestingly, cells that are c-kit-positive but negative for hematopoietic markers have also been identified in human pediatric liver disease (Baumann et al. 1999).

Until recently, it has been difficult to induce oval cell proliferation in the mouse and thus take advantage of the powerful genetics in this organism. Using transgenic mice, it would be possible to determine whether factors known to be important in liver regeneration after partial hepatectomy are also required for oval cell-driven regeneration.

Now, however, two protocols have been developed that result in progenitor-dependent hepatocyte regeneration in the mouse (Preisegger et al. 1999). One regimen utilizes cocaine + phenobarbital (Rosenberg et al. 2000) and the other 3,5-diethoxycarbonyl-1,4-dihydrocollidine (DDC) (Preisegger et al. 1999). Mouse "oval cells" differ from their rat and human counterparts in not expressing AFP. The OV6 antibody does also not react with murine oval cells, and to date only one oval-cell-specific antibody, termed A6, has been developed for the mouse (Faktor et al. 1990). Nonetheless, work on the genetics of oval cell proliferation is now possible. An example is the recent discovery, using transgenic mice, that TGFβ1 inhibits oval cell proliferation (Preisegger et al. 1999).

Table 4 shows a list of conditions that result in oval cell proliferation in the rat and mouse.

Table 4 Induction of progenitor-dependent liver regeneration

Chemical/Manipulation	Reference
Rat	
2-Acetylaminofluorene (AAF)	Teebor and Becker (1971)
Diethylnitrosamine (DEN)	Schwarze et al. (1984)
Solt-Farber model	Solt et al. (1977)
DEN + AAF + p.H.	
Modified Solt-Farber model	Evarts et al. (1990)
AAF + p.H.	
Choline-deficient diet + DL-ethionine	Shinozuka et al. (1978)
D-Galactosamine + p.H.	Lemire et al. (1991)
Lasiocarpine + p.H.	Laconi et al. (1995)
Retrorsine + p.H.	Laconi et al. (1998); Gordon et al. (2000)
Mouse	
Dipin	Factor et al. (1994)
3,5-Diethoxycarbonyl-1,4-dihydro-collidine (DDC)	Preisegger et al. (1999)
Phenobarbital + cocaine + p.H.	Rosenberg et al. (2000)

p.H. = Partial hepatectomy.

Non-oval-cell Progenitors

Oval cells are defined by their morphologic appearance in the rat, but there is variability in the marker genes they express at different times after induction of their proliferation. The different induction regimens also result in variability of the phenotype. Therefore, it is not clear whether oval cells are all equivalent or whether different subclasses exist. Recently, another class of hepatocyte progenitors has been described after treatment of rats with retrorsine and partial hepatectomy (Gordon et al. 2000). Retrorsine blocks the division of mature hepatocytes but does not result in the emergence of classic oval cells, which are α-fetoprotein- and OV6-positive. Instead, foci of small hepatocyte-like cells emerge and eventually result in organ reconstitution. These small cells express both hepatocyte and bile duct markers. At this time, their origin (dedifferentiated hepatocytes, transitional cells in the canal of Hering, bone marrow) is unknown.

LIVER REPOPULATION BY TRANSPLANTED CELLS

The hematopoietic stem cell was defined primarily by its ability to repopulate and rescue hematopoiesis in lethally irradiated hosts. In the 1990s, similar repopulation assays were developed for the liver in several animal models (Rhim et al. 1994; Overturf et al. 1996; Laconi et al. 1998). In liver repopulation, a small number of transplanted donor cells engrafted in the liver expand and replace >50% of the liver mass (Grompe et al. 1999). Thus, it has now become possible to perform experiments analogous to those done in the hematopoietic system, including cell sorting, competitive repopulation, serial transplantation, and retroviral marking. Hepatic stem cells can now be defined by their ability to repopulate the liver. It should be emphasized that liver repopulation refers to replacement of only the hepatocytes by transplanted cells since efficient repopulation of the biliary system by transplanted cells has not yet been reported.

Models for Liver Repopulation

Three main animal models for liver repopulation studies are briefly described below. The first two are transgenic mice and the third is a chemical liver injury model in the rat.

Urokinase Plasminogen Activator Transgenic Mice

In 1991, Sandgren et al. developed mice transgenic for the urokinase plasminogen activator (uPA) gene under control of the albumin promoter.

These animals displayed liver inflammation with necrosis and a paucity of mature hepatocytes. Most animals died, but some survivors showed spontaneous development of nodular regions of liver containing normal hepatocytes. These nodules were found to be clonal and to have originated from a spontaneous loss of the uPA transgene. The reverted cells had a selective growth advantage and thus repopulated the transgenic liver. Similarly, transplanted wild-type cells (hepatocytes) also have a powerful selective advantage and can repopulate these mice (Rhim et al. 1994).

Fumarylacetoacetate Knockout Mice

The enzyme fumarylacetoacetate hydrolase (FAH) catalyzes the last reaction in the tyrosine catabolic pathway (Knox and Edwards 1955). FAH deficiency results in accumulation of a hepatotoxic metabolite and causes the human liver disease tyrosinemia type I (HT1) (Lindblad et al. 1977; Mitchell et al. 1999). Similar to the uPA transgenic mice, human HT1 patients frequently develop clonal hepatocyte nodules derived from reverted cells, which have lost the disease-causing mutation and express FAH (Kvittingen et al. 1993, 1994). This finding suggested that transplanted FAH-positive donor cells could be used to repopulate FAH mutant liver. Indeed, it was shown that as few as 1000 donor cells could completely repopulate the liver of an FAH knockout mouse within 6 weeks (Overturf et al. 1996). In mice, FAH deficiency is lethal in the neonatal period (Grompe et al. 1993) unless the animals are treated with 2(2-nitro-4-trifluoromethylbenzoyl)-1,3 cyclohexane dione (NTBC), a pharmacological inhibitor of tyrosine catabolism upstream of FAH (Lindstedt et al. 1992; Grompe et al. 1995). NTBC blocks the hepatocyte injury, thus allowing the propagation of mutant animals and control of the selective pressure that drives repopulation by transplanted cells.

Retrorsine-treated Rats

Both murine models for liver repopulation utilize genetically modified animals. In contrast, Laconi et al. (1995) developed an approach to liver repopulation by chemically blocking the regenerative capacity of host cells using lasiocarpine or retrorsine, structurally similar pyrrolizidine alkaloids. These compounds are selectively metabolized to their active form by hepatocytes, where they alkylate cellular DNA and cause proliferation arrest of hepatocytes in the G_2 phase of the cell cycle (Samuel and Jago 1975; Mattocks et al. 1986). Gordon et al. (2000) have shown recently that partial hepatectomy of retrorsine-treated animals induces proliferation of endogenous, small, hepatocyte-like progenitor cells. Retrorsine followed by partial hepatectomy can also be used to achieve near-total liver repopulation by transplanted donor cells. Typically, genetically marked rat hepatocytes that are positive for the bile canalicular membrane protein dipeptidyl peptidase IV (DPPIV) are injected into the spleen of a congenic strain of mutant rats not expressing DPPIV enzyme activity. Within 2 months, there was 40–60% replacement by transplanted hepatocytes in female rats and >95% replacement in male rats (Laconi et al. 1998).

LIVER-REPOPULATING CELLS

The animals described above have been utilized to determine the nature of transplantable liver-repopulating cells and to determine whether undifferentiated stem cells are driving this process. The stem cell hypothesis was strengthened by the observation that liver-repopulating cells could be serially transplanted without loss of functionality (Overturf et al. 1997). Male wild-type hepatocytes were serially transplanted at limiting dilution through seven rounds of female FAH knockout recipients. Complete repopulation was achieved in each round, and it was estimated that the repopulating cells in the seventh-round recipients had undergone at least 100 cell doublings, similar to what has been seen in serial transplantation of hematopoietic stem cells (Overturf et al. 1997). Interestingly, the only donor-derived cells in this experiment were hepatocytes. No biliary epithelium or other cell types of donor origin were found, thus raising the possibility of a "unipotential" stem cell.

Hepatocytes as Liver-repopulating Cells

In most liver repopulation experiments reported to date, only unfractionated cell suspensions from whole liver were used, and thus, it remained unclear whether the hepatocytes themselves or only a rare subpopulation(s) participates in the process. It would seem reasonable to hypothesize that adult liver cells are not homogeneous in their capacity for cell division and that subpopulations with high repopulation capacity might exist. The highly regenerative capacity of serially transplantable cells in particular has raised the question whether liver stem cells may be responsible for liver repopulation.

In the hematopoietic system, repopulation experiments with purified fractions of total bone marrow were used to identify stem cells (Spangrude et al. 1988; Baum et al. 1992). Similar experiments have now been performed with liver cells.

In the FAH mutant mouse model, three sets of experiments were performed to address whether differentiated hepatocytes or putative stem cells were responsible for the repopulation (Overturf et al. 1999). First, cell fractionation by centrifugal elutriation was used to identify and purify three major-size fractions of hepatocytes (16 µm, 21 µm, and 27 µm). Each fraction was transplanted in competition with unfractionated liver cells carrying a distinct genetic marker, which serves as a baseline reference for liver repopulation. The larger hepatocytes, which represented ~70% of the population, were primarily responsible for liver repopulation. In contrast, small diploid hepatocytes were inferior to the larger cells in competitive repopulation experiments. Second, competitive repopulation was performed between naive liver cells and those that had been serially transplanted up to seven times. Importantly, serial transplantation neither enhanced nor diminished the liver repopulation capacity. If serial liver repopulation were stem cell-dependent, this result would suggest that the ratio of progenitors to differentiated hepatocytes was kept constant during a 10^{20}-fold cell expansion. More likely, this result means that virtually all the original input cells (>95% hepatocytes) were capable of serial transplantation. The third set of experiments involved retroviral marking of donor hepatocytes in vitro and in vivo. Again, no evidence for a rare stem cell responsible for liver repopulation was detected. Together, these experiments strongly suggested that fully differentiated hepatocytes, which constitute the majority of liver cells, were responsible for liver repopulation and have a stem-cell-like capacity for cell division.

LIVER REPOPULATION BY NON-HEPATOCYTES

Despite the evidence that hepatocytes themselves are serially transplantable liver-repopulating cells, other cell types are also capable of repopulating the liver. This finding is analogous to the situation in liver regeneration where hepatocytes themselves, as well as undifferentiated hepatocyte progenitors, are capable of reconstituting the organ. In the following, we describe transplantation experiments that demonstrate the capacity of five non-hepatocyte cell types to differentiate into hepatocytes in vivo: (1) fetal hepatoblasts, (2) oval cells, (3) pancreatic liver progenitors, (4) hematopoietic stem cells, and (5) neurospheres.

Fetal Hepatoblasts

During embryonic development, the fetal liver bud contains hepatoblasts, cells that express α-fetoprotein as well as hepatocyte (albumin) and biliary (CK19) markers. These cells therefore may represent fetal liver stem cells capable of hepatocyte repopulation and, potentially, also reconstitution of the biliary system.

Only one report on transplantation of hepatoblasts has been published (Dabeva et al. 2000). This study, using fetal rat liver cells in the retrorsine model, indicated that there were at least three distinct subpopulations of hepatoblasts at ED 12–14. One population appeared to be bipotential on the basis of histochemical markers, and the other two had either a unipotent hepatocyte or biliary epithelial cell phenotype (Dabeva et al. 2000). After transplantation, the bipotential cells were able to proliferate in retrorsine-treated cell transplantation recipients, whereas the unipotent cells grew even in untreated rats. However, none of the fetal liver cell populations proliferated spontaneously, partial hepatectomy or thyroid hormone treatment being required to augment proliferation of the transplanted cells (Dabeva et al. 2000). Nonetheless, fetal liver cells proliferated more readily than adult cells. Finally, the transplanted fetal cells gave rise to both hepatocyte cords and mature bile duct structures. It was not formally proven, however, that both of these cell lineages originated clonally from a common precursor. Together, these results indicated that transplanted fetal hepatoblasts proliferate more readily than adult hepatocytes, and some fetal liver cells may remain bipotential.

Oval Cells

Oval cells are similar to fetal hepatoblasts in that they are also bipotential. These cells have, therefore, been of interest in liver repopulation experiments. Hepatocyte progenitor (or oval) cells can be isolated from the liver of rats treated with D-galactosamine (Lemire et al. 1991) or the pancreas of rats treated with a copper-deficient diet (Rao et al. 1986). Copper depletion causes atrophy of pancreatic acini and proliferation of duct-like oval cells expressing genes in the hepatocyte lineage (Rao et al. 1986, 1988). Transplantation of both hepatic- and pancreatic-derived oval cells has been reported in the rat (Dabeva et al. 1997). Upon transplantation, these cells proliferated modestly and differentiated into mature hepatocytes (Dabeva et al. 1997), even under nonselective conditions. However, because no in vivo selection model was used, their true capacity for liver repopulation was not demonstrated in these experiments. Thus, oval cells can become hepatocytes (by morphological criteria) upon transplantation into the liver, but their proliferative capacity remains unknown.

Pancreatic Hepatocytes

During embryogenesis, the main pancreatic cell types, including ducts, ductules, acinar cells, and the endocrine α, β, and δ cells, develop from a common endodermal precursor located in the ventral foregut (Spooner et al. 1970; Rutter 1980). Importantly, the main epithelial cells of the liver, hepatocytes and bile duct epithelium (BDE), are also thought to arise from the same region of the foregut endoderm (Shiojiri et al. 1991; Gerber and Thung 1992). The hepatic anlage develops ventrally toward the cardiac mesenchyme, which induces the hepatoblast differentiation pathway. The pancreas buds from the same region, with its ventral lobe growing anteriorly in the same direction as the liver and its larger dorsal lobe growing posteriorly. Thus, the ventral lobe of the pancreas is particularly closely related anatomically to the liver. The signals that govern the respective developmental pathways are only beginning to be understood (Gittes and Rutter 1992; Rudnick et al. 1994).

This tight relationship between liver and pancreas in embryonic development has raised the possibility that a common hepato-pancreatic precursor/stem cell may persist in adult life in both the liver and pancreas. Indeed, several independent lines of evidence suggest that adult pancreas contains cells which can give rise to hepatocytes. The best-known example is the emergence of hepatocytes in copper-depleted rats after re-feeding of copper (Rao et al. 1986, 1988). In this system, weanling rats are fed a copper-free diet for 8 weeks, which leads to complete acinar atrophy, and then are re-fed copper. Within weeks, cells with multiple hepatocellular characteristics emerge from the remaining pancreatic ducts. This work has been interpreted to suggest the presence of a pancreatic liver stem cell (Reddy et al. 1991). This notion is also supported by the appearance of hepatocellular markers in human pancreatic cancers (Hruban et al. 1987). More recently, a specific cytokine has been identified as a candidate to drive this process. Transgenic mice in which the keratinocyte growth factor (KGF) gene is driven by insulin promoter consistently develop pancreatic hepatocytes (Krakowski et al. 1999a,b). Thus, the existence of pancreatic liver precursors has been shown in several different mammalian species and under multiple experimental conditions. Both adult liver and adult pancreas may continue to harbor a small population of primitive hepato-pancreatic stem cells with the potential to give rise to the same differentiated progeny as during embryogenesis.

Transplantation experiments have verified the pancreatic liver stem cell hypothesis. As mentioned above, pancreatic oval cells induced by copper depletion were shown to give rise to morphologically normal hepatocytes in vivo (Dabeva et al. 1997). To determine whether pancreatic hepatocyte precursors also exist in normal pancreas without the use of toxic induction regimens, repopulation experiments were performed in the FAH knockout mouse model. Pancreatic cell suspensions from adult wild-type mice on a normal diet were transplanted into FAH mutant recipients, and selection was induced by NTBC withdrawal. Extensive liver repopulation (>50%) was observed in about 10% of transplant recipients, and another 35% had histological evidence for donor-derived hepatocyte nodules (Wang et al. 2001). Thus, adult murine pancreas contains hepatocyte precursors, even under normal, nonpathologic conditions. It remains to be determined whether these pancreatic liver stem cells also harbor other differentiation potential, particularly toward the pancreatic endocrine lineage.

Bone Marrow-derived Hepatocytes

Recent work has documented that the adult bone marrow of mammals contains cells with a variety of differentiation capacities. The hematopoietic stem cell (HSC) giving rise to all blood cell lineages has been known to reside in this compartment for many years. However, bone marrow also contains mesenchymal stem cells (MSC) capable of differentiating into chondrocytes, osteoblasts, and other connective tissue cell types (Pereira et al. 1995, 1998; Kopen et al. 1999; Pittenger et al. 1999; Chapter 16). Although HSCs are nonadherent, MSCs adhere to plastic dishes in tissue culture and can be expanded there. A population of primitive, nonadherent cells characterized by their ability to expel the DNA-staining Hoechst dye can give rise to both muscle and hematopoietic cells (Gussoni et al. 1999; Jackson et al. 1999). Thus, adult bone marrow produces a variety of tissue types of mesodermal origin. Petersen et al. (1999) first suggested that bone marrow also contained epithelial precursors. Cross-sex or cross-strain bone marrow and whole liver transplantation were used to trace the origin of the repopulating liver cells. Transplanted rats were treated with 2-acetylaminofluorene, to block hepatocyte proliferation, and then hepatocyte injury to induce oval cell proliferation. Markers for Y chromosome, dipeptidyl peptidase IV enzyme, and L21-6 antigen were used to identify liver cells of bone marrow origin, and a proportion of the regenerated hepatocytes were shown to be donor-derived. Next, Theise et al. (2000a) showed that bone marrow-derived hepatocytes also exist in the mouse and that oval cell induction was not required for this phenomenon. Female mice that had received lethal irradiation and bone marrow transplantation from a male donor displayed 1–2% Y-chromosome-positive epithelial cells in their livers. Most recently, two reports demonstrated that donor-derived epithelial cells are also present in human patients who have undergone a gender-mismatched bone marrow transplantation

(Alison et al. 2000; Theise et al. 2000b). In all these studies, the epithelial nature of the cells was demonstrated morphologically and by the expression of hepatocyte-specific markers. The nature of the bone marrow cell responsible for repopulation was not shown (adherent versus nonadherent, etc.).

Most recently, the FAH mutant model has been utilized to identify the nature of the bone marrow-derived hepatocyte precursor. Cell-sorting experiments and transplantation of purified hematopoietic stem cells of the KTLS phenotype (c-kit^{high}Thy^{lo}Lin^{neg}Sca-1^{+}) at limiting dilution showed that the primitive HSC is also capable of giving rise to hepatocytes (Lagasse et al. 2000). HSC not only gave rise to cells morphologically similar to hepatocytes, but also formed repopulation nodules and resulted in extensive organ reconstitution.

Thus, it now has been shown that the population of primitive bone marrow cells with the KLTS phenotype contains both hematopoietic and hepatocyte precursors. Although it seems likely, it has not yet been formally shown that the same clonal precursor is responsible for both lineages. The physiologic significance of bone marrow-derived hepatocytes in the response to liver injury is not known at this time. However, it is possible that circulating hepatocyte precursors are an important contributor to progenitor-dependent liver regeneration.

Neurosphere-derived Liver Precursors

In the mouse, neuronal stem cells cultured in neurospheres can give rise to many different cell lineages (Bjornson et al. 1999). Cultured neurospheres can effect repopulation of the hematopoietic system after transplantation (Bjornson et al. 1999). More recently, cultured neurospheres were injected into the blastocyst of a recipient embryo. Upon analysis of adult mice derived from such injections, the donor cells were found in many different tissues, including liver. Donor-derived cells were thought to express the hepatocyte phenotype (Clarke et al. 2000).

IN VITRO MODELS OF HEPATIC STEM CELLS

Several in vitro models for hepatic stem cell growth and differentiation have been developed. Putative liver progenitors from several mammalian species, including mouse, rat, pig, and human, have been isolated and propagated in primary tissue culture. In addition, immortal cell "liver progenitor" lines have been developed. Generally speaking, in vitro culture of liver progenitor cells is based on the growth of epithelial cells that are liver-derived but express either no hepatocyte markers or markers of both bile duct epithelium and hepatocytes. These in vitro systems have both medical and scientific goals. The medical purpose is to generate large numbers of hepatocytes in vitro for therapeutic transplantation. The scientific aims are to understand the factors that control the differentiation of these cells into hepatocytes and biliary duct epithelium. To date, the only cell lines that have had documented therapeutic effects have been cell lines or primary cultures derived from hepatocytes themselves (Gupta and Chowdhury 1994; Fox et al. 1995; Kobayashi et al. 2000a,b). Despite the availability of a variety of good in vitro model systems, surprisingly little is known about the molecular mechanisms that govern the transition of progenitor cells to hepatocytes and/or bile duct epithelium.

A complete review of in vitro systems is beyond the scope of this chapter. However, the most important in vitro systems are briefly described below.

Rat Cell Lines

WB-344 Cells

This cell line was clonogenically derived from non-parenchymal rat liver cells (Grisham 1980) and is probably the most intensely studied liver stem cell line (Coleman et al. 1993, 1997; Dees and Travis 1996; Grisham and Coleman 1996). WB3-44 cells are likely derived from canal of Hering cells (Grisham 1980). Although WB-344 cells can be cultured indefinitely in vitro, they retain the ability to differentiate into morphologically normal hepatocytes after transplantation without forming tumors (Coleman et al. 1997). To date, WB-344 cells are the only cells to fulfill this stringent criterion necessary to represent a true liver stem cell line. Nonetheless, little is known about the molecular mechanisms regulating the stem cell-to-hepatocyte transition, and liver repopulation with this cell line has not yet been reported.

Oval Cell Lines

Multiple laboratories have isolated oval cell lines from carcinogen treated rats (Sells et al. 1981; Yoshimura et al. 1983; Braun et al. 1988; Pack et al. 1993). Consistent with the proposed role of oval cells in the formation of hepatocarcinoma, these cell lines form tumors upon transplantation into immunodeficient recipients. The isolation, culture, and transplantation of these cells has been well reviewed (Sirica et al. 1990). Although the phenotypic properties of these cell lines have been described in great detail, the molecular mechanisms regulating phenotypic transitions are not well understood.

Mouse Cell Lines

Although it is normally difficult to establish permanent cell lines from mouse liver, such lines can be established routinely from transgenic mice that overexpress a constitutively active form of c-met (Amicone et al. 1997; Spagnoli et al. 1998). Two morphologically distinct types of cells emerge from such cultures, both of which grow extensively in culture under certain media conditions, but can be induced to differentiate with the appropriate signals. Clonal cell lines with "epithelial" morphology resemble hepatocytes and give rise to only hepatocyte-like offspring. In contrast, "palmate" clones can give rise to two distinct lineages, depending on the differentiation conditions used. Some general conditions that can cause differentiation of palmate cells in either direction have been discovered. Acidic FGF or DMSO induces hepatocytic differentiation, whereas culture in matrigel induced the formation of bile-duct-like structures (Spagnoli et al. 1998). In vivo transplantation and differentiation of these cells has not yet been reported.

HBC-3 cells are a novel bipotential cell line derived from day-9.5 mouse embryonic liver (Rogler 1997; Ott et al. 1999). This clonal cell line can be induced to differentiate into hepatocytes by DMSO or sodium butyrate (Rogler 1997). Again, matrigel induces the formation of duct structures, but the details of the differentiation process are not understood at the molecular level.

Pig Cell Lines

An interesting cell line was established from cultured pig epiblast (Talbot et al. 1993, 1994, 1996). PICM-19 cells are bipotential, similar to the murine cell lines reported above. In contrast to other cell lines, however, PICM-19 cells were derived from a very early embryo prior to the formation of a liver primordium (Talbot et al. 1993).

Human Cell Lines

Only a single human cell line, AKN-1, which may have liver progenitor characteristics, has been described (Nussler et al. 1999).

CONCLUDING REMARKS

The liver is one of the few organs amenable to repopulation by transplanted cells. Therefore, the subject of liver stem cells is not only of scientific,
but also of medical, interest. Current evidence shows that both endogenous
liver regeneration and repopulation by transplanted, exogenous cells can be
effected by more than one cell type. Hepatocytes themselves have a very
high capacity for cell division and can be considered unipotential stem
cells, which are used for most tissue repair. In addition, however, facultative liver stem cells distinct from hepatocytes exist and are important in the
response to some forms of liver injury. Hepatocyte progenitors have been
found in the liver itself, in the pancreas, and most recently in bone marrow.
It is unclear whether these are distinct cell types or whether the same cell
has been isolated from several different anatomical locations. It also has
not yet been conclusively shown in vivo that hepatocyte precursors can differentiate into bile duct epithelium. Oval cells can be viewed as committed progenitors, a transitional phenotype between self-renewing stem cells
and differentiated hepatocytes. Figure 6 depicts our current knowledge
about lineage relationships of hepatocytes during embryogenesis and adult
life. The molecular mechanisms controlling the phenotypic transitions are
not well understood and will be the subject of future research.

ACKNOWLEDGMENTS

The authors are supported by a National Institiues of Health grant,
NIDDK DK-51592.

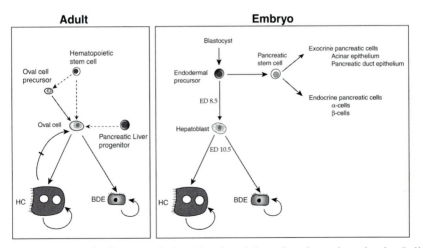

Figure 6 Hepatic lineage relationships in adult and embryonic animals. Solid
arrows indicate the differentiation of one cell type into another. Dashed lines
mark possible but not proven relationships.

REFERENCES

Alison M.R., Golding M.H., and Sarraf C.E. 1996. Pluripotential liver stem cells: Facultative stem cells located in the biliary tree. *Cell Prolif.* **29**: 373–402.

———. 1997. Liver stem cells: When the going gets tough they get going. *Int. J. Exp. Pathol.* **78**: 365–381.

Alison M.R., Poulsom R., Jeffery R., Dhillon A.P., Quaglia A., Jacob J., Novelli M., Prentice G., Williamson J., and Wright N.A. 2000. Hepatocytes from non-hepatic adult stem cells. *Nature* **406**: 257.

Amicone L., Spagnoli F.M., Spath G., Giordano S., Tommasini C., Bernardini S., De Luca V., Della Rocca C., Weiss M.C., Comoglio P.M., and Tripodi M. 1997. Transgenic expression in the liver of truncated Met blocks apoptosis and permits immortalization of hepatocytes. *EMBO J.* **16**: 495–503.

Ang S.L. and Rossant J. 1994. HNF-3 beta is essential for node and notochord formation in mouse development. *Development* **120**: 2979–2989.

Ang S.L., Wierda A., Wong D., Stevens K.A., Cascio S., Rossant J., and Zaret K.S. 1993. The formation and maintenance of the definitive endoderm lineage in the mouse: Involvement of HNF3/forkhead proteins. *Development* **118**: 139–149.

Arber N., Zajicek G., and Ariel I. 1988. The streaming liver. II. Hepatocyte life history. *Liver* **8**: 80–87.

Baum C.M., Weissman I.L., Tsukamoto A.S., Buckle A.M., and Peault B. 1992. Isolation of a candidate human hematopoietic stem-cell population. *Proc. Natl. Acad. Sci.* **89**: 2804–2808.

Baumann U., Crosby H.A., Ramani P., Kelly D.A., and Strain A.J. 1999. Expression of the stem cell factor receptor c-kit in normal and diseased pediatric liver: Identification of a human hepatic progenitor cell? *Hepatology* **30**: 112–117.

Beg A.A., Sha W.C., Bronson R.T., Ghosh S., and Baltimore D. 1998. Embryonic lethality and liver degeneration in mice lacking the RelA component of NF-kappa B. *EMBO J.* **17**: 2846–2854.

Bjornson C.R., Rietze R.L., Reynolds B.A., Magli M.C., and Vescovi A.L. 1999. Turning brain into blood: A hematopoietic fate adopted by adult neural stem cells in vivo. *Science* **283**: 534–537.

Bladt F., Riethmacher D., Isenmann S., Aguzzi A., and Birchmeier C. 1995. Essential role for the c-met receptor in the migration of myogenic precursor cells into the limb bud. *Nature* **376**: 768–771.

Bottaro D.P., Rubin J.S., Faletto D.L., Chan A.M., Kmiecik T.E., Vande Woude G.F., and Aaronson S.A. 1991. Identification of the hepatocyte growth factor receptor as the c-met proto-oncogene product. *Science* **251**: 802–804.

Bouwens L., Wang R.N., De Blay E., Pipeleers D.G., and Kloppel G. 1994. Cytokeratins as markers of ductal cell differentiation and islet neogenesis in the neonatal rat pancreas. *Diabetes* **43**: 1279–1283.

Bralet M.P., Branchereau S., Brechot C., and Ferry N. 1994. Cell lineage study in the liver using retroviral mediated gene transfer. Evidence against the streaming of hepatocytes in normal liver. *Am. J. Pathol.* **144**: 896–905.

Braun L., Goyette M., Yaswen P., Thompson N.L., and Fausto N. 1988. Growth in culture and tumorigenicity after transfection with the ras oncogene of liver epithelial cells from carcinogen-treated rats. *Am. J. Pathol.* **130**: 91–102.

Bucher N.L.R. and Malt R.A. 1971. *Regeneration of liver and kidney,* 1st edition. Little Brown, Boston, Massachusetts.

Bucher N.L.R. and Swaffield M.N. 1964. The rate of incorporation of labeled thymidine into the deoxyribonucleic acid of regenerating rat liver in relation to the amount of liver excised. *Cancer Res.* **240:** 1611–1625.

Cascio S. and Zaret K.S. 1993. Hepatocyte differentiation initiates during endodermal-mesenchymal interactions prior to liver formation. *Development* **119:** 1301–1315.

Cereghini S. 1996. Liver-enriched transcription factors and hepatocyte differentiation. *FASEB J.* **10:** 267–282.

Cereghini S., Blumenfeld M., and Yaniv M. 1988. A liver-specific factor essential for albumin transcription differs between differentiated and dedifferentiated rat hepatoma cells. *Genes Dev.* **2:** 957–974.

Cereghini S., Ott M.O., Power S., and Maury M. 1992. Expression patterns of vHNF1 and HNF1 homeoproteins in early postimplantation embryos suggest distinct and sequential developmental roles. *Development* **116:** 783–797.

Chen W.S., Manova K., Weinstein D.C., Duncan S.A., Plump A.S., Prezioso V.R., Bachvarova R.F., and Darnell Jr., J.E. 1996. Disruption of the HNF-4 gene, expressed in visceral endoderm, leads to cell death in embryonic ectoderm and impaired gastrulation of mouse embryos. *Cancer Lett.* **101:** 205–210.

Ciruna B.G., Schwartz L., Harpal K., Yamaguchi T.P., and Rossant J. 1997. Chimeric analysis of fibroblast growth factor receptor-1 (Fgfr1) function: A role for FGFR1 in morphogenetic movement through the primitive streak. *Development* **124:** 2829–2841.

Clarke D.L., Johansson C.B., Wilbertz J., Veress B., Nilsson E., Karlstrom H., Lendahl U., and Frisen J. 2000. Generalized potential of adult neural stem cells. *Science* **288:** 1660–1663.

Coffinier C., Barra J., Babinet C., and Yaniv M. 1999. Expression of the vHNF1/HNF1β homeoprotein gene during mouse organogenesis. *Mech. Dev.* **89:** 211–213.

Coleman W.B., Wennerberg A.E., Smith G.J., and Grisham J.W. 1993. Regulation of the differentiation of diploid and some aneuploid rat liver epithelial (stemlike) cells by the hepatic microenvironment. *Am. J. Pathol.* **142:** 1373–1382.

Coleman W.B., McCullough K.D., Esch G.L., Faris R.A., Hixson D.C., Smith G.J., and Grisham J.W. 1997. Evaluation of the differentiation potential of WB-F344 rat liver epithelial stem-like cells in vivo. Differentiation to hepatocytes after transplantation into dipeptidylpeptidase-IV-deficient rat liver. *Am. J. Pathol.* **151:** 353–359.

Costa R.H., Grayson D.R., and Darnell Jr., J.E. 1989. Multiple hepatocyte-enriched nuclear factors function in the regulation of transthyretin and alpha 1-antitrypsin genes. *Mol. Cell. Biol.* **9:** 1415–1425.

Cressman D.E., Greenbaum L.E., DeAngelis R.A., Ciliberto G., Furth E.E., Poli V., and Taub R. 1996. Liver failure and defective hepatocyte regeneration in interleukin-6-deficient mice. *Science* **274:** 1379–1383.

Crosby H.A., Hubscher S.G., Joplin R.E., Kelly D.A., and Strain A.J. 1998. Immunolocalization of OV-6, a putative progenitor cell marker in human fetal and diseased pediatric liver. *Hepatology* **28:** 980–985.

Cruise J.L. 1991. Alpha 1-adrenergic receptors in liver regeneration. *Dig. Dis. Sci.* **36:** 485–488.

Cruise J.L., Houck K.A., and Michalopoulos G. 1988. Early events in the regulation of hepatocyte DNA synthesis: The role of alpha-adrenergic stimulation. *Scand. J. Gastroenterol. Suppl.* **151:** 19–30.

Dabeva M.D., Petkov P.M., Sandhu J., Oren R., Laconi E., Hurston E., and Shafritz D.A. 2000. Proliferation and differentiation of fetal liver epithelial progenitor cells after transplantation into adult rat liver. *Am. J. Pathol.* **156:** 2017–2031.

Dabeva M.D., Hwang S.G., Vasa S.R., Hurston E., Novikoff P.M., Hixson D.C., Gupta S., and Shafritz D.A. 1997. Differentiation of pancreatic epithelial progenitor cells into hepatocytes following transplantation into rat liver. *Proc. Natl. Acad. Sci.* **94:** 7356–7361.

Dees C. and Travis C. 1996. Phenotypic and genotypic analysis of rat liver epithelial cells infected with retroviral shuttle vectors. *Cancer Lett.* **107:** 19–28.

Descombes P. and Schibler U. 1991. A liver-enriched transcriptional activator protein, LAP, and a transcriptional inhibitory protein, LIP, are translated from the same mRNA. *Cell* **67:** 569–579.

Desmet V.J. 1994. Organizational principles. In *The liver—Biology and pathobiology* (ed. I.M. Arias), pp. 3–14. Raven Press, New York.

Digernes V. and Bolund L. 1979. The ploidy classes of adult mouse liver cells. A methodological study with flow cytometry and cell sorting. *Virchows Arch. B Cell Pathol. Includ. Mol. Pathol.* **32:** 1–10.

Drolet D.W., Scully K.M., Simmons D.M., Wegner M., Chu K.T., Swanson L.W., and Rosenfeld M.G. 1991. TEF, a transcription factor expressed specifically in the anterior pituitary during embryogenesis, defines a new class of leucine zipper proteins. *Genes Dev.* **5:** 1739–1753.

Duncan S.A., Nagy A. and Chan W. 1997. Murine gastrulation requires HNF-4 regulated gene expression in the visceral endoderm: Tetraploid rescue of *Hnf-4*$^{(-/-)}$ embryos. *Development* **124:** 279–287.

Duncan S.A., Manova K., Chen W.S., Hoodless P., Weinstein D.C., Bachvarova R.F., and Darnell Jr., J.E. 1994. Expression of transcription factor HNF-4 in the extraembryonic endoderm, gut, and nephrogenic tissue of the developing mouse embryo: HNF-4 is a marker for primary endoderm in the implanting blastocyst. *Proc. Natl. Acad. Sci.* **91:** 7598–7602.

Dunsford H.A. and Sell S. 1989. Production of monoclonal antibodies to preneoplastic liver cell populations induced by chemical carcinogens in rats and to transplantable Morris hepatomas. *Cancer Res.* **49:** 4887–4893.

Engelhardt N.V., Factor V.M., Yasova A.K., Poltoranina V.S., Baranov V.N., and Lasareva M.N. 1990. Common antigens of mouse oval and biliary epithelial cells. Expression on newly formed hepatocytes. *Differentiation* **45:** 29–37.

Evarts R.P., Nakatsukasa H., Marsden E.R., Hsia C.C., Dunsford H.A., and Thorgeirsson S.S. 1990. Cellular and molecular changes in the early stages of chemical hepatocarcinogenesis in the rat. *Cancer Res.* **50:** 3439–3444.

Factor V.M., Radaeva S.A., and Thorgeirsson S.S. 1994. Origin and fate of oval cells in dipin-induced hepatocarcinogenesis in the mouse. *Am. J. Pathol.* **145:** 409–422.

Faktor V.M., Engel'gardt N.V., Iazova A.K., Lazareva M.N., Poltoranina V.S., and Rudinskaia T.D. 1990. Common antigens of oval cells and cholangiocytes in the mouse. Their detection by using monoclonal antibodies. *Ontogenez* **21:** 625–632.

Fausto N. 1994. Liver stem cells. In *The liver—Biology and pathobiology* (ed. I.M. Arias), pp. 1501–1518. Raven Press, New York.

———. 2000. Liver regeneration. *J. Hepatol.* **32:** 19–31.

Fausto N., Lemire J.M., and Shiojiri N. 1993. Cell lineages in hepatic development and the identification of progenitor cells in normal and injured liver. *Proc. Soc. Exp. Biol. Med.* **204:** 237–241.

Fox I.J., Chowdhury N.R., Gupta S., Kondapalli R., Schilsky M.L., Stockert R.J., and Chowdhury J.R. 1995. Conditional immortalization of Gunn rat hepatocytes: An ex vivo model for evaluating methods for bilirubin-UDP-glucuronosyltransferase gene transfer. *Hepatology* **21:** 837–846.

Friedman S.L. 1996. Hepatic stellate cells. *Prog. Liver Dis.* **14:** 101–130.

Fujio K., Evarts R.P., Hu Z., Marsden E.R., and Thorgeirsson S.S. 1994. Expression of stem cell factor and its receptor, c-kit, during liver regeneration from putative stem cells in adult rat. *Lab. Invest.* **70:** 511–516.

Gauldie J., Lamontagne L., Horsewood P., and Jenkins E. 1980. Immunohistochemical localization of alpha 1-antitrypsin in normal mouse liver and pancreas. *Am. J. Pathol.* **101:** 723–735.

Gebhardt R. and Mecke D. 1983. Heterogeneous distribution of glutamine synthetase among rat liver parenchymal cells in situ and in primary culture. *EMBO J.* **2:** 567–570.

Gebhardt R., Burger H.J., Heini H., Schreiber K.L., and Mecke D. 1988. Alterations of hepatic enzyme levels and of the acinar distribution of glutamine synthetase in response to experimental liver injury in the rat. *Hepatology* **8:** 822–830.

Gerber M.A. and Thung S.N. 1992. Cell lineages in human liver development, regeneration and transplantation. In *The role of cell types in hepatocarcinogenesis* (ed. A.E. Sirica), pp. 209–226. CRC Press, Boca Raton, Florida.

Giroux S. and Charron J. 1998. Defective development of the embryonic liver in N-myc-deficient mice. *Dev. Biol.* **195:** 16–28.

Gittes G.K. and Rutter W.J. 1992. Onset of cell-specific gene expression in the developing mouse pancreas. *Proc. Natl. Acad. Sci.* **89:** 1128–1132.

Golding M., Sarraf C.E., Lalani E.N., Anilkumar T.V., Edwards R.J., Nagy P., Thorgeirsson S.S., and Alison M.R. 1995. Oval cell differentiation into hepatocytes in the acetylaminofluorene-treated regenerating rat liver. *Hepatology* **22:** 1243–1253.

Gordon G.J., Coleman W.B., Hixson D.C., and Grisham J.W. 2000. Liver regeneration in rats with retrorsine-induced hepatocellular injury proceeds through a novel cellular response. *Am. J. Pathol.* **156:** 607–619.

Grisham J.W. 1980. Cell types in long-term propagable cultures of rat liver. *Ann. N.Y. Acad. Sci.* **349:** 128–137.

Grisham J.W. and Coleman W.B. 1996. Neoformation of liver epithelial cells: Progenitor cells, stem cells, and phenotypic transitions. *Gastroenterology* **110:** 1311–1313.

Grompe M., Laconi E. and Shafritz D.A. 1999. Principles of therapeutic liver repopulation. *Semin. Liver Dis.* **19:** 7–14.

Grompe M., al-Dhalimy M., Finegold M., Ou C.N., Burlingame T., Kennaway N.G., and Soriano P. 1993. Loss of fumarylacetoacetate hydrolase is responsible for the neonatal hepatic dysfunction phenotype of lethal albino mice. *Genes Dev.* **7:** 2298–2307.

Grompe M., Lindstedt S., al-Dhalimy M., Kennaway N.G., Papaconstantinou J., Torres-Ramos C.A., Ou C.N., and Finegold M. 1995. Pharmacological correction of neonatal lethal hepatic dysfunction in a murine model of hereditary tyrosinaemia type I. *Nat. Genet.* **10:** 453–460.

Gualdi R., Bossard P., Zheng M., Hamada Y., Coleman J.R., and Zaret K.S. 1996. Hepatic specification of the gut endoderm in vitro: Cell signaling and transcriptional control. *Genes Dev.* **10:** 1670–1682.

Gupta S. and Chowdhury J.R. 1994. Hepatocyte transplantation. In *The liver—Biology and pathobiology* (ed. I.M. Arias), pp. 1519–1536. Raven Press, New York.

Gussoni E., Soneoka Y., Strickland C.D., Buzney E.A., Khan M.K., Flint A.F., Kunkel L.M., and Mulligan R.C. 1999. Dystrophin expression in the mdx mouse restored by stem cell transplantation. *Nature* **401:** 390–394.

Hall R.K., Sladek F.M., and Granner D.K. 1995. The orphan receptors COUP-TF and HNF-4 serve as accessory factors required for induction of phosphoenolpyruvate carboxykinase gene transcription by glucocorticoids. *Proc. Natl. Acad. Sci.* **92:** 412–416.

Haruna Y., Saito K., Spaulding S., Nalesnik M.A., and Gerber M.A. 1996. Identification of bipotential progenitor cells in human liver development. *Hepatology* **23:** 476–481.

Haussinger D., Lamers W.H., and Moorman A.F. 1992. Hepatocyte heterogeneity in the metabolism of amino acids and ammonia. *Enzyme* **46:** 72–93.

Hentsch B., Lyons I., Li R., Hartley L., Lints T.J., Adams J.M., and Harvey R.P. 1996. Hlx homeo box gene is essential for an inductive tissue interaction that drives expansion of embryonic liver and gut. *Genes Dev.* **10:** 70–79.

Hilberg F., Aguzzi A., Howells N., and Wagner E.F. 1997. c-jun is essential for normal mouse development and hepatogenesis. *Nature* **365:** 179–181.

Hixson D.C. and Allison J.P. 1985. Monoclonal antibodies recognizing oval cells induced in the liver of rats by N-2-fluorenylacetamide or ethionine in a choline-deficient diet. *Cancer Res.* **45:** 3750–3760.

Hixson D.C., Faris R.A., and Thompson N.L. 1990. An antigenic portrait of the liver during carcinogenesis. *Pathobiology* **58:** 65–77.

Hixson D.C., Affigne S., Faris R.A., and McBride A.C. 1996. Delineation of antigenic pathways of ethionine-induced liver cancer in the rat. *Pathobiology* **64:** 79–90.

Hixson D.C., Chapman L., McBride A., Faris R., and Yang L. 1997. Antigenic phenotypes common to rat oval cells, primary hepatocellular carcinomas and developing bile ducts. *Carcinogenesis* **18:** 1169–1175.

Houssaint E. 1980. Differentiation of the mouse hepatic primordium. I. An analysis of tissue interactions in hepatocyte differentiation. *Cell Differ.* **9:** 269–279.

Hruban R.H., Molina J.M., Reddy M.N. and Boitnott J.K. 1987. A neoplasm with pancreatic and hepatocellular differentiation presenting with subcutaneous fat necrosis. *Am. J. Clin. Pathol.* **88:** 639–645.

Inaba T., Shapiro L.H., Funabiki T., Sinclair A.E., Jones B.G., Ashmun R.A., and Look A.T. 1994. DNA-binding specificity and *trans*-activating potential of the leukemia-associated E2A-hepatic leukemia factor fusion protein. *Mol. Cell. Biol.* **14:** 3403–3413.

Jackson K.A., Mi T., and Goodell M.A. 1999. Hematopoietic potential of stem cells isolated from murine skeletal muscle. *Proc. Natl. Acad. Sci.* **96:** 14482–14486.

Jacquemin P., Durviaux S.M., Jensen J., Godfraind C., Gradwohl G., Guillemot F., Madsen O.D., Carmeliet P., Dewerchin M., Collen D., Rousseau G.G. and Lemaigre F.P. 2000. Transcription factor hepatocyte nuclear factor 6 regulates pancreatic endocrine cell differentiation and controls expression of the proendocrine gene ngn3. *Mol. Cell. Biol.* **20:** 4445–4454.

Jirtle R.L., Carr B.I., and Scott C.D. 1991. Modulation of insulin-like growth factor-II/mannose 6-phosphate receptors and transforming growth factor-beta 1 during liver regeneration. *J. Biol. Chem.* **266:** 22444–22450.

Jung J., Zheng M., Goldfarb M., and Zaret K.S. 1999. Initiation of mammalian liver development from endoderm by fibroblast growth factors. *Science* **284:** 1998–2003.

Jungermann K. and Katz N. 1989. Functional specialization of different hepatocyte populations. *Physiol. Rev.* **69:** 708–764.

Jungermann K. and Kietzmann T. 1996. Zonation of parenchymal and nonparenchymal metabolism in liver. *Annu. Rev. Nutr.* **16:** 179–203.

Kaestner K.H., Hiemisch H., and Schutz G. 1998. Targeted disruption of the gene encoding hepatocyte nuclear factor 3γ results in reduced transcription of hepatocyte-specific genes. *Mol. Cell. Biol.* **18:** 4245–4251.

Kaestner K.H., Hiemisch H., Luckow B., and Schutz G. 1994. The HNF-3 gene family of transcription factors in mice: Gene structure, cDNA sequence, and mRNA distribution. *Genomics* **270:** 30029–30035.

Kaestner K.H., Katz J., Liu Y., Drucker D.J., and Schutz G. 1999. Inactivation of the winged helix transcription factor HNF3α affects glucose homeostasis and islet glucagon gene expression in vivo. *Genes Dev.* **13:** 495–504.

Kennedy S., Rettinger S., Flye M.W., and Ponder K.P. 1995. Experiments in transgenic mice show that hepatocytes are the source for postnatal liver growth and do not stream. *Hepatology* **22:** 160–168.

Kim T.H., Mars W.M., Stolz D.B., Petersen B.E., and Michalopoulos G.K. 1997. Extracellular matrix remodeling at the early stages of liver regeneration in the rat. *Hepatology* **26:** 896–904.

Kimura A., Nishiyori A., Murakami T., Tsukamoto T., Hata S., Osumi T., Okamura R., Mori M., and Takiguchi M. 1993. Chicken ovalbumin upstream promoter-transcription factor (COUP-TF) represses transcription from the promoter of the gene for ornithine transcarbamylase in a manner antagonistic to hepatocyte nuclear factor- 4 (HNF-4). *J. Biol. Chem.* **268:** 11125–11133.

Knox W.E. and Edwards S.W. 1955. Enzymes involved in conversion of tyrosine to acetoacetate. *Methods Enzymol.* **2:** 287–300.

Kobayashi N., Ito M., Nakamura J., Cai J., Gao C., Hammel J.M., and Fox I.J. 2000b. Hepatocyte transplantation in rats with decompensated cirrhosis. *Hepatology* **31:** 851–857.

Kobayashi N., Fujiwara T., Westerman K.A., Inoue Y., Sakaguchi M., Noguchi H., Miyazaki M., Cai J., Tanaka N., Fox I.J., and Lebouch P. 2000a. Prevention of acute liver failure in rats with reversibly immortalized human hepatocytes. *Science* **287:** 1258–1262.

Kopen G.C., Prockop D.J., and Phinney D.G. 1999. Marrow stromal cells migrate throughout forebrain and cerebellum, and they differentiate into astrocytes after injection into neonatal mouse brains. *Proc. Natl. Acad. Sci.* **96:** 10711–10716.

Krakowski M.L., Kritzik M.R., Jones E.M., Krahl T., Lee J., Arnush M., Gu D., and Sarvetnick N. 1999a. Pancreatic expression of keratinocyte growth factor leads to differentiation of islet hepatocytes and proliferation of duct cells. *Am. J. Pathol.* **154:** 683–691.

Krakowski M.L., Kritzik M.R., Jones E.M., Krahl T., Lee J., Arnush M., Gu D., Mroczkowski B., and Sarvetnick N. 1999b. Transgenic expression of epidermal growth factor and keratinocyte growth factor in beta-cells results in substantial morphological changes. *J. Endocrinol.* **162:** 167–175.

Kuo C.T., Morrisey E.E., Anandappa R., Sigrist K., Lu M.M., Parmacek M.S., Soudais C., and Leiden J.M. 1997. GATA4 transcription factor is required for ventral morphogenesis and heart tube formation. *Genes Dev.* **11:** 1048–1060.

Kvittingen E.A., Rootwelt H., Berger R., and Brandtzaeg P. 1994. Self-induced correction of the genetic defect in tyrosinemia type I. *J. Clin. Invest.* **94:** 1657–1661.

Kvittingen E.A., Rootwelt H., Brandtzaeg P., Bergan A., and Berger R. 1993. Hereditary tyrosinemia type I. Self-induced correction of the fumarylacetoacetase defect. *J. Clin. Invest.* **91:** 1816–1821.

Laconi E., Sarma D.S., and Pani P. 1995. Transplantation of normal hepatocytes modulates the development of chronic liver lesions induced by a pyrrolizidine alkaloid, lasiocarpine. *Carcinogenesis* **16:** 139–142.

Laconi E., Oren R., Mukhopadhyay D.K., Hurston E., Laconi S., Pani P., Dabeva M.D., and Shafritz D.A. 1998. Long-term, near-total liver replacement by transplantation of isolated hepatocytes in rats treated with retrorsine. *Am. J. Pathol.* **153:** 319–329.

Lagasse E., Connors H., Al-Dhalimy M., Reitsma M., Dohse M., Osborne L., Wang X., Finegold M., Weissman I.L., and Grompe M. 2000. Purified hematopoietic stem cells can differentiate to hepatocytes in vivo. *Nat. Med.* **6:** 1229–1234.

Lavery D.J. and Schibler U. 1993. Circadian transcription of the cholesterol 7 alpha hydroxylase gene may involve the liver-enriched bZIP protein DBP. *Genes Dev.* **7:** 1871–1884.

Lazennec G., Kern L., Valotaire Y., and Salbert G. 1997. The nuclear orphan receptors COUP-TF and ARP-1 positively regulate the trout estrogen receptor gene through enhancing autoregulation. *Mol. Cell. Biol.* **17:** 5053–5066.

Lee Y.H., Sauer B., and Gonzalez F.J. 1998. Laron dwarfism and non-insulin-dependent diabetes mellitus in the *Hnf-1α* knockout mouse. *Mol. Cell. Biol.* **18:** 3059–3068.

Lee Y.H., Sauer B., Johnson P.F., and Gonzalez F.J. 1997. Disruption of the *c/ebpα* gene in adult mouse liver. *Mol. Cell. Biol.* **17:** 6014–6022.

Legraverend C., Eguchi H., Strom A., Lahuna O., Mode A., Tollet P., Westin S., and Gustafsson J.A. 1994. Transactivation of the rat CYP2C13 gene promoter involves HNF-1, HNF-3, and members of the orphan receptor subfamily. *Biochemistry* **33:** 9889–9897.

Lemire J.M., Shiojiri N., and Fausto N. 1991. Oval cell proliferation and the origin of small hepatocytes in liver injury induced by D-galactosamine. *Am. J. Pathol.* **139:** 535–552.

Li J., Ning G., and Duncan S.A. 2000. Mammalian hepatocyte differentiation requires the transcription factor HNF-4α. *Genes Dev.* **14:** 464–474.

Lindblad B., Lindstedt S. and Steen G. 1977. On the enzymic defects in hereditary tyrosinemia. *Proc. Natl. Acad. Sci.* **74:** 4641–4645.

Lindroos P.M., Zarnegar R., and Michalopoulos G.K. 1991. Hepatocyte growth factor (hepatopoietin A) rapidly increases in plasma before DNA synthesis and liver regeneration stimulated by partial hepatectomy and carbon tetrachloride administration. *Hepatology* **13:** 743–750.

Lindstedt S., Holme E., Lock E.A., Hjalmarson O., and Strandvik B. 1992. Treatment of hereditary tyrosinaemia type I by inhibition of 4-hydroxyphenylpyruvate dioxygenase. *Lancet* **340:** 813–817.

Mall F.P. 1906. A study of the structural unit of the liver. *Am. J. Anat.* **5:** 227–308.

Mattocks A.R., Driver H.E., Barbour R.H., and Robins D.J. 1986. Metabolism and toxicity of synthetic analogues of macrocyclic diester pyrrolizidine alkaloids. *Chem. Biol. Interact.* **58:** 95–108.

Mead J.E. and Fausto N. 1989. Transforming growth factor alpha may be a physiological regulator of liver regeneration by means of an autocrine mechanism. *Proc. Natl. Acad. Sci.* **86:** 1558–1562.

Medvedev Z.A. 1988. Age-related polyploidization of hepatocytes: The cause and possible role. A mini-review. *Mech. Ageing Dev.* **46:** 159–174.

Michalopoulos G.K. 1994. Control mechanisms of liver regeneration. *J. Gastroenterol.* **7:** 23–29.

Michalopoulos G.K. and DeFrances M.C. 1997. Liver regeneration. *Science* **276:** 60–66.

Michalopoulos G., Houck K.A., Dolan M.L., and Leutteke N.C. 1984. Control of hepatocyte replication by two serum factors. *Cancer Res.* **44:** 4414–4419.

Mitchell G.A., Grompe M., Lambert M., and Tanguay R.M. 1999. Hypertyrosinemia. In *The metabolic basis of inherited disease* (ed. C.R. Scriver et al.), pp. 1077–1106. McGraw-Hill, New York.

Molkentin J.D., Lin Q., Duncan S.A., and Olson E.N. 1997. Requirement of the transcription factor GATA4 for heart tube formation and ventral morphogenesis. *Genes Dev.* **11:** 1061–1072.

Moorman A.F., Vermeulen J.L., Charles R., and Lamers W.H. 1989. Localization of ammonia-metabolizing enzymes in human liver: Ontogenesis of heterogeneity. *Hepatology* **9:** 367–372.

Morrisey E.E., Tang Z., Sigrist K., Lu M.M., Jiang F., Ip H.S. and Parmacek M.S. 1998. GATA6 regulates HNF4 and is required for differentiation of visceral endoderm in the mouse embryo. *Genes Dev.* **12:** 3579–3590.

Motoyama J., Kitajima K., Kojima M., Kondo S., and Takeuchi T. 1997. Organogenesis of the liver, thymus and spleen is affected in jumonji mutant mice. *Mech. Dev.* **66:** 27–37.

Motta P., Fujita T., and Muto M. 1978. *The liver: An atlas of scanning electron microscopy*, 1st edition. Igaku-Shoin, Tokyo, Japan.

Mueller C.R., Maire P., and Schibler U. 1990. DBP, a liver-enriched transcriptional activator, is expressed late in ontogeny and its tissue specificity is determined posttranscriptionally. *Cell* **61:** 279–291.

Nishina H., Vaz C., Billia P., Nghiem M., Sasaki T., De la Pompa J.L., Furlonger K., Paige C., Hui C., Fischer K.D., Kishimoto H., Iwatsubo T., Katada T., Woodgett J.R., and Penninger J.M. 1999. Defective liver formation and liver cell apoptosis in mice lacking the stress signaling kinase SEK1/MKK4. *Development* **126:** 505–516.

Noguchi S., Ohba Y., and Oka T. 1991. Influence of epidermal growth factor on liver regeneration after partial hepatectomy in mice. *J. Endocrinol.* **128:** 425–431.

Nussler A.K., Vergani G., Gollin S.M., Dorko K., Morris Jr., S.M., Demetris A.J., Nomoto M., Beger H.G., and Strom S.C. 1999. Isolation and characterization of a human hepatic epithelial-like cell line (AKN-1) from a normal liver. *In Vitro Cell. Dev. Biol. Anim.* **35:** 190–197.

Ott M., Ma Q., Li B., Gagandeep S., Rogler L.E., and Gupta S. 1999. Regulation of hepatitis B virus expression in progenitor and differentiated cell types: Evidence for negative transcriptional control in nonpermissive cells. *Gene Expr.* **8:** 175–186.

Overturf K., al-Dhalimy M., Finegold M., and Grompe M. 1999. The repopulation potential of hepatocyte populations differing in size and prior mitotic expansion. *Am. J. Pathol.* **155:** 2135–2143.

Overturf K., al-Dhalimy M., Ou C.N., Finegold M., and Grompe M. 1997. Serial transplantation reveals the stem-cell-like regenerative potential of adult mouse hepatocytes. *Am. J. Pathol.* **151:** 1273–1280.

Overturf K., al-Dhalimy M., Tanguay R., Brantly M., Ou C.N., Finegold M., and Grompe M. 1996. Hepatocytes corrected by gene therapy are selected in vivo in a murine model of hereditary tyrosinaemia type I. *Nat. Genet.* **12:** 266–273.

Pack R., Heck R., Dienes H.P., Oesch F., and Steinberg P. 1993. Isolation, biochemical characterization, long-term culture, and phenotype modulation of oval cells from carcinogen-fed rats. *Exp. Cell Res.* **204:** 29–33.

Pereira F.A., Qiu Y., Zhou G., Tsai M.J., and Tsai S.Y. 1999. The orphan nuclear receptor COUP-TFII is required for angiogenesis and heart development. *Genes Dev.* **13:**

1037–1049.

Pereira R.F., Halford K.W., O'Hara M.D., Leeper D.B., Sokolov B.P., Pollard M.D., Bagasra O., and Prockop D.J. 1995. Cultured adherent cells from marrow can serve as long-lasting precursor cells for bone, cartilage, and lung in irradiated mice. *Proc. Natl. Acad. Sci.* **92:** 4857–4861.

Pereira R.F., O'Hara M.D., Laptev A.V., Halford K.W., Pollard M.D., Class R., Simon D., Livezey K., and Prockop D.J. 1998. Marrow stromal cells as a source of progenitor cells for nonhematopoietic tissues in transgenic mice with a phenotype of osteogenesis imperfecta. *Proc. Natl. Acad. Sci.* **95:** 1142–1147.

Petell J.K., Quaroni A., Hong W.J., Hixson D.C., Amarri S., Reif S., and Bujanover Y. 1990. Alteration in the regulation of plasma membrane glycoproteins of the hepatocyte during ontogeny. *Exp. Cell Res.* **187:** 299–308.

Petersen B.E., Bowen W.C., Patrene K.D., Mars W.M., Sullivan A.K., Murase N., Boggs S.S., Greenberger J.S., and Goff J.P. 1999. Bone marrow as a potential source of hepatic oval cells. *Science* **284:** 1168–1170.

Pittenger M.F., Mackay A.M., Beck S.C., Jaiswal R.K., Douglas R., Mosca J.D., Moorman M.A., Simonetti D.W., Craig S., and Marshak D.R. 1999. Multilineage potential of adult human mesenchymal stem cells. *Science* **284:** 143–147.

Plenat F., Braun L., and Fausto N. 1988. Demonstration of glucose-6-phosphatase and peroxisomal catalase activity by ultrastructural cytochemistry in oval cells from livers of carcinogen-treated rats. *Am. J. Pathol.* **130:** 91–102.

Poli V., Mancini F.P., and Cortese R. 1990. IL-6DBP, a nuclear protein involved in interleukin-6 signal transduction, defines a new family of leucine zipper proteins related to C/EBP. *Cell* **63:** 643–653.

Ponder K.P. 1996. Analysis of liver development, regeneration, and carcinogenesis by genetic marking studies. *FASEB J.* **10:** 673–682.

Pontoglio M., Barra J., Hadchouel M., Doyen A., Kress C., Bach J.P., Babinet C., and Yaniv M. 1996. Hepatocyte nuclear factor 1 inactivation results in hepatic dysfunction, phenylketonuria, and renal Fanconi syndrome. *Cell* **84:** 575–585.

Pontoglio M., Sreenan S., Roe M., Pugh W., Ostrega D., Doyen A., Pick A.J., Baldwin A., Velho G., Froguel P., Levisetti M., Bonner-Weir S., Bell G.I., Yaniv M., and Polonsky K.S. 1998. Defective insulin secretion in hepatocyte nuclear factor 1alpha-deficient mice. *J. Clin. Invest.* **101:** 2215–2222.

Preisegger K.H., Factor V.M., Fuchsbichler A., Stumptner C., Denk H., and Thorgeirsson S.S. 1999. Atypical ductular proliferation and its inhibition by transforming growth factor beta1 in the 3,5-diethoxycarbonyl-1,4-dihydrocollidine mouse model for chronic alcoholic liver disease. *Lab. Invest.* **79:** 103–109.

Qiu Y., Pereira F.A., DeMayo F.J., Lydon J.P., Tsai S.Y., and Tsai M.J. 1997. Null mutation of mCOUP-TFI results in defects in morphogenesis of the glossopharyngeal ganglion, axonal projection, and arborization. *Genes Dev.* **11:** 1925–1937.

Rao M.S., Subbarao V., and Reddy J.K. 1986. Induction of hepatocytes in the pancreas of copper-depleted rats following copper repletion. *Cell Differ.* **18:** 109–117.

Rao M.S., Dwivedi R.S., Subbarao V., Usman M.I., Scarpelli D.G., Nemali M.R., Yeldandi A., Thangada S., Kumar S., and Reddy J.K. 1988. Almost total conversion of pancreas to liver in the adult rat: A reliable model to study transdifferentiation. *Biochem. Biophys. Res. Commun.* **156:** 131–136.

Rappaport A.M., Borowy Z.J., Lougheed W.M., and Lotto W.N. 1954. Subdivision of hexagonal liver lobules into a structural and functional unit: Role in hepatic physiology and pathology. *Anat. Rec.* **119:** 11–34.

Reddy J.K., Rao M.S., Yeldandi A.V., Tan X.D., and Dwivedi R.S. 1991. Pancreatic hepatocytes. An in vivo model for cell lineage in pancreas of adult rat. *Dig. Dis. Sci.* **36:** 502–509.

Rey-Campos J., Chouard T., Yaniv M., and Cereghini S. 1991. vHNF1 is a homeoprotein that activates transcription and forms heterodimers with HNF1. *EMBO J.* **10:** 1445–1457.

Rhim J.A., Sandgren E.P., Degen J.L., Palmiter R.D., and Brinster R.L. 1994. Replacement of disease mouse liver by hepatic cell transplantation. *Science* **263:** 1149–1152.

Rogler L.E. 1997. Selective bipotential differentiation of mouse embryonic hepatoblasts in vitro. *Am. J. Pathol.* **150:** 591–602.

Rosenberg D., Ilic Z., Yin L., and Sell S. 2000. Proliferation of hepatic lineage cells of normal C57BL and interleukin-6 knockout mice after cocaine-induced periportal injury. *Hepatology* **31:** 948–955.

Rudnick A., Ling T.Y., Odagiri H., Rutter W.J., and German M.S. 1994. Pancreatic beta cells express a diverse set of homeobox genes. *Proc. Natl. Acad. Sci.* **91:** 12203–12207.

Rutter W.J. 1980. The development of the endocrine and exocrine pancreas. *Monogr. Pathol.* **21:** 30–38.

Samuel A. and Jago M.V. 1975. Localization in the cell cycle of the antimitotic action of the pyrrolizidine alkaloid, lasiocarpine and of its metabolite, dehydroheliotridine. *Chem. Biol. Interact.* **10:** 185–197.

Sandgren E.P., Palmiter R.D., Heckel J.L., Daugherty C.C., Brinster R.L., and Degen J.L. 1991. Complete hepatic regeneration after somatic deletion of an albumin-plasminogen activator transgene. *Cell* **66:** 245–256.

Schmidt C., Bladt F., Goedecke S., Brinkmann V., Zschiesche W., Sharpe M., Gherardi E., and Birchmeier C. 1995. Scatter factor/hepatocyte growth factor is essential for liver development. *Nature* **373:** 699–702.

Schwarze P.E., Pettersen E.O., Shoaib M.C., and Seglen P.O. 1984. Emergence of a population of small, diploid hepatocytes during hepatocarcinogenesis. *Carcinogenesis* **5:** 1267–1275.

Sell S. 1994. Liver stem cells. *Mod. Pathol.* **7:** 105–112.

Sell S. and Ilic Z. 1997. *Liver stem cells.* Landes Bioscience, Austin, Texas.

Sells M.A., Katyal S.L., Shinozuka H., Estes L.W., Sell S., and Lombardi B. 1981. Isolation of oval cells and transitional cells from the livers of rats fed the carcinogen DL-ethionine. *J. Natl. Cancer Inst.* **66:** 355–362.

Shinozuka H., Lombardi B., Sell S., and Iammarino R.M. 1978. Early histological and functional alterations of ethionine liver carcinogenesis in rats fed a choline-deficient diet. *Cancer Res.* **38:** 1092–1098.

Shiojiri N., Lemire J.M., and Fausto N. 1991. Cell lineages and oval cell progenitors in rat liver development. *Cancer Res.* **51:** 2611-2620.

Shiojiri N., Imai H., Goto S., Ohta T., Ogawa K., and Mori M. 1997. Mosaic pattern of ornithine transcarbamylase expression in spfash mouse liver. *Am. J. Pathol.* **151:** 413–421.

Shiojiri N., Sano M., Inujima S., Nitou M., Kanazawa M. and Mori M. 2000. Quantitative analysis of cell allocation during liver development, using the spf(ash)-heterozygous female mouse. *Am. J. Pathol.* **156:** 65–75.

Short J., Klein K., Kibert L., and Ove P. 1980. Involvement of the Iodothyronines in liver and hepatoma cell proliferation in the rat. *Cancer Res.* **40:** 2417–2422.

Sirica A.E. 1995. Ductular hepatocytes. *Histol. Histopathol.* **10:** 433–456.

Sirica A.E., Mathis G.A., Sano N., and Elmore L.W. 1990. Isolation, culture, and transplantation of intrahepatic biliary epithelial cells and oval cells. *Pathobiology* **58:** 44–64.

Sladek F.M., Zhong W.M., Lai E., and Darnell Jr., J.E. 1991. Liver-enriched transcription factor HNF-4 is a novel member of the steroid hormone receptor superfamily. *Genes Dev.* **4:** 2353–2365.

Smith D.D.J. and Campbell J.W. 1988. Distribution of glutamine synthetase and carbamoyl-phosphate synthetase I in vertebrate liver. *Proc. Natl. Acad. Sci.* **85:** 160–164.

Solt D.B., Medline A., and Farber E. 1977. Rapid emergence of carcinogen-induced hyperplastic lesions in a new model for the sequential analysis of liver carcinogenesis. *Am. J. Pathol.* **88:** 595–618.

Sosa-Pineda B., Wigle J.T., and Oliver G. 2000. Hepatocyte migration during liver development requires prox1. *Nat. Genet.* **25:** 254–255.

Spagnoli F.M., Amicone L., Tripodi M., and Weiss M.C. 1998. Identification of a bipotential precursor cell in hepatic cell lines derived from transgenic mice expressing cyto-Met in the liver. *J. Cell Biol.* **143:** 1101–1112.

Spangrude G.J., Heimfeld S. and Weissman I.L. 1988. Purification and characterization of mouse hematopoietic stem cells. *Science* **241:** 58–62.

Spooner B.S., Walther B.T., and Rutter W.J. 1970. The development of the dorsal and ventral mammalian pancreas in vivo and in vitro. *J. Cell Biol.* **47:** 235–246.

Stocker E. and Pfeifer U. 1965. On the manner of proliferation of the liver parenchyma after partial hepatectomy. Autoradiography studies using 3H-thymidine. *Naturwissenschaften* **52:** 663.

Stocker E., Wullstein H.K., and Brau G. 1973. Capacity of regeneration in liver epithelia of juvenile, repeated partially hepatectomized rats. Autoradiographic studies after continous infusion of 3H-thymidine. *Virchows Arch. B Cell Pathol.* **14:** 93–103.

Sucov H.M., Dyson E., Gumeringer C.L., Price J., Chien K.R., and Evans R.M. 1994. RXR alpha mutant mice establish a genetic basis for vitamin A signaling in heart morphogenesis. *Genes Dev.* **8:** 1007–1018.

Talbot N.C., Rexroad Jr., C.E., Pursel V.G., Powell A.M., and Nel N.D. 1993. Culturing the epiblast cells of the pig blastocyst. *In Vitro Cell Dev. Biol. Anim.* **29A:** 534–554.

Talbot N.C., Caperna T.J., Lebow L.T., Moscioni D., Pursel V.G., and Rexroad C.J. 1996. Ultrastructure, enzymatic, and transport properties of the PICM-19 bipotent liver cell line. *Exp. Cell Res.* **225:** 22–34.

Talbot N.C., Rexroad Jr., C.E., Powell A.M., Pursel V.G., Caperna T.J., Ogg S.L., and Nel N.D. 1994. A continuous culture of pluripotent fetal hepatocytes derived from the 8-day epiblast of the pig. *In Vitro Cell Dev. Biol. Anim.* **30A:** 843–850.

Tanaka T., Yoshida N., Kishimoto T., and Akira S. 1997. Defective adipocyte differentiation in mice lacking the C/EBPβ and/or C/EBPδ gene. *EMBO J.* **16:** 7432–7443.

Taub R. 1996. Liver regeneration 4: Transcriptional control of liver regeneration. *FASEB J.* **10:** 413–427.

Teebor G.W. and Becker F.F. 1971. Regression and persistence of hyperplastic hepatic nodules induced by N-2-fluorenylacetamide and their relationship to hepatocarcinogenesis. *Cancer Res.* **31:** 1–3.

Theise N.D., Badve S., Saxena R., Henegariu O., Sell S., Crawford J.M., and Krause D.S. 2000a. Derivation of hepatocytes from bone marrow cells in mice after radiation-induced myeloablation. *Hepatology* **31**: 235–240.

Theise N.D., Nimmakayalu M., Gardner R., Illei P.B., Morgan G., Teperman L., Henegariu O., and Krause D. 2000b. Liver from bone marrow in h umans. *Hepatology* **32**: 11–16.

Theise N.D., Saxena R., Portmann B.C., Thung S.N., Yee H., Chiriboga L., Kumar A., and Crawford J.M. 1999. The canals of Hering and hepatic stem cells in humans. *Hepatology* **30**: 1425–1433.

Thorgeirsson S.S. 1996. Hepatic stem cells in liver regeneration. *FASEB J.* **10**: 1249–1256.

Thurman R.G. and Kauffman F.C. 1985. Sublobular compartmentation of pharmacologic events (SCOPE): Metabolic fluxes in periportal and pericentral regions of the liver lobule. *Hepatology* **5**: 144–151.

Timchenko N.A., Wilde M., Nakanishi M., Smith J.R., and Darlington G.J. 1996. CCAAT/enhancer-binding protein alpha (C/EBP alpha) inhibits cell proliferation through the p21 (WAF-1/CIP-1/SDI-1) protein. *Genes Dev.* **17**: 7353–7361.

Van Eyken P., Sciot R., and Desmet V. 1988. Intrahepatic bile duct development in the rat: A cytokeratin-immunohistochemical study. *Lab. Invest.* **59**: 52–59.

Wagenaar G.T., Geerts W.J., Chamuleau R.A., Deutz N.E., and Lamers W.H. 1994. Lobular patterns of expression and enzyme activities of glutamine synthase, carbamoylphosphate synthase and glutamate dehydrogenase during postnatal development of the porcine liver. *Biochim. Biophys. Acta* **1200**: 265–270.

Wals P.A., Palacin M., and Katz J. 1988. The zonation of liver and the distribution of fructose 2,6-bisphosphate in rat liver. *J. Biol. Chem.* **263**: 4876–4881.

Wang N.D., Finegold M.J., Bradley A., Ou C.N., Abdelsayed S.V., Wilde M.D., Taylor L.R., Wilson D.R., and Darlington G.J. 1995. Impaired energy homeostasis in C/EBP alpha knockout mice. *Science* **269**: 1108–1112.

Wang X., Al-Dhalimy M., Lagasse E., Finegold M., and Grompe M. 2001. Therapeutic liver reconstitution by transplanted adult mouse pancreatic cells. *Am. J. Pathol.* (in press).

Weinstein D.C., Ruiz i Altaba A., Chen W.S., Hoodless P., Prezioso V.R., Jessell T.M., and Darnell Jr., J.E. 1994. The winged-helix transcription factor HNF-3 beta is required for notochord development in the mouse embryo. *Cell* **78**: 575–588.

Wisse E. 1970. An electron microscopic study of the fenestrated endothelial lining of rat liver sinusoids. *J. Ultrastruct. Res.* **31**: 125–150.

Wu H., Wade M., Krall L., Grisham J., Xiong Y., and Van Dyke T. 1996. Targeted in vivo expression of the cyclin-dependent kinase inhibitor p21 halts hepatocyte cell-cycle progression, postnatal liver development and regeneration. *Genes Dev.* **10**: 245–260.

Yamada Y. and Fausto N. 1998. Deficient liver regeneration after carbon tetrachloride injury in mice lacking type 1 but not type 2 tumor necrosis factor receptor. *Am. J. Pathol.* **152**: 1577–1589.

Yamada Y., Kirillova I., Peschon J.J., and Fausto N. 1997. Initiation of liver growth by tumor necrosis factor: Deficient liver regeneration in mice lacking type I tumor necrosis factor receptor. *Proc. Natl. Acad. Sci.* **94**: 1441–1446.

Yang L., Faris R.A. and Hixson D.C. 1993. Characterization of a mature bile duct antigen expressed on a subpopulation of biliary ductular cells but absent from oval cells. *Hepatology* **18**: 357–366.

Yin L., Ghebranious N., Chakraborty S., Sheehan C.E., Ilic Z., and Sell S. 1998. Control of mouse hepatocyte proliferation and ploidy by p53 and p53ser246 mutation in vivo. *Hepatology* **27**: 73–80.

Yoshimura H., Harris R., Yokoyama S., Takahashi S., Sells M.A., Pan S.F., and Lombardi B. 1983. Anaplastic carcinomas in nude mice and in original donor strain rats inoculated with cultured oval cells. *Am. J. Pathol.* **110:** 322–332.

Zajicek G., Oren R., and Weinreb Jr., M. 1985. The streaming liver. *Liver* **5:** 293–300.

Zaret K.S. 1996. Molecular genetics of early liver development. *Annu. Rev. Physiol.* **58:** 231–251.

———. 1998. Early liver differentation: Genetic potentiation and multilevel growth control. *Curr. Opin. Genet. Dev.* **8:** 526–553.

———. 2000. Liver specification and early morphogenesis. *Mech. Dev.* **92:** 83–88.

21

Pancreatic Stem Cells

Marcie R. Kritzik and Nora Sarvetnick
Department of Immunology
The Scripps Research Institute
La Jolla, California 92037

β-CELL LOSS: A TERMINAL PROCESS

Insulin-dependent, or type I, diabetes mellitus (IDDM) is a devastating disease in which affected individuals depend on daily injections of exogenous insulin for regulation of glucose homeostasis and survival. The lifetime dependency on insulin invariably leads to a variety of debilitating complications that threaten quality of life and significantly shorten life expectancy of IDDM patients. Insulin-producing cells in the pancreatic islets of Langerhans are the targets for selective inflammatory destruction in IDDM. This loss of the pancreatic islets is a terminal process, since the pancreas lacks any significant ability to regenerate insulin-producing cells. Indeed, pancreatic islet cells have a very low rate of growth in adults, and knowledge of the factors that regulate islet growth is lacking. Increased knowledge of islet stem cells and potential islet regeneration could allow critical advances in the development of new therapies for IDDM. Knowledge regarding pancreatic stem cells has grown dramatically in recent years, but continued progress is still hampered by the lack of in vitro and in vivo assay systems for stem cell activity and function. In this review, we focus on pancreatic stem cells during morphogenesis and regeneration, as well as on the molecular markers associated with these cells.

ONTOGENY OF PANCREATIC ENDOCRINE CELLS

During embryogenesis, the pancreas arises from the foregut, initially as two distinct bulges on either side of the duodenum, termed the dorsal and ventral buds (for review, see Slack 1995). The two buds grow independently, with both endocrine and exocrine tissue components present in each bud. As development proceeds, the stomach and duodenum rotate, bringing the two buds into contact, at which point they fuse to form the pancreas. Endocrine cells in the pancreas are organized into clusters of cells referred to as the islets of Langerhans. The endocrine cells develop from the pancreatic ducts, and stem cells responsible for endocrine cell formation are thought to reside in the fetal pancreatic ducts (Pictet and Rutter 1972; Pictet et al. 1972; Githens 1988). The neogenesis of islets from duct epithelial cells occurs during normal embryonic development and in very early postnatal life. By 2 to 3 weeks of age, the pancreatic islets are well defined and distinct from duct structures, as they are in the adult mouse. From this point on, endocrine cells are not observed in the ducts, and the mitotic index of duct and islet cells is very low (Githens 1988). Therefore, following the early postnatal period, the normal developmental process that generates islets ceases. Islet growth and the maintenance of islet mass are under strict regulatory controls (for review, see Hellerstrom and Swenne 1985; Hellerstrom et al. 1988). Thus, little if any stem cell activity is observed in the normal adult pancreas.

Endocrine gene expression occurs prior to the appearance of the pancreatic diverticulum during pancreatic organogenesis (Gittes and Rutter 1992). All four endocrine cell types are thought to arise through progressive differentiation from a common pluripotent stem cell (Alpert et al. 1988; for review, see Peshavaria and Stein 1997). The endocrine cells first appear as single cells in the duct wall (Dubois 1975). These cells migrate to form clusters, which grow and become islets during the course of pancreatic development. The glucagon-secreting α cells are typically the first endocrine cell type observed during normal ontogeny (Rall et al. 1973). However, the earliest emergence of this endocrine cell type is controversial. In some studies insulin- (β cells), somatostatin- (δ cells), or pancreatic polypeptide-secreting cells (PP cells) are observed prior to or coincidental with the appearance of α cells (Adesanya et al.1966; Clark and Rutter 1972).

During endocrine cell formation, cells producing more than one hormone are often observed, with cells producing glucagon and insulin arising first (Alpert 1988; Herrera et al. 1991; de Krijger et al. 1992; Gittes and Rutter 1992; Teitelman 1993). The identification of multiple hormone-expressing cells in the pancreatic ducts during development, as well as in many pancreatic endocrine tumors, has led to the proposal that these multi-hormone-bearing cells represent a transient phase during the differentiation of endocrine cell precursors to the single hormone-expressing phenotype found in mature endocrine cells. However, the derivation of endocrine cell types is not well defined, and controversy remains as to whether or not multi-hormone-expressing cells represent true transitional cell types during endocrine cell formation (Herrera et al. 1994; Pang et al. 1994; Jensen et al. 2000a).

As described above, the pancreas arises from the outpouching of the gut endoderm in the region of the duodenum during development. However, heterotopic formation of pancreatic tissue, including mature endocrine cells, can arise from other regions of the gut endoderm, including the stomach and additional regions of the small intestine (de Castro Barbosa et al. 1946; Dolan et al. 1974). Recent studies in chicks have revealed that inhibition of the intercellular signaling protein Sonic hedgehog (SHH) promotes heterotopic formation of pancreatic tissue from regions of the stomach and duodenum (Kim and Melton 1998). Thus, in addition to "pancreatic stem cells" in the region of posterior foregut evagination that normally forms the pancreas, other cells of similar embryonic derivation indeed have the capacity to form pancreatic cells.

PANCREATIC ISLET REGROWTH AND REGENERATION

In general, adult pancreatic β cells are known to have a poor growth capacity (Lazarow 1952) and, in pathogenic states where islet destruction occurs, such as IDDM, regeneration is not detected. In animal models of IDDM, such as the non-obese diabetic (NOD) mouse or the biological breeding (BB) rat, where the islet cells are lost by presumed immunological mechanisms, islet regeneration is not observed (Like 1985). Furthermore, streptozotocin (Sz) injection of adult rats, which results in destruction of β cells and produces a diabetic condition, does not induce islet regeneration (Steiner et al. 1970; Logothetopoulos 1972). However, under certain conditions of pancreatic regeneration, new islet cells can arise postnatally and later in adult life. For example, limited islet regeneration has been reported under several experimental conditions, such as after partial pancreatectomy of young rats (Setalo et al. 1972; Bonner-Weir et al. 1981, 1983). In this case, new islets have been shown to differentiate from ductal epithelium, recapitulating islet formation during embryogenesis and suggesting that stem cells in the adult pancreas can be activated during regeneration (Bonner-Weir et al. 1993). Some islet cell regeneration has also been reported following ligation of pancreatic arteries (Adams and Harrison 1953), in steroid diabetes (Kern and Logothetopoulos 1970), following injection of insulin antibody (Logothetopoulos and Bell 1966), after alloxan administration (Johnson 1950; Hughes 1956; House 1958; Bunnag et al. 1967; Boquist 1968; Korcakova 1971; Jacob 1977), and after cellophane wrapping (Rosenberg and Vinik 1989). The most impressive regeneration can be found in newborn and neonatal animals following islet destruction. Thus, studies have shown that after treatment of newborn rats with Sz, the pancreas is able to repair itself, and new islet formation is observed (Portha et al. 1974, 1979; Cantenys et al. 1981; Dutrillaux et al. 1982).

New islet cells are thought to arise through two distinct processes. One mechanism involves the regeneration of islets through division of existing terminally differentiated islet cells. A second mechanism involves the differentiation of new islet cells from stem cells residing in the pancreatic ducts. In the latter case, quiescent stem cells in the adult are thought to be "reactivated" under particular conditions of regeneration, leading to new endocrine cell and islet formation. Clearly, much work needs to be done to define the precise factors ultimately responsible for the induction of stem cell activity during pancreatic regeneration.

Transdifferentiation of pancreatic cells to nonpancreatic cell types is also found under certain conditions, highlighting the plasticity of the pancreatic cell phenotype (Rao et al. 1986, 1989, 1990; Reddy et al. 1991). In the db/db mouse, proliferating duct cells give rise to ciliated cells, mucous or Paneth secretory cells (Like and Chick 1970a,b). In addition, there are instances of human pancreatic metaplasia in which well-differentiated goblet cells (Walters 1965) and other mucous cells (Oertel 1989) have been reported to have a ductal origin. In rats, hepatocytes develop in the pancreas after maintenance of the animals on a copper-deficient diet, apparently arising from ductal and interstitial pancreatic cells (Scarpelli and Rao 1981; Rao et al. 1989). Additionally, pancreatic hepatocytes are found in a number of other models of experimental destruction of the exocrine pancreas (Sirica 1995). These latter two observations suggest a possible common stem cell, or at least the potential for plasticity between these two terminally differentiated cell types, implying they may share a closely connected lineage.

EXPERIMENTAL MODELS OF β-CELL LOSS AND REPOPULATION OF PANCREATIC ISLETS

Many transgenic mouse models for studying IDDM have been described previously (Sarvetnick et al. 1988; Lund et al. 1990; Oldstone et al. 1991; Allison et al. 1992; Heath et al. 1992). These transgenic mice have, to different degrees, been successful in duplicating various stages of human IDDM and have provided valuable tools for elucidating mechanisms that lead to IDDM. Clearly, the ability of pancreatic stem cells to reactivate islet development in the adult would provide a powerful basis for treatment of IDDM. However, regeneration of islet cells has not been reported among these many transgenic mouse strains, with the exception of a report describing expression of the tumor necrosis factor (TNFα) transgene under control of the insulin promoter (Higuchi et al. 1992). In this case, expression of TNFα caused insulitis, disorganization of islet structure, and proliferation of pancreatic ductules; little regeneration of endocrine cells was observed.

We have developed a unique model system in which new pancreatic growth and islet formation are clearly evident throughout adult life (Sarvetnick et al. 1988; Gu and Sarvetnick 1993; Gu et al. 1994). These Ins-IFNγ mice, who express IFNγ in the β cells of the pancreatic islets, display unusually high proliferative activity in ductal epithelial cells. We have demonstrated that new endocrine cells derive from pancreatic ducts in these transgenic mice, suggesting that a well-defined and functional stem cell population exists in the ducts of the Ins-IFNγ mice (Gu et al. 1994). Much of our work has since focused on further defining the stem cell population active in these mice.

The regeneration and differentiation observed in the Ins-IFNγ mouse is very aggressive, with cells showing substantially higher mitotic indices than are normally found in the pancreatic ducts (Gu and Sarvetnick 1993). Interestingly, the pancreases of these mice also display ductal hyperplasia and destruction of islets by infiltrating lymphocytes, characteristic of that seen in type I diabetes mouse models. The most intriguing phenotype of these mice is the balance between regeneration of "new" islets and the destruction of the preexisting islets in the acinar tissue. The newly formed islets bud into the lumen of the ducts, where they are protected from infiltration and destruction. The aggressive expansion of ducts, and the continuous formation of new endocrine cells in the pancreas during adult life, are important characteristics of the remarkable regrowth occurring in the transgenic pancreas. In these animals, new islet cells are formed continuously from duct cells, without a requirement for T cells, B cells, or macrophages.

On the basis of the expression of endocrine, exocrine, and duct cell markers, endocrine cells are thought to derive from duct cells in the Ins-IFNγ mouse through a defined pathway involving a number of transitional cell types, including those bearing a multi-hormone-expressing phenotype (Gu et al. 1994). In addition, we have recently demonstrated the expression of a number of molecules known to be critical for normal pancreatic development in the ducts of the Ins-IFNγ transgenic mouse (see below), including PDX-1, HNF3β, Isl-1, and Pax-6 (Kritzik et al. 1999, 2000). The striking expression of PDX-1 in the pancreatic ducts of the transgenic mouse is illustrated in Figure 1. As seen in this figure, significant PDX-1 expression is detected in the ducts of the transgenic but not the nontransgenic mouse. We believe that these PDX-1-expressing ductal cells represent endocrine precursor cells from which new islets derive. Comparison in this case is also made with insulin expression, which is also observed, albeit to a lesser extent than PDX-1, in the ducts of the transgenic mouse. Thus, two distinct populations of PDX-1-expressing cells are observed: one population expressing only PDX-1 and one population expressing both PDX-1 and insulin. These data lead us to speculate that those cells expressing PDX-1 but not insulin represent an earlier precursor cell type than those synthesizing both PDX-1 and insulin.

There are a number of similarities between new islet formation during development and IFNγ-mediated pancreatic regeneration. These similarities include the derivation of new endocrine cells from ductal cells, the presence of multi-hormone-expressing cells in the pancreatic ducts, and the ductal expression of relevant molecules such as PDX-1 and Isl-1 during both processes. These similarities suggest that new endocrine cell formation likely proceeds through similar pathways in both these process-

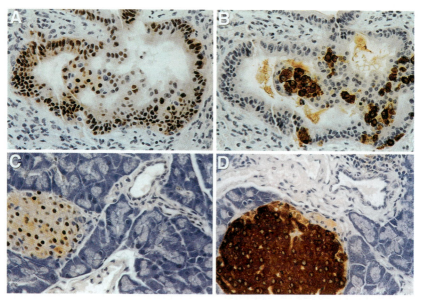

Figure 1 PDX-1 immunostaining in the IFNγ transgenic pancreas. Serial pancreatic sections from an adult IFNγ transgenic mouse (*A, B*) and an adult nontransgenic mouse (*C, D*) were stained with antibody to either PDX-1 (*A, C*) or insulin (*B, D*). Note the presence of both insulin-positive and insulin-negative PDX-1-expressing ductal cells. Magnification 50×. (Reprinted, with permission, from Kritzik et al. 1999 [© Society for Endocrinology].)

es, with new endocrine cells arising from stem cells residing in the pancreatic ducts. Thus, the IFNγ transgenic mouse provides a valuable system for further analysis and characterization of endocrine stem cells. However, it is important to note that the differentiation of pancreatic islets in this model may not be exactly identical to that which occurs during ontogeny. Indeed, it is possible that there is more than one type of islet stem cell and more than one developmental lineage for the differentiation of mature islet cells. For example, Gittes and colleagues have demonstrated that isolated pancreatic epithelium grown under the renal capsule forms pure clusters of mature islets, without any acinar or ductal components (Gittes et al. 1996). This contrasts with a number of other studies indicating that islets arise from ducts, and it suggests that there might be alternate pathways leading to the formation of mature islets.

STEM CELL-ASSOCIATED MARKERS

The field of pancreatic islet cell ontogeny enjoyed comparative solitude until the fascinating discovery that factors regulating insulin transcription were required for the differentiation of the mature pancreas. This and related discoveries have fueled the rapid expansion of the pancreas ontogeny field, the discovery of a variety of potential islet stem cells, and new theories on the ontogeny of mature islet cells. Indeed, several proteins associated with pancreatic stem cells have been defined, and studies have shown that a number of transcription factors are important in pancreas differentiation (for review, see Sander and German 1997; Edlund 1998). Significantly, the homeodomain protein PDX-1, which is important in regulating insulin gene expression, plays a critical role in the development of endocrine and exocrine compartments of the pancreas. In mice genetically deficient for the PDX-1 gene, no pancreas develops (Ohlsson et al. 1993; Jonsson 1994; Offield et al. 1996). HNF3β is an important regulator of PDX-1 gene transcription in the pancreas and is required for endodermal cell lineage development (Zaret 1996; Wu et al. 1997). The exact role of HNF3β in pancreatic islet development has not been resolved, since mice lacking this transcription factor die early in embryogenesis, but given the importance of this molecule in PDX-1 gene expression, HNF3β may be critical for this process as well (Ang et al. 1993; Weinstein et al. 1994). We have recently demonstrated striking expression of HNF3β in the ducts of the IFNγ transgenic mouse, suggesting a role for this molecule during endocrine cell formation (Kritzik 2000). Studies using knockout mice have also shown that Isl-1 is required for the differentiation of islet cells (Ahlgren et al. 1997). Interestingly, although the dorsal bud does not develop in Isl-1-deficient mice, the ventral bud does form. However, endocrine cells, but not exocrine cells, are lacking in the ventral bud. Thus, whereas Isl-1 clearly contributes to endocrine cell formation, its expression is also important for development of exocrine tissue in the dorsal bud.

Two other homeodomain proteins, PAX 4 and PAX 6, are expressed in the embryonic gut and the adult pancreas as well. Interestingly, gene deletion studies have demonstrated that mature endocrine cells do not develop in the absence of PAX 4 and PAX 6. PAX 4 is essential for the generation of insulin-producing β cells and somatostatin-producing δ cells (Sosa-Pineda et al. 1997), whereas PAX 6 is required for the differentiation of glucagon-producing α cells (St-Onge et al. 1997). Analysis of mutants lacking Nkx2.2 has demonstrated a role for this homeobox transcription factor in the development of pancreatic β cells as well (Sussel et al. 1998).

A number of basic helix-loop-helix (bHLH) proteins have also been implicated in endocrine cell development. For example, neurogenin 3 (Ngn3), a bHLH transcription factor, has recently been shown to be required for the development of all four endocrine cell types (Gradwohl et al. 2000). In addition, the bHLH protein BETA2/NeuroD, a transcription factor important in expression of the insulin gene, is involved in proper pancreas development. Mice lacking this protein display significantly reduced numbers of β cells. Reduction in the numbers of other islet endocrine cell types, as well as defective islet and exocrine tissue morphology, is also observed in these mice (Naya et al. 1997). Analysis of mice deficient in Hes1 has also demonstrated a role for this bHLH transcriptional repressor in maintenance of the pancreatic precursor pool during development (Jensen et al. 2000b). Hes1 has been proposed to inhibit endocrine cell differentiation mediated by Ngn3 (Jensen et al. 2000b). In addition, expression of Hes1 is regulated through the Notch signaling pathway, which has been implicated in endocrine cell development (Apelqvist et al. 1999; Jensen et al. 2000a). Notch signaling is discussed in Chapter 3.

Several other proteins are thought to be associated with pancreatic stem cells. For example, studies of the distribution of Nkx 6.1 during early development of the rat pancreas suggest that this molecule may be important in pancreatic development (Oster et al. 1998). In addition, the pancreatic and intestinal hormone peptide YY is thought to be expressed by endocrine stem cells during development (Upchurch et al. 1994). Early embryonic endocrine cells in the duct wall also transiently express tyrosine hydroxylase (TH), the rate-limiting enzyme of the catecholamine biosynthetic pathway, suggesting that this molecule serves as a marker for early endocrine progenitor cells (Teitelman et al. 1981a,b, 1987; Teitelman and Lee 1987). In addition, there is a report that acid β-galactosidase expression, which occurs at significantly higher levels in islet-like clusters from the fetal pancreas than in adult islets, might serve as a marker for endocrine stem cells as well (Beattie et al. 1994). Glut-2 (glucose transporter type 2)-expressing cells have also been proposed as stem cells in the developing pancreas (Pang et al. 1994). Additionally, Bouwens and De Blay (1996) have reported on the expression of CK20, vimentin, and Bcl-2 as markers for islet stem cells. We have recently found that Msx-2, a homeobox-containing transcription factor involved in tissue growth and patterning during the development of diverse organs (such as teeth and limb buds), is also expressed at sites of endocrine stem cell activity (Davidson 1995; Kritzik et al. 1999).

DEVELOPMENTAL LINEAGES

The identification of molecules associated with pancreatic stem cells will be valuable in defining intermediate cell types involved in the developmental progression from multipotent precursor cell to mature endocrine cell types. For example, PDX-1, expressed in the early pancreatic primordia, prior to the formation of the dorsal and ventral buds, is thought to be expressed by the earliest pancreatic stem cells that give rise to both endocrine and exocrine tissues. Development of intermediate progenitor cell types involves the subsequent expression of molecules such as Ngn3 and Isl-1 (although not necessarily at the same time; Jensen et al. 2000a), which are required for the derivation of all four endocrine cell types. Clearly, continued and progressive differentiation of islet cell types would involve the specific expression of a number of additional molecules in the correct temporal sequence, such as Pax4 (required for β and δ cell formation), Pax6 (required for α cell formation), and Nkx2.2 (required for β cell formation).

PERSPECTIVES

The identification of islet stem cells, the development of new antigenic markers for these cells, and the establishment of an assay system to monitor stem cell activity will be of critical importance in advancing our knowledge of pancreatic islet stem cell ontogeny. Such knowledge could enable critical advances in the development of new therapies for IDDM, a debilitating disease that severely compromises pancreatic function in affected individuals. For example, new pancreatic islet cells could be dif-

Herrera P.L., Huarte J., Zufferey R., Nichols A., Mermillod B., Philippe J., Muniesa P., Sanvito F., Orci L., and Vassalli J.D. 1994. Ablation of islet endocrine cells by targeted expression of hormone-promoter-driven toxigenes. *Proc. Natl. Acad. Sci.* **91:** 12999–123003.

Higuchi Y., Herrera P., Muniesa P., Huarte J., Belin D., Ohashi P., Aichele P., Orci L., Vassalli J.-D., and Vassalli P. 1992. Expression of a tumor necrosis factor in murine pancreatic β cells results in severe and permanent insulitis without evolution towards diabetes. *J. Exp. Med.* **176:** 1719–1731.

House E.L. 1958. A histological study of the pancreas, liver and kidney both during and after recovery from alloxan diabetes. *Endocrinology* **62:** 189–200.

Hughes H. 1956. An experimental study of regeneration in the islets of Langerhans with reference to the theory of balance. *Acta Anat.* **27:** 1–61.

Jacob S. 1977. Regeneration of the islets of Langerhans in the guinea pig. *Cell Tissue Res.* **181:** 277–286.

Jensen J., Heller R.S., Funder-Nielsen T., Pedersen E.E., Lindsell C., Weinmaster G., Madsen O.D., and Serup P. 2000a. Independent development of pancreatic α- and β-cells from neurogenin3-expressing precursors: A role for the Notch pathway in repression of premature differentiation. *Diabetes* **49:** 163–176.

Jensen J., Pedersen E.E., Galante P., Hald J., Heller R.S., Ishibashi M., Kegeyama R., Guillemot F., Serup P., and Madsen O.D. 2000b. Control of endodermal endocrine development by Hes-1. *Nat. Genet.* **24:** 36–44.

Johnson D.D. 1950. Alloxan administration in the guinea pig. A study of regenerative phase in the islands of Langerhans. *Endocrinology* **47:** 393–398.

Jonsson J., Carlsson L., Edlund T., and Edlund H. 1994. Insulin-promoter-factor 1 is required for pancreaas development in mice. *Nature* **371:** 606–609.

Kern H. and Logothetopolous J. 1970. Steroid diabetes in the guinea pig studies on islet-cell ultrastructure and regeneration. *Diabetes* **19:** 145–154.

Kim S.K. and Melton D.A. 1998. Pancreas development is promoted by cyclopamine, a hedgehog signaling inhibitor. *Proc. Natl. Acad. Sci.* **95:** 13036–13041.

Korcakova L. 1971. Mitotic division and its significance for regeneration of granulated B-cells in the islets of Langerhans in alloxan-diabetic rats. *Folia Morphol.* **14:** 24–30.

Kritzik M.R., Krahl T., Good A., Krakowski M., St.-Onge L., Gruss P., Wright C., and Sarvetnick N. 2000. Transcription factor expression during pancreatic islet regeneration. *Mol. Cell. Endocrinol.* **164:** 99–107.

Kritzik M.R., Jones E., Chen Z., Krakowski M., Krahl T., Good A., Wright C., Fox H., and Sarvetnick N. 1999. PDX-1 and Msx-2 expression in the regenerating and developing pancreas. *J. Endocrinol.* **163:** 523–530.

Lazarow A. 1952. Spontaneous recovery from alloxan diabetes in rats. *Diabetes* **1:** 363–370.

Like A.A. 1985. Spontaneous diabetes in animals. In *The diabetic pancreas,* 2nd edition (ed. B.W. Volk), pp. 385–413. Plenum Press, New York.

Like A.A. and Chick W.L. 1970a. Studies on the diabetic mutant mouse. I. Light microscopy and radioautography of pancreatic islets. *Diabetologia* **6:** 207–215.

Like A.A. and Chick W.L. 1970b. Studies in the diabetic mutant mouse. II. Electron microscopy of pancreatic islets. *Diabetologia* **6:** 216–242.

Logothetopoulos J. 1972. Islet regeneration and neogenesis. In *Handbook of Physiology: Endocrinology* (ed. N. Freinkel), vol. 1, pp. 67–76. Weverly Press, Baltimore, Maryland.

Logothetopoulos J. and Bell E.A. 1966. Histological and autoradiographic studies of the islets of mice injected with insulin antibody. *Diabetes* **15:** 205–211.

Lund T., O'Reilly L., Hutchings R., Kanagawa W., Simpson E., Gravely R., Chandler P., Dyson J., and Edwards A. 1990. Prevention of insulin-dependent diabetes mellitus in non-obese diabetic mice by transgenes encoding modified I-A B-chain or normal I–E A-chain. *Nature* **345:** 727–729.

Naya F.J., Huang H.-P., Qui Y., Mutoh H., DeMayo F.J., Leiter A.B., and Tsai M.-J. 1997. Diabetes, defective pancreatic morphogenesis, and abnormal enteroendocrine differentiation in BETA2/NeuroD-deficient mice. *Genes Dev.* **11:** 2323–2334.

Oertel J.E. 1989. The pancreas, nonneoplastic alterations. *Am. J. Sur. Pathol.* **13:** 50–65.

Offield M.F., Jetton T.L., Lobosky P.A., Ray M., Stein R.W., Magnuson M.A., Hogan B.L.M., and Wright C.V.E. 1996. PDX-1 is required for development of the pancreas and differentiation of the rostral duodenum. *Development* **371:** 983–995.

Ohlsson H., Karlsson K., and Edlund T. 1993. IPF-1, a homeodomain-containing transactivator of the insulin gene. *EMBO J.* **12:** 4251–4259.

Oldstone M.B.A., Nerenberg M., Southern P., Price J., and Lewicke H. 1991. Virus infection triggers insulin-dependent diabetes mellitus in a transgenic model: Role of anti-self virus immune response. *Cell* **65:** 319–331.

Oster A., Jensen J., Serup P., Galante P., Madsen O.D., and Larson L.I. 1998. Rat endocrine pancreatic development in relation to two homeobox gene products (Pdx-1 and Nkx 6.1). *J. Histochem. Cytochem.* **46:** 707–715.

Pang K., Mukonoweshuro C., and Wong G.G. 1994. Beta cells arise from glucose transporter type 2 Glut2-expressing epithelial cells of the developing rat pancreas. *Proc. Natl. Acad. Sci.* **91:** 9559–9563.

Peshavaria M. and Stein R. 1997. PDX-1: An activator of genes involved in pancreatic development and islet gene expression. In *Pancreatic growth and regeneration* (ed. N. Sarvetnick), pp. 96–107. Karger S, Basel, Switzerland.

Pictet R.L. and Rutter W.J. 1972. Development of the embryonic endocrine pancreas. *Handbook Physiol.* 25–66.

Pictet R.L., Clark W.R., Williams R.H., and Rutter W.J. 1972. An ultrastructural analysis of the developing embryonic pancreas. *Dev. Biol.* **29:** 436–467.

Portha B., Picon L., and Rosselin G. 1979. Chemical diabetes in the adult rat as the spontaneous evolution of neonatal diabetes. *Diabetologia* **17:** 371–377.

Portha B., Levacher C., Picon L., and Rosselin G. 1974. Diabetogenic effect of streptozotocin in the rat during the perinatal period. *Diabetes* **23:** 889–895.

Rall L.B., Pictet R.L., Williams R.H., and Rutter W.J. 1973. Early differentiation of glucagon-producing cells in embryonic pancreas: A possible developmental role for glucagon. *Proc. Natl. Acad. Sci.* **71:** 3478–3482.

Rao M.S., Scarpelli D.G., and Reddy J.K. 1986. Transdifferentiated hepatocytes in rat pancreas. *Curr. Top. Dev. Biol.* **20:** 63–78.

Rao M.S., Yeldandi A.V., and Reddy J.K. 1990. Stem cell potential of ductular and periductular cells in the adult rat pancreas. *Cell Differ. Dev.* **29:** 155–163.

Rao M.S., Dwivedi R.S., Yeidandi A.V., Subbarao V., Tan X., Usman M.I., Thangada S., Neimali M.R., Kumar S., Scarpelli D.G., and Reddy J.K. 1989. Role of periductal and ductal epithelial cells of the adult rat pancreas in pancreatic hepatocyte lineage: A change in the differentiation commitment. *Am. J. Pathol.* **134:** 1069–1086.

Reddy J.K., Rao M.S., Yeldandi A.V., Tan X., and Dwivedi S. 1991. Pancreatic hepatocytes: An in vivo model for cell lineage in pancreas of adult rat. *Dig. Dis. Sci.* **36:**

22

Stem Cells in the Epithelium of the Small Intestine and Colon

Douglas J. Winton
CRC Department of Oncology
Cambridge Institute for Medical Research
University of Cambridge
Cambridge CB2 2XY, United Kingdom

The inner lining of the colon and small intestine is a simple columnar epithelium that is constantly renewed by cellular migration from pockets of proliferative activity or crypts. Small intestinal cells leave the crypt and migrate onto villi that protrude into the gut lumen. Only at the point of exit from the crypt do villus epithelial cells become fully mature with respect to biochemical markers of differentiation. These cells are principally epithelial columnar cells, goblet cells, and enteroendocrine cells. Within the crypt, immature proliferative forms are morphologically identifiable as being precursors to these mature cell types. Near the crypt base, immature cells lacking the morphological characteristics of mature types are found and coexist with a fourth differentiated cell type, the Paneth cell (Fig. 1). These features present as a gradient with progressively higher positions being associated with a more developed morphological appearance. Cell kinetic experiments have determined the cycling characteristics of epithelial cells within the crypt, the time of appearance of identifiable differentiated cells from proliferative precursors, and the turnover times of crypt and villus populations. Studies of this kind, in both small intestine and colon, analyzed as a function of cellular position within the crypt (from position 1 at the crypt base), have led to the central tenet of gut stem cell biology: that cells originate from, and therefore stem cells reside near, the crypt base (Fig. 2). Proliferating cells at higher locations in the crypt may have the potential to divide 1, 2, 3, 4, and possibly 5 or 6 times, with the actual number being determined by distance from the crypt base stem cell pool. Consequently, these cells are an amplifying transit population capable of up to 6 transit divisions. Many

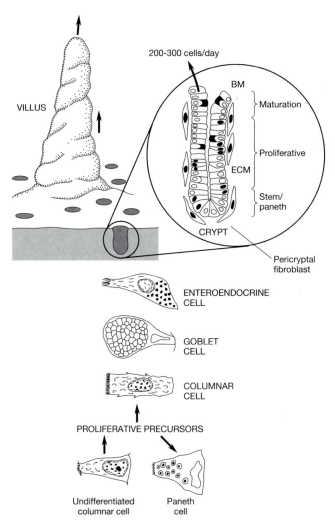

Figure 1 Schematic representation showing clockwise, from top, the relationship between small intestinal villi and crypts; the organization of crypts into discrete functional compartments with the likely cellular (pericryptal fibroblasts) and extracellular (extracellular matrix [ECM] and basement membrane [BM]) regulators of epithelial function; the four principal intestinal cell types. Fully mature and nonproliferative enteroendocrine, mucous (goblet), and columnar cells are located in the villus epithelium, whereas Paneth cells share the same distribution in the crypt base as undifferentiated columnar (presumptive stem) cells.

aspects of gut biology support the concept of a graded change with progressive loss of proliferative and regenerative potential accompanying the acquisition of a differentiated phenotype (for review, see Potten et al.

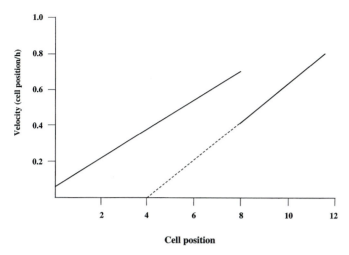

Figure 2 Location of the region of cellular genesis in colon and small intestine by cell migration velocity plotted as a function of cell position in the crypt. Following treatment with [³H]thymidine, the rate of migration of percentiles of radiolabeled cells can be measured. In colon (*upper plot*) the solid line is based on the best fit to actual data points and indicates that cellular genesis originates in the very base of the crypt. For small intestine (*lower plot*), extrapolation (*dotted line*) is required from cell position 8 to indicate a region of cellular genesis at or below position 4.

1997). This organization creates tremendous opportunities to analyze pathways of differentiation and to examine the consequences of perturbation within proliferating populations, for example, by manipulating signaling or adhesion molecules. In terms of stem cell biology, there is a down side. No cell-specific markers have yet been identified to permit the isolation and characterization of intestinal stem cells. Furthermore, no truly robust tissue culture method yet allows the primary culture of the intestinal epithelium to explore colony forming potential, pluripotentiality, and long-term versus short-term growth. Hence, intestinal stem cells are never analyzed in functional assays and there is an undue reliance on determining the characteristics and behavior of cells based on their topographical distribution.

CRYPT STEM CELL NUMBER

A cross-section of flask-shaped crypts identifies a circumference occupied by about 16 cells. At cell position 4, indicated as the approximate location of the stem cells in small intestine (Fig. 2), many of the cells around the circumference would be Paneth cells. On functional grounds it has been argued that in a column of cells stretching from the crypt base, any resident stem cell would reside above the highest Paneth cell position and could therefore occupy any position between 2 and 7 (Potten et al. 1997). If this argument is questioned, an additional 10 or so undifferentiated columnar cells are mixed with the Paneth cells. Thus, the number of undifferentiated crypt base columnar cells available to contain the stem cell population is in the range of 20–30 per crypt with 16 in an "undulating annulus" centered on cell position 4 and the remainder mixed with Paneth cells. Integration of cell kinetic data within a mathematical simulation (which assumes the annulus model) suggests that around 4–6 stem cells per crypt could most easily maintain the epithelium.

Other evidence comes from clonality studies in which clones of marked cells are induced following mutagen exposure. Mutation affects one allele of a polymorphic locus. Two detection systems have been used extensively. One involves loss of lectin-binding ability for Dolichos biflorus agglutinin (DBA) following mutation of the Dlb-1^b allele (Dolichos lectin-binding locus) which in Dlb-$1^b/Dlb$-1^a heterozygous mice determines the expression of the lectin-binding site in intestinal epithelia (Winton et al. 1988). The other clonal marker involves detection of loss of glucose 6-phosphate dehydrogenase (G6PD) activity in mice functionally hemizygous for a wild-type $G6PD$ allele (Griffiths et al. 1988). Such hemizygosity arises in male mice or in females homozygous for the wild-type allele after X-inactivation. These studies demonstrate that with time following chemical mutagenesis, intra-crypt epithelial clones are first detected, and subsequently, whole mutant crypts. In the small intestine, the Dlb-1 assay indicates that the time taken for such monoclonal crypts to appear is up to 8–12 weeks, whereas in the colon using the G6PD assay the equivalent time is around 4 weeks (Winton and Ponder 1990; Williams et al. 1992). The differences between the two tissues are probably real, but direct comparison is impossible due to the differences in the mutagens used and the likely cytotoxic effects (Winton 1993).

In mice, the total transit time of cells from crypt base to villus tip is around 5 days. Analysis of Dlb-1 mutant clones at 10 days (and therefore assaying a progenitor population from within the stem cell region of the crypt) demonstrates that the vertical clones of mutant cells present on the villus epithelium following migration from the crypt are some 2 cells wide (Winton 1997). This equates to 20–25% of the average cellular output of the crypt and indicates that 4–5 stem cells per crypt have survived mutagenesis. Similar numbers are indicated by a gain-of-function version of the *Dlb-1* assay (Bjerknes and Cheng 1999). For the colon, the estimate is 2–3 stem cells (Williams et al. 1992). Whether the cell death induced by mutagen exposure makes this calculation an underestimate is not known at present. These results indicate that there is a mechanism whereby several stem cells in each crypt are supplanted by the progeny of only one. The progression to crypt monoclonality in adult animals has been confirmed by the accumulation of spontaneous whole crypt mutations in small intestine and colon in mice and humans (Fuller et al 1990; Winton and Ponder 1990; Campbell et al. 1994; Novelli et al. 1996). Thus, stem cell turnover is a physiological process. The mechanism by which an estimated 4–6 stem cells per small intestinal crypt and 2–3 per colonic crypt are replaced has been the subject of some debate (see below).

Extrapolation of survival curves for regenerating foci of small intestinal epithelium (microcolonies) following irradiation has allowed estimates of the number of clonogenic cells to be made under different experimental conditions. Although the method can be criticized for the assumptions made and a high degree of observed variability (Wright and Alison 1984), a general picture of the radiosensitivity of the stem and proliferative cells has emerged from split dose protocols and different dosage regimens (for review, see Potten et al. 1997). The steady-state stem cells may be radiosensitive and rarely contribute to regeneration. An additional population of around 6 clonogenic cells per crypt with intermediate sensitivity regenerates the epithelium at low doses (less than 9 Gy). Above 9 Gy, a larger population of 16–24 radioresistant clonogens contributes to regeneration. Adaptation of the method to the colon gives qualitatively similar findings. The results imply a gradient of radiosensitivity among stem cells and their first, second, and third generation progeny which are normally destined to enter, or are actually in, the transit amplifying population. Apparently cells normally destined for differentiation can be called back to regenerate a functional stem cell compartment, although from these acute studies it is unclear how long they can continue to fulfill this role.

MODES OF DIVISION

There is no unequivocal evidence that indicates whether intestinal stem cells divide asymmetrically or symmetrically. The progression to monoclonality described above implies different fates for stem cells within the crypt. However, there is no evidence that this asymmetry in fate is determined prior to division. Different models for self-renewal of the stem cell population and which might explain the progression to monoclonality have been proposed. In one model, a probabilistic maintenance of the steady-state stem cell pool arises through purely symmetrical division with two stem cells or two committed cells arising at each stem cell division (Bjerknes 1986). This might create monoclonal crypts through progressive clonal expansions and extinctions. In this model, problems associated with complete stem cell extinction in a proportion of crypts (for which there is little evidence) due to small stem cell numbers are resolved by postulating that increased stem cell numbers in other crypts provide a signal for crypt replication through fission. Certainly there is evidence for a crypt cycle, and this might provide a route for the propagation of stem cells. However, it seems speculative to conclude that fluctuations in stem cell numbers are the driving force for crypt fission. The relative contribution of clonal expansion due to the nature of stem cell division and of segregation of clones into crypts by fission in explaining the monoclonality of the crypt epithelium is unknown. Bifurcating crypts (intermediate fission forms) are present in the steady state, and their numbers are increased by mutagen/cytotoxic treatments (Park et al. 1995). Hence, there may be a substantially greater contribution from fission events following chemical mutagenesis. This model denies any regulatory role for control of stem cell divisions through feedback mechanisms. In contrast, a multifactorial mathematical model indicates that a working crypt could be maintained by mainly asymmetrical stem cell division (95% of mitoses) with occasional division (5% of mitoses) being symmetrical and generating two stem cell daughters. Here again, it is the symmetrical divisions that allow clonal expansion (and extinctions) and might therefore account for monoclonality (Loeffler et al. 1993).

It is generally agreed that, in contrast to invariant asymmetrical divisions, symmetrical stem cell divisions are regulatable by environmental factors, because the probability of self-renewing divisions can be controlled (Morrison et al. 1997). Indeed, the gut epithelium is greatly influenced by environmental signals, and the ability of its stem cells to regenerate a normal epithelium following irradiation amply demonstrates that symmetrical self-renewing divisions can be triggered under conditions of regeneration. However, if the converse applies and there is little need to modulate the size of the stem cell pool in the steady state, in theory asymmetrical division could be the norm. There is no published evidence in intestinal stem cells for an asymmetrical cellular distribution of mammalian homologs of molecular determinants of asymmetry as described in other tissues and species. Consequently, asymmetrical divisions in the intestinal epithelium may be dictated immediately subsequent to mitosis by the relative vertical displacement of the two daughters. If so, this is not due to an inbuilt planar orientation of each mitotic event in the crypt as a whole, which can be at almost any orientation except at right angles to the epithelial sheet (Bjerknes and Cheng 1989), but even very small vertical displacements might determine fate. Supporting evidence for nonrandom cell deletion, and therefore asymmetrical divisions in intestinal epithelium, comes from computer simulations of the amount of genetic diversity affecting microsatellite repeats in small samples of around 200 epithelial cells in mismatch-repair-deficient mice (Tsao et al. 1997,1998). Higher levels of genetic diversity are predicted when one daughter of stem cell division is selected for extinction than when both daughters have the opportunity to be retained. Nonrandom cell death is compatible with the different fates of two daughters being determined prior to division (intrinsic asymmetry) or as a consequence of cell position.

NICHE

The concept of a unique microenvironment or niche maintaining the intestinal stem cell population first came from cell marking studies in which crypt base columnar cells that had taken up phagosomes after exposure to [³H]thymidine were tracked over time. These experiments demonstrate that prior to the acquisition of differentiated characteristics, stem cells first leave the crypt base (Bjerknes and Cheng 1981a,b). For example, Paneth cells colocalize within the stem cell zone, but their precursors are only recognized immediately above the stem cell zone and subsequently migrate downward. This implies that undifferentiated cells first have to leave the stem cell zone to enter an environment permissive for differentiation.

The nature of the niche in terms of its composition and in the aspects of stem cell behavior it regulates is still not understood. The above observation seems to require that niche determinants are localized to the crypt base, and consequently, attention has focused on the Paneth cells themselves and on molecular determinants with the appropriate distribution.

Paneth cells are long-lived and could therefore maintain a stable environment in the crypt base. They produce a number of factors that could regulate proliferation and differentiation in neighboring cells, including epidermal growth factor, tumor necrosis factor α, guanglin, and matrilysin, as well as other factors thought to be involved in the regulation of bacterial populations. However, ablation of the Paneth cell population in mice transgenic for an attenuated diphtheria toxin expressed from an upstream Paneth cell promoter (cryptidin 2) causes no change in the rate of crypt to villus migration or in the ordered differentiation of enteroendocrine, columnar, or goblet cells, or any change in the relative numbers of these cells (Garabedian et al. 1997). Furthermore, species lacking Paneth cells, such as pigs and dogs, have in other respects a similar crypt architecture and organization to that found in mice and humans.

There is ample evidence that the maintenance of a functional gut epithelium results from extensive regulation by and interaction with components of the extracellular matrix (ECM). Retention and loss of stem cells from the crypt base may be best achieved by regulating their adhesion to the ECM. Regulation of proliferation and commitment by the ECM is also likely to be of major importance. Gene deletion experiments in mice have demonstrated that both positive and negative regulators of growth are provided to the intestinal endoderm during development. *Hlx*, a divergent murine homeobox gene, is expressed in the mesenchyme underlying the mid- and hindgut and is required for gut elongation, and is a positive regulator of growth (Hentsch et al. 1996). In contrast, *Fkh6*, a winged helix transcription factor with a similar mesenchymal distribution, is a negative regulator. Mice deficient in *Fkh6* show intestinal overgrowth and severe dysregulation of proliferation both during development and in the adult (Kaestner et al. 1997). In the adult, the number of dividing cells is increased fourfold and the crypt morphology is altered.

The distribution of components of the ECM underlying the intestine in both mouse and humans has been investigated by immunohistochemistry, and clear patterns of differential expression have been recognized (see Fig. 3). The composition of the basement membrane immediately juxtaposed to the epithelium could be particularly important in regulation. One major component of the basement membrane that shows high molecular variability is the laminin (LN) group. These are heterotrimeric proteins composed of α, β, and γ chains. LN1 ($\alpha1$, $\beta2$, $\gamma1$)and LN2 ($\alpha2$, $\beta1$, $\gamma1$) are of particular interest because in humans they show a reciprocal pattern of villus and crypt expression, respectively (Beaulieu and Vachon 1994; Simon-Assmann et al. 1994). LN1 appears to be involved in triggering intestinal differentiation (Kedinger et al. 1998); LN2 is concentrated around the base of the crypt, suggesting a possible role in regulating the stem cell population (Fig. 4). However, *dy* mice lacking the $\alpha2$ chain (due to a natural mutation) appear to have no obvious intestinal abnormality, leaving the role of LN2 equivocal (Simon-Assmann et al. 1994).

Integrin receptors of ECM components can also show spatially distinct patterns of intestinal expression (Fig. 3). Integrin $\alpha2\beta1$ and $\alpha3\beta1$ show reciprocal expression in the crypt and villus, respectively (Beaulieu 1992). Determining the nature and consequence of interactions between the crypt

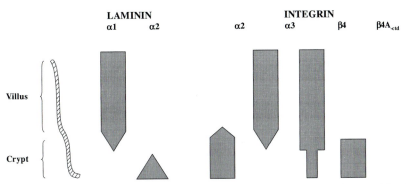

Figure 3 Schematic of crypt:villus pattern of expression of laminin 1 and laminin 2 (subchains α1 and α2) and of integrin α2, α3, and β4 chains in human intestine. The width of the stippled region gives an indication of the relative amounts of each molecule expressed along the crypt:villus axis as determined by the intensity of immunostaining. The reciprocal pattern of laminin α1 and α2 and of integrin α1 and α3 chains is shown. The integrin β4 chain is expressed at highest levels in the villus epithelium. A posttranslation cleavage event (which removes only the cytoplasmic tail of the predominant A isoform) in the crypt generates an inactive complex on association with α6.

epithelium and the ECM can be complicated by varying degrees of binding specificity. In this respect, α2β1 is promiscuous and binds both laminins and collagen. Not surprisingly, α2β1 has been implicated in diverse effects, including gland branching in breast, adhesion, motility, maintenance of differentiation, and cell cycle progression (Zutter et al. 1999). More detailed analysis of variant molecules can reveal underlying spatial differences. For example, the β4 chain is present in the intestinal basement membrane throughout the crypt-to-villus axis, but in the crypt epithelium it is proteolytically cleaved to remove the cytoplasmic tail (Basora et al. 1999). This modification renders integrin α6β4 functionally inactive in terms of its ability to bind LN5. Again, the functional significance of this modification is unclear, but in addition to conformational changes on adhesion, could affect the ability of α6β4 to signal through the Ras/map kinase pathways and to modulate cyclin-dependent kinase inhibitors.

No unequivocal molecular determinant of the stem cell niche has yet been identified, but there is an enormous potential for cross-talk between crypt stem cells and the ECM. It is likely that an effect at a given cell position will be mediated by multiple determinants/signals, and consequently, the composition of the niche will be complex. More problematic is discriminating whether an effect, such as the intestinal overgrowth and dysregulation observed in *Fkh6* null mice, involves or requires a stem cell

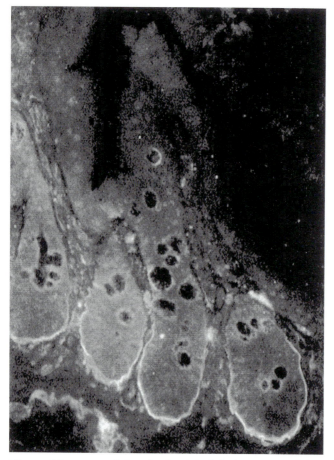

Figure 4 Immunostaining for laminin-2 in human small intestine. Note that the fluorescence is concentrated at the basement membrane at the crypt base. (Photomicrograph courtesy of M. Kedinger and P. Simon-Assmann.)

defect or whether changes in the transit population are sufficient. Similarly, with integrin-mediated interactions, the regulated function may involve a general effect on proliferation or differentiation.

Subepithelial fibroblasts and myofibroblasts may play a crucial role in defining the stem cell niche. Isolation of cloned sublines has shown that these are heterogeneous and differ in their ability to induce phenotypic changes in intestinal endoderm from day 14 fetal rats. In particular, one line stimulates proliferation, and development of an undifferentiated glandular structure. Another induces differentiation markers and supports the development of a normal crypt/villus structure (Fritsch et al. 1997). Additional lines isolated from different geographical positions along the longitudinal axis of the gut (proximal and distal small intestine and proximal colon) appear to retain the characteristics of their site of origin (Plateroti et al. 1998). Similar heritable differences in phenotype in myofibroblasts localized along the vertical axis of the crypt could help maintain a favorable environment for intestinal stem cells.

SECRETED FACTORS

Systemic or localized production of growth factors and cytokines must regulate intestinal stem cells, and their localized sequestering may limit availability at the niche. Their effects may extend to altering ECM–epithelial interaction through an effect on stromal fibroblasts (Fritsch et al. 1997; Burgess 1998). Due to difficulties in maintaining normal cells, the effects of candidate cytokines and growth factors have mainly been assayed using colon cancer lines. Molecules with general stimulating or inhibitory effects on cell proliferation in such systems include interleukins (IL-2, IL-4, IL-10, IL-11), epidermal growth factor (EGF) and EGF family members, insulin-like growth factor (IGF), and prostaglandins (for review, see Potten et al. 1997; Burgess 1998). In some cases, in vivo stimulatory effects are indicated by association with gut pathologies (e.g., the association of IL-4 and IL-10 expression in inflammatory bowel disease). Many of the molecules may be primarily involved in wound healing. It is unclear even within well-characterized gene families such as the EGF family whether a given factor is regulating specific aspects of intestinal epithelium behavior such as differentiation, survival, or cell proliferation. Equally, which cell compartment—stem or proliferative cells—is responding is unclear. Only for a few molecules has an effect on the intestinal stem cell population been demonstrated either by a change in stem cell survival following radiation or by measurement of cell kinetics by cell position following in vivo administration. Thus, transforming growth factor β (TGFβ), which is thought to be a negative regulator of epithelial proliferation, is expressed within the crypt. Furthermore, its administration reduces cell proliferation, alters cell cycle characteristics within the stem cell region, and protects stem cells from radiation induced-death as determined by the microcolony assay (Potten et al. 1997). Exposure to keratinocyte growth factor (a member of the FGF family) stimulates proliferation and affects crypt fission and also protects stem cells from radiation-induced death (Khan et al. 1997; Goodlad et al. 2000). Stem cell factor (SCF) and FGF-2 have also been shown to protect intestinal stem cells from the effects of ionizing radiation (Leigh et al. 1995; Houchen et al. 1999), and subepithelial intestinal myofibroblasts express the SCF receptor c-kit. Whether radiation protection arises directly from an effect of the cytokine/growth factor or indirectly through stimulating other cell populations is unclear. For example, keratinocyte growth factor is induced by serum factors in cultured dermal fibroblasts by two distinct pathways involving protein kinase C or cyclin-dependent kinases (Brauchle et al. 1994). Furthermore, KGF is inducible from such fibroblasts by treatment with IL-6, IL-1, or TNFα (Brauchle et al. 1994). Thus, production of growth factors and cytokines may regulate the stem cell compartment. Paneth cells, although not essential for stem cell maintenance, may still play a role in more subtle ways and certainly produce TNFα. Lymphoid cells may also be able to regulate stem cell behavior by the localized production of cytokines.

Tcf-4

Recently, it has been shown that germ-line deletion of the high-mobility group transcription factor Tcf-4 causes a failure to lay down the adult pattern of stem (and proliferative) cells in small intestinal epithelium (Korinek et al. 1998). Proliferating cells in the intervillus region (from which crypts will form after birth) of Tcf-4 null mice are completely absent from E16.5 stage embryos onward. In colon, where Tcf-4 is also expressed, the phenotype is not evident, presumably due to the activity of another member of the Tcf family. The relevance of this finding is that it implicates by association several of the molecular partners of Tcf-4, which are involved in the neoplastic transformation of colonic cells, in the establishment of intestinal stem cells. Thus, β-catenin complexes with Tcf-4 to generate an active transcription factor but is normally found in low concentrations associated with the product of the adenomatous polyposis coli (APC) gene (for review, see Roose and Clevers 1999). APC acts to suppress signaling via the Tcf-4/β-catenin complex. Key events in transcriptional activation include: signaling through the wingless/Wnt pathway; stabilization of β-catenin as a cytoplasmic monomer that no longer forms a complex with APC; and translocation of β-catenin to the nucleus where it associates with Tcf-4. Constitutively active Tcf-4/β-catenin complexes are present in Apc$^{-/-}$ colon carcinoma cell lines and in Apc$^{+/+}$ cell lines containing a dominant mutation affecting the amino terminus of β-catenin (Korinek et al. 1997; Morin et al. 1997). One interpretation of these observations is that neoplastic transformation as a consequence of activation of Tcf-4 results in a maintenance of stem cell characteristics (Korinek et al. 1998): In effect, cells that should undergo terminal differentiation continue to divide and to persist.

The link between colon cancer and stem/proliferative behavior has been taken further: CD44, which is often overexpressed early in the development of colorectal cancers, is restricted to the crypt epithelium in normal mice. This family of glycoproteins is believed to link ECM components to the cytoskeleton and, through an interaction with heparin sulfate, to bind growth factors that may promote receptor signaling. CD44 expression appears to be controlled by the Tcf-4/β-catenin pathway (Wielenga et al. 1999).

The role of Tcf-4 in maintaining functional stem cells in adult epithelium is unknown. In situ hybridization indicates expression of Tcf-4 message throughout the crypt (CD44 has a similar pattern of expression), although no detailed expression studies have determined the pattern of expression of the protein. Other factors may serve to maintain the stem cell zone in conjunction with the Tcf-4-mediated pathway. The requirement for Wnt signaling implicates the mesenchymal cells underlying the crypt epithelium as the probable source. Identification of a crypt-specific Wnt receptor might yet define a stem-cell-specific marker. Overall, the need for cross-talk between cells of the ECM and developing and presumably established stem cell population is demonstrated both by the requirement for Wnt signaling and the action of its downstream target CD44.

HOMEOSTASIS

In the steady stage, the small intestine shows a background of apoptosis which in the crypt is coincident with the stem cell position. Up to 10% of crypt base columnar cells may be dying at any time. It has been suggested that such spontaneous apoptosis acts to remove excess stem cells after symmetrical stem cell division (Potten et al. 1997). If correct, this appears to be a small-intestine-specific strategy, as spontaneous apoptosis in the colon is not associated with the stem cell region. This may relate to the expression of Bcl-2 in the latter and not the former. Currently, there are no functional data to indicate the nature of the deleted cells.

Apoptosis as a homeostatic mechanism is supported by experiments causing crypt hyperplasia. Following small bowel resection (SBR), both proliferation and apoptosis are increased to a similar degree as part of an adaptive response (Shin et al. 1999). Similarly, chimeric mice in which one parental component is directed to overexpress an amino-truncated β-catenin in intestinal epithelium show a fourfold increase in cell division and "spontaneous" apoptosis in affected crypt epithelium (Wong et al. 1998). Qualitatively equivalent findings have been described in the overgrown crypt epithelium in *Fkh6* null mice (Kaestner et al. 1997). These observations would be in accord with establishment of new steady state with increased numbers of stem cells being deleted. Longer-term study of the proliferation and apoptotic changes accompanying SBR in rabbits shows that 3 weeks post-surgery, crypt cell apoptosis levels are returned to normal while crypt cell proliferation remains stimulated (Thompson and Barent et al. 1999). This dissociation is interesting: Can a steady state be established in which an increased proliferative compartment is maintained by a normal number of stem cells?

Regulation of spontaneous apoptosis by specific gene products has been investigated (for review, see Potten et al. 1997; Potten 1998; Watson and Pritchard 2000). p53 and Bax null mice show no difference in the levels of spontaneous apoptosis. (p53 deletion also has no effect on the elevated levels of apoptosis observed following SBR [Shin et al. 1999]). Bcl-2 null mice show elevated levels of spontaneous apoptosis in colonic epithelium (at the putative stem cell location) but not in the small intestine, and overexpression of Bcl-2 in the latter does not affect the frequency of spontaneous apoptosis (Coopersmith et al. 1999). These last observations indicate that Bcl-2 may be involved in homeostasis of normal colonic stem cells but indicate that it is not involved in the small intestine.

Following γ irradiation, there is an increase in the level of apoptosis at the stem cell position that is p53-dependent. In p53 null mice, the peak of apoptosis normally observed at 3–4 hours postirradiation is absent (there is a later p53-independent peak of apoptosis that probably arises due to aberrant mitoses). In colon (and not small intestine) irradiated Bcl-2 null mice show increases in apoptosis over wild-type animals, and again this is linked to cell position 1–2. It has been proposed that the lack of a homeostatic mechanism for spontaneous deletion of excess cells in colon due to Bcl-2 may explain the greater susceptibility of the colonic, as compared to the small intestinal, epithelium to neoplastic induction.

COMMITMENT

There is evidence for proliferative and self-maintaining progenitors committed to maintaining different cell types within the small intestine. Cell marking studies using a gain-of-function modification of the *Dlb-1* mutation assay have identified DBA-positive clones composed only of goblet/oligomucous cells (Bjerknes and Cheng 1999). These are induced by high doses of chemical mutagen and persist for up to 154 days postmutagenesis. Cell ablation studies in which enteroendocrine cells expressing secretin are deleted have also been supportive of a committed precursor

(Rindi et al. 1999). Secretin is expressed in a subset of small intestinal enteroendocrine cells, which are identified by the coexpression of multiple hormones. Hence, cholecystokinin- and glucagon-expressing cells also express secretin. Gancyclovir, in mice transgenic for a secretin promoter linked to herpes simplex virus thymidine kinase, ablates some 95% of secretin cells (S cells) and reduces cholecystokinin-, glucagon-, and peptide YY-expressing cells to a comparable degree. Cells expressing gastric-inhibitory peptide, substance P, somatostatin, and serotonin are only partially ablated (45–59%), and gastrin cells are reduced by ~13%. Ablation takes about 5 days as mature villus forms are not killed by the treatment. Rather, proliferative precursors within the middle region crypt are susceptible and are observed to apoptose. Furthermore, after a 5-week posttreatment recovery period, there is complete recovery of all cell types, indicating that earlier progenitors (or stem cells) are spared because the secretin promoter is not active. The relative reductions in numbers reflect the closeness of the lineage relationship with S cells (Fig. 5).

Commitment of S-cell precursors seems to require BETA2, a basic helix-loop-helix protein (Mutoh et al. 1998). BETA2, in association with

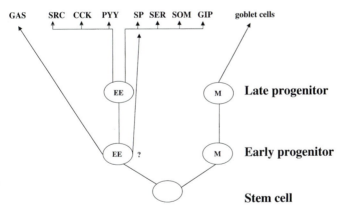

Figure 5 Model for differentiation pathways in mouse small intestine. Multipotent stem cells can give rise to early progenitors committed to the enteroendocrine (EE) or oligomucous/goblet cell (M) lineage. Intermediate/late progenitors for the different enteroendocrine subtypes indicated by cell ablation studies also suggest that gastrin-producing cells arise from a unique precursor and that distinct routes for the differentiation of substance P (SP), serotonin (SER), somatostatin (SOM), and gastric inhibitory peptide (GIP) subtypes must exist from that giving rise to the secretin (SEC) peptide YY (PYY) and cholecystokinin (CCK) subtypes. Evidence for the mucous cell pathway comes from mutation-induced marker experiments (see text).

the coactivator p300, can coordinate transcription of the secretin gene, cell cycle arrest, and apoptosis. Mice deficient for BETA2 due to gene targeting lack enteroendocrine cells expressing both secretin and chole- cystokinin, providing additional support for the model shown in Figure 5.

Evidence for selective versus instructional mechanisms for stem cell commitment is lacking. Long-term (e.g., goblet cell) precursors and short-term precursors may be regulated by different mechanisms, pre- sumably because they occupy different crypt positions. Inhibition of upward migration of proliferating cells due to overexpression of E-cad- herin does not affect the normal pattern of differentiation (Hermiston et al. 1996). Hence, differentiation is not cell-autonomous and relates to cell position rather than to actual age of cells from "birth" among the stem cells. It is unclear whether this also applies to commitment of stem cells as well as the differentiation process itself.

Little is known about molecular mediators of the commitment process. Members of the Cdx family of homeobox genes may be involved. In the adult gut, Cdx-2 mRNA is present in the undifferentiated crypt base cells, but the protein is expressed at highest levels in the villus epithelium (James et al. 1994). The bulk of work carried out to date sug- gests that, in fully differentiated intestine, Cdx-2 is primarily involved in the final maturation of enterocytes (Lorentz et al. 1997). Cdx-1 is expressed in small intestine and colon throughout the crypt–villus axis in a graded manner, with the highest levels of expression in the crypt base. In comparison to Cdx-2, rather less is known about the properties of Cdx-1, although it too appears to be able to regulate transcription of intestinal brush-border enzymes and may be able to regulate progression through the cell cycle (Lynch et al. 2000). However, Cdx-1 is also associ- ated with the transition of normal gastric and esophageal epithelium to intestinal metaplasia, and this may play an important role in maintaining the intestinal phenotype (Silberg et al. 1997). What, if any, role Cdx-1, or indeed Cdx-2, plays in establishing lineage-committed precursors from the multipotential stem cell pool is currently unknown.

CONCLUDING REMARKS

Progress in unraveling the mystery of stemness in intestinal epithelium has been impaired by the limited usefulness of tissue culture systems. As it currently stands, primary cultures can be established from epithelial aggregates and not from completely dissociated cells (Evans et al. 1994; Perrault and Beaulieu 1998; Booth et al. 1999). Transplantation experi- ments show that such aggregates can reconstitute normal epithelium (Tait et al. 1994; Slorach et al. 1999). However, the methods do not allow the self-renewing potential of isolated and defined cell populations to be assessed. It is unclear whether this is a resolvable technical problem.

The lack of stem-cell-specific markers is also limiting: Do they exist for intestinal stem cells? It may be that intestinal stem cells are defined by the absence of such markers. Quantitative differences in integrin expression seem to be an important factor in determining the self-renewing capacity of keratinocytes. The emphasis on highly localized crypt base "stem cell" markers may be misplaced, and gradients of expression of such molecules may better relate to self-renewal. Considerable thought will be required on how to validate any such markers in the absence of appropriate in vitro assay systems.

Despite these limitations, the intestinal epithelium still attracts due to the clear separation of functional compartments and the ability to detect changes in these following genetic manipulation in transgenic experiments, or to establish what is required for their maintenance in transplantation/restitution experiments. These approaches are powerful, but it is unclear even in the most refined transgenic experiment the extent to which genetic redundancy or adaptive responses in vivo mask important interactions that could be teased apart in a more defined, in vitro, setting. Furthermore, subtle changes in stem cell behavior may not be detected because ultimately in vivo analyses depend on determining the spatial distribution of cells and differentiation markers in descendants of the entire crypt stem cell pool and not in the stem cells themselves.

Given the evident plasticity of a variety of apparently tissue-specific stem cells to transdifferentiate, the question arises: Do intestinal stem cells show this ability? The limitations described above do not allow the establishment of experimental conditions under which such behavior could be defined. However, a number of in vivo observations do imply considerable versatility of small intestinal stem cells. Most dramatic is the ability of crypts adjacent to areas of ulceration to generate a novel ulcer-associated cell lineage (UACL, Fig. 6) (Wright 1998). Originating from the stem cell zone of individual crypts, these new cell lineages form complicated networks, change their pattern of gene expression, and establish new proliferative patterns as part of an adaptive response. Crypt epithelium surrounding lymphoid Peyer patches shows adaptation to produce M cells, a minor epithelial cell type found on the mucosal surface overlying the lymphoid follicles (Gebert et al. 1999). Intestinal metaplasia in the stomach and esophagus is a common pathological observation. Conversely, metaplasia of normally caudal intestine into rostral squamous-type epithelium in haplo-insufficient Cdx-2 $^{+/-}$ mice suggests a molecular candidate involved

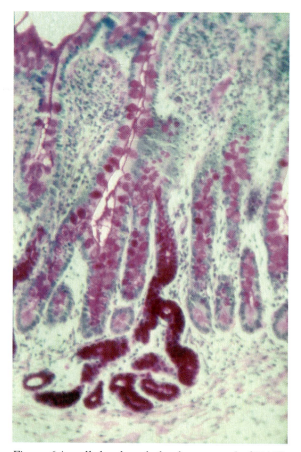

Figure 6 A well-developed gland composed of UACL cells (*darker red staining*) in human intestine is revealed by staining for neutral mucins using the diastase periodic acid Schiff method. These complex glands arise initially from the stem cell region of individual crypts and are part of an adaptive response in the epithelium adjacent to areas of ulceration.

in the programming to generate intestinal phenotypes (Beck et al. 1999). Before fully testing the limits of intestinal stem cell plasticity, the requirement for the future is to devise appropriate assay systems for establishing the normal criteria for maintaining stem properties in intestinal cells.

ACKNOWLEDGMENTS

The author is supported by a program grant from The Cancer Research Campaign.

REFERENCES

Basora N., Herring-Gillam F.E., Boudreau F., Perrault N., Pageot L.-P., Simoneau M., Bouatross Y., and Beaulieu J.F. 1999. Expression of functionally distinct variants of the $\beta_4 A$ integrin subunit in relation to the differentiation state in human intestinal cells. *J. Biol. Chem.* **274:** 29819–29825.

Beaulieu J.-F. 1992. Differential expression of the VLA family of integrins along the crypt-villus axis in the human small intestine. *J. Cell. Sci.* **102:** 427–436.

Beaulieu J.-F. and Vachon P.H. 1994. Reciprocal expression of laminin A-chain isoforms along the crypt-villus axis in the human small intestine. *Gastroenterology* **106:** 829–839.

Beck F., Chawengsaksophak K., Waring P., Playford R.J., and Furness J.B. 1999. Reprogramming of intestinal differentiation and intercalary regeneration in Cdx-2 mutant mice. *Proc. Natl. Acad. Sci.* **96:** 7318–7323.

Bjerknes M. 1986. A test of the stochastic theory of stem cell differentiation. *Biophys. J.* **49:** 1223–1227.

Bjerknes M. and Cheng H. 1981a. The stem cell zone of the mouse small intestinal epithelium. I. Evidence from Paneth cells in the adult mouse. *Am. J. Anat.* **160:** 51–64.

———. 1981b. The stem cell zone of the mouse small intestinal epithelium. III. Evidence from columnar, enteroendocrine and mucous cells in the adult mouse. *Am. J. Anat.* **166:** 77–92.

———. 1989. Mitotic orientations in three dimensions determined from multiple projections. *Biophys. J.* **55:** 1011–1015.

———. 1999. Clonal analysis of mouse intestinal epithelial progenitors. *Gastroenterology* **116:** 7–14.

Booth C., O'Shea J.A., and Potten C.S. 1999. Maintenance of functional stem cells in isolated and cultured adult intestinal epithelium. *Exp. Cell Res.* **249:** 359–366.

Brauchle M., Angermeyer K., Hubner G., and Werner S. 1994. Large induction of keratinocyte growth factor expression by serum growth-factors and pro-inflammatory cytokines in cultured fibroblasts. *Oncogene* **9:** 3199–3204.

Burgess A.W. 1998. Growth control mechanisms in normal and transformed intestinal cells. *Philos. Trans. R. Soc. Ser. B Biol. Sci.* **353:** 903–909.

Campbell F., Fuller C.E., Williams G.T., and Williams E.D. 1994. Human colonic stem cell mutation frequency with and without radiation. *J. Pathol.* **174:** 175–182.

Coopersmith C.M., O'Donnell D., and Gordon J.I. 1999. Bcl-2 inhibits ischemia-reperfusion-induced apoptosis in the intestinal epithelium of transgenic mice. *Am. J. Physiol.* **276:** G677–G686.

Evans G.S., Flint N., and Potten C.S. 1994. Primary cultures for studies of cell regulation and physiology in intestinal epithelium. *Annu. Rev. Physiol.* **56:** 399–417.

Fritsch C., Simon-Assmann P., Kedinger M., and Evans G.S. 1997. Cytokines modulate fibroblast phenotype and epithelial-stroma interactions in rat intestine. *Gastroenterology* **112:** 826–838.

Fuller C.E., Davies R.P., Williams G.T., and Williams E.D. 1990. Crypt restricted heterogeneity of goblet cell mucus glycoprotein in histologically normal human colonic mucosa: A potential marker of somatic mutation. *Br. J. Cancer* **61:** 382–384.

Garabedian E.M., Roberts L.J.J., McNevin M.S., and Gordon J.I. 1997. Examining the role of Paneth cells in the small intestine by lineage ablation in transgenic mice. *J. Biol. Chem.* **272:** 23729–23740.

Gebert A., Fassbender S., Werner K., and Weissferdt A. 1999. The development of M cells in Peyer's patches is restricted to specialized dome-associated crypts. *Am. J. Pathol.* **154:** 1573–1582.

Goodlad R.A., Mandir N., Meeran K., Ghatei M.A., Bloom S.R., and Playford R.J. 2000. Does the response of the intestinal epithelium to kerartinocyte growth factor vary according to the method of administration? *Regul. Pept.* **87:** 1–3.

Griffiths D.F.R., Davies S.J., Williams D., Williams G.T., and Williams E.D. 1988. Demonstration of somatic mutation and colonic crypt clonality by X-linked enzyme histochemistry. *Nature* **333:** 461–463.

Hentsch B., Lyons I., Li R., Hartley L., Lints T.A., Adams, J.M., and Harvey R.P. 1996. *Hlx* homeobox gene is essential for an inductive interaction that drives expansion of embryonic liver and gut. *Genes Dev.* **10:** 70–79.

Hermiston M.L., Wong M.H., and Gordon J.I. 1996. Forced expression of E-cadherin in the mouse intestinal epithelium slows cell migration and provides evidence for nonautonomous control of cell fate in a self-renewing system. *Genes Dev.* **10:** 985–996.

Houchen C.W., George R.J., Sturmoski M.A., and Cohn S.M. 1999. FGF-2 enhances intestinal stem cell survival and its expression is induced after radiation injury. *Am. J. Physiol.* **276:** G249–G258.

James R., Erler T., and Kazenwadel J. 1994. Structure of the murine homeobox gene cdx-2. Expression in embryonic and adult intestinal epithelium. *J. Biol. Chem.* **269:** 15229–15237.

Kaestner K.H., Silberg D.G., Traber P.G., and Schultz G. 1997. The mesenchymal winged helix transcription factor *Fkh6* is required for the control of gastrointestinal proliferation and differentiation. *Genes Dev.* **11:** 1583–1595.

Kedinger M., Lefebvre O., Duluc I., Freund J.N., and Simon-Assmann P. 1998. Cellular and molecular partners involved in gut morphogenesis and differentiation. *Philos. Trans. R. Soc. Ser. B Biol. Sci.* **353:** 847–856.

Khan W.B., Shui C.X., Ning S.C., and Knox S.J. 1997. Enhancement of murine intestinal stem cell survival after irradiation by keratinocyte growth factor. *Radiat. Res.* **148:** 248–253.

Korinek V., Barker N., Moerer P., van Donselaar E., Huls G., Peters P.J., and Clevers H. 1998. Depletion of epithelial stem-cell compartments in the small intestine of mice lacking Tcf-4. *Nat. Genet.* **19:** 379–383.

Korinek V., Barker N., Morin P.J., vanWichen D., deWeger R., Kinzler K.W., Vogelstein B., and Clevers H. 1997. Constitutive transcriptional activation by a β-catenin-Tcf complex in APC$^{-/-}$ colon carcinoma. *Science* **275:** 1784–1787.

Leigh B.R., Khan W., Hancock S.L., and Knox S.J. 1995. Stem-cell factor enhances the survival of murine intestinal stem cells after photon irradiation. *Radiat. Res.* **142:** 12–15.

Loeffler M., Birke A., Winton D., and Potten C. 1993. Somatic mutation, monoclonality and stochastic models of stem cell organization in the intestinal crypt. *J. Theor. Biol.* **160:** 471–491.

Lorentz O., Duluc I., DeArcangelis A., Simon-Assmann P., Kedinger M., and Freund J.N. 1997. Key role of the cgx-2 homeobox gene in extracellular matrix-mediated intestinal cell differentiation. *J. Cell Biol.* **139:** 1553–1565.

Lynch J., Suh E-R., Silberg D.G., Rulyak S., Blanchard N., and Traber P.G. 2000. The caudal-related homeodomain protein Cdx1 inhibits proliferation of intestinal epithelial cells by down regulation of D-type cyclins. *J. Biol. Chem.* **275:** 4499–4506.

Morin P.J., Sparks A.B., Korinek V., Barker N., Clevers H., Vogelstein B., and Kinzler

K.W. 1997. Activation of β-catenin-Tcf signalling in colon cancer by mutations in β-catenin or APC. *Science* **275:** 1787–1790.

Morrison S.J., Shah N.M., and Anderson D.J. 1997. Regulatory mechanisms in stem cell biology. *Cell* **88:** 287–298.

Mutoh H., Naya F.J., Tsai M.-J., and Leiter A.B. 1998. The basic helix-loop-helix protein BETA2 interacts with p300 to coordinate differentiation of secretin-expressing enteroendocrine cells. *Genes Dev.* **12:** 820–830.

Novelli M.R., Williamson J.A., Tomlinson I.P.M., Elia G., Hodgson S.V., Talbot I.C., Bodmer W.F., and Wright N.A. 1996. Polyclonal origin of colonic carcinoma in an XO/XY patient with FAP. *Science* **272:** 1187–1190.

Park H.S., Goodlad R.A., and Wright N.A. 1995. Crypt fission in the small intestine and colon: A mechanism for the emergence of G6PD locus-mutated crypts after treatment with mutagens. *Am. J. Pathol.* **147:** 1416–1427.

Perreault N. and Beaulieu J-F. 1998. Primary cultures of fully differentiated and pure human intestinal epithelial cells. *Exp. Cell Res.* **245:** 34–42.

Plateroti M., Rubin D.C, Duluc I., Singh R., Foltzer-Jourdainne C., Freund J.N, and Kedinger M. 1998. Subepithelial fibroblast cell lines from different levels of gut axis display regional characteristics. *Am. J. Physiol.* **274:** G945–G954.

Potten C.S. 1998. Stem cells in gastrointestinal epithelium: Numbers characteristics and death. *Philos. Trans. R. Soc. Lond. B Biol. Sci.* **353:** 821–830.

Potten C.S., Booth C., and Pritchard D.M. 1997. The intestinal epithelial stem cell: The mucosal governor (review). *Int. J. Exp. Pathol.* **78:** 219–243.

Rindi G., Ratineau C., Ronco A., Candusso M.E., Tsai M.-J., and Leiter A.B. 1999. Targeted ablation of secretin-producing cells in transgenic mice reveals a common differentiation pathway with multiple enteroendocrine cell lineages in the small intestine. *Development* **126:** 4149–4156.

Roose J. and Clevers H. 1999. TCF transcription factors: Molecular switches in carcinogenesis. *Biochim. Biophys. Acta* **1424:** M23–M37.

Shin C.E., Falcone Jr., R.A., Kemp C.J., Erwin C.R., Litvak D.A., Evers B.M., and Warner B.W. 1999. Intestinal adaptation and enterocyte apoptosis following small bowel resection is p53 independent. *Am. J. Physiol.* **277:** G717–G724.

Silberg D.G., Furth E.E., Taylor J.K., Schuck T., Chiou T., and Traber P.G. 1997. CDX1 protein expression in normal, metaplastic, and neoplastic human alimentary tract epithelium. *Gastroenterology* **113:** 478–486.

Simon-Assmann P., Duclos B., Orian-Rousseau V., Arnold C., Mathelin C., Engvall E., and Kedinger M. 1994. Differential expression of laminin isoforms and α6-β4 integrin subunits in the developing human and mouse intestine. *Dev. Dyn.* **201:** 71–85.

Slorach E.M., Campbell F.C., and Dorin J.R. 1999. A mouse model of intestinal stem cell function and regeneration. *J. Cell Sci.* **112:** 3029–3038.

Tait I.S., Flint N., Campbell C.F., and Evans G.S. 1994. Generation of neomucosa in vivo by transplantation of dissociated rat postnatal small intestinal epithelium. *Differentiation* **56:** 91–100.

Thompson J.S. and Barent B. 1999. Effects of intestinal resection on enterocyte apoptosis. *J. Gastrointest. Surg.* **3:** 672–677.

Tsao J.-L., Davies S.D., Baker S.M., Liskay R.M., and Shibata D. 1997. Intestinal stem cell division and genetic diversity: A computer and experimental analysis. *Am. J. Pathol.* **151:** 573–579.

Tsao J.-L., Zhang J., Salovaara R., Li Z.-H., Jarvinen H.J., Mecklin J.-P., Aaltonen L.A., and Shibata D. 1998. Tracing cell fates in human colorectal tumors from somatic microsatellite mutations: Evidence of adenomas with stem cell architecture. *Am. J. Pathol.* **153:** 1189–1200.

Watson A.J.M. and Pritchard D.M. 2000. Lessons from genetically engineered animal models. VII. Apoptosis in intestinal epithelium: Lessons from transgenic and knockout mice. *Am. J. Physiol. Gastrointest. Liver Physiol.* **278:** G1–G5.

Wielenga V.J.M., Smits R., Korinek V., Smit L., Kielman M., Fodde R., Clevers H., and Pals S.T. 1999. Expression of CD44 in Apc and Tcf mutant mice implies regulation by the Wnt pathway. *Am. J. Pathol.* **154:** 515–523.

Williams E.D., Lowes A.P., Williams D., and Williams G.T. 1992. A stem cell niche theory of intestinal crypt maintenance based on somatic mutation in colonic mucosa. *Am. J. Pathol.* **141:** 773–776.

Winton D.J. 1993. Mutation induced clonal markers from polymorphic loci: Application to stem cell organization in the mouse intestine. *Semin. Dev. Biol.* **4:** 293–302.

———. 1997. Intestinal stem cells and clonality. In *The gut as model in cell and molecular biology- Falk symposium 94.* (eds Halter F., Wright N.A., and Winton D.), pp. 3–13. Kluwer, London, United Kingdom.

Winton D.J. and Ponder B.A.J. 1990. Stem-cell organisation in mouse small intestine. *Proc. R. Soc. Lond. B Biol. Sci.* **241:** 13–18.

Winton D.J., Blount M.A., and Ponder B.A.J. 1988. A clonal marker induced by somatic mutation in mouse intestinal epithelium. *Nature* **333:** 463–466.

Wong M.H., Rubinfield B., and Gordon J.I. 1998. Effects of forced expression of an NH_2-terminal truncated β-catenin on mouse intestinal epithelial homeostasis. *J. Cell Biol.* **141:** 765–777.

Wright N.A. 1998. Aspects of the biology of regeneration and repair in the human gastrointestinal tract. *Philos. Trans. R. Soc Lond. B Biol. Sci.* **353:** 925–933.

Wright N.A. and Alison M. 1984. The theory of renewing cell populations. In *The biology of epithelial cell populations,* vol. 1, pp. 21–90. Clarendon Press, Oxford, United Kingdom.

Zutter M.M., Santoro S.A., Wu J.E., Wakatsuki T., Dickeson S.K., and Elson E.L. 1999. Collagen receptor control of epithelial morphogenesis and cell cycle progression. *Am. J. Pathol.* **155:** 927–940.

Index